Chest Radiographic Analysis

Chest Radiographic Analysis

Norman Blank, M.D.

Professor Emeritus, Active
Department of Diagnostic Radiology and Nuclear Medicine
Stanford University School of Medicine
Stanford, California

Churchill Livingstone
New York, Edinburgh, London, Melbourne

Library of Congress Cataloging-in-Publication Data

Blank, Norman.
    Chest radiographic analysis.

    Includes bibliographies and index.
    1. Chest—Radiography. I. Title.   [DNLM: 1. Lung—
radiography.   WF 600 B642c]
RC941.B65   1989   617.5′407572   89-9885
ISBN 0-443-08658-3

Distributed in the United Kingdom by Churchill Livingstone, Robert Stevenson House, 1–3 Baxter's Place, Leith Walk, Edinburgh EH1 3AF, and by associated companies, branches, and representatives throughout the world.

The Publishers have made every effort to trace the copyright holders for borrowed material. If they have inadvertently overlooked any, they will be pleased to make the necessary arrangements at the first opportunity.

Acquisitions Editor: *Bob Hurley*
Copy Editor: *Margot Otway*
Production Supervisor: *Sharon Tuder*

Production Services provided by Bermedica Production

Printed in the United States of America

First published in 1989

Preface

My aim in writing *Chest Radiographic Analysis* was to help both medical students and residents in radiology or chest medicine to master the principles of chest film interpretation and to develop their ability to extract information from imaging studies. In contrast to many elegant texts that emphasize chest disease per se, this work is organized to function primarily as a "how-to" source — how to analyze radiographic data, how to decide whether findings are normal or abnormal, how to integrate radiographic data with other clinical findings and with one's knowledge of disease processes to formulate a differential diagnosis.

Each chapter is accompanied by an atlas of illustrations, which are chosen to serve as examples of classes of diseases and disorders. The organization of the material into sets and subsets makes it easier to remember than if it were presented as a long series of individual diagnoses. The extensive legends include the information and concepts that students are most likely to find useful in clinical work. Therefore, each chapter can effectively be reviewed by studying the illustrations and the chapter summary rather than by rereading the entire text.

Because my aim was to concentrate on principles of chest film interpretation, I decided to omit some topics. For example, congenital and developmental abnormalities and the pulmonary problems of infancy are not covered, and only certain of the relevant bone lesions and cardiac disorders are illustrated. A comprehensive coverage would have required a text of twice the size.

Choosing suitable illustrations was the most time-consuming and frustrating part of this effort. It is extremely difficult — impossible — to reproduce in a book illustration the subtleties visible on a chest radiograph. I have done my best.

Careful attention was given to substantiating the individual diagnoses by correlation with bacteriologic, pathologic, physiologic, and follow-up clinical studies. In a few older cases in which the radiographic findings were classic for the diagnosis, I relied on the original teaching file designation.

There is no doubt that newer imaging modalities, such as CT and MRI, have materially altered the approach to the study of chest disease. In this text, CT and MRI scans are used when they augment the understanding of the plain film findings or when they show details of anatomy and pathology that are not displayed well on chest films. Both CT and MRI are expensive and time-consuming, so, for the present, plain films remain the primary roentgenologic method for examination of the chest. Moreover, when digital radiographic and other image-manipulation techniques come into common use, they will employ some modification of the chest film format as hard copy or video terminal display. Expertise in chest film analysis is likely to remain important for a long time to come.

Norman Blank, M.D.

Acknowledgments

I am grateful to my teachers from the full-time and voluntary faculty of the University of Minnesota and the Veterans Administration Hospital of Minneapolis, and to all of my colleagues at Stanford University Hospital who have contributed to my continuing education. It has been my good fortune to be a member of the Fleischner Society since its inception, and no brief note can adequately express my gratitude to all of the members who have shared their expertise with me.

The technologist staff and the film-library staff of the Department of Diagnostic Radiology and Nuclear Medicine at Stanford Medical Center have borne my incessant invasions with remarkable grace. The students, residents and fellows who have passed through the department in the last 25 years have helped me to become a better teacher and hopefully a better radiologist — sometimes at no little pain to themselves.

My entire family has been nothing short of spectacular in their tolerance of my obsession, but the greater burden has been borne gracefully by my wife, Donna.

Over the years several secretaries have typed and re-typed this manuscript with forbearance, but Mrs. Marie Miller has faithfully helped me to bring it to completion.

The illustrative material has come largely from patients and employees examined at Stanford University Hospital, but colleagues at other imaging centers have been generous in giving their permission to use those illustration which are acknowledged. The bibliographic references purposely include many review articles for the sake of brevity, but the bibliographies of the review articles allow the reader to find the source of the original work they cite.

Contents

1

A Method of Chest Film Analysis

The chest film is an information system, and the task of the interpreter is to retrieve, analyze, and successfully communicate the available information.[6,10] The most significant contribution that you can make to the patient's welfare is to decide first whether the chest film is normal or abnormal. No matter how brilliant you may be in elaborating differential diagnoses based on chest film abnormalities, the patient's needs will not be served unless you first find the abnormality that needs to be defined. In fact, if you perform this task successfully, you can then at least seek counsel among your medical colleagues as to how to proceed to a definitive diagnosis, whereas if you fail, the abnormality may not come to light until another time, often at a stage less favorable for successful intervention.

CHEST RADIOGRAPHIC ANATOMY

Recognition of an abnormality on a chest film depends on a critical knowledge of the details of chest radiographic anatomy — normal anatomy as well as congenital and developmental variants and harmless departures from normal.

Figures 1-1 to 1-4 show annotated details of pulmonary and nonpulmonary structures visible on posteroanterior (PA) and lateral views of the chest. The commonly accepted important landmarks of radiographic anatomy, such as the costophrenic angles, the diaphragmatic contours, the hilar structures, and the margins of the cardiomediastinal silhouette, are identified and present no recognition problem when they are normal. However, there are many nonpulmonary soft tissue and bony shadows whose images are superimposed on the lungs. It is important to understand these shadows so as not to confuse them with abnormalities. Fortunately, they can all be recognized once you are familiar with their appearance and if you remember to consider them when analyzing chest films (Table 1-1).

TABLE 1-1. Some Normal Structures and Configurations Not To Be Confused With Intrathoracic Lesions

Transverse and spinous processes of thoracic vertebrae (Figs. 1-1A to C, 1-2A).

Pedicles and articulating processes of thoracic vertebrae (Figs. 1-1A and C, 1-2D, 1-3A)

Calcified costal cartilages (Figs. 1-2C and D, 1-6A and E)

Variations in rib contours (Figs. 1-2A, D, and G)

Images of scapulae superimposed on lungs (Figs. 1-1C_1, 1-3)

Rib companion shadows — soft tissue shadows seen along the inferior margins of the upper ribs posteriorly and along the course of the lower ribs laterally (Fig. 1-6F)

Deformities of the chest, e.g., secondary to scoliosis (Fig. 1-2D and F)

Azygos lobe fissure (Fig. 1-2I and J)

PA AND LATERAL VIEWS OF THE CHEST

The data from both the PA and the lateral view should be correlated and integrated before reaching conclusions about any chest radiographic examination. The lateral view deserves as careful an analysis as the PA view. If you find that you have a tendency to pay maximum attention to the PA view and minimum attention to the lateral view, you might practice analyzing the lateral view before the PA view.

Figures 1-3 and 1-4 show many anatomic landmarks seen on the lateral view of the chest and on acceptable slight variations off of the true lateral projection. The article by Proto and Speckman[8] is a valuable source of anatomic-radiologic correlations for those who wish to study this subject in more detail.

THE MEDIASTINUM

Many features of radiographic anatomy of the mediastinum[9] are included in the illustrations already presented (Figs. 1-1A and 1-3A). In Chapter 7 the normal mediastinum is discussed and illustrated in detail as a prelude to a discussion of the deviations from normal caused by mediastinal masses.

THE HILA

There are no measurements that reliably separate hila into normal and abnormal categories. Strictly speaking, a lung hilum is an area in a plane of the medial portions of the lungs through which vessels, bronchi, and nerves pass into the lung from the mediastinum. As applied to the chest film, however, the term denotes the central shadows of the lung roots, which are comprised of larger vessels and bronchi. Hilar images represent individual but superimposed anatomic structures, and it is useful to think of them in those terms rather than consider them as solitary structures.

The Right Hilum

The right upper lobe bronchus and the bronchus intermedius serve as landmarks for evaluating the right hilum. With practice, both can be recognized on films exposed using modern techniques. Since the right pulmonary artery (RPA) gives off its upper division branch while inside the mediastinum, the origin of this branch is not recognizable on plain films. The vessel becomes visible, with varying degrees of clarity from individual to individual, when it passes into the right upper lobe at approximately the level of the right upper lobe bronchus. Usually the superior pulmonary vein presents a more prominent image at this level of the hilum and is projected obliquely in a position lateral and inferior to the upper division artery. Branch vessels of both this artery and the accompanying vein are partly superimposed on one another in the lung beyond their major trunks.

The interlobar branch of the RPA carries blood to pulmonary arterial branches supplying the right middle and lower lobes. After the interlobar artery exits the mediastinum it is projected roughly parallel to the bronchus intermedius (Figs. 1-1A and 1-3A). Measurements of the width of this vessel on radiographs have been based on this relationship (see Chapter 9).

The Left Hilum

The left main and left upper lobe bronchi serve as convenient landmarks for evaluating the left hilum (Figs. 1-1A and 1-3A). As the left pulmonary artery (LPA) passes from anterior to posterior, it passes over these airways and presents as a mass of variable size interposed between the image of the transverse portion of the aortic arch and these subjacent airways. The upper walls of these bronchi form a sharp interface with the lower edge of the LPA. (This image of the LPA is commonly interpreted as a tumor by neophyte students.) Branch vessels to the left upper lobe can be identified as they emerge beyond the central portion of the LPA, but frequently their precise site of origin from the parent vessel cannot be recognized on either the PA or the lateral view. The intermediate portion of the LPA, known as the left interlobar artery, passes obliquely and caudally out into the lung, where branches to the lingula can be identified. The basal branch of the vessel then is projected lateral to the left lower lobe bronchus and gives off branches to the segments of this lobe. Some of these branches pass lateral to the air shadow of the left lower lobe bronchus, whereas others cross the image of the bronchus and pass medially toward the base of the lung.

In the vast majority of people, the left hilum is projected higher than the right, because the LPA is projected as a unit above the left main and upper lobe bronchi whereas the RPA has divided into upper and lower divisions while inside the mediastinum. Only the lower division, which is projected below the right upper lobe bronchus, accounts for the bulk of the right hilum on both PA and lateral views.

The details of hilar arterial and venous anatomy along with examples of hilar pathology are illustrated in Chapter 8.

Bronchial arteries and veins are not recognizable on chest films under normal circumstances. In patients with certain congenital heart lesions, bronchial arteries may play such an important role in collateral circulation that they become large enough to project as discrete images.

FILM SEARCH TECHNIQUE

There is no scientific evidence that a systematic approach to chest film analysis is any better than a "gestalt" approach in terms of retrieving significant information from the film, but it appears that part of the problem lies in confusing our belief that we are using a systematic analysis when, in practice, we are not.

"Seeing" is learned, but cannot even begin until one develops the self-discipline necessary to "look." Successful looking requires that no portion of the film escapes attention. Any technique that ensures complete study of the film will serve you well. You must then develop the discipline to apply the technique in each case and not consciously become enmeshed in the details of execution while forgetting the purpose.

I have tried to develop a search technique applicable to chest film analysis (Fig. 1-5). I do not make any claims of originality for this technique, I do not remember its origins and I have modified it many times. You may find it useful, or you may choose to use only some parts of it in developing your own search methods. Whatever technique you eventually develop, bear in mind two key principles:

1. The vast majority of "water-density" shadows (i.e., those produced by any of the body's natural liquids or tissues other than fat and bone) seen in radiographs of normal lungs are produced by blood vessels. If you see an image that does not conform to your concept of a blood vessel in the lung, you must think about it carefully, for it is almost always abnormal. Do not, however, confuse "in the lung" with "in the chest."

2. There is relative bilateral symmetry of form and density in normal images of the lungs. The number of small vessels seen and the overall degree of blackening of a square centimeter of lung area on one side of the chest film will be closely comparable to those of a corresponding area on the opposite side, *barring technical flaws.* This principle does not apply to the hila, to the larger pulmonary vessels, or to lung superimposed on the heart.

The search technique presented in Figure 1-5 requires a lot of words to describe and demands more time to read than to do. Most students will be able to perform the whole sequence in a minute and a half after considerable practice. However, there is seldom a legitimate need to rush film analysis. At first, you will get bogged down in the mechanics of the search and miss observations because you are concentrating on the technique rather than its purpose. This burden will recede markedly with time, and yet you may never achieve a perfect search pattern. The challenge is in the trying.

If you simply cannot put up with such a seemingly laborious technique, you might try to scan the film in successive horizontal bands from top to bottom (or vice versa), with supplemental search of each hilum, the mediastinal contours, and the retrocardiac region.

Horizontal eye movements are recommended for search of the lungs on the frontal view of the chest because that technique encourages comparison of one side with the other. Vertical eye movements are used for inspection of the lateral view because side-to-side comparison serves no purpose in the analysis.

Eventually, those who persevere will find a technique that suits their needs. Do not be discouraged if you feel you are inconsistent for a longer period than you like. No one interprets chest films with complete success all of the time.

Using a Variety of Maneuvers

Try to view all projections of the chest from varying distances and angles or, alternatively, experiment with the use of a minifying lens in order to enhance the visibility of subtle lesions. Do not be satisfied with viewing films only when mounted on the viewer panel; instead, remove them (being careful to put your fingers only on noncritical areas of the film) in order to use a bright light. There are details present in the blacker regions that are not detectable with the intensity of light coming from the average viewer. In addition, use of the bright light encourages you to scan smaller areas of the film at one time. If a bright light is not available, a rolled-up piece of dark paper or black film can be used like a child's toy spyglass to focus on dark areas of the film. This maneuver will enhance details surprisingly well. When digitized images replace conventional filming techniques it will be possible to manipulate the gray scale of the images electronically and thus eliminate the need for brightlighting.

Try to view films in a quiet area where you can concentrate on the task. Eliminate all unnecessary light, and particularly avoid light to either side of the films being studied as well as light shining on the film from behind your viewing position.

The Use of "Left" and "Right"

Whenever the terms "left" and "right" are used to locate pathologic or anatomic structures on a radiographic, computed tomographic, or magnetic resonance examination, they refer to the *patient's* left or right side. It often takes several weeks before beginning students and residents become accustomed to the fact that imaging studies are usually viewed in a manner that places the patient's left side on the observer's right side and vice versa.

Whenever the terms "left" and "right" are used to designate the position of an illustration in a series, they refer to the *observer's* left or right side.

Causes of Differences in Film Density From Side To Side

Technical Flaws

Technical flaws account for the majority of instances in which differences in film density are noted between the right and left sides of the frontal view (PA or AP). The most common of these flaws occurs when the patient's position is actually slightly oblique rather than squarely perpendicular to the x-ray beam. This causes the beam to pass through the soft tissues (mainly paraspinal muscles) for a greater distance on one side than the other. This longer path through water-density absorbers results in more x-ray absorption and an overall lighter gray appearance than on the opposite side. Rotation can be recognized by noting the relative positions of the medial ends of the clavicles in reference to the spine.

In chest radiography, a grid is commonly interposed between the patient and the x-ray film to reduce the image degradation caused by scatter radiation from the patient reaching the film. When the x-ray tube is off-center to the grid, both laterally and in the focus-to-grid distance, an uneven exposure of the film occurs. This causes one side of the film to be lighter than the other. (See Ch. 8 of reference 3 for a discussion of grids.) A similar technical flaw occurs when the heel of the tube's anode is placed so that more x-rays pass through one side of the patient than the other.[3] These flaws can be recognized because the soft tissues along the lateral chest wall and the bones of the shoulder girdle participate in the film density discrepancy rather than the lungs along.

Structural Differences

An absence of soft tissues on one side (e.g., as a result of mastectomy) or an increase in the amount of soft tissues on one side (e.g., due to hematoma or a chest wall mass) will also cause film density differences. These tissue discrepancies can usually be recognized by careful attention to the appearance of the soft tissues on the film and can be confirmed by physical examination.

Air Trapping, Hypoperfusion, and Compensatory Overexpansion of the Lung

Differences in the overall opacity of one lung, or even a lung zone, compared to its counterpart, when accompanied by a reduction in the number of small vessels visible per unit area, are abnormal findings. Hypoperfused zones will appear darker gray. (To estimate and compare vessel deficiencies in one zone to its opposite you may have to use a bright light.) This indicates that there is either (1) air trapping in the involved lung and hypoxic vasoconstriction; (2) vascular obstruction due to disease, or vascular deficiency due to an anatomic anomaly; or (3) compensatory overexpansion (compensatory "emphysema") of the involved region due to collapse or removal of other lobes.

A film made during expiration will accentuate the film density discrepancy when it is due to air trapping. Bronchoscopy can be used to assess the possibility of central bronchial obstruction as the cause. On the other hand, vascular lesions do not cause air trapping, so that there will be no associated accentuation of density differences on films made during expiration. Pulmonary arteriography or radioisotope perfusion lung scans may be used to evaluate the cause in these cases. Compensatory overexpansion due to atelectasis of the adjacent lung is usually apparent because the atelectatic portion is seen on the chest film. Compensatory expansion due to prior surgical removal of an adjacent lobe or lobes can usually be inferred by recognizing the effects of surgery (e.g., rib resection or deformity) and confirmed by history and physical examination. Illustrations of these conditions will be found in Chapters 4, 6, and 9.

Comparing Current and Prior Examinations

Comparison of a current chest examination with any prior chest imaging studies that are available should be made a principle of operation. Even when the current films are considered to be normal, such comparisons are valuable. Changes from a previous appearance are often early indications of abnormality, even though the overall appearance of the mediastinum or hila or diaphragm or lung is still within the broad range of normal for a population.

When several prior studies are available, comparison with the current study should be made with those that are more remote as well as with those that are recent. Often the determination of a "stable finding" versus a "significant interval change" will strongly influence the diagnosis, course of action, and treatment planning.

NOW THAT YOU ARE "LOOKING," WHAT SHOULD YOU "SEE"?

The Costophrenic Angles

Since you are starting the search at the left costophrenic angle (Fig. 1-5), you ought to become familiar with the normal range of variation in the contours of the costophrenic angles. In general, the costophrenic angles can be accepted as normal when there is a relatively sharp angle between the lateral aspects of the hemidiaphragm and the adjacent rib. One or two millimeters medial to the rib the diaphragm may intersect with a crescentic soft tissue "companion" shadow paralleling the course of the bone (Fig. 1-6A to F).

When the costophrenic angle assumes a shallow "U" shape, it is considered blunted, and when flattened out it is considered obliterated. These alterations in contour are almost always manifestations of pleural abnormalities, either acute or chronic, and will be discussed in Chapter 3.

In some patients, several curved, short, "edge" shadows are seen to constitute the margins of the costophrenic angles. These represent slips of origin of diaphragmatic muscle bundles from adjacent ribs. (If the muscular slips of the diaphragm originate from the ribs, where do they insert?) These muscular slips and their pleural covering are exaggerated in people whose lungs are large in volume. In adulthood these edge shadows occur in patients who suffer from some form of obstructive lung disease, such as emphysema, chronic bronchitis, or asthma (during attacks). On the other hand, they may also be seen in people who are healthy, particularly those who are capable of very deep inspiration. Knowing the patient's age will separate these two groups in the majority of cases, and even a modest appraisal of the patient's exercise tolerance (from the history) will separate all but a very few of the remainder.

The Diaphragm

The variability in the contour of the diaphragm often surprises students and beginning residents. The convenient conception is that of a continuous, smooth arch that is convex upward, extending from the costophrenic angle to the spine (Fig. 1-6A). In fact, the contour spectrum is quite variable (Fig. 1-6B to L).

In the majority of people, the high point of the right hemidiaphragm will be projected at a higher level than that of the left hemidiaphragm on a PA view. In approximately 10 percent of normal people, however, the left will be projected at the same level or slightly higher than the right. The high point of either hemidiaphragm may be located along the middle third of its arc or may be located medially, adjacent to the spine. The high points of the diaphragm shadows are never adjacent to the costophrenic angle in the normal individual.

Since the hemidiaphragms are water-density structures in close approximation to normally air-containing lung, you should expect to see a sharp diaphragm surface wherever these juxtaposed, different-density absorbers present a sufficient tangent to the beam. However, if the truly subcardiac portion of the diaphragm is tangential to the beam, that segment will not be seen as a distinct image, since the tangent will present a water density (heart) against a water density (diaphragm).

In addition, when any liquid, such as blood, pus, or edema fluid, occupies a portion of lung or pleural space adjacent to the lung-diaphragm tangent, the sharp interface will be lost. That segment of the diaphragm shadow will be effaced or replaced by a pseudodiaphragm image. A pseudodiaphragm image can also appear when subpulmonic pleural fluid, layered over the diaphragm, produces a fortuitous sharp interface with adjacent lung.

There are circumstances in which a segment of the diaphragm is not sharply defined in the normal individual (Fig. 1-6D). On either the right or the left side, a short segment of the diaphragm may appear unsharp and slightly tented (Fig. 1-6E). This is the point at which the major interlobar fissure reaches the level of the diaphragm, or it may represent the point at which the inferior pulmonary ligament or inferior accessory fissure[5] reaches the diaphragm.

The combination of a flattened diaphragm and an angled x-ray beam may prevent recognition of a distinct diaphragm surface, because the interface between the diaphragm and the adjacent normal lung is not tangential to the beam under these circumstances. This is especially troublesome on AP chest films made with the patient supine. Likewise, in children who have a sharply downward-sloping diaphragm from anterior to posterior, there may not be a lung-diaphragm tangent long enough to produce a good image on the PA projection.

Free air or gas in the abdomen can accumulate under the diaphragm when the patient is erect, and even small amounts can be seen on chest films made when the patient is upright or sitting (Fig. 1-6H). Care must be exercised to avoid mistaking large volumes of air in a distended stomach, gas in a distended colon, or a high right colon for free abdominal air (Fig. 1-6G and I). Occasionally fat under the diaphragm or a Mach effect[7] can cause confusion, but correlation with the clinical status of the patient will usually resolve doubts. A left lateral decubitus film of the abdomen can be used whenever doubt remains, since free abdominal gas should move up to the right flank when the patient is in that position.

Details

After the study of the diaphragm, the search pattern calls for an evaluation of mediastinal structures, lung, bones, and soft tissues. The details shown in Figures 1-1 through 1-4 now must be understood so that your scan can be completed knowledgeably. Throughout the remainder of this book, emphasis will be placed on understanding the radiographic spectrum of these anatomic landmarks and the variety of ways in which they may become altered by intrathoracic disease.

SUMMARY

1. Two key principles can be used to govern the interpretation of chest radiographs:
   a. The vast majority of water-density images seen in radiographs of normal lungs represent blood vessels. Blood vessels are tubular structures that taper and branch as they extend peripherally. Any water-density image in a lung zone that does not conform to your expectation of a blood vessel should be suspected as abnormal.
   b. There is relative symmetry of form (number and size of blood vessels) and film density (average opacity) between equivalent zones of the right and left lungs. Violations of this principle should raise the consideration of abnormality, barring common technical flaws.
2. The correct interpretation of chest imaging studies requires the discipline to develop and use a search technique that ensures that all portions of the display will be *looked* at. *Seeing* requires *looking* and learning.
3. A major obligation of the interpreter is to recognize departures from normal. This requires the continual study of normal and harmless variations in any given population to develop a thorough understanding of radiographic anatomy.
4. Knowledge of anatomy per se must be augmented by knowledge of how the images of anatomic structures are altered by differences in radiographic projection, technique, and imaging methods.
5. Comparison of current imaging studies with prior examinations is critically important.

BIBLIOGRAPHY

1. Some general texts that are extremely helpful and can be used to explore further all of the subjects covered in this text are:
   a. Felson B: Chest Roentgenology. WB Saunders, Philadelphia, 1973
   b. Fraser RB, Pare JAP: Diagnosis of Diseases of the Chest. 2nd Ed. WB Saunders, Philadelphia, 1979
   c. Heitzman ER: The Lung: Radiologic-Pathologic Correlations, 2nd Ed. CV Mosby, St. Louis, 1984
   d. Simon G: Principles of Chest X-Ray Diagnosis. 4th Ed. Butterworths, London, 1978
   These will not be referenced again, but generally they could be included as part of the bibliography at the end of each chapter.
2. Bachman DM, Ellis K, Austin JHM: The effects of minor degrees of obliquity on the lateral chest radiograph. Radiol Clin North Am 16:465–485, 1978
3. Curry TS III, Dowdey JE, Murry RC: Christensen's Introduction to the Physics of Diagnostic Radiology. 3rd Ed. Lea & Febiger, Philadelphia, 1984
4. Gale MC, Grief LW: Intrafissural fat: CT correlation with chest radiographs. Radiology 160:333, 1986
5. Godwin JD, Tarver RD: Accessory fissures of the lung. AJR 144:39, 1985
6. Kundel HL, La Follette PS Jr: Visual search patterns and experience with radiologic images. Radiology 103:523, 1972
7. Lane EJ, Proto AV, Phillips TW: Mach bands and density perceptions. Radiology 121:9, 1976
8. Proto AV, Speckman JM: The lateral radiograph of the chest. Medical Radiography and Photography 55:30–74, 1979; 56:38–62, 1980 (Those who intend to make chest radiographic interpretation a significant part of their work may wish to write the Eastman Kodak Co. to obtain these issues for the library. They are worth reading more than once.)
9. Proto AV: Mediastinal anatomy: emphasis on conventional images with anatomic and computed tomographic correlations. J Thorac Imaging 2(1):1–48, 1987
10. Tuddenham WJ: Visual search, image organization and reader error in roentgen diagnosis: studies of the psychophysiology. Radiology 78:694, 1962

Atlas

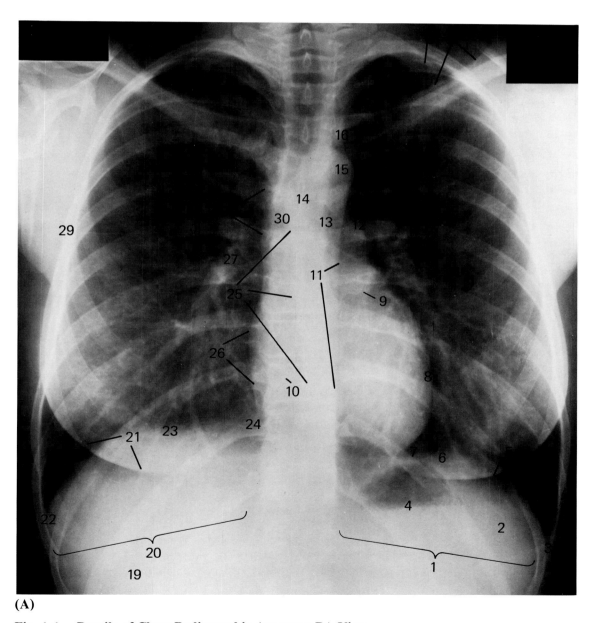

(A)

Fig. 1-1. Details of Chest Radiographic Anatomy: PA View

(A,B) Posteroanterior (PA) chest radiographs of a normal individual. *(Figure continues.)*

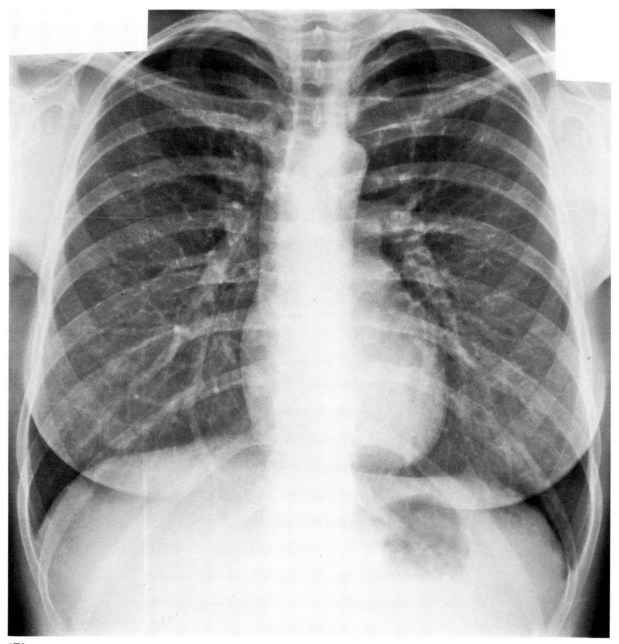

(B)

Fig. 1-1. *(Continued).* **(B)** Another PA view, with the radiographic and photographic techniques adjusted to emphasize the details of the pulmonary vessels. All of the structures labeled in Fig. A can still be seen, but those in the retrocardiac region are barely identifiable. A light exposure technique will enhance the visibility of the pulmonary vessels at the expense of detail of retrocardiac structures, and in more heavily built patients there will be loss of lung detail below the diaphragmatic domes.

The details of pulmonary vessels in the upper lungs of a film exposed as in Fig. A can be brought out by transilluminating those portions of the film with a bright light. However, there is no convenient way to resurrect the details lost in a film that is too light. One must constantly strive for an optimum technique that balances these trade-offs in any given patient. The technique here is acceptable.

Identify as much anatomical detail as you can before referring back to Fig. A. *(Figure continues.)*

Key (Fig. 1-1A,B)

1. Lung projecting below the left diaphragm dome, recognizable because of images of blood vessels extending well toward the periphery
2. Spleen
3. Left costrophrenic angle
4. Air in the stomach
5. Margin of the left breast
6. Left hemidiaphragm
7. Left cardiophrenic angle
8. Edge of the left ventricle
9. Transverse process of a lower vertebra behind the heart and beneath the medial end of its corresponding rib
10. Pedicle of a lower vertebra seen end-on
11. Left lateral margin of the descending thoracic aorta
12. Left pulmonary artery
13. Left main bronchus
14. Carina of the trachea
15. Aortic arch (notice its impression on the adjacent trachea; the "aortic knob" is the posterior turn of the aortic arch, which is seen as a prominent image on a PA view)
16. Left subclavian artery
17. Supraclavicular soft tissue companion shadow
18. Companion shadow of the second rib
19. Liver
20. Lung projecting below the right diaphragm dome, recognizable because of images of blood vessels extending well toward the periphery
21. Margin of the right breast
22. Right costophrenic angle
23. Right hemidiaphragm
24. Right cardiophrenic angle
25. Azygoesophageal pleural reflection, prespinal; medial edge of the right lung
26. Edge of the right atrium (right heart border)
27. Interlobar branch of the right pulmonary artery (the branch beyond the origin of the pulmonary artery trunk that is the main supply of the upper lobe)
28. Superior vena cava
29. Minor interlobar fissure
30. Right main bronchus

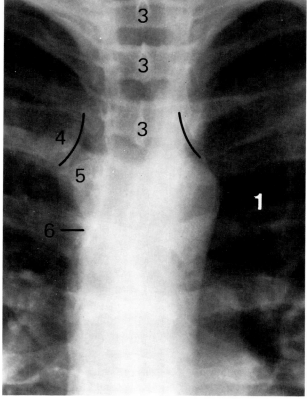

(C)

Fig. 1-1. *(Continued).* **(C)** PA coned view of the upper chest.

Key (Fig. 1-1C)

1. Lateral edge of the left side of the manubrium. The cortex is visible as a fine line shadow superimposed on the aortic arch (it mimics a calcific plaque in the aortic arch).
2. Medial end of the left clavicle
3. Spinous processes of upper thoracic vertebrae seen end-on
4. Medial end of the right clavicle
5. Right side of the manubrium
6. A diminutive azygos vein image

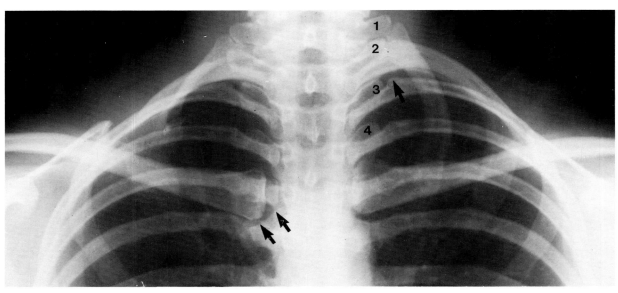

(A)

Fig. 1-2. Features Visible on PA Chest Views

(A) PA film. Note the following details:

1. **Rib Anomaly.** There is an anomaly of the right first and second ribs. The right first rib is thin and short and joins the second anteriorly. The anterior portion of the right second rib is wider than its opposite.
2. **Articulation of Clavicle and Manubrium.** This person is fairly well positioned in that the spinous processes of the vertebrae are projected in the midline of the tracheal air column. The medial end of the right clavicle, however, is projected a little further from the edge of the vertebra than is that of the left, indicating a slight degree of rotation. Similarly, the manubrial fossa for the right clavicular head (paired black arrows) is seen over a slightly greater extent than is the left.
3. **Transverse processes.** The transverse processes (1–4) of the thoracic vertebrae are projected so that a considerable portion of their mass is seen above the level of the pos-teromedial ends of the corresponding ribs at the upper thoracic levels (T1 through T4 in this person). On films exposed with a high-kilovoltage technique, these relatively thin bony structures may be mistaken for nodules in the lung, particularly when their lateral edges are sharply defined. When their bulk is projected behind the rib end (T5–T7) they do not cause confusion. More inferiorly (see Fig. 1-1A), they are projected below the corresponding rib ends, and any one may be mistaken for a lung nodule, particularly when located in the left retrocardiac region.
4. **Costotransverse articulations.** The joints of the costotransverse articulations may be quite conspicuous at some levels. The tubercle (black arrow on left third rib) along the superior aspect of the ribs at this joint may develop spurs that can be confused with small pulmonary nodules by the unwary. *(Figure continues.)*

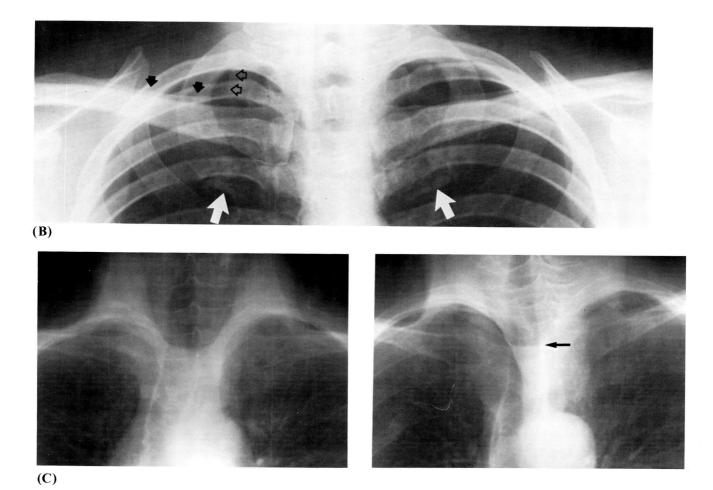

(B)

(C)

Fig. 1-2. *(Continued).*   **(B,C)** Films of a different patient. On film B, note the following details:

1. **Calcified cartilages of the first rib.** There is moderately extensive calcification or ossification of the costal cartilages of both first ribs (white arrows). These cartilages are the first to calcify and frequently are visible as early as the third decade. Here they are relatively symmetric and bandlike, and therefore unlikely to cause confusion or be mistaken for pulmonary lesions.
2. **Sternocleidomastoid muscle and supraclavicular companion shadow.** The edge of the sternocleidomastoid muscle on the right is seen superimposed on the pulmonary apex (open arrows) and blends with the soft tissue companion shadow over the superior surface of the right clavicle (black arrows). Similar findings are present on the left, but they are less conspicuous. If you stand in front of a mirror with your hands on your hips, your shoulders rotated forward, and your chin raised — the position assumed for the PA chest film — you will see how these soft tissues can project enough of a tangent to the x-ray beam to cast radiographic images.

A soft tissue mass in the neck or the supraclavicular fossa will alter or efface these contours. However, such a mass would also be evident simply by looking at the patient.

(C) In this thin patient the medial margins of the sternocleidomastoid muscles are well defined and joined by a suprasternal fold of skin, which imparts a U-shaped lower margin to the space between these muscles.

On the next film the patient is seen to have rotated into a slight left anterior oblique position. The suprasternal skin fold is foreshortened and superimposed on the trachea. It could be mistaken for a fluid level in the esophagus. *(Figure continues.)*

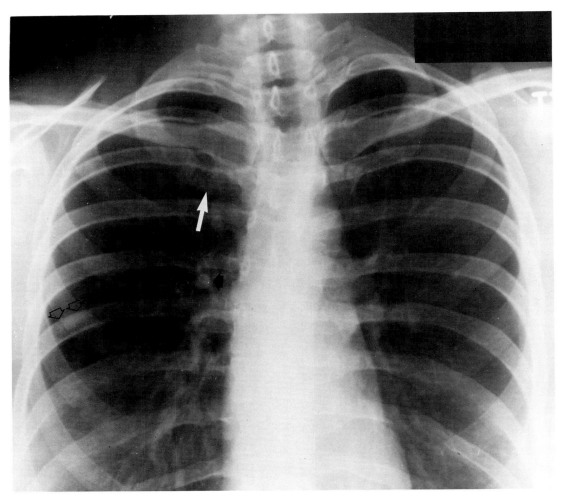

(D)

Fig. 1-2. *(Continued).*   **(D,E)** Films of a different patient. On film D, the following details can be seen:

1. There is irregular calcification or ossification) of the right first rib cartilage (arrow) and costochondral junction. Calcification is present to a lesser extent on the left side in the cartilage adjacent to the manubrium. When asymmetrical, a calcified cartilage can be mistaken for a noncalcified pulmonary lesion on a film made with modern high-kilovoltage techniques. An asymmetrical spur at the costochondral junction may also be mistaken for a pulmonary nodule.

2. A focal area of sclerosis is present in the posterior right seventh rib (paired open arrows). This may be produced by focal benign sclerosis, comparable to a compact bone island. In patients with carcinoma, especially of the prostate or the breast, such foci may be confused with osteoblastic metastases if old films are not available to show their stability over long periods.

3. Notice the bronchus seen end-on and its adjacent artery in the superior aspect of the right hilum (opposing open and black arrows).

4. The asymmetry in the conformation of the apices is due to scoliosis of the thoracic spine.

5. The right pedicles of T5 – T7 are easily seen in the lower portion of the scoliotic curve. They are projected clear of mediastinal structures.

6. Count the posterior ribs. Notice that the inferior cortex of the posterior right eighth rib appears to be interrupted over a long midsegment (compare to the appearance of the inferior cortex of the rib above). This is a normal appearance and a common occurrence in many ribs. It should not be confused with a destructive process. The shape of the rib at this site (find a skeleton to study) accounts for this appearance, and usually you see a thin flange of bone bridging this site inferiorly. *(Figure continues.)*

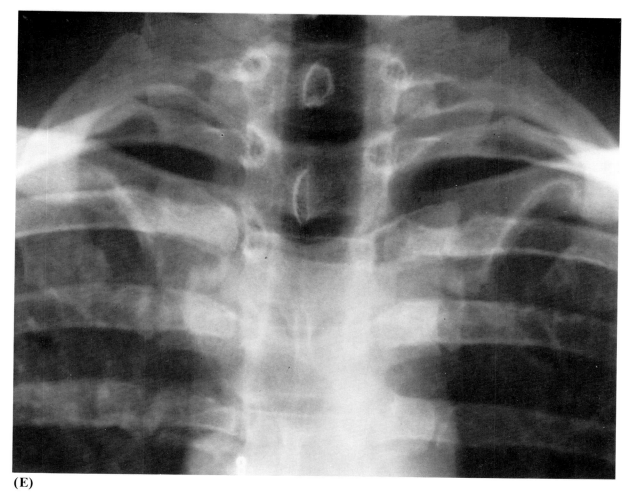

(E)

Fig. 1-2. *(Continued).* **(E)** There is a large, sharply defined defect in the medial end of each clavicle at the site of the rhomboid fossa. This is the location of the ligamentous attachment to the first rib. These anatomic defects are quite variable and may be much more prominent on one side than the other. They should not be mistaken for destructive bone lesions when asymmetrical. *(Figure continues.)*

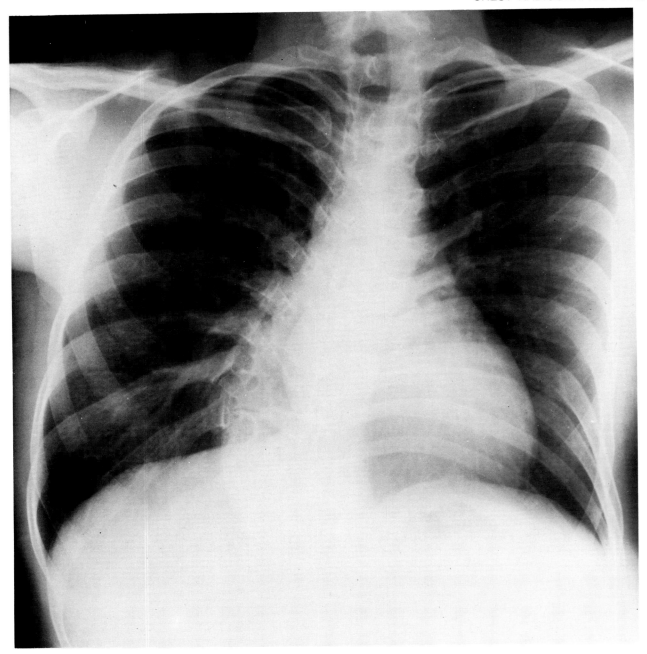

(F)

Fig. 1-2. *(Continued).* **(F)** Patient with thoracic scoliosis. Note the following points:

1. The scoliosis is moderately severe, so that the lower thoracic vertebrae are projected to the right of the right heart border. The trachea is projected to the right of the midline of the superimposed vertebrae, and the medial end of the right clavicle is projected farther away from the adjacent vertebral margin than is the left.

2. The trunk of a large right inferior pulmonary vein is superimposed on the ninth posterior rib and causes its posteromedial end to appear dense.

3. Even though it is superimposed on the spine, the right heart border is sharply defined since it maintains an interface with adjacent aerated lung. *(Figure continues.)*

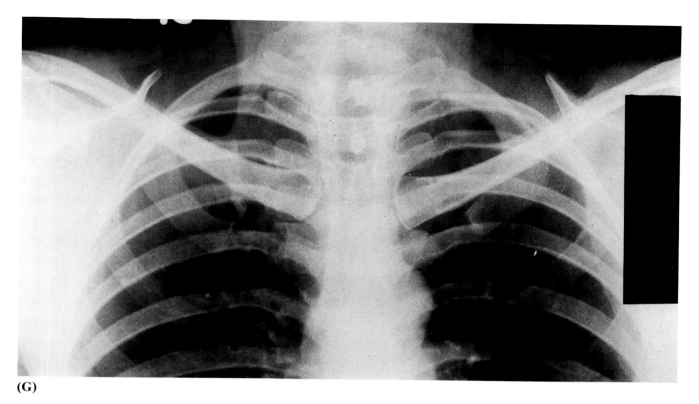

(G)

Fig. 1-2. *(Continued).* **(G,H)** Patient with an anomalous cervical rib on the right. **(G)** In this film, compare the right and left pulmonary apices. There is an image in the right apical and subclavicular region that has no counterpart on the left. It is oval and has irregular margins.

1. It violates the principle of relative symmetry of form and density and therefore should be considered abnormal (or its absence on the left is abnormal).
2. It absorbs the x-ray beam as though it were of greater density than nearby vessels, and it appears similar in radiodensity to the adjacent clavicle and ribs.

The following incidental details are also visible:

1. There are shallow notches (scalloping) of the inferior cortices of the posteromedial ends of the fifth and sixth ribs on the right and on the left. These are normal. Rib notching due to tortuous intercostal arteries serving as collateral flow channels, as in patients with coarctation of the aorta, occurs more laterally. There are many other causes of rib notching.[1a]
2. Both lateral margins of the manubrium are seen. They are asymmetrical, but normal.
3. A small granuloma is seen adjacent to the eighth rib in the right axillary line. It is too big to be a vessel seen end-on, but its density (due to calcium) is similar. The small round dots in the right lower lung zones are vessels and appear dense because they are produced by a relatively long column of blood projected end-on.
4. The small, white, zigzag opacity beneath the posterior left fifth rib is an artifact. A small metallic foreign body could present the same appearance. *(Figure continues.)*

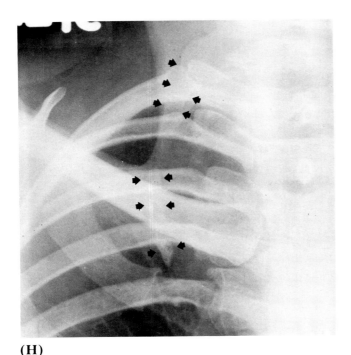

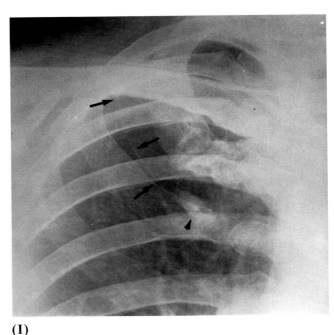

(H)   **(I)**

Fig. 1-2. *(Continued).* **(H)** Coned view of the right apex and subclavicular region of the same patient seen in G. With great diligence and a little imagination, you can see a small nubbin projecting inferiorly from the right transverse process of C7 (upper arrows). It is difficult to appreciate because it is superimposed on the posterior first rib for most of its course. Once you have made the observation, you could deduce that this and the apparently unconnected elongated structure projected medial to the first rib (lower arrows) are all part of an imperfect cervical rib. They are probably connected by a nonopaque fibrous bridge.

Notice that the soft tissues over the right sternocleidomastoid muscle are sharply defined all the way down to the supraclavicular companion shadow. On the left (see Fig. G), the lower portion of the sternocleidomastoid muscle is not as sharp, probably because of a slight rotation of the neck, making it less tangential to the beam. The sharply defined lateral cortical margin of the manubrium is seen extending well below the medial end of the right clavicle.

(I) The azygos lobe. The azygos lobe fissure is formed by anomalous descent of the azygos vein through the substance of the right upper lobe. As it descends from an extrapleural location, the vein creates a sling consisting of four layers of pleura, two parietal and two visceral. These pleural surfaces become apposed and cast an image of a fine line. The degree of obliquity of the line varies with the degree of lateral displacement from which the vein began its descent, whereas the curvature of the line depends on the course of descent toward the superior vena cava. The elliptical shadow at the lower end of the arc represents the azygos vein (arrow).

Because it does not have a separate dedicated bronchus, the azygos lobe is not a true lobe of the lung. Lung medial to the fissure may appear slightly more opaque than adjacent lung even though normal. Uncommonly, however, an area of pulmonary consolidation appears limited to the azygos lobe.

Notice the marked calcification and ossification of the costal cartilage of the right first rib. *(Figure continues.)*

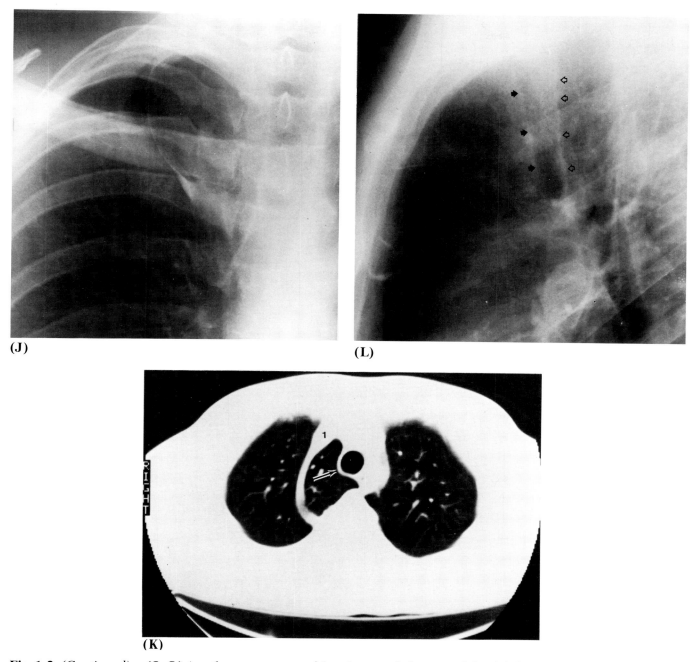

(J)

(L)

(K)

Fig. 1-2. *(Continued).* **(J – L)** Another young man with a characteristic azygos lobe. **(J)** Coned view of the right upper chest. This view differs from the one in Fig. I in that the fissure at the apex is more medial in position and the pleural boundaries (which account for the white line) are more bowed. Again, the elliptical shadow at the lower end is produced by the azygos vein. **(K)** CT section through the bottom of the azygos lobe fissure to show its anteroposterior relationships. The vein courses anteriorly to empty into the superior vena cava (1). Notice how much lung is interposed between the mediastinum and the azygos fissure. This lung has interfaces with the right lateral and posterolateral walls of the trachea (arrow) and with the posterior wall of the vena cava.

(L) Coned lateral view of the upper chest. A faint edge (black arrows) is projected anterior to the anterior tracheal wall (open arrows). This edge is produced by the interface of the posterior wall of the superior vena cava with the azygos lobe and is a more conspicuous shadow than is seen in most people who do not have an azygos lobe.

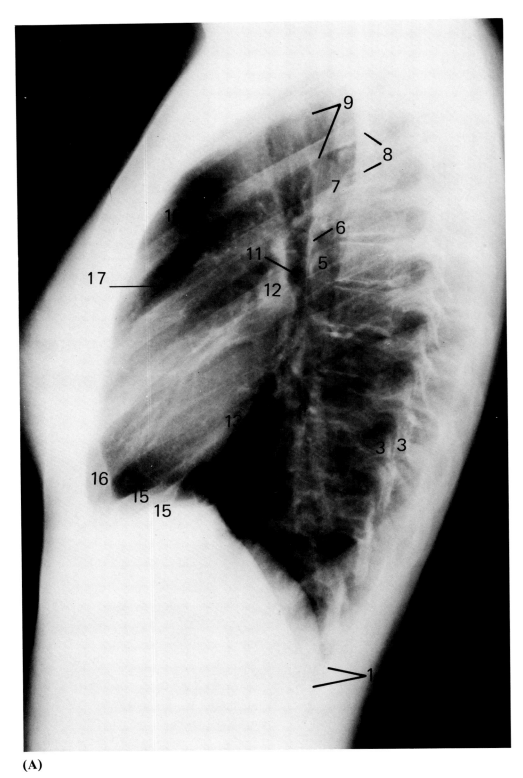

(A)

Fig. 1-3. Details of Chest Radiographic Anatomy: Lateral View

(A) Orienting the lateral view. Since we look at the PA view as though we are facing the patient from behind the film holder, it is reasonable to look at the lateral view in the same manner. A left lateral view (patient's left side against the film holder) will be mounted on the viewer so that the patient is facing to the observer's left. Nevertheless, this viewpoint is not shared by all, and in many other texts and articles you will find the left lateral view shown as though the patient is facing to the observer's right.

Note that there is a gradation of the gray tones over the posterior third of the chest such that the image becomes darker gray as you proceed caudally. This gradation is most marked in films of muscular and heavy-set individuals and will be less conspicuous in films of thin individuals or films that are heavily exposed. In this example the gradation is definite.

Search the film from top to bottom, over the region of the spine and the intervertebral foramina, to appreciate the gradual change from lighter to darker gray. The shape of the thoracic cage and the relatively large amount of overlying soft tissue in the path of the beam superiorly, as compared to the lesser thickness of soft tissues about the larger chest cage caudally, account for this appearance.

Assessment of this gray tone range is very useful. When it is uniform or lighter caudally you know that some additional absorber has to be in the beam path, either in the lung (a lower lobe mass or atelectasis), in the pleura (fluid or mass), in the chest wall (hematoma or mass), or even in the esophagus, the posterior mediastinum, or the spine. Correlation with the PA view usually permits localization of the abnormality, but fluoroscopy or CT scan can resolve doubts in most questionable cases. *(Figure continues.)*

Key (Fig. 1-3A,B)

1. Posterior costophrenic angles
2. A lower thoracic vertebral body (the pedicles are seen extending posteriorly, and the intervertebral foramina are easily recognized)
3. Articulations of superior and inferior articulating processes of adjacent vertebrae
4. Superimposition of arteries and veins supplying the lower portions of the lungs
5. Left pulmonary artery
6. Posterior wall of the right main bronchus and the bronchus intermedius
7. Posterior portion of the aortic arch
8. Scapula
9. Posterior wall of the trachea
10. Anterior wall of the ascending aorta
11. Left upper lobe bronchus seen end-on
12. Interlobar branch of the right pulmonary artery (the branch beyond the origin of the main supply trunk of the upper lobe)
13. Posterior margin of the left ventricle
14. Inferior vena cava
15. Individual images of right and left hemidiaphragms
16. Extrapulmonary soft tissue anterior to the heart (the prominence of this shadow varies tremendously from patient to patient and is markedly affected by slight degrees of rotation off true lateral).
17. Outflow tract of right ventricle in continuity with the main pulmonary artery.

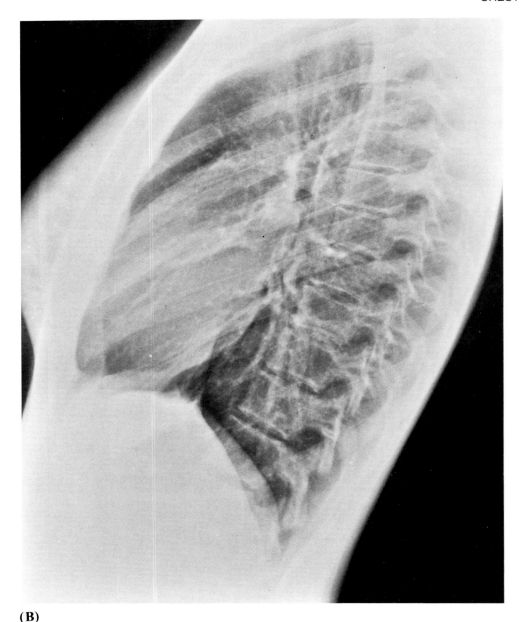

(B)

Fig. 1-3. *(Continued).* **(B)** Another lateral view of the patient in Fig. A. It has been reproduced using a logetronographic technique, which narrows the gray scale and provides edge enhancement so that the pulmonary vessels are seen better. When digital imaging techniques become widely used, this type of image enhancement will be commonly employed.

Distinguishing Right Diaphragm from Left Diaphragm on Lateral View

In radiography, it is a general principle to place the part being studied as close to the film as possible in order to achieve sharpest image definition. Therefore, if one suspected a lesion in the left lung, a left lateral view would serve best, whereas a right lateral view would be preferred for a lesion suspected in the right lung. However, in most radiologic practices, a left lateral view is obtained whenever a particular side is not specified.

A left lateral view of the chest is made with the patient standing with the left side against the film holder. The x-ray beam thus traverses the chest from right to left. Even though the x-ray tube is usually at a distance of 6 feet from the film, the rays in the beam will diverge. In the left lateral position, the portion of the beam that "sees" the posterior tangent of the ribs on the right side will traverse a longer path to the film than will those rays that "see" the posterior tangent of the ribs on the left side.

Therefore, in a true left lateral projection, the posterior tangents of the right ribs will be projected as slightly larger images posterior to the corresponding tangents of the left ribs (see Fig. 1-4B). At times it may be difficult to decide which set of rib images is really larger, because the ribs are not uniform in size along their entire course and a wider portion of a rib may be projected on one side than on the other.

Unfortunately, patients are not built in squares and rectangles, so that a true lateral projection is difficult to achieve consistently. If you cannot be certain the film was made with the patient in the true left lateral position, what other generalizations can you use to decide which posterior gutter is which, and which hemidiaphragm shadow is which?

1. If you can clearly see that gas in the fundus of the stomach or the splenic flexure of the colon is projected *under* one hemidiaphragm and *above* the other, then you can confidently identify the high diaphragm, with which it is associated, as the left. You also have to check the PA view to be sure that the stomach or colon gas is on the left side to avoid the pitfall presented by the rare patient with situs inversus or with hepatocolonic interposition.

2. The anterior third of the right hemidiaphragm commonly can be identified as a sharp shadow on the lateral view, whereas the left is often obscured by the overlying heart. This generalization is only of limited use. In fact, whether or not you will see any portion of either hemidiaphragm depends on the interface between the diaphragm and the adjacent lung. When they produce a tangential interface parallel to the x-ray beam that is long enough to produce a radiographic image, you will see a clear contour of the diaphragm on the film. Therefore, you will be able to see the left hemidiaphragm extending as far anteriorly as the right in normal subjects when the interface between the diaphragm and the lung lateral to the heart happens to be tangential to the beam on the lateral view.

3. The image of the anterior aspect of the right hemidiaphragm will be higher than the left on the left lateral view in the majority of instances.

4. The right posterior gutter is projected caudal to the left posterior gutter on the left lateral view of the chest. This is a very reliable sign in the absence of gross pleural disease provided the relative relationships of the right and left diaphragm images on the accompanying PA view are the usual ones (right dome slightly higher than the left). Therefore, the caudal posterior gutter on a left lateral view will almost always identify the right hemidiaphragm.

The only one of these generalizations that will work flawlessly in identifying a hemidiaphragm on the lateral view is clear identification of the gastric bubble or splenic flexure gas under the higher hemidiaphragm shadow. If these gas shadows are seen inferior to both hemidiaphragm images, tempting as it may be to assume that the hemidiaphragm in closer relationship to the gas shadows is the left, this conclusion will not always be correct.

There is yet another pitfall to consider. Often, in the lateral view, the images of the right and left hemidiaphragm surfaces cross one another, and sometimes it is quite easy to mistake the posterior portion of one hemidiaphragm as belonging to the anterior portion of the other, and vice versa.

How does one finally decide which is the right hemidiaphragm and which is the left on the lateral view? First, try to decide how "lateral" the lateral view you are analyzing really is (see Fig. 1-4). Then make a mental tally of the points discussed, see how many are concordant, how many discordant, and reach a decision therefrom. This can be done literally in seconds. When the films are completely normal, the decision becomes unimportant. When there is a diaphragmatic or posterior gutter abnormality identified only on the lateral view, fluoroscopy or oblique projections of the chest will readily resolve any dilemma. These techniques permit clear separation of one hemidiaphragm from the other. CT scans also permit clear lateralization of lesions involving or closely approximated to the diaphragm on a lateral view of the chest.

Usually, when only one hemidiaphragm shadow is seen on the lateral view, a gross abnormality of lung or pleura is apparent on the PA view to explain it. However, there are rare occasions when large segments of the right and left diaphragm may fortuitously be projected as a single image because they are superimposed.

Infrequently, pulmonary lesions also are seen only on the lateral view and cannot be localized with confidence. This problem, too, is solvable by fluoroscopic or oblique film studies. If CT scans are indicated for other reasons, the problem of side localization can be resolved by that examination. Some pulmonary lesions can be accurately localized on lateral view when they interface with and efface the margins of known anatomic structures such as the aortic arch, the posterior heart border, the inferior vena cava, or the diaphragm.

Fig. 1-4. Appearance of Small Variations in Projection Off True Lateral

Frequently, a patient may be positioned so that the right side (the side away from the film holder in the left lateral view) is anterior (about 10°) or slightly posterior to the true lateral plane. These minor degrees of obliquity may not be recognized by the technologist taking the film, but the influence on the image is predictable, although not absolutely constant.[2]

This figure shows a series of left lateral views of the chest of the same individual. There is blunting of the left posterior gutter, which is old and unchanged in comparison with other films made over the last five years. The films are otherwise normal. The orientations of the films are given below. Figs. D, E, and F are coned views of the orientations in Figs. A, B, and C, respectively.

(A) Right side is anterior to true lateral (RATL) by an estimated 10°.

(B) True lateral (TL)

(C) Right side is posterior to true lateral (RPTL) by an estimated 10°.

(D) Coned view of the hilar region of an RATL variant.

(E) Coned view of the hilar region of a left TL view.

(F) Coned view of the hilar region of an RPTL variant. *(Figure continues.)*

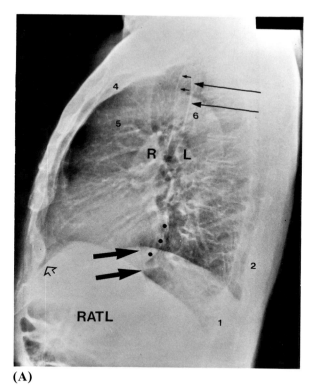

(A)

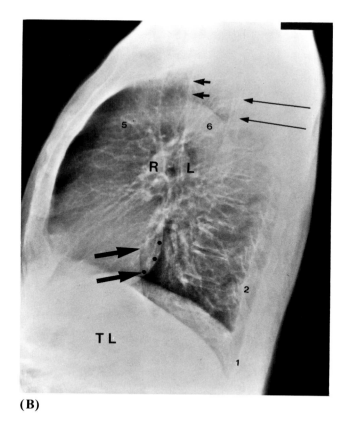

(B)

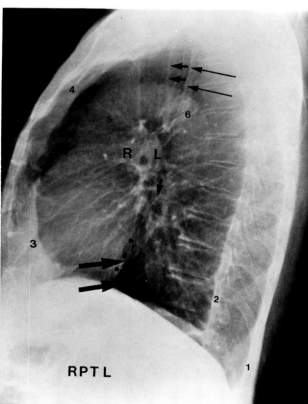

(C)

Key (Fig. 1–4A through C)

1. Posterior portions of the right ribs above the right posterior costophrenic sulcus (gutter)
2. Posterior portions of the left ribs above the left posterior costophrenic sulcus (note that this posterior gutter is slightly blunted)
3. The soft tissues of the lower anterior chest wall, which became very prominent in the RPTL variant, where they are shown sharply interfaced with the anterior surface of the lung
4. Soft tissues of the high retrosternal region
5. Ascending aorta
6. Posterior portion of the aortic arch

R: Interlobar branch of the right pulmonary artery
L: Left pulmonary artery after it has passed over the left upper lobe (LUL) bronchus
Short black arrows: Posterior wall of the trachea
Long black arrows: Anterior margins of the scapula (right scapula in RATL, both scapulae in TL, and left scapula in RPTL.
Thick black arrows: Pleural reflections over the posterior wall of the inferior vena cava
Dots: Posterior heart border (left ventricle).

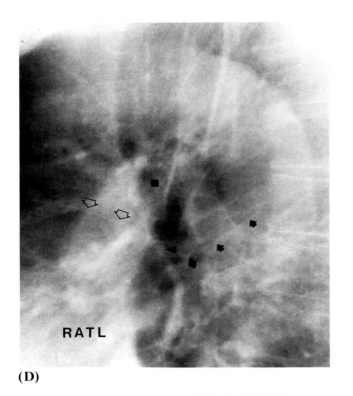

(D)

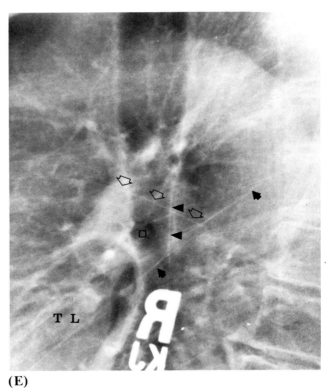

(E)

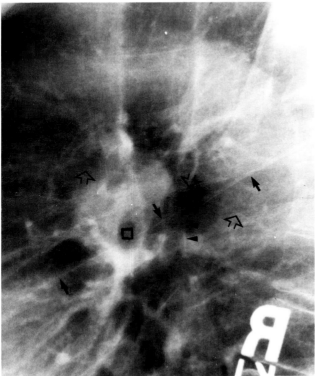

(F)

Key **(Fig. 1-4D through F)**

Short black arrows: A major interlobar ("oblique") fissure

Short open arrows: The minor interlobar ("horizontal") fissure

Solid black square: The RUL bronchus seen end-on (seen only in the RATL variant in this case)

Open black square: The LUL bronchus seen end-on

Black diamond: The LLL bronchus in profile (seen separate from other bronchi only in the RATL variant)

Arrowheads: Back wall of the bronchus intermedius

Comparative Observations for Fig. 1-4A through F

	Right Side Anterior of True Lateral (RATL)	Right Side Posterior of True Lateral (RPTL)
1. Effect on apparent heart size	The posterior wall of the left ventricle is projected closer to the thoracic spine and more posterior to the projected image of the IVC than on a TL view. If one uses those relationship to predict left heart enlargement, a false positive judgment may result.	The distance between the posterior wall of the left ventricle and the spine is increased compared to a TL view. The projected relationship of the posterior wall of the left ventricle and the IVC is such as to cause underestimation of left ventricular enlargement, were it present. The soft tissues of the anterior chest wall are superimposed on and obscure the anterior (right ventricular) heart margin. In a minority of subjects the overall heart size may appear enlarged unless relations to the spine and the IVC are taken into account.
2. Effect on posterior gutters and posterior rib tangents	With very slight RATL variation, the ribs may nearly superimpose posteriorly, and one posterior costophrenic angle (gutter) may be difficult to see. With moderate RATL variation (Fig. A), the right posterior gutter is projected anterior to the left. The right posterior ribs (slightly magnified) are projected anterior to those on the left. This is a reversal of the relationships seen on TL or RPTL variants.	The right posterior gutter is projected posterior to the left (Fig. C) to a greater degree than on a TL view. The right posterior ribs are projected behind the left posterior ribs—the opposite of the relationships seen on RATL variants and an exaggeration of the relationships as seen on a TL view (Fig. B).
3. Effect on cephalocaudad relationships of posterior gutters	In the normal subject in whom the right hemidiaphragm is higher than the left on a PA view, it is usual for the right posterior gutter to project caudal to the left on a lateral view, regardless of which variant is obtained.	
4. Effect on high retrosternal soft tissues	The prominence of soft tissues anteriorly high in the chest is least in a TL view (Fig. B) and increases with either RATL (Fig. A) or RPTL variants (Fig. C). Pleural undulations over regions of costal cartilage and costochondral junctions, with posterior projections of soft tissue, can be prominent and confused with internal mammary adenopathy or extrapleural masses in any of these variants.	
5. Effect on soft tissues of the anterior chest wall and the anterior aspects of the diaphragm (variable but most commonly as described here)	Appearances are similar to those of a TL view. The higher diaphragm arc seen anteriorly is usually the right. With moderate RATL, the anterior costophrenic angle on the right is sharply defined (Fig. A). The anterior margin of the right lung is projected anterior to the left. The lower anterior chest wall-lung interface is well defined on the right, but not on the left.	The left lung is projected anterior to the right. Part of the heart and adjacent soft tissues on the left are projected in front of the sharp anterior margin of the lower right lung producing a wedge-shaped, prominent soft tissue shadow that can be mistaken as abnormal (Fig. C), particularly if compared with a previous lateral view of the TL or RATL variant.
6. Effect on the appearance of the anterior edge of the ascending aorta	The anterior edge of the ascending aorta may be seen as a relatively sharp image in approximately half of all subjects in at least one of the three variants. In this subject it is seen on all three projections (Figs. A–C). Recall that the anterior wall of the ascending aorta has an interface with the right lung, not the left.	
7. Effect on visibility of the posterior wall of the trachea	The posterior wall of the trachea may be seen in all three variants, as in this subject, or in none. The visibility of the posterior wall probably depends on how much lung occupies the mediastinal recess behind the trachea.	

(Table continues.)

Comparative Observations for Fig. 1-4A through F *(continued)*

	Right Side Anterior of True Lateral (RATL)	Right Side Posterior of True Lateral (RPTL)
8. Effect on appearance of hila and bronchi	Separates the images of the right and left hilar vessels (Fig. D) and makes the hila appear larger than seen on the TL view (Fig. E) or the RPTL variant (Fig. F).	Frequently causes main hilar vessles to appear smaller than on the TL view or the RATL variant, and right and left hilar vessels ae projected closer to one another (Fig. F).
	The RUL bronchus may be seen end-on, superimposed on the airway in the same coronal plane as the anterior aspect of the arch of the left pulmonary artery (Fig. D). It is clearly seen, however, in fewer than half of all subjects.	The RUL bronchus is seen less frequently than in the RATL variant.
	The LUL bronchus may be seen end-on in the majority of (but not all) subjects, with its upper wall sharply defined by the left pulmonary artery, which passes over it. It is usually seen best in the RATL variant (Fig. A).	May make the lumen of the LUL bronchus look narrow in its AP dimension (Fig. F).The LUL bronchus is seen less often than in the RATL variant.
	The LLL bronchus is projected more posteriorly than on TL or RPTL views, and may lead to erroneous assessment of left atrial enlargement or decrease in LLL volume (Fig. D).	
	The posterior wall of the bronchus intermedius may be seen best in this variant, but can be seen in all three views.	
9. Effects on fissures	In general, the junction of the right major and minor fissures may be seen more often, but the major fissure of one or both sides frequently may not be visible in any of these views. In this subject the junction of the major and minor fissures happens to be more difficult to see on the RATL view than on the TL or the RPTL view.	The posterolateral end of the minor fissure may be projected far posterior to the intersection of the major fissure and posterior to the plane of the hilum, spuriously suggesting a superior accessory fissure of the RLL (Fig. F). This is only an exaggeration of these relationships as seen on a TL view (Fig. E).

You might consider a film off true lateral as a technically bad lateral view, but actually these variations can be correctly interpreted, if properly understood. Serious problems of interpretation arise, however, when one is comparing a series of lateral views in order to assess changes from a previous condition and does not recognize that the projections are not comparable. For example, it is easy to make an erroneous assessment of change in cardiac size if one compares an RATL variant with an RPTL variant of the same patient unless the differences in projection are considered. Similarly, an extrapleural mass along either the anterior or the posterior chest wall may be seen best on a lateral view; changes in its size may be incorrectly assessed when comparing views made in different degrees of rotation off TL. These are only a few of the errors in interpretation that may result from comparing lateral views that are not strictly comparable. They can be avoided by recognizing those key anatomic configurations that reveal that what is labeled as a "lateral" view is indeed a variant.

IVC, inferior vena cava.

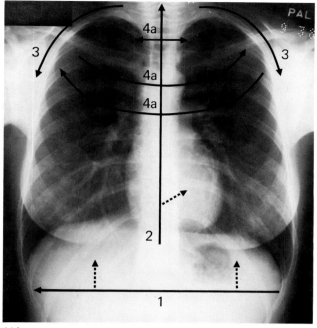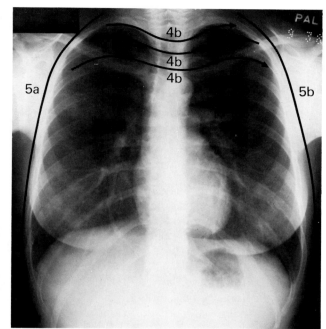

(A)

Fig. 1-5. Scanning Techniques

(A) Technique for scanning the PA view of the chest.

A. Check the film identification markers and the date to be sure you are analyzing the correct film. In this figure the film identification data have been replaced by a black box at the top left corner of the film.

B. Assess the degree of rotation off a strict frontal (PA or AP) view by determining the relative distance between the medial end of each clavicle and the margin of the adjacent vertebra. Assess whether there is any major degree of scoliosis or chest wall deformity that deserves special consideration.

C. Conduct a preliminary overview of the film. This overview is important because in this period of "free search" many lesions may be seen. Although free search may be the most common technique used by experienced observers, it has the potential of leaving significant areas of the film unexamined. For the novice, free search alone will result in missing many important lesions.

D. After the free search proceed as follows:

1. Start at the left costophrenic angle (there is nothing special about this site; it is simply an identifiable place to begin) and move from left to right, searching all that band of the film that projects below the level of the dia-

phragmatic domes. Specifically search the lung bases that project below the domes. To be sure that you have done this, seek out the shadows of pulmonary vessels that extend caudal to the dome on the right and often to a lesser extent on the left. Other landmarks to be sought and evaluated are:

(a) The conformation of the left costophrenic angle

(b) The spleen (you may see no image of the spleen, part of it, or all of it)

(c) The splenic flexure of the colon when it contains gas

(d) The gastric fundus when it contains air

(e) The conformation of the left hemidiaphragm

(f) The conformation of the left cardiophrenic angle

(g) The conformation of the right cardiophrenic angle

(h) The conformation of the right hemidiaphragm

(i) The liver and whatever portion of gas-filled or contrast-filled gut is visible in the upper abdomen

(j) The conformation of the right costophrenic angle *(Figure continues.)*

Fig. 1-5 *(continued)* 2. Move back to the region of the cardiomediastinal silhouette and scan upward toward the larynx. Evaluate:

(a) The contour of the right heart border

(b) The contour of the left heart border

(c) Overall heart size

(d) Make a detour and examine that portion of the lung that occupies the left retro-cardiac area. If the film is exposed well enough to permit even faint visualization of an intervertebral space behind the heart, then it is adequately exposed to show images of pulmonary vessels in the retrocardiac portion of the LLL.* If you leave this area unexamined, as is easy to do, you will miss not only nodular lesions but large areas of consolidation or atelectasis and even pleural effusion. Understand that not all lung that is projected over the heart represents lower lobes; portions of the middle lobe on the right and the lingula on the left also are superimposed on the heart (Fig. B). The volume of lung anterior to the heart, however, is less than the volume posterior to the heart.

(e) Analyze the right and left hila, including the air-filled major bronchi.

(f) Evaluate the mediastinal pleural reflections over the superior vena cava, the right brachiocephalic vein, the left subclavian artery, the aortic arch, and the space between the aortic arch and the left pulmonary artery (see Ch. 7).

(g) Locate the carina of the trachea and follow the air column of the trachea as far cephalad as possible. Identify the larynx whenever you can.

3. Now that you are at the top of the film, remove it from the viewer so that you can examine structures hidden by the film holders. Examine the soft tissues of the neck, the supraclavicular fossae, and the shoulder girdles. Examine those bony portions of the shoulder girdles included on the film.

4. Rehang the film and compare the right pulmonary apex to the left. Proceed down the film, using arclike horizontal eye movements, as follows:

(a) Study the anterior ribs, the underlying lung, and the part of the lung projected into the anterior interspaces, comparing one side to the other as you proceed all the way down the film. You can use the ribs as "picture frames," but remember to analyze both that which projects inside the frame and the frame itself.

(b) Go back to the apices and, with the same horizontal eye movements, study the posterior ribs, the underlying lung, and the part of the lung projected into the posterior interspaces. Compare one side to the other as you proceed caudally.

(c) You have now looked at the anterior ribs, the posterior ribs, and all the visible pulmonary parenchyma. (You have actually studied the parenchyma twice, since a lung zone projected into an anterior interspace must also be projected, at some level, into a posterior interspace or over a posterior rib.)

5. You have yet to finish looking at the ribs. A large segment of the axillary portions of the middle and lower ribs is foreshortened in projection along the lateral chest wall. (Look at the ribs on a mounted skeleton in order to obtain an appreciation of this phenomenon.) Analyze these portions of the ribs using a descending eye movement that encompasses them sequentially. Scan the ribs on the right and then repeat the scan on the left. These axillary rib segments have their lateral and medial cortices projected in profile, providing a good opportunity to seek out osteoblastic or osteolytic metastases or rib fractures that may otherwise be very subtle. Remember to examine those ribs that are projected below the level of the diaphragm.

Simultaneously, or separately, examine the soft tissues lateral to all the ribs.

6. Finish with an overview of the film. *(Figure continued.)*

---

* Many illustrations throughout this book were photographed and printed to emphasize specific regions, and in these you often will not see retrocardiac vessels in the LLL even though they were seen on the original films. Nevertheless, you can follow the same principle; if you can see an intervertebral space behind the heart on the illustration then you should also be able to see pulmonary vessels in the left lung base superimposed on the heart.

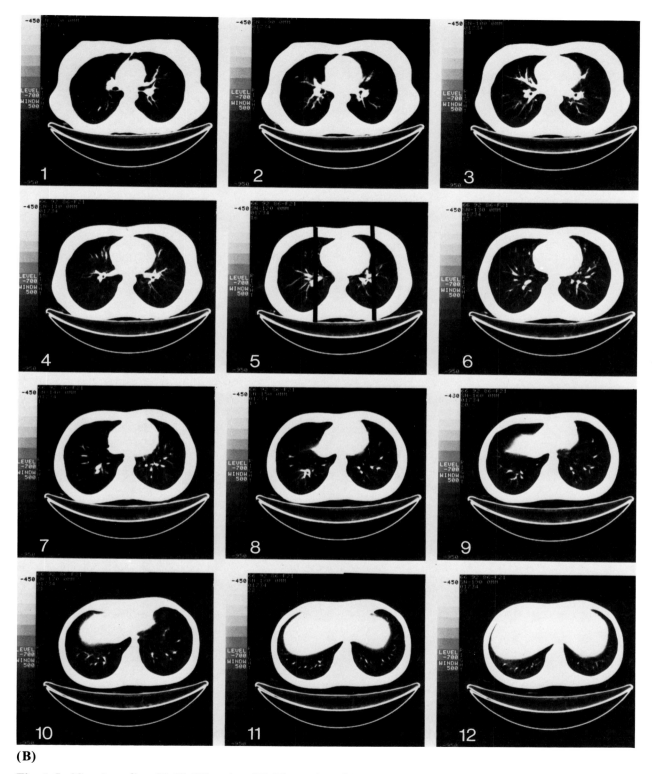

(B)

Fig. 1-5. *(Continued).* **(B,C)** CT series. **(B)** The series of CT scans of the chest was taken at 1.0-cm intervals, starting 2.0 cm caudal to the carina and proceeding caudad. The gray scale chosen for filming (see window width and level data on the left of each scan) accentuates the blackness of the lungs and eliminates details of the chest wall, heart, and mediastinum. This information remains in the computer, however, and can be displayed by changing the gray scale.

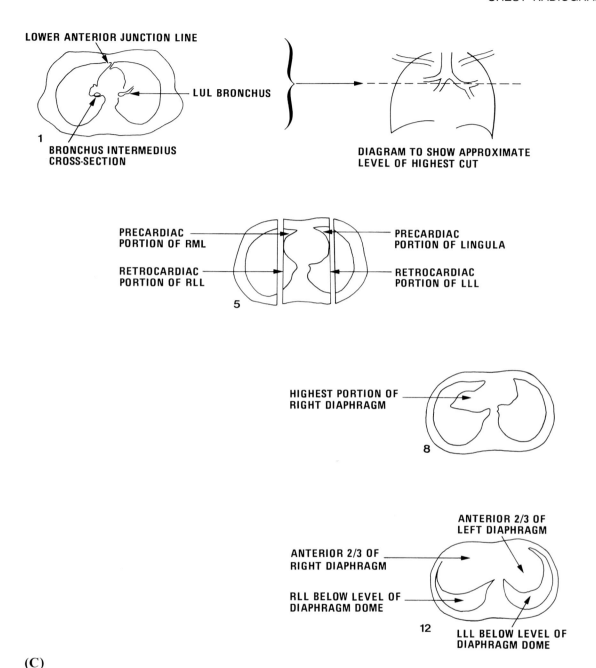

(C)

Fig. 1-5. *(Continued).* **(C)** Diagrams showing structures visible in some of the CT scans in Fig. B.

In frame 1 **(B,C)** (2.0 cm caudal to the carina), the right and left lungs are visible closely approximated anterior to the heart. The lungs themselves are separated only by a thin band of tissue—the juxtaposed pleurae of the two lungs, here constituting the lower portion of the anterior junction line. Lung is seen both in front of and behind the heart, but at the lung bases there is much more lung behind the heart, especially on the left side. In frame 5, bars mark the heart margins and show the lung zones that would be superimposed on the heart on a PA chest film. In the bottom row, the white areas in the anterior portions of the sections are images of the diaphragm, whereas the white wedge seen posteriorly consists largely of the spine and paraspinal tissues, which show no detail at the gray scale chosen for filming. Notice how much more caudally you can see the lung (black) in the posteroinferior and lateral portions of the chest, because of the slope of the diaphragm. The posterior portions of the diaphragm are not seen in this series. *(Figure continues.)*

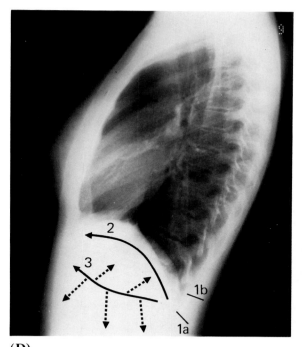 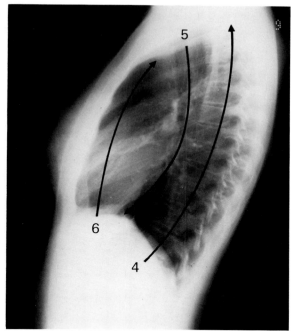

(D)

Fig. 1-5. *(Continued).* **(D)** Technique for scanning the lateral view of the chest. After a preliminary overview:

1. Begin the search at the posterior costophrenic angles. There is nothing special about beginning here, except that important information, easily overlooked, may be found in one or both posterior gutters. This information (e.g., a small effusion) may not be at all apparent on the PA view. Identify both posterior costophrenic angles (gutters) and analyze their shapes. Try to distinguish right from left.
2. Follow the contours of each hemidiaphragm as far anteriorly as you can. Assess the integrity of the interface between the diaphragm surface and the adjacent lung.
3. Examine the portion of the film inferior to the diaphragm domes to seek out abdominal abnormalities that may be present, such as abnormal gas shadows, abnormal fluid levels, or abnormal calcifications.
4. Start posteriorly and use a vertical eye movement to search the film from the level of the lowest vertebra visible upward to the thoracic inlet. Evaluate the vertebral bodies, their interspaces, and their posterior arches; include the visible portions of the posterior tangents of the ribs and the soft tissues of the posterior chest wall. That portion of the lungs which projects behind the extended coronal plane of the trachea should also be incorporated in this

sweep. Follow each lung all the way back to the corresponding posterior ribs; superiorly this usually cannot be done because of the superimposition of the shoulder girdles.
5. Using a descending eye movement, search a band extending from the thoracic inlet to the lung base that incorporates the trachea, both hila, the retrocardiac portions of the lung, and the posterior heart margins. Identify the image of the pleural reflection over the inferior vena cava.
6. In a vertical sweep commencing at the anteriorinferior portion of the film, search that portion of the film that encompasses the cardiac shadow, the retrosternal soft tissues, the superimposed portions of the lingula and the right middle lobe, and the retrosternal lung extending up to the thoracic inlet. It is important to include the image of the sternum and the manubrium and the soft tissues of the anterior chest wall in this sweep. It is worthwhile to remove the film from the film hanger to see what portion of the upper airway — the larynx and the hypopharynx — as well as the cervical and upper thoracic spine are visible on the upper portions of the film.
7. Conclude the examination with a final overview.

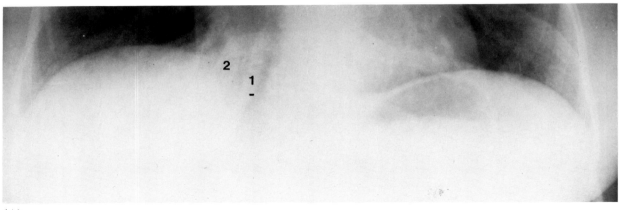

(A)

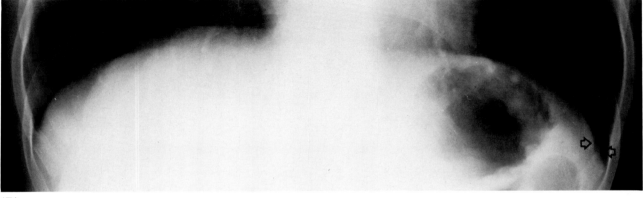

(B)

Fig. 1-6. Diaphragm

(A) In this individual, both hemidiaphragms project as smooth continuous arcs. The costophrenic angles are both sharp. The subcardiac, medial segment of the right hemidiaphragm is effaced. The left hemidiaphragm is well defined even medially, where it appears subcardiac. To be so well defined, however, this segment of the hemidiaphragm must interface with aerated lung and thus cannot be truly subcardiac. It must be a projection of a diaphragm-lung tangent either behind or in front of the heart. Since the hemidiaphragm appears as a sharp image as far medially as the spine, this lung-diaphragm tangent must be retrocardiac, as lung anterior to the heart does not extend this far medially in the normal individual.

The high points of both hemidiaphragms are along their middle thirds. Air is seen in the fundus of the stomach on the left side. Notice the short distance from the air in the fundus to the lung over the diaphragm.

Obliquely vertical band shadows superimposed on the right heart are due to calcified costal cartilages (1 and 2).

(B) The right hemidiaphragm presents as two large arcs with the highest point located in the middle third of the medial arc. The hemidiaphragm edge can be followed medially to the spine.

The left hemidiaphragm presents as one arc up to a few centimeters medial to its lateral end, where two slightly separated arcs are seen (arrows). The slope of the left side is such that the high point is adjacent to the spine. A small pericardial fat pad imparts a short, laterally convex bulge to the left cardiophrenic angle.

Notice the prominent rugae in the air-filled gastric fundus; some of them project as nodular shadows, which can be confused with nodular lesions in the lung base. *(Figure continues.)*

(C)

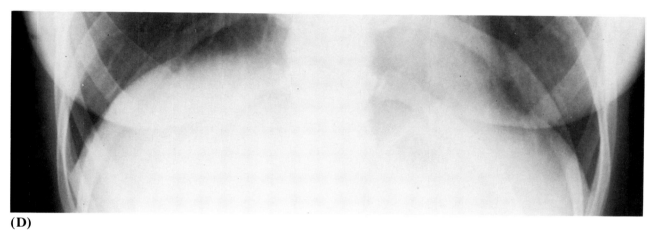

(D)

Fig. 1-6. *(Continued).* **(C)** The right hemidiaphragm is projected as three arcs laterally, but they appear to overlap one another rather than appear in linear continuity (arrows). These represent slips of origin of diaphragm muscle from the lower ribs.

The left hemidiaphragm is projected as two arcs laterally (arrows); each arc of diaphragm is seen to extend to its rib of origin. The medial segment of the left hemidiaphragm is fairly sharp, but a small segment under the left pericardial fat pad is not. The left hemidiaphragm slopes downward laterally from the spine and then has a slight curve upward toward a higher dome lateral to the cardiac apex.

The edges of breast shadows are seen as caudally convex arcs superimpsed on both lung bases.

(D) The medial segments of both hemidiaphragms are not sharp images. The unsharp segment on the left is subcardiac; the unsharp segment on the right is not. There is no apparent reason why this portion of the right diaphragm should not appear sharp. By inference, this segment does not present a tangent to the beam comparable to that presented by the larger segment lateral to it. Another possible explanation is that extrapleural accumulations of fat prevent sharp approximation of the lung with the diaphragm in these regions.

Note the faint collection of gas in the fundus of the stomach. The edges of breast shadows are seen on both sides. *(Figure continues.)*

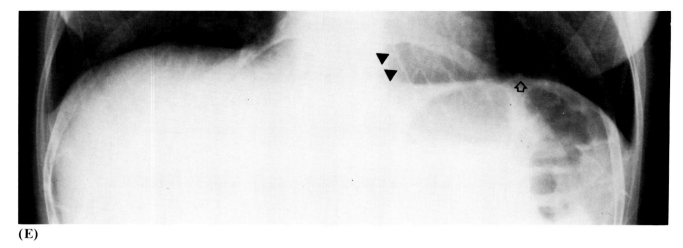

(E)

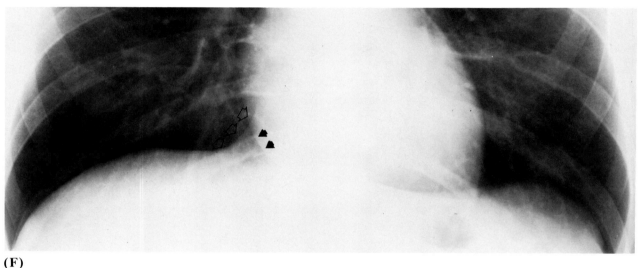

(F)

Fig. 1-6. *(Continued).* **(E)** There is a small, tentlike projection of the superior surface of the midportion of the left hemidiaphragm, about 1 cm lateral to the heart margin (arrow). Frequently, tentlike peaks are seen over the hemidiaphragms at sites where either an accessory intersegmental fissure[5] or the major interlobar fissure or the inferior pulmonary ligament is expected to meet the diaphragm. These peaks may be seen on either side and on PA or lateral views or both. They correspond to accumulations of interfissural fat seen on CT scans. Pleural fluid extending into a major fissure can produce a similar appearance on a lateral chest film but is accompanied by other signs of pleural effusion.[4]

The high point of this right hemidiaphragm is a dome in the middle third. Oblique, linear shadows over the left heart are produced by the projection of calcified costal cartilages (arrowheads). Gas is seen in the stomach (medially) and the splenic flexure of the colon (laterally) in the left upper quadrant of the abdomen.

(F) There is a well-defined pleural reflection over the inferior vena cava (probably a complex of inferior vena cava and hepatic vein) in the right cardiophrenic angle (open arrows). The edge of the right atrium (black arrows) can still be identified through the image of the vena cava, testifying to the fact that the edges — that is, the air-water interfaces of these structures — must be in different planes. **Exercise.** Go back and look at Figs. A through F. Search along the lower lateral chest walls. Notice that, in addition to the shadows of ribs, you can see subtle but well-defined edges that nearly parallel the ribs but often have a steeper inclination. These represent so-called "companion shadows," that is, interfaces between pleural reflections over extrapleural muscles and the adjacent lung. They are not visible in everyone at these levels, and they are frequently not symmetrical in appearance or extent on the two sides. It is important to recognize a rib companion shadow as a normal structure so as not to confuse it with a pleural plaque in a patient with a history of asbestos exposure, or a small extrapleural metastasis in a patient with a malignant neoplasm. *(Figure continues.)*

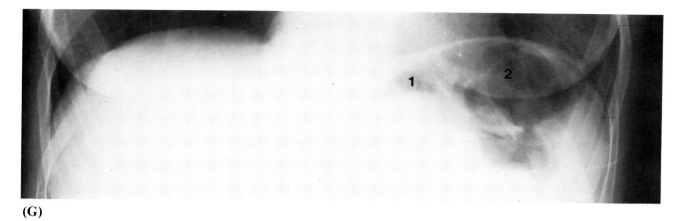

(G)

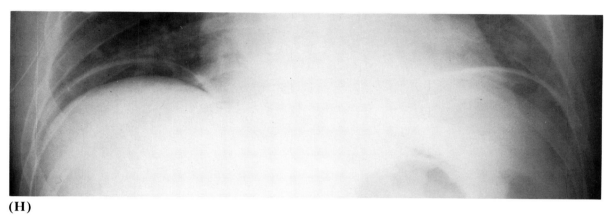

(H)

Fig. 1-6. *(Continued).* **(G)** Air is seen in the stomach medially (1), and considerable gas is seen in a redundant splenic flexure of the colon (2), under the left hemidiaphragm.

The dome of the left hemidiaphragm is projected slightly higher than the right. This is not unusual when considerable gas is seen in stomach or bowel high in the left upper quadrant, and the elevation of the hemidiaphragm may be more marked than is seen here. The arguable point is whether the hemidiaphragm is high because of distended gut below, or whether gas collects in this portion of the gut because the hemidiaphragm is elevated from another cause.

(H) There is a large crescent of air under the right hemidiaphragm. A similar collection is seen under the left diaphragm. Free intraperitoneal air is commonly seen following abdominal surgery when chest films are obtained with the patient upright.

More importantly, free gas in the abdomen may come from a perforated viscus. There are numerous causes of free gas in the abdomen, but usually the associated history and clinical signs and symptoms will permit recognition of those that are due to an abdominal catastrophe.

Very small amounts of subdiaphragmatic free air or gas may not be visible on chest films of an erect patient unless the x-ray beam is centered at the diaphragm level.

An AP chest film obtained with the patient supine is totally inadequate for the purpose of evaluating the presence or absence of free intra-abdominal, gas even though on occasion free abdominal gas in large quantities may be seen on such films. *(Figure continues.)*

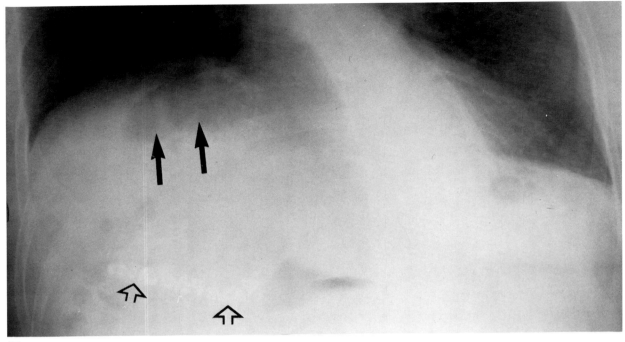

(I)

(J)

Fig. 1-6. *(Continued).* **(I)** The right hemidiaphragm is high, and a gas-filled loop of the hepatic flexure of the colon (black arrows) is located high under the anterior portions of the diaphragm in this PA view. The haustral markings identify this as a loop of colon rather than a collection of free air. This is the position of a portion of the right colon interposed between the anterior wall and the liver high under the right hemidiaphragm.

There is severe scoliosis of the lower thoracic and upper lumbar spine, which is convex to the left.

Air is seen in the fundus of the stomach. A cluster of calcified stones (open arrows) is seen in the gallbladder in the right upper quadrant, although difficult to recognize.

(J) This is a lateral view of the patient seen in (I). The black arrow points to the gas in the right colon interposed between the liver and abdominal wall. The open arrow identifies the location of the gallstones which were seen faintly on the original film but which are not visible on the reproduction. *(Figure continues.)*

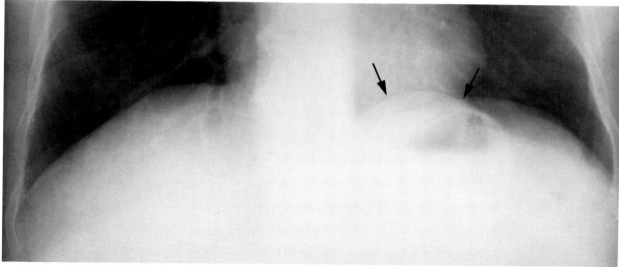

(K)

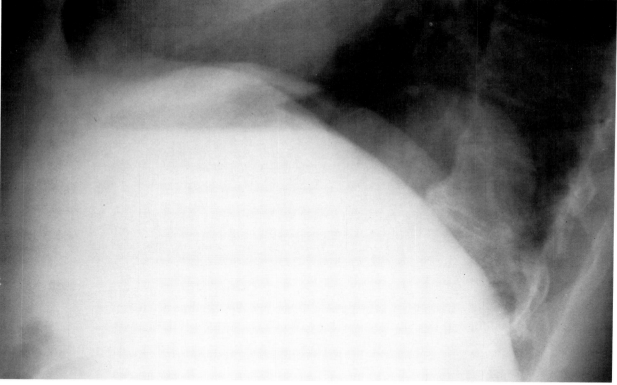

(L)

Fig. 1-6. *(Continued).* **(K–M)** Patient with herniation through the diaphragm. **(K)** PA view. The left hemidiaphragm has a lobulated contour, and medially a well-defined arc can be seen. **(L)** It simulates a lobulation of the diaphragm (arrows). Lateral view. A large soft tissue mound with a sharply defined superior surface is seen projected posteriorly partly superimposed on the spine and partly projected anterior to the spine. The superior edge of the posterior one-fourth of the left hemidiaphragm is effaced, whereas the right hemidiaphragm can be traced all the way to its junction with the right posterior chest wall. *(Figure continues.)*

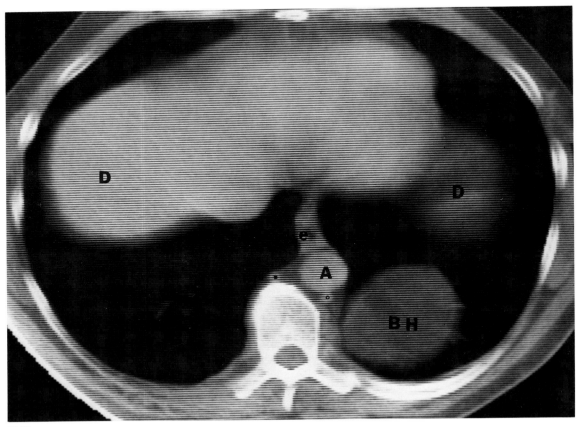

(M)

Fig. 1-6 *(Continued).* The location and appearance of this abnormality are characteristic of herniation of abdominal contents through the foramen of Bochdalek. The majority of Bochdalek hernias occur on the left side, and in the adult these hernias are asymptomatic. These hernias commonly contain fat, or a portion of the left kidney, or the spleen.

(M) The patient had no symptoms referable to this hernia, but a CT scan was done for other reasons. This slice was made through the contents of the Bochdalek hernia (BH), and the Hounsfield number of the contents was indicative of fat. Notice the similarity of the gray scale of the omental fat in the hernia to that of the subcutaneous fat. (A, aorta; D, diaphragm dome; e, esophagus; *, azygos vein; ◇, hemiazygos vein.)

Although this is not strictly a normal variant of diaphragmatic contour, it is a relatively common cause of an asymptomatic posterior supradiaphragmatic mass. Theoretically, a lipoma or a mesothelioma of the pleura could be found in this location and have this plain film appearance, as could a metastasis to the pleura from an intrathoracic or extrathoracic primary tumor. A cyst could also cause this appearance on chest films. A CT scan or an MRI examination permits distinction between fat, non-fat soft tissue, and cystic masses.

2

Why Do We See What We See? How Should We Describe It?

To understand the normal and abnormal images seen on a chest film, it is necessary to have at least a simple knowledge of the basics of image formation using film as a recording device. *Christensen's Introduction to the Physics of Diagnostic Radiology*[1] is an enjoyable readable text that covers pertinent basic principles. You may want to review the theories of x-ray production, beam attenuation through interaction with tissues, and the effects of different technical factors, especially kilovoltage and milliampere-seconds, on film images. Some will also enjoy the more detailed coverage of these subjects in *The Physical Aspects of Diagnostic Radiology* by Michel M. Ter-Pogossian.[7]

TISSUE DENSITY AND ATTENUATION OF X-RAYS

The attenuation of a beam of x-rays depends on the energy spectrum of the incident x-rays and the density, effective atomic number, and electrons per gram of the absorber through which the beam passes. The higher the values of the last three variables for a given absorber, the greater its attenuation capabilities.

Modern radiographic techniques are such that for the lung (normal or abnormal) differences in tissue density (g/cm^3) play the major role in differential attenuation of the x-ray beam. The amount (or path length) of a particular attenuator in the beam is also critical. This is a property of the orientation of the attenuator to the beam, rather than a physical property of the matter itself, but it does govern the average density of all the absorbers in the beam path.

To grossly simplify matters, we will assign muscle, pleura, blood, lymph, transudates, exudates, and all soft tissues other than fat a density of 1. We can think of them as "water-like" absorbers or, simply, water absorbers. Fat is assigned a density of less than one (<1), whereas air is assigned a density of much less than one ($\ll 1$), simply to indicate that air is less dense than both fat and water. Bone density, of course, is greater than one (>1), and the density of calcified tissues is likewise greater than one.

In addition, the presence of calcium results in a significantly higher effective atomic number for bone and calcified lesions than for other tissues in the lung and thus further increases their attenuation of incident x-rays.

An x-ray beam will traverse the chest, from posterior to anterior, in the following sequence:

Structure	Relative density
Skin	1
Subcutaneous fat	< 1
Muscle	1
Bone	> 1
Pleura	1
Lung	
"Air"	≪ 1
Vessels	1

The sequence is reversed as the beam exits.

When film or film-screen combinations are used as recording devices, we usually (and, much of the time, only) recognize distinctions among water, fat, and air densities when at least part of the interface between them is tangent to the beam. For example, if you made a muscle-fat-muscle sandwich and radiographed it en face, you would not recognize the fat, whereas if you oriented it so the layers were tangential to the beam, the fat layer would show on the film as a darker gray stripe between the lighter gray muscle stripes.

A SIMPLE MODEL

A set of thin Plexiglas sheets separated by a few centimeters of air serves as a useful model (Figs. 2-1 and 2-2). If the model is placed on an x-ray film that is smaller than the Plexiglas sheets and the system is radiographed, nothing will show on the developed film (Fig. 2-3). If instead a film that is larger than the model is used, we can easily recognize the presence of the model because we can see its edges. That is, we have recorded the interface between two different absorbers (room air and Plexiglas) where their interface is perpendicular to the beam (Fig. 2-4). Since the sheets are thin, the tangential interface is short and the edges are faint. Next, the model is placed so that the sheets are perpendicular to the beam while resting on the film (Fig. 2-2B). Now the image is seen as two *dense* lines (Fig. 2-5). We have not changed the density (g/cm³) of the plastic, of course, but we have changed markedly the distance through the plastic that is traversed by the beam.

Thus, for example, you can see how small vessels that project end-on on a chest film may produce images that can be difficult to distinguish from small, calcified granulomata. Such a long column of blood can produce an image comparable to that of a much shorter column of

calcium. (If you had a fluoroscope at your disposal, how could you distinguish a vessel seen end-on from a small, calcified granuloma in a second?)

EDGES VERSUS LINES

An "edge" image is a record of the interface of two different absorbers (Fig. 2-4). It is an important concept. Detection of many lesions depends on recognition of their edges. The silhouette sign of Felson is also based on understanding the nature of edge images. That is, an edge of a structure, such as a heart border, the aortic arch, or the descending aorta, will be seen when its tangential interface with normal lung is preserved. Its edge will be lost whenever a process significantly increases the density of the adjacent lung and eliminates the sharp density gradient across the interface.

A "line" or "band" image is produced by three different absorbers in continuity: the absorber producing the line itself, bordered on either side by absorbers that are different from it, although they may be equal to each other. Air-plastic-air, lung-pleura-lung, and lung-pleura-pneumothorax are examples of such sequences (Fig. 2-5).

FILM DENSITY

When we refer to the density of matter, we usually think of mass per unit volume (g/cm³). Unfortunately, in radiology *density* is also used to refer to photographic density and film blackening. You can think of a chest film as a continuum of gray tones, with high attenuators such as bone or calcified structures producing low-density film images (toward the white end of the gray tones), and low attenuators such as air and fat producing high-density images (toward the black end of the gray tones). It requires more incident light to see through dense areas of the film.

FILM IMAGES

In the normal chest film we see intrapulmonary blood vessels because of the interface between these water absorbers and the air content of adjacent alveoli. When this interface is sharp, the vessel shadows are sharp (Figs. 2-6A, 2-7A and B); when this interface loses its integrity because of abnormalities in adjacent air spaces or interstitium, the vessel shadows become unsharp, and the smaller caliber vessel images may become indistinguishable from their background (Figs. 2-6C and D, 2-7C and D).

When this focal loss of vessel shadows is accompanied by a lightening of the gray tone, we can assume a concomitant increase in either the fluid or the cellular content (or both) of the surrounding tissues. When this loss of vessel shadows is accompanied by a darkening of the gray tone, we can assume a loss of tissue density such as may occur in zones of emphysema or of air trapping and decreased perfusion, or in areas of lung peripheral to a vascular obstruction.

Vigilance is required to avoid the erroneous assumption that these changes are always due to technical flaws. Technical defects may indeed produce similar appearances in film density but are usually distinguishable from true tissue density changes (see Ch. 1).

Lesions of low tissue density may be seen on chest films when they are large enough to cause differential absorption of x-rays in comparison to surrounding tissues (tissue contrast) and when the radiographic and filming techniques used reflect those differences as film contrast. Film contrast influences the amount of light transmitted through neighboring areas of the roentgenogram.

A noncalcified nodule less than 3.0 mm in diameter can be seen when surrounded by normal lung if optimum radiographic technique is used. Whether or not such a nodule is recognized as an abnormality is another matter, since in all but the very peripheral lung zones it would probably not be distinguishable from a vessel.

Recognition of low-density lung lesions may be extraordinarily difficult when the lesion's orientation to the beam does not provide sufficient tangents to produce edge images; under such circumstances even lesions several centimeters in diameter may not be recognized (Figs. 2-8A and B). Lesions that *taper* toward an interface with normal lung are often not seen in a single projection. Films obtained through multiple angles can prevent errors in interpretation because longer tangents of the lesion-lung interface may be projected in profile, and the length of the absorber traversed by the beam may be increased. This is particularly true of lesions located adjacent to pleural surfaces either in the lung or in the pleural or extrapleural space (Fig. 2-8C). Fluoroscopy is also useful to position patients so that suspect lesions can be filmed in optimum projection.

The chest film is the product of a compromise in that it is an attempt to display images of bone, bulky soft tissue structures such as the heart and great vessels, and the low tissue densities of the lungs on film with a single technique. Ideally one would use different techniques to display these structures on different films; however, that cannot be done routinely for economic reasons. Individualized techniques can and should be used whenever there is a need to clarify suspect abnormalities seen on routine films.

ANATOMIC NOISE

If we want to see details of ribs, it would be best if we could display their images devoid of overlapping lung vessels and soft tissues. When we want to see details of lung structure, it would be best if we could eliminate the images of overlying ribs, vertebrae, mediastinal structures, and even soft tissues of the chest wall. If we want to see small pulmonary nodules, it would be extremely useful to be able to eliminate all pulmonary vessels from the display.

Any anatomic structure that interferes with seeing a specific structure or pathologic process can be considered "anatomic noise." This is a formidable problem in chest radiology. We have some ability to mitigate technical noise but a very limited ability to control anatomic noise. Stereoscopic views, tomographic studies, and variations in technique (such as the use of very high kilovoltages and the nascent techniques of line-scanned digital radiography in conjunction with dual kVp) all attempt to solve this problem, with limited success so far.

APPEARANCES AND DESCRIPTIONS OF PULMONARY ABNORMALITIES

Even if we all see the same abnormal patterns on a chest film, unless we agreed on terminology beforehand we would not likely choose the same words to describe them. When I ask students to choose common words that they think appropriate to describe various patterns of lung disease, diversity reigns. Invariably, three, four, or five descriptions of the same lesions come from even a small group of students. After discussion and compromise we agree on some mutually acceptable, although still inadequate, set of descriptors.

In practice, no common agreement on terminology has yet been reached. Experienced radiologists have disagreements on the validity of the terms "interstitial," "alveolar," "acinar," or "air-space disease" when used as descriptive modifiers of radiographic abnormalities. In the bibliography at the end of this chapter you will find expositions by authors who have strong feelings about the usefulness of separating patterns of lung disease into "interstitial" or "alveolar" (or "acinar" or "airspace") categories whenever possible.[2-4]

Other authors, however, feel that more descriptive terms such as "reticular" or "reticulonodular" or "consolidation with air bronchograms" are more appropriate. These terms describe what is actually seen rather than make assumptions about the histopathology.

Nevertheless, certain correlations between the descriptive terms and their histopathologic counterparts are strongly implied. For example, discrete diffuse nodules, whether microscopic ($<$1 mm), small (1 to 5 mm), medium-sized (6 to 10 mm), or large ($>$10 mm), are considered by some to be part of the pattern of interstitial lung disease. Others consider nodules under a separate classification.[4] Reticular patterns, septal line patterns, and peribronchial and perivascular patterns are also associated with abnormalities in the interstitium of the lung.

Other patterns such as acinar nodules (poorly marginated, inhomogeneous nodules 4 to 8 mm in diameter), air bronchograms, or air bronchiolograms (radiolucencies measuring 1 to 5 mm within a background of consolidation, due to residual air in peripheral airways) are considered primarily representative of air-space patterns with or without features of coalescence and segmental or lobar distribution. Frequently mixed patterns are seen; that is, patterns associated with interstitial lesions may be seen mixed with each other or with patterns of air-space lesions.

TERMS USED IN THIS TEXT

In general, descriptive rather than inferential terms are used throughout this text. There are times, however, when the presence of septal lines (Kerley-A, -B, or -C lines) correlates rather specifically with interstitial abnormalities, and other times when consolidation with air bronchograms correlates well with acinar or air-space disease. The latter finding, however, is not absolutely specific in that there are occasions when extensive disease in the pulmonary interstitium can obliterate alveoli to such an extent that an air bronchogram pattern can be seen on the radiographs.

WHAT IS TO BE SEEN?

Loss of Vessel Sharpness

Any type of water-like absorber (e.g., edema fluid, inflammatory exudate, abnormal collections of benign or malignant cells, or hemorrhage), in either the interstitium or the peripheral air spaces, or both, interrupts the normal air-water interface of pulmonary vessels. The earliest radiographic sign of pulmonary abnormality is often the loss of sharp detail of the margins of small

vessels in the involved area. The assessment is subjective, and comparison with films of the same individual prior to the illness is extremely useful whenever possible (Fig. 2-6B). Interzonal comparison is helpful when the abnormality is focal, but may be deceptive when the process is diffuse.

Factors other than pulmonary parenchymal disease, however, do affect the clarity of vessel images. Motion of the part being examined can seriously impair image detail, as can poor film-screen contact within the cassette used to hold the film (see ref. 1 for a discussion of film-screen contact). Whenever you suspect that a technical flaw is responsible for an abnormality it is best to repeat the examination (at no expense to the patient) to prove that contention.

Moderate reduction in the degree of inspiration can also cause degradation of vessel images at the lung bases, since there will be less adjacent alveolar air. The assessment is complicated by the fact that, as pulmonary disease reduces lung compliance, the same inspiratory effort produces a lesser degree of lung expansion. Thus, for a patient who has developed restrictive lung disease, the diaphragm will be projected higher on a chest film made after the development of the disease than it was before. Now we have a dilemma. Are the vessels in the lung bases unsharp and is the diaphragm high because the patient has inadvertently not taken a deep breath, or because the patient has developed a restrictive pulmonary disease process? It is surprising how faithfully most healthy patients will reproduce the volume of their lungs, and hence the position of their diaphragm at maximum inspiration, under the guidance of a good radiologic technologist. A sick patient, however, may fatigue and not do as well. The dilemma is resolved by knowing the status of the patient at the time of filming, by performing a clinical evaluation of diaphragmatic motion, and by repeating the chest film with special attention to achieving maximum inspiration before filming or fluoroscoping the diaphragm when doubt persists.

Soft tissues of the chest wall act as additional x-ray-scattering media, and portions of lung projected behind heavy breast shadows or thick pectoral muscles can show loss of vessel detail even though there is no lung abnormality. Any mass in a patient's soft tissues close to the film can cause similar image degradation. Scatter radiation is reduced by the use of grids or air-gap techniques, but not entirely eliminated. Film blackening is increased by scatter radiation, but film contrast and image quality are reduced.[1]

In a patient with clinically suspect lung disease but questionable radiographic abnormalities, the question can frequently be resolved by obtaining repeat films at short intervals and by comparing current films with earlier radiographs.

Granularity

Certain pulmonary abnormalities cause a finely stippled or granular radiographic appearance of the involved lung. This is sometimes referred to as a micronodular pattern. It may also be part of the pattern that some observers describe as "ground glass," but I am never quite sure what others expect me to see when they talk of a ground glass appearance. I believe "ground glass" is used sometimes in reference to frank consolidation.

Film mottle or system noise may impart a background pattern of granularity, and at times it may be difficult to know whether you are looking at film mottle or lung disease. The appearance of the film in the region of extrathoracic soft tissue can be used as a control. If the granularity of the lung zones exceeds that in regions of soft tissue along the lateral chest wall, lung disease is the likely cause. Practice comparing these film zones in order to experience the range of relative appearances that may be found in patients who have no pulmonary disease. With practice, the granular or stippled appearance of lung disease can be recognized even when it is only a minimal departure from normal. There is no sharp point where granularity ends and miliary nodulation begins.

Nodules

Nodular opacities are common components of both focal and diffuse lung disease. It is convenient to think of two types of nodular lung disease. One is composed of nodules whose size and separation are such that you could count them if you so chose. The other consists of myriad nodules on the order of 3 to 5 mm in size that you would not choose to count even though it might not be impossible to do so. Most of the time these two categories are distinct, but occasionally there is an overlap, for example, in an occasional patient with numerous nodular metastases.

The separation of nodular lesions into "countable" and "uncountable" classes is for purposes of description and understanding, not to imply the existence of mutually exclusive differential diagnoses. Multiple, diffusely distributed, countable nodules may be produced, for example, by pulmonary metastases, by infectious granulomatous disease, or by noninfectious granulomatous disease or even nongranulomatous infections. These same abnormalities may also produce multiple uncountable nodules. Yet, in fact, if you saw multiple countable nodules in the lung of a patient about whom you knew nothing else, probabilities alone would indicate metastases as first choice among diagnoses. If you saw miliary lesions (uncountable nodules) in the lung of a patient about whom you knew nothing else, probabilities would indi-

cate not metastases as the first choice, but rather an infection such as tuberculosis. In neither case, however, could you eliminate the other choices from the differential diagnosis. The radiographic appearance alone only allows you to consider the possibilities in order of likelihood; it does not allow any of the possibilities to be eliminated entirely from consideration. The rank-ordering of possibilities will be best served by integrating the radiographic findings with all available clinical data.

Lines

Short straight, curved, or irregular line shadows are frequent components of the radiographic image of lung disease. Interlobular septa comprise a significant part of the interstitium of lung, even though they are not uniformly distributed. Whenever abnormal quantities of fluid or of cells accumulate in interlobular septa, they may be seen as line shadows. Those most easily recognized are seen laterally in the lung bases and were called Kerley B-lines after the radiologist who first described them. Elsewhere in the lung, these septal images may line up and project longer shadows, originally called Kerley A-lines. Others, randomly distributed and producing superimposed images, present a reticular appearance when viewed en face; these have been called Kerley C-lines. It is most convenient and anatomically appropriate to consider all of these as abnormally thick interlobular septa. They are important constituents of the pathologic anatomy of diffuse lung disease, and radiographically they are reliable evidence that excess fluid or abnormal accumulation of cells are in the interstitium of the lung.

The interlobar fissures may be considered analogous to giant interlobular septa. Sometimes fluid in the subpleural interstitium adjacent to fissures accumulates to the point at which the image simulates fluid in the fissure itself.

Thick lines and thick bands, bearing no resemblance to septal lines, can be produced by peripheral areas of atelectasis; these are discussed in Chapter 4.

Reticulonodular Patterns

Often the appearance of short, irregular line shadows is accompanied by ill-defined, irregularly contoured, small nodular shadows to constitute a reticulonodular pattern. Some of these nodular shadows have been shown to be the product of superimposition of intersecting images of thickened interlobular septa, and thus are called "false" nodules, whereas others are considered to be due to true nodular foci mixed with thickened interlobular septa. Radiographically these distinctions often are not possible to make.[4]

Peribronchial and Perivascular Thickening

Fluid or cells accumulating in the perivascular and peribronchial interstitial spaces cause thickening and effacement of the boundaries of bronchovascular bundles and loss of sharpness of vascular shadows.

These abnormalities appear as irregular zones of opacity along the distribution of the bronchi and vessels. Pooling of secretions in bronchi can produce a similar appearance, although it is unlikely that the adjacent parenchyma is entirely normal under circumstances in which intrabronchial pooling occurs.

Honeycombing

"Honeycombing" is a popular term used to describe a radiographic image consisting of rounded lucencies 5 to 10 mm in diameter, jacketed by relatively thick walls. The gross pathology consists of markedly distorted lung tissue with small cystic spaces surrounded by zones of fibrosis. Histopathologically, both interstitial and alveolar compartments are involved.

Honeycomb lung has been considered a pattern of end-stage lung disease. This does not imply a prognosis, but rather that the histopathologic changes are those that may be found in the late (end-stage) phases of many chronic or subacute lung diseases. Thus, you may encounter a biopsy specimen that, were it truly representative of the patient's entire lungs, would not be compatible with life, yet no specific diagnosis can be deduced. Often it is necessary to obtain biopsies from lung outside most severely affected areas in order to find histopathologic features that permit recognition of the etiology.

Although the term "honeycomb lung" is commonly used, it is not clear that everyone uses it to describe the same lesions. Small foci of relatively normal lung interspersed with fluid-filled alveoli or small air spaces ringed by fluid or cells may closely mimic honeycomb lung, as in an unusual case of alveolar proteinosis. If you considered honeycomb lung a pattern of predominant interstitial disease, you would omit consideration of the correct diagnosis in such cases. In some patients a pattern of cystic bronchiectasis may resemble honeycomb lung as well.

Consolidation

When a portion of lung has much of its air content replaced by fluid or cells, so that the overall density changes to that of water, the term "consolidation" applies. Consolidation may be patchy, segmental, or lobar in distribution, and homogeneous or inhomogeneous in appearance. When the distribution is patchy, the lesions can appear as poorly marginated nodules or clusters of "acinar nodules." Some examples of consolidation are termed "lobar" in distribution, although seldom is the lobar consolidation complete.

In this text "consolidation" does not imply the presence of infection. Although pneumonia is one of the common causes of lung consolidation, hemorrhage, edema, chronic inflammation, or even severe airspace or interstitial infiltration by cells and fluid can cause zones of consolidation.

Air Bronchograms

Air bronchograms are seen when air-filled segmental and peripheral bronchi remain contrasted against surrounding regions of consolidation. It is common to see the relatively large air-filled proximal trunks of the major bronchi on normal chest films once you learn to seek them out. These should not be confused with air bronchograms, since that term is ordinarily reserved to indicate an abnormality.

The relatively narrow bands of lung seen between images of blood vessels at the lung bases can be mistaken for air bronchograms. With practice the error is avoided. Since the blood vessels diverge as they extend to the periphery, the bands of lung seen between them become wider distally, whereas with true air bronchograms they do not (except in cases of bronchiectasis).

Air bronchogram patterns may be seen in areas of atelectasis, pneumonia, pulmonary edema or hemorrhage, pulmonary sarcoid, malignant lymphoma, bronchoalveolar neoplasm, Wegener's granulomatosis, and even some chronic interstitial pneumonias.

Infiltrates

Many radiologists deplore the use of the term "infiltrate" to describe any pulmonary lesion. However, almost every descriptive term in use, including "consolidation," is considered poor by some and acceptable by others. "Infiltrate" seems to be commonly used as a nonspecific descriptor of almost any pulmonary abnormality of greater tissue density than normal lung. This term is easy to use but implies that the observer will not or cannot find the words to describe the lesion accurately. Thus, often out of frustration with the lack of commonly accepted descriptive terminology, or perhaps out of laziness, one takes refuge in misuse of the term. The ideal description of an abnormality permits a knowledgeable person receiving only the description to visualize the abnormality accurately. "Infiltrate" simply does not permit accurate visualization.

Mass

The term "mass" is ordinarily applied to a circumscribed region of water density. No rules exist to say when a nodule achieves sufficient size to be designated a mass. Hence, descriptions of lesions should include measurements indicating size in at least two dimensions, and three when possible. It is also common and useful to include modifiers describing shape and marginal contours. A mass may be composed of cells (e.g., neoplasm or fibrosis), or fluid (e.g., a cyst), or a combination of cells and fluid (e.g., pneumonia or abscess). You cannot determine the specific constituents of a mass from chest films alone. Distinctions between masses and consolidations may be arbitrary in that opacity is a property of both. Masses are usually identified by rounded or oval contours that do not ordinarily correspond to segmental or lobar boundaries.

Blebs, Bullae, Air Cysts, and Pneumatoceles

Blebs are small air spaces on the order of 1 cm in diameter located in the pleura. Bullae are air spaces in the lung substance and may vary from very small (about 1 cm) to very large (approaching the volume of a hemithorax). Bullae are common lesions in the lungs of patients with emphysema due to breakdown of alveolar walls and loss of the vascular bed. However, many patients who have symptomatic emphysema will not have detectable bullae on radiographic examination. Furthermore, not all patients with bullae have diffuse airway obstruction. In other words, patients with emphysema may have bullae, but not all patients with bullae have emphysema.

On chest films, bullae frequently are demarcated by pencil-point-thin curvilinear walls, which are seldom seen through 360 degrees of arc. More commonly only short arc segments are seen. The thin walls seen on chest films are probably due to projection of adjacent atelectatic lung.

As opposed to blebs or bullae, true developmental pulmonary air cysts are uncommon. Although theoretically they may be congenital, they are rarely found at autopsy in infants. In radiology, however, the term "air cyst" is frequently used to denote any thin-walled, air-containing space not found in normal lung. Thus, bullae and pneumatoceles may also be called air cysts. Air cysts may also result from cystic bronchiectasis.

Patients may have one or more air cysts of indeterminate cause and have no symptoms related to them. A cyst may not become visible radiographically until a pulmonary infection causes a fluid level to appear within it.

Cystic hamartomas are rare.

Pneumatoceles are circumscribed pockets of air that result from ball-valve-like obstruction of peripheral airways. These air spaces may arise acutely in children with staphylococcal pneumonia and may also develop from lung damage following hydrocarbon aspiration pneumonitis. In some patients with blunt chest trauma there may be tears of the pulmonary parenchyma, and sizeable focal air collections may develop in the interstitium of the lung. They may also result from barotrauma in patients on respirators. These focal air pockets may be referred to as post-traumatic pneumatoceles.

Cavities

Cavities are holes in the lung that occur when necrotic tissue, discharged through bronchial communications, is replaced by air. Cavities may be of any size, thick or thin walled, regular or irregular in either inner or outer marginal contour, benign or malignant. They may or may not show fluid levels or other cavitary contents. Characteristics that favor a benign or a malignant etiology are discussed in subsequent chapters.

Rarely, as benign cavities resolve they leave behind thin-walled, cystic-appearing spaces that cannot be distinguished from bullae. Ordinarily when a cavity resolves there is only a nonspecific linear scar or no telltale radiographic clue to its former presence.

Other Terms

Many other terms have been proposed as descriptors of radiographic pulmonary abnormalities. The International Labor Organization (ILO) has developed a set of descriptors for use in the study of pneumoconiosis that includes not only terms used to describe radiographic abnormalities but also terms to describe their distribution and the degree of involvement.

For example, nodules are designated as "small rounded opacities" and classified as to predominant size: up to 1.5 mm (p), 1.6 to 3 mm (q), and 3.0 to 10.0 mm (r). Small linear or irregular opacities are further classified as to thickness: fine (s), medium (t), and coarse or blotchy (u). The degree of involvement, designated as the "profusion," is classified as either normal (0), slight (1), moderate (2), or advanced (3).

Carrington, Gaensler, and co-workers have added another designation of small, rounded opacities of varying sizes similar to those of the ILO classification, but having short linear or curvilinear extensions about their peripheries. This was an attempt to make the classification applicable to a larger group of interstitial lung diseases, particularly those noninfectious granulomatous diseases such as sarcoidosis and berylliosis.

Mach Bands

Mach bands create an edge enhancement effect at the interface of regions of different contrast.[6] They are visual phenomena. The functioning of the neural networks in the retina is such that while certain receptor signals are transmitted, adjacent ones are inhibited. Thus, although Mach bands are quite real to you and me, they are not recognized by a densitometer and therefore are classified as illusions.

A negative Mach band is a narrow band of black seen where a light image with a convex edge interfaces with a darker image having a corresponding concave edge. A positive Mach band is a narrow band of white seen where a darker image with a convex edge interfaces with a lighter image having a corresponding concave edge.

Apparently there is interindividual variation in the ability to see Mach bands, but they are visible on illustrations throughout this text. When edge images are effaced by adjacent disease processes, the accompanying Mach band will also be effaced.

It is important not to confuse Mach bands with abnormalities. Fat surrounding viscera, (e.g., epicardial fat) may also produce dark bands similar to negative Mach bands, and at times it is difficult to distinguish between the two.

COMPUTED TOMOGRAPHY OF THE CHEST

Computed tomography (CT) is a process that uses a computer to reconstruct an image of a portion (slice) of an object or a part of the body. The reconstruction is based on a series of x-ray absorption measurements obtained by rotating an x-ray source (the tube), coupled with a series of radiation detectors (the collector array), about the object being studied (Figs. 2-9 and 2-12). Some units use a rotating x-ray source and a fixed ring of radiation detectors.

A narrow beam of x-rays can be produced by collimating the output of the tube. Collimation devices are also used at the level of the detectors to eliminate the scatter radiation that results from interaction of the primary beam with the parts being studied. The collimation can be adjusted within the width of the detectors. In modern scanners, the beam can be made broad enough (fan beam) to encompass the entire object of study by using hundreds of detectors in the collector array. For each exposure cycle, the computer is programmed to calculate a myriad of linear attenuation coefficients of a matrix of small blocks of tissue, and to display this data as a matrix of numbers (CT numbers or Hounsfield units) or to create a gray-scale image based on these numbers. Each picture element (pixel) of the two-dimensional display on the cathode ray tube actually represents data derived from a small volume of tissue (voxel). The thickness of this slice is commonly on the order of 10 mm but varies with the machine used. On more modern units, one can also choose to reduce the thickness of a given slice or slices to as little as 1.5 mm in order to study selected anatomic sites more critically.

By minimizing the influence of scattered radiation, and by the use of sensitive detectors, CT scans permit the manipulation of data so as to make it possible to recognize differences of tissue density of less than 1 percent. With conventional chest film radiography, differences in radiation transmission of less than 10 percent go unrecognized. CT examinations thus allow for much greater discrimination between structures of different density than do chest film examinations, and thereby permit recognition of body parts and organ structures not possible with conventional x-ray techniques.

The simple assignment of relative tissue densities that we use in thinking about the formation of conventional chest film images is not applicable to the formation of CT images. The densities of various tissues and fluids must be considered in units closer to their true values. Furthermore, since CT examinations are conducted in such a fashion that all structures within a small band of tissue are traversed by the x-ray beam through a multiplicity of angles, interfaces between tissues of different density in the horizontal plane of the slice may be recognized regardless of their orientation to the beam at any one position (Figs. 2-10 to 2-14).

CT images are usually displayed in the form of axial cross sections and hence require a detailed knowledge of cross-sectional anatomy. If slices are obtained at close intervals, it is also possible to use the computer to create coronal, sagittal, or even multiple oblique planar reconstructions of the same data. However, commonly these reconstructions result in very rough images.

The display and recording systems of the CT format permit more sensitive distinctions between regions of different tissue density. The ability to distinguish solid tissue such as neoplasm from low-density fluid as in a simple cyst, or to distinguish fat from higher density solid tissue, is made possible by CT. CT makes small amounts of calcification within tissues much easier to recognize than with routine chest film techniques. Iodine-containing contrast material is also recognized in tissues in much smaller amounts and at lesser concentrations with CT. The intravenous administration of contrast agents may allow one to make reliable deductions concerning the blood supply of neoplasms and thus distinguish them from avascular cysts. Comparable deductions, utilizing routine filming techniques, would require catheterization of the vessels supplying the structure. The catheterization of vessels, injection of contrast, and the use of appropriate filming techniques, however, still offer the advantage of displaying small vessels that are beyond the abilities of CT to display as discrete entities.

Because the viewing and filming conditions can be manipulated, it is critical that each CT section be surveyed over different gray scales; otherwise some lesions will not be recognized, and normal anatomic structures may be mistaken for abnormalities.

You can obtain a much better appreciation of the functioning of a CT scanner and the ability to manipulate the gray scale by sitting with the radiologist or technologist while performing and analyzing the studies. Try to arrange to do this wherever you can. The experience will enhance your understanding of the technique more than any number of words in a textbook.

MAGNETIC RESONANCE IMAGING

Magnetic resonance imaging (MRI) has many similarities to CT and some important differences (Fig. 2-15). Both imaging methods depend on signals derived from the interaction of radiant energy with tissue. In the case of CT, the diagnostic signal depends on attenuation of high energy x-rays by the tissues and organ contents under study. In MRI the diagnostic signal depends on the interaction of low-energy radio waves with the tissues and organ contents under study in a strong static magnetic field. Both methods require computers for conversion of the energy-dependent signals (received by special detectors) into a matrix of numerical values, which in turn are converted into gray-scale images.

The diagnostic signal in both CT and MRI studies is manipulated by sophisticated computer programs; the actual acquisition of the signal, however, is quite different. The manner in which the signals are obtained for MRI images is much more complex than that for CT.

Nuclear Spin

Data acquisition for MRI is based on the physical principles of nuclear magnetic resonance. Theory holds that elementary particles such as protons and neutrons rotate on their central axes and thus possess angular momentum, or spin. Atomic nuclei with even numbers of protons and neutrons have no net spin because of mutual cancellation of spin by these particles. Atomic nuclei with odd numbers of protons or neutrons have a net spin, and because they also have a net charge they behave as small bar magnets. In conventional MRI of the chest, the hydrogen nucleus, a single proton, is the source of the diagnostic signal. When placed in a strong magnetic field, the individual magnetic fields of the protons become aligned either parallel or antiparallel (180 degrees opposite) to the external magnetic field. At a point of equilibrium, however, a slightly greater number of protons (a few per million) are aligned in the direction of the applied magnetic field than are aligned in the opposite direction, and thus there is a small net magnetic vector in the direction of the external magnetic field. The spinning motion of the proton about its axis does not align exactly with the main magnetic field, but has a gyroscopic or "wobbling" motion like a spinning top. The frequency of this wobble or precession, the Larmor frequency, varies with the type of nucleus and is increased with stronger external magnetic fields.

Radiofrequency Pulse and T_1 and T_2 Relaxation Times

When a radiofrequency (RF) pulse having the exact frequency of the precessing protons is introduced into the volume of tissue being studied, additional energy is imparted to a portion of the protons, and they are tipped as a group away from their prestimulus (equilibrium) orientation. When the RF signal is turned off, this group of precessing nuclei returns to its original orientation, and in so doing gives off energy in the form of an RF signal that can be measured and recorded. It is this signal that is used for image formation. By convention, the time required for this return to equilibrium is called the T_1 (or longitudinal) relaxation time. The T_2 relaxation time is another constant derived from measurement of the rate at which this group of precessing protons becomes less coherent, or dephases, in the xy plane. Thus, T_2 is a measure of the rate at which the RF signal emitted from the protons decays after cessation of stimulation. T_1 and T_2 are important in MRI because tissues are characterized by these relaxation times. For example, fat has short T_1 and T_2 relaxation times whereas water has long T_1 and T_2 relaxation times. The signal intensity in

MRI depends on the amplitude of the RF signal that is emitted from the tissues under study. The amplitude in turn depends on the proton density of the tissues under study and their T_1 and T_2 relaxation times. In addition, the signal intensity depends on the phenomenon of "flow," or the rate at which moving fluids (e.g., blood) enter and leave the section being imaged.

In addition to these characteristics of the tissue being studied, other variables that are operator dependent influence signal intensity. These are referred to as TR, TE, and TI. The variable TI is not critical to the following discussion, but its significance is covered elsewhere.[8,9]

RF Pulse Sequences: TE and TR

A 90-degree pulse is an RF pulse of sufficient magnitude or duration to "flip" precessing protons 90 degrees from the parallel alignment with the external magnetic field. A 180-degree RF pulse is one that is of sufficient magnitude or duration to increase the flip angle to 180 degrees. Thus, the power of the RF pulse is a function of its amplitude and duration at a given frequency. The frequency of the RF pulse capable of producing these changes in the net magnetic field must be equal to the frequency of the precessing protons, which in turn depends on the strength of the magnetic field.

In the pulse sequence known as "spin echo," in which a 90-degree RF pulse is followed by a 180-degree RF pulse, TE refers to the time in milliseconds between the 90-degree pulse and the "spin-echo" produced by the 180-degree pulse (two times the 90-degree to 180-degree pulse interval). After the decay of the first echo, a second 180-degree RF pulse may be transmitted and a second echo can be generated. Likewise, successive 180-degree RF pulses will generate echo number three, and so on. In the spin-echo pulse sequences, TR refers to the time in milliseconds between successive 90-degree RF pulses. Other pulse sequences may be used in obtaining MRI images, and new pulse sequences are being developed as more experience is gained in MRI.

Gray Scale Assignment in MRI

The gray scale assigned to MRI images is such that the stronger the signal intensity from any point in the section under study, the lighter that point will be depicted on the MRI image. The weaker the signal intensity from any point, the darker it will be on the gray scale.

An image created from a pulse sequence using a short TR (e.g., 300 msec) and a short TE (e.g., 25 msec) is considered to be "T_1 weighted." Matter that has a short T_1 relaxation time will have a high signal intensity and appear on the white end of the gray scale on T_1-weighted images. Matter that has a long T_1 relaxation time will be

of low signal intensity and appear on the dark end of the gray scale on T_1-weighted images.

A T_2-weighted image is one acquired after a long TE (e.g., 60 to 90 msec) and a long TR (e.g., 2,500 to 3,000 msec). Tissue with a short T_2 will appear dark, and tissue with a long T_2 will appear bright on T_2-weighted images.

Spin-echo images that are produced from pulse sequences having a long TR interval (e.g., 2,000 msec) and a short TE (30 msec or less) are considered to be of indeterminate weighting with contrast due to both T_1 differences and T_2 differences as well as proton density differences between tissues. The comparison of T_1-weighted and T_2-weighted images in the study of a specific body part allows you to recognize different tissues within the studied volume.

In general, major blood vessels seen on the MRI in this text will appear to have black lumens (Fig. 2-15B), because stimulated protons in the flowing blood move out of the area being imaged before signal acquisition takes place. The phenomenon may also be due to rapid dephasing caused by motion. The precise explanation for the appearance of flowing blood on individual MRI scans is complicated, but a detailed discussion can be found in the references.[8,9] Flowing blood within vessels does not have a low signal intensity under all circumstances of MRI, and thus it becomes important to have a working knowledge of the signal intensity to be expected from blood vessels under different examination circumstances.

CT and MRI scanners are quite similar in external appearance, although the shape of the gantry opening differs. In a CT scanner the gantry houses the x-ray tube and detector array. In an MRI scanner the gantry houses a powerful magnet, an RF transmitter and receiver, and magnetic gradient coils, which permit localization of the section under study.

CT and MRI have in common the ability to produce cross-sectional (axial) images (Fig. 2-15). Multiplanar images can also be directly accessed by electronically switching the plane of orientation on MRI. Multiplanar images can be obtained in CT by reconstruction of the data obtained from multiple axial slices at close intervals. In general, however, the spatial resolution of axial images obtained using CT is similar to that of MRI, whereas coronal and other planar images of MRI studies have superior spatial resolution compared to those reconstructed from CT data.

Bone and Bone Marrow on MRI

The protons in cortical bone are immobile in a crystalline lattice. Thus, cortical bone appears as a rim of black (signal void) about the marrow contents of bone on

MRI. Fatty bone marrow has high signal intensity on T_1-weighted images and is displayed on the near-white end of the gray scale. Cellular marrow, as in the ribs, the sternum, and the vertebrae, contains less fat and therefore has less signal intensity on T_1-weighted images and appears darker on the gray scale.

ON COUNTING RIBS

PA View

You would think that counting ribs should be a simple task. It usually is, but many errors can be made if you do not use care. A common error, when counting the posterior portions of the ribs on a PA view, is to miss the first. This can be avoided by locating the first rib anteriorly, following it back to its costotransverse articulation, and counting downward from there. When there is a high spinal kyphosis, several posterior ribs may be superimposed on one another and miscounted, unless you pay attention to their costotransverse articulations when counting. Counting the anterior portions of ribs is usually simple but may be complicated by variations in the position of the first rib when there is a cervical rib present or when anomalous bifid anterior ribs are present. Counting of ribs in their axillary course depends on correctly aligning them with their posterior or anterior portions. It is surprising how easy it is to miscount those along the lower axillary regions, where they can be superimposed in confusing fashion.

You may be tempted to count ribs from the bottom up on some films. Avoid this temptation; not everyone has 12 ribs.

Lateral View

Ribs can also be counted on a lateral view if done with care. Find the sternal angle of Louis—the gap between the manubrium and the body of the sternum. The second rib articulates at this level. Once you have identified the second ribs, you have a base from which to count the others. Follow the second ribs back to their vertebra and use that as a base for counting vertebral levels. Again, counting from the bottom up is tempting but less reliable, because of the uncertainty as to which rib is number 12. The right and left ribs will be projected at slightly different levels, but the pair usually will be superimposed over part of their course.

If you take into account beam divergence and assume that centering is approximately at the hilar level, which set of ribs (right or left) would you expect to project above the other in the upper and lower regions of the chest in a left lateral view?

Oblique Views

Counting ribs on oblique views is usually simple, as long as you count the first, which may present a subtle image on the narrow side (right side on the right anterior oblique view, left side on the left anterior oblique view), because it is high on the film and may not be seen with a sharp lung interface (Fig. 2-8C).

SUMMARY

1. Most water-density images seen in the lung on normal chest films are produced by blood vessels. The imaging of these vessels depends on the integrity of the air-water interface between the vessels and adjacent air-containing structures, mainly alveoli.*
2. An edge image is produced by projecting the interface of two different absorbers tangential to the beam. A line or band image is produced by the interfaces of three different absorbers, two of which may be of the same density whereas the third, which separates them, is different.
   a. The interface between absorbers of low density (g/cm^3), such as between muscle and fat, or between air and a water-density absorber, is recognized on routine films only when that interface projects a sufficient tangent perpendicular to the beam.
   b. The visibility of low-density tissue structures or lesions can be enhanced by obtaining projections that increase the path length of the x-ray beam through that structure, and by attempting to position the lesion-lung interface tangential to the beam so that an edge is seen. Peripheral low-density lesions with tapered margins may go unrecognized when projected en face.
3. Images are displayed on film over a continuum of gray tones. Black areas of film are dense in terms of film density but are produced by remnant radiation that has traversed low-density matter such as air or fat. Areas on the white end of the gray tones are considered light in terms of film density, but are produced by remnant radiation that has traversed either high-density matter such as bone or calcium or a long path through near-water-density matter such as muscle mass, heart and great vessels, or pulmonary vessels projected end-on. The technical fac-

---

* You know that alveoli are not simply little bags of air, but are surrounded by a capillary bed whose individual constituents are below the resolving power of radiographic imaging systems. This tissue does, however, contribute to the density of the lungs; therefore, even those portions of lung not traversed by recognizable vessels have a density slightly in excess of air alone.

tors used (kilovoltage and milliampere-seconds) as well as overexposure or underexposure techniques will also greatly influence these appearances.

4. More incident light is needed to see details that may be present in the blacker regions of the film. Hence the need to have a good bright light available next to your viewer. There are no practical techniques for resurrecting information that may be lost in too light areas of the film. (Viewing through a minifying lens helps.)

5. Pulmonary abnormalities produce a variety of patterns on chest films. These patterns can be used in the formulation of differential diagnoses but are not specific for any given diagnosis.

6. It is difficult to describe certain radiographic images in a universally acceptable manner, regardless of whether descriptive or inferential terms are used, because a common nomenclature has not been agreed upon.

7. Compared to chest films, CT and MRI scans provide significantly increased ability to distinguish differences in tissue density. This is extremely useful. For example, depositions of fat in the mediastinum, the cardiophrenic angles, and even the extrapleural space commonly cannot be recognized as such on chest films and may be mistaken for more ominous soft tissue masses. CT or MRI scans make the distinctions clear. CT scans are more sensitive than plain films in detecting calcification in tissues, but MRI scans do not detect calcification specifically.

8. CT and MRI scans permit recognition of different tissue interfaces regardless of their orientation to one another because of the multiplicity of angles through which the imaging data are obtained. Lesions that often are cryptic on chest films may be easy to see on CT scans. The price paid for this gain, however, is that often on CT inconsequential scars in the lung may be seen that may not be distinguishable from more ominous lesions such as metastases.

9. CT scans are usually displayed as axial cross-sectional images, and MRI scans are commonly displayed in this format. Their interpretation requires a detailed knowledge of cross-sectional anatomy. The multiplanar images of MRI have superior spatial resolution compared to multiplanar images reconstructed from CT data acquired in axial cross section.

10. CT scans should be viewed over different gray-scale ranges to take advantage of the details that are available in images viewed at both narrow and wide gray-scale windows.

11. MRI scans can be obtained using different pulse sequences to aid in distinguishing different tissues. The tissue contrast resolution capabilities of MRI are superior to those of CT.

12. MRI scans permit recognition of major blood vessels without the use of intravenous contrast material because of the signal void created by flowing blood.

BIBLIOGRAPHY

1. Curry TS III, Dowdey JE, Murry RC: Christensen's Introduction to the Physics of Diagnostic Radiology. 3rd Ed. Lea & Febiger, Philadelphia, 1984

2. Felson B: A new look at pattern recognition of diffuse pulmonary disease. AJR 133:183, 1979

3. Genereux GP: Pattern recognition in diffuse lung disease. A review of theory and practice. Med Radiogr Photogr 61:2, 1985

4. Hetizman ER: Pattern recognition in pulmonary radiology. In *The Lung.* 2nd Ed. CV Mosby Co, St. Louis, 1984

5. Kattan KR, Felson B, Eyre JT. The silhouette sign revisited experimentally. Appl Radiol 113:36, 1984

6. Lane EJ, Proto AV, Phillips TW: Mach bands and density perception. Radiology 121:9, 1976

7. Ter-Pogossian MM: The Physical Aspects of Diagnostic Radiology. Harper & Row, Hagerstown, MD, 1967

8. Weinreb JC, Redman HC: Magnetic Resonance Imaging of the Body. WB Saunders Co, Philadelphia, 1987

9. Young SW: Magnetic Resonance Imaging: Basic Principles. 2nd Ed. Raven Press, New York, 1988

Atlas

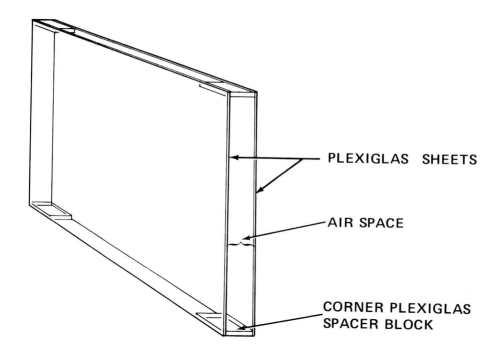

PLEXIGLAS SHEETS

AIR SPACE

CORNER PLEXIGLAS
SPACER BLOCK

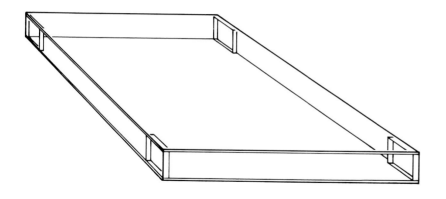

**Fig. 2-1. Plexiglas Sand-
wich Model**

Two thin sheets of Plexiglas
of the same size are separated by an air space. The
separation is maintained
by small Plexiglas spacer
blocks along the long axis at
each corner.

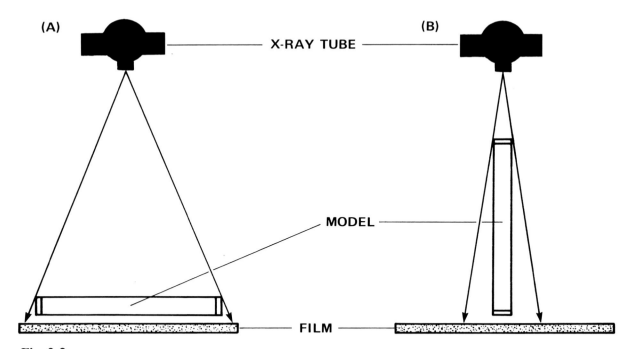

Fig. 2-2.

Diagrams of the relationships of the x-ray tube, the Plexiglas model, and the film used in making Figs. 2-3, 2-4, and 2-5.

Fig. 2-3. **Radiograph of the Plexiglas Model Coned So Edges of the Model Are Not Included in the Field of View**

The field has been coned so that the edges of the model are not included, and it appears that nothing is in the path of the x-ray beam. In fact, a film exposed with the model in place and another exposed without the model in place show differences very difficult for the eye to distinguish. It is only recognition of the edges—the interface of the margins of the Plexiglas sheets with room air—that allows one to recognize their presence in Fig. 2-4.

Fig. 2-4. **Radiograph of the Plexiglas Model with Edges Included**

The corner spacer blocks are projected as dense bands, because they are standing on edge and present long paths and long tangents to the x-ray beam. The Plexiglas sheets, however, lying flat, provide only a short path for the beam to traverse. The inclusion of their edges in the field allows one to recognize the presence of the Plexiglas sheets. However, there is no way to recognize the air *between* the sheets.

Notice that one set of edges projects slightly beyond the other, in spite of the sheets being the same size and positioned precisely one above the other. The divergence of the x-ray beam accounts for this magnification: The sheet farthest from the film is projected as being larger than the sheet next to the film.

Fig. 2-5. **Radiograph of Plexiglas Model Standing On Edge**

Now one can easily see the black air space between the plastic sheets, because the interface between the air and the plastic is tangential to the beam. The plastic sheets project as lines because there are three different absorbers in tangent (air, plastic, air) for each sheet. The vertical orientation of the model does not permit recognition of the dimension of the sheets perpendicular to the plane of the film. Hence, a sheet is projected as a line. The black areas outside as well as in between the plastic sheets are simply images of room air. Can you figure out why the spacer blocks at the ends of the image appear as they do?

Fig. 2-6.   Changes in Clarity of Pulmonary Vessels Due to Disease

(A) Coned view of the right lower zone of a normal chest film shows small vessel detail.

(B) Coned view of the right lower lung of a young woman with known acute myelogenous leukemia, who is also toxic and febrile. Is the lung normal or abnormal? Do not concern yourself here with the relative size of the smaller vessel images but only with their clarity or sharpness of outline. Do you think this appearance is within the spectrum of normal variation? The decision is subjective and difficult to make. Comparison with previous films, even if they are slightly different in technique, may convince you that the subtle loss of vessel detail is abnormal or at least that follow-up films are indicated within a short time to reassess your decision.

(C) Coned view of the right lower lung of the same patient as in Fig. B, only one day later. The exposure technique is different and the film is lighter. Is the small vessel detail degraded in comparison to Fig. B, or is the difference in technique enough to explain the change in appearance? The further loss of sharp small vessel outlines indicates that the lung is abnormal, even though the lighter exposure makes some of the larger vessels more conspicuous. (D) Coned view of the right lower lung of the same patient only one day after Fig. C was taken. The exposure is comparable, although not precisely the same as for C. There is almost total effacement of small vessel detail by the inflammatory exudate of varicella-zoster pneumonitis. The pneumonia is diffuse throughout both lungs, but coned views were used here to facilitate comparison of details.

Differences in exposure technique from film to film can account for changes in gray tones, but unless the differences are extreme they should not alter the relative sharpness of vessel outlines. Thus, true pulmonary disease should be suspected when vessel clarity is altered, as in Figs. B and C, although Fig. B may be more easily considered abnormal in retrospect than in prospect.

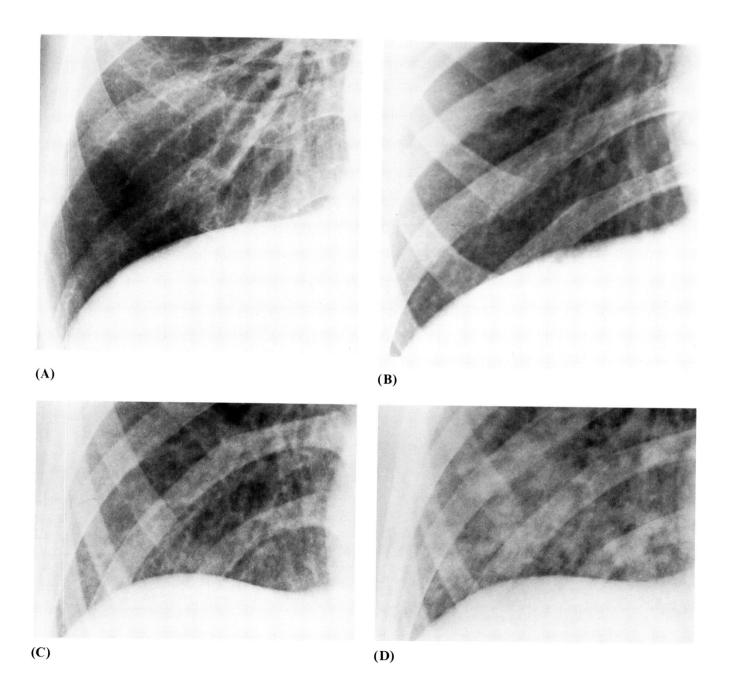

(A)

(B)

(C)

(D)

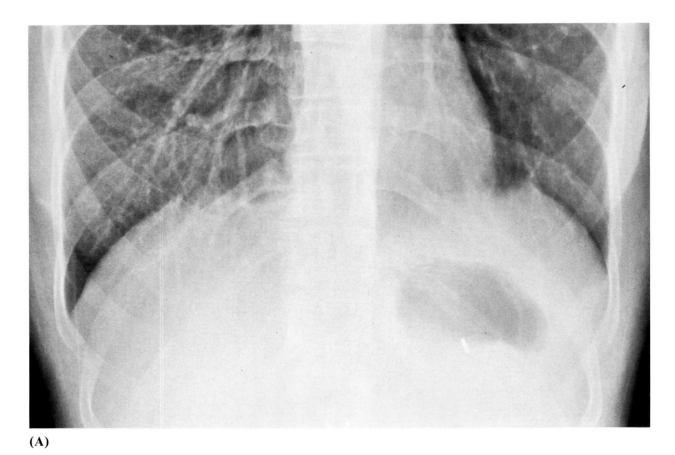

(A)

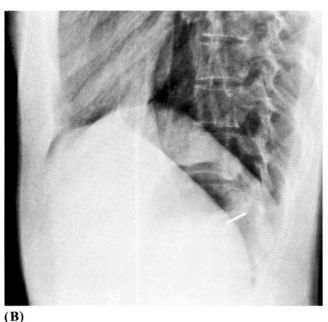

(B)

Fig. 2-7. Changes in Pulmonary Vessel Clarity at the Lung Bases

(A) Coned view of the lung bases of a young woman who had previously been treated for Hodgkin's disease and was doing well at the time of this film. Blood vessels are clearly seen even in that portion of lung that is projected below the level of the diaphragmatic domes and behind the left heart. With proper exposure, this amount of detail can be achieved in most thin individuals. Notice the wide separation of the stomach bubble and the left diaphragm on this PA view.

(B) Lateral view taken at the same time as Fig. A. The stomach bubble is actually quite close to the posterior slope of the left diaphragm in this patient, who has had a splenectomy. The apparent separation on the PA view is due to projection of the high tangent of the diaphragm, which is anterior to the position of the stomach. Understanding these relationships is important to avoid confusion with a left subpulmonic effusion or left upper quadrant mass (see Ch. 3). *(Figure continues.)*

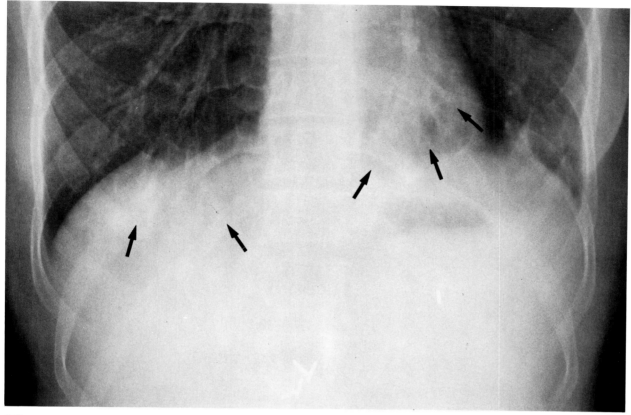

(C)

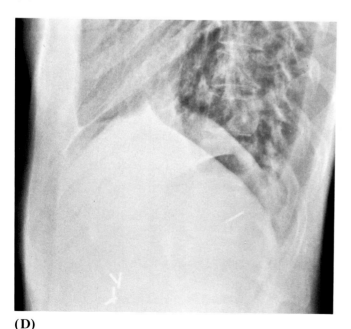

(D)

Fig. 2-7. *(Continued).* **(C)** Coned view of the lung bases of the same woman at a later date. She is now febrile, has a cough productive of green sputum, and on physical examination has basilar rales.

The vessels that were visible at the bases below the diaphragm domes and in the left retrocardiac area in Fig. A have lost their sharp margins. Peripherally, the vessel shadows have been replaced by bands of ill-defined opacities, as though accompanying bronchi and their marginating lung were stuffed with exudate. These findings are important in establishing that the patient has pneumonia rather than just an upper respiratory infection.

(D) Lateral view taken on the same day as Fig. C. There is a marked loss of clarity of the vessels in the lower lobes compared to Fig. B.

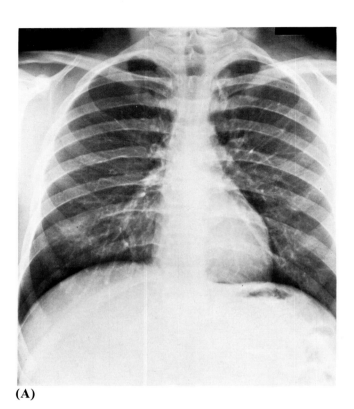

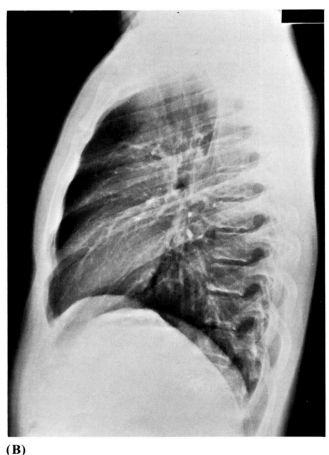

(A)

(B)

Fig. 2-8. Small Extrapleural Mass

PA, lateral, and right anterior oblique views of the chest of a young man with a small extrapleural mass due to recurrent Hodgkin's disease. All the films are of the same date.

(A) PA view shows a focal area of increased tissue density at the level of the superimposed images of the posterior right eighth and anterior fifth ribs in the midclavicular line. (Compare this area with its counterpart on the left side.)

This abnormality has no distinct edges. It is a subtle and easily overlooked finding. Could it be a patchy area of pneumonitis? Could it be a focus of Hodgkin's disease in the lung? In other words, could it be a pulmonary parenchymal lesion? The answer is yes. However, whenever you see an ill-defined lesion in one projection, consider at least the possibility of the lesion being pleural or extrapleural or even in or upon the surface of the chest wall.

(B) No lesion is seen on this lateral view. Does this rule out the possibility of a parenchymal lesion? Does it indicate that the subtle finding seen on the PA view is not a lesion at all? Unfortunately not. The fact that a lesion is not visible in both projections does not indicate that it is not in the parenchyma or that it is not real. Under these circumstances, however, we should again consider sites such as the extrapleural space or chest wall. *(Figure continues.)*

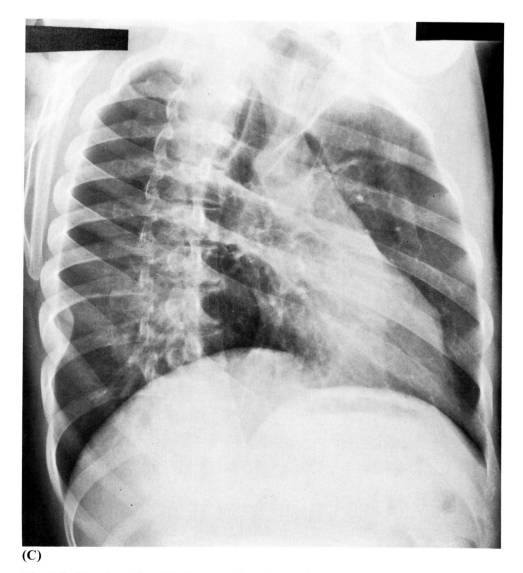

(C)

Fig. 2-8. *(Continued).* **(C)** An extrapleural mass is clearly seen on this right anterior oblique projection between the right eighth and ninth ribs. Why is it so much easier to recognize here than on the PA view? First, the interface between the extrapleural mass and the adjacent lung is now tangential to the beam and presents a sharp edge and contrast gradient. Second, we have probably increased the length of the absorber in the beam path.

Incidentally, note how well the right and left hemidiaphragms are seen on the oblique view. Slightly oblique views are also useful for separating the posterior gutters from one another when necessary.

The second rib is easy to identify, but the arc of the right first rib is not seen as well as those below. It must be included in the rib count, or the location of the lesion will not be identified correctly.

Exercise. Go back to the lateral view (Fig. B). A portion of the stomach bubble is projected under the higher diaphragm. This identifies the left diaphragm. However, the high diaphragm anteriorly (in the region of the heart) is the right. The images of the right and left diaphragms cross one another beneath the image of the inferior vena cava.

The right posterior gutter is at the very lower border of the film. Follow the lung along the inner aspect of the posterior right ribs up to the ninth rib. Above that level, the posterior arcs of the right and left ribs project so close together that any lesion along the posterior wall would be obscured. If, by chance, the lateral view had been obtained in the RPTL (right side posterior to true lateral) variant, the lesion probably would have been seen (see Fig. 3-20B).

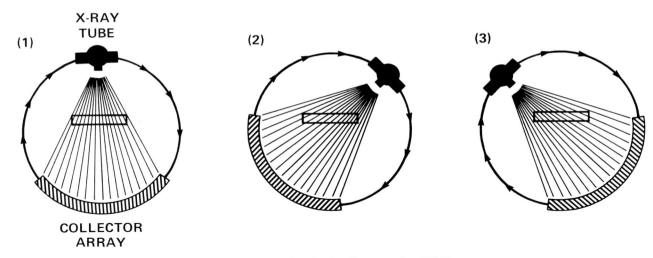

Fig. 2-9. Diagram of Plexiglas Model Lying Flat in the Gantry of a CT Scanner

The model is placed in the gantry so that it is lying flat in relation to the tube and collector array during rotation of the scanner.

Fig. 2-10. CT Section Through the Middle of the Plexiglas Model Lying Flat

The CT image is produced after one 360-degree rotation of the scanner. This slice is taken through the middle of the model, where there are no spacer blocks. The model appears as two lines separated by a layer of air. From this image you could calculate the width of the model and its height, but not its length, which is perpendicular to the plane of the image. We know from the technical settings at the time of the scan that the image was created from data collected over 1.0 cm of this unregistered dimension, but you cannot deduce that from the image.

It is easy to recognize the air space (black) between the plastic sheets in this image; contrast this with the inability to do so in Fig. 2-4.

The model is sitting on a large sponge on top of the gantry table. The sponge is barely visible between the tabletop and the model. The surface of the gantry table is seen as a sharp white line. Notice that a small cluster of dirt in the bottom of the sponge is also recorded in the image.

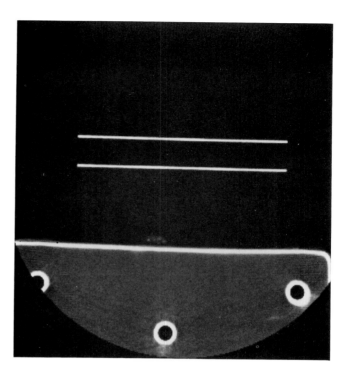

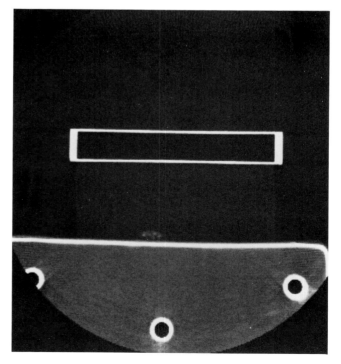

Fig. 2-11. CT Section Through the End of the Plexiglas Model Lying Flat

This image is similar to that in Fig. 2-10 except that now the slice is made through an end of the model, where the spacer blocks are located, and their position is faithfully recorded.

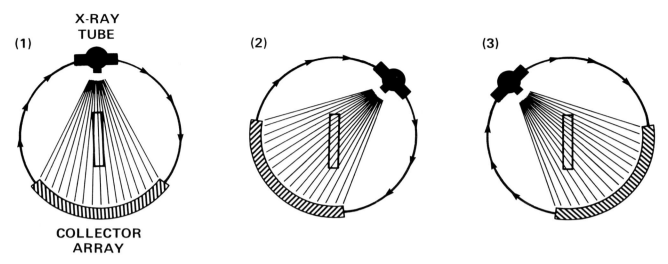

Fig. 2-12. Plastic Model Lying Vertical in the Gantry of a CT Scanner

The model is placed in the gantry so that it is standing vertical in relationship to the tube and the collector array.

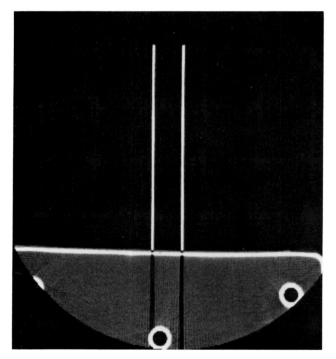

Fig. 2-13. CT Section Through the Middle of the Plexiglas Model Standing Vertical

The image is produced by a cut through the model standing on the gantry table. Again, the image results from examining a 1.0-cm-thick (in the plane perpendicular to the page) segment of the model. Since this CT slice was made where there are no spacer blocks, none is recorded.

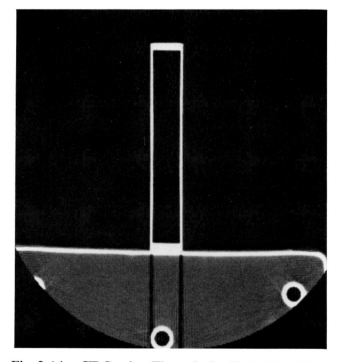

Fig. 2-14. CT Section Through the End of the Plexiglas Model Standing Vertical

The model is positioned as in Fig. 2-13, except that the slice is now made through an end section with spacer blocks, so that they are recorded.

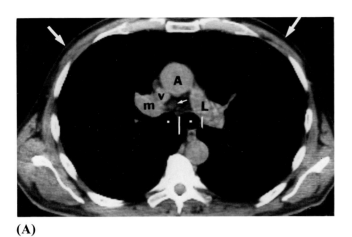

(A)

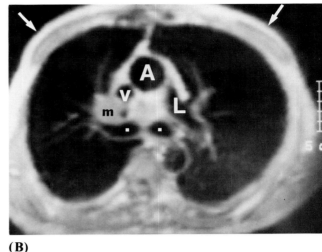

(B)

Fig. 2-15. Tissue Characterization With MRI

CT and MRI scans of a patient with a right hilar mass.

(A) On the CT scan the mass (m) has a gray-scale image that is indistinguishable from that of the ascending aorta (A) and the left pulmonary artery (L). Therefore, it is not possible to distinguish this mass from an abnormal vessel or even a partial-volume effect due to having a portion of the right pulmonary artery in the plane of the slice.

(B) On the MRI scan, however, it is clear that the mass (m) is not a vessel because it does not show the characteristic black signal void of flowing blood in the aorta (A), the left pulmonary artery (L), and the vena cava (V), which are also shown in this scan. The right and left main bronchi (small squares) also appear on the black end of the gray scale on both the CT and MRI scans. The main bronchi are separated by the tracheal carina (the longer bar on the CT scan), which appears thinner on CT than on MRI (unmarked space between the major bronchi) because of the filming technique used for the CT scan and the fact that the two scans are not at exactly the same level. For purposes of scale, the left main bronchus on the CT scan measures approximately 2.2 cm between the vertical bars. The scale (in centimeters) is seen along the right side of the MRI scan.

The MRI scan was gated to the cardiac cycle so that TR was dependent on the heart rate. In this case TR was 500 msec. TE was 15 msec. With this pulse sequence, fat gives a high-intensity signal (on the white end of the gray scale), just as it should on a T_1-weighted image.

Notice that on the CT scan the subcutaneous fat (oblique arrows) is on the black end of the gray scale, whereas on the MRI scan the subcutaneous fat, with a short T_1 relaxation time, is on the white end of the gray scale.

The fat seen anterior to the tracheal carina (longer vertical bar) and posterior to the ascending aorta (A) is black on the CT scan but contains a few small lymph nodes that are lighter gray (small arrow). On the MRI scan the fat in front of the carina is on the white end of the gray scale, but there are some dark gray zones within it that represent the lymph nodes, which are also seen on the CT scan.

On CT examinations, blood vessels can usually be distinguished from nonvascular masses by obtaining scans after intravenous bolus injection of contrast agent in coordination with the timing of the scans. On MRI studies the flow void signal in major blood vessels makes it possible to distinguish these vessels from nonvascular masses without injection of contrast agents. Thus, MRI study of the mediastinum and hila is preferred over CT examination when the use of contrast agents is contraindicated or refused by the patient.

On this MRI scan, the sternum, ribs, and vertebrae (cellular marrow) have low signal intensity, and their images are further degraded by the blur artifact on this cut. The bone cortices produce a signal void (see text) and are not seen.

On the CT scan, bones appear as bright images. Cortical bone is a relatively strong absorber of x-rays because of its density and calcium content.

3

The Pleura

Imaging studies are important in detecting and defining pleural abnormalities because:

1. The abnormalities are often clinically occult or underestimated, and symptoms are nonspecific.
2. Defining pleural lesions powerfully influences formulation of (a) the differential diagnosis, (b) the staging, (c) the treatment, and (d) the prognosis of the responsible disease or condition.

Uncommonly, history and physical findings alone may lead one to the diagnosis of acute pleurisy without effusion, since there may be no chest film abnormalities until pleural fluid accumulates. Far more commonly, radiographs serve as the principal method by which the presence and physical characteristics of pleural lesions are detected and evaluated. The pleura may also be studied by means of ultrasonography, computed tomography (CT), and magnetic resonance imaging (MRI). CT and MRI may discriminate more accurately between fluid collections and tissue masses, and are more sensitive in recognizing small pleural effusions and lesions such as plaques resulting from asbestos exposure.

From the radiographic standpoint, five principal ends are served in the evaluation of pleural disease:

1. The detection of pleural fluid and discrimination among free-flowing components, loculated pockets, and areas of chronic pleural thickening
2. The detection of chronic pleural thickening, either focal or diffuse
3. The detection and localization of pleural and extra-pleural masses, including pleural plaques and pleural neoplasms
4. The detection and localization of air in the pleural space, not only in pneumothorax, but also in air-fluid pockets consequent to bronchopleural fistula or to gas-producing organisms in infected pleural pockets
5. The detection of calcification within pleural lesions.

DETECTION AND EVALUATION OF PLEURAL FLUID

Pleural effusion is the most significant pleural abnormality encountered in day-to-day practice. Unfortunately, there are no radiographic techniques that permit distinction between exudates and transudates, or between one type of fluid and another, such as blood, chyle,[1] serum, or pus.

TABLE 3-1. Distinguishing Pleural Exudates From Transudates

Exudate
  Ratio of pleural fluid protein to serum protein > 0.5
  Ratio of pleural fluid LDH to serum LDH > 0.6
  Pleural fluid LDH > two-thirds normal upper limit of serum LDH
  Fluid may be clear, pale yellow, and odorless, or turbid, bloody, brownish, viscid, and odoriferous

Transudate
  None of the above chemical ratios are elevated
  Fluid is usually clear, pale yellow, and odorless

LDH, Lactic dehydrogenase.
(Data from Light et al.[6,7])

65

**TABLE 3-2. Conditions That May Be Associated
With Elevated Pleural Fluid Amylase**

Pancreatic disease
Esophageal perforation (salivary amylase)
Malignant neoplasm (Although neoplastic involvement of the pleura
  may cause effusions with high amylase content (> 160 U/dl), most
  neoplastic effusions do not have high amylase levels.)
Rarely parapneumonic

(Data from Light et al.[6,7])

TABLE 3-4. Causes of Chylothorax[a]

Neoplasm — involvement of mediastinal lymph nodes, obstruction of
  the thoracic duct (lymphoma most commonly, metastases less com-
  mon)
Surgical trauma
Penetrating trauma
Idiopathic
Others (e.g., lymphangioleiomyomatosis, filariasis, superior vena cava
  obstruction)

[a] May require distinction from pseudochylothorax by analysis of
triglyceride levels in the pleural fluid.

It is seldom necessary to employ imaging modalities to perform successful thoracentesis, but ultrasound guidance can be useful when difficulties are anticipated, because of the presence of small volumes of fluid, or the presence of small loculated pockets.

Frequently it is necessary to obtain samples of the pleural fluid for chemical, physical, cytologic, and bacteriologic study. A variety of determinations both provide the data on which diagnostic probabilities are based and are critical in treatment planning (Tables 3-1 to 3-4).[6-8] Biopsy of the pleura is often necessary to diagnose tuberculous pleurisy and some malignant effusions when cytologic or bacteriologic analysis of pleural fluid specimens is inconclusive.

One can attempt to memorize long lists of causes of pleural effusions, but they can be divided into five subsets of basic disturbances for easier recall:

1. Any pathophysiologic process that results in increased pulmonary or systemic capillary pressure or severe hypoproteinemia. Generally, these effusions will have the properties of transudates. Examples include:

   Congestive heart failure from any cause
   Constrictive pericarditis
   Lesions of the left atrium or mitral valve sufficient to cause partial obstruction of venous return
   Cirrhosis
   Nephrotic syndrome
   Some cases of pulmonary embolism.[6]

2. Any pathophysiologic process that alters pleural capillary or lymphatic permeability. Generally these

**TABLE 3-3. Conditions That May Be Associated
With Decreased Pleural Fluid Glucose[a]**

Parapneumonic effusion with emyema
Tuberculous pleuritis
Malignant effusion
Rheumatoid pleural effusion

[a] Glucose <60 mg/dl.
(Data from Light et al.[6,7])

will cause exudates and include:
   Infections and infestations
   Inflammation (e.g., secondary to adjacent pulmonary infarction or radiation therapy)
   Pulmonary embolism
   Neoplasm, metastatic or primary, including malignant lymphomas and leukemias
   Conditions known to be associated with serositis (e.g., lupus erythematosus, rheumatoid arthritis, uremia)
   Immunologic disorders (e.g., postmyocardial infarction and pericardiectomy syndromes, drug and hypersensitivity reactions).

3. Any process that can obstruct or interrupt thoracic vascular or lymphatic pathways can also cause pleural exudates or hemorrhage:

   Lymphadenopathy or other hilar or mediastinal lesions that impair flow through central vascular channels (e.g., superior vena cava obstruction, pulmonary vein obstruction)
   Obstruction of the thoracic duct due to neoplasms or other masses
   Obstruction of the thoracic duct due to inflammation
   Hypoplasia of lymphatic vessels (e.g., yellow nail syndrome)
   Interruption of lymphatic or vascular channels due to trauma or surgery, or tearing of pleural adhesions.

4. Abnormalities within the abdomen that affect diaphragmatic peritoneal and pleural surfaces are another general cause of pleural effusions:

   Acute or chronic pancreatitis
   Subphrenic abscesses
   Hepatic abscesses
   "Urinomas" associated with urinary tract obstruction or disruption
   Benign solid tumors of the ovary (Meigs' syndrome) and other benign and malignant tumors of the ovaries and uterus, even in the absence of manifest peritoneal spread[11,12]
   Peritonitis

Ascites
Nonspecific changes following abdominal surgery.
Peritoneal dialysis
5. Asbestos-related pleural disease.

The same pathophysiologic mechanisms that cause pleural effusion may also cause pericardial effusion, and it is important to consider that association regardless of the appearance of the cardiac silhouette on the chest film. Echocardiography has greatly simplified the detection of pericardial effusions and can be employed under most clinical circumstances.

In general, the radiographic appearance of pleural effusion per se gives no clues as to its etiology. The chest film, however, may show evidence that the patient has features of congestive heart failure, or hilar or mediastinal adenopathy, or pulmonary or pleural masses, or signs of trauma, that permit valid deductions as to the likely cause of the effusion. Knowledge of common events is also useful in the evaluation of pleural effusions. For example, small effusions, unilateral or bilateral, may frequently be seen following abdominal surgery, and these effusions usually regress without any special treatment. Therefore, small pleural effusions alone cannot be assumed to be a reflection of upper abdominal infection in these patients; rather, their significance in any individual must be evaluated in correlation with other clinical signs and symptoms.

Once you suspect, for any reason, that pleural abnormalities are present, it is useful to determine how much of the abnormality is due to a free fluid component and how much is fixed. This determination not only helps in the differential diagnosis but is equally important in deciding how to proceed with the investigation. A lateral decubitus view with the patient lying on the suspect side is usually feasible, even in very ill patients, and will demonstrate even small amounts of free-flowing fluid (less than about 25 ml). However, a small percentage of normal people may also show very small amounts of pleural fluid on lateral decubitus views.[5]

RADIOGRAPHIC SIGNS OF PLEURAL FLUID

The Meniscoid Arc

The radiographic manifestations of pleural effusion are easy to recognize when the fluid is abundant, as fortunately it often is. Instead of the lung extending to the chest wall or to its diaphragmatic or mediastinal boundaries, an absorber of uniform water density is interposed. Classically, the upper limits of this water absorber appear in the shape of an arc concave toward the visible lung with the lateral aspects of the high point of the arc adjacent to the chest wall. This is not a true meniscus but a meniscoid phenomenon of projection (Fig. 3-1A and B). This classic appearance may be seen on either the PA or the lateral view but often not on both (Fig. 3-2).

There are, however, enough instances of pleural effusions that either are minimal in volume or depart sufficiently from classic expectations to present diagnostic challenges almost daily. Exactly why these departures from expectations occur is seldom known in any given case. However, we are often not privy to details of local physical conditions, and, undoubtedly, local differences in lung compliance, chest wall compliance, pleural space continuity, and other physiologic variables dictate these configurations.

Other Configurations for Pleural Fluid

Fluid usually first accumulates in the pleural space in a dependent position and may be totally unrecognized on conventional upright chest views. As the volume of fluid increases and fills in the costophrenic recesses, the chest film may show blunting of the costophrenic sinuses, either laterally on the PA view or posteriorly on the lateral view, or both (Fig. 3-3A and B). The volume of fluid necessary to show these changes may vary greatly from patient to patient. As little as 200 ml may cause recognizable change, or as much as 1,000 ml may hide in subpulmonic recesses. It is a guessing game to predict the volume of pleural effusion from routine views. The head-down, lateral decubitus view of the side involved allows a much better estimate of the amount of pleural fluid (Fig. 3-3C).

Radiographic signs other than blunted gutters[5,15] can be used to predict the presence of a subpulmonic effusion on upright chest films. For example:

1. Apparent elevation of a "hemidiaphragm" without other evident cause. The subpulmonic fluid can mimic the appearance of a high diaphragm (Fig. 3-3A). The lung may be displaced from the lateral chest wall by a thin layer of fluid. A relatively sharp angle may be maintained between this fluid layer and the apparent diaphragm. This can mimic a sharp costophrenic angle except that it is located medially (Fig. 3-4H).
2. Alteration of the expected contour of a hemidiaphragm on a PA view, such that the high point of the contour occurs in the lateral third. Often the

slope of the contour from that point to the costophrenic angle is steeper than one would expect. (Compare Fig. 3-4G with 3-4A, and 3-4H with 3-4I.)

3. Alteration of the contour of a hemidiaphragm on the lateral view, such that the slope of that portion extending anterior to the point of intersection of the major interlobar fissure is more steeply inclined than usual. This finding is most reliable when it represents a change from previous films or when there is evident projection of fluid up into a visible major fissure (Fig. 3-4D and F; compare with Fig. 3-4B).

4. Separation of the stomach bubble from the top of the apparent left hemidiaphragm by 2.0 cm or more on a PA view[5] (Fig. 3-4C). This sign is very useful but must be considered with care to avoid a false-positive interpretation (Fig. 3-4A and B).

5. Loss of definition of the usually sharp diaphragm-lung interface (Fig. 3-4E and F). This sign also requires most judicious use in order to avoid false-positive interpretations. Abnormal lung sitting on the diaphragm can mimic this appearance, and in some patients, segments of the diaphragm image may appear unsharp because of variations in projection. In those adults who have abundant extrapleural fat anteriorly over the left hemidiaphragm, lordotic variations in projection may cause substitution of the irregular image of this fat pad for the sharper image of the lung-diaphragm interface, and hence loss of sharp definition of the diaphragm.

Whenever you compare films made in significantly different projections, you run the risk of making erroneous judgments that abnormalities are improving or worsening when in fact they are not. Projections of different tangents and different lengths of absorber in the beam account for these discrepancies (Fig. 3-4J and K) as well as different distributions of pleural fluid when it is present.

Perilobar Effusion

Occasionally, pleural fluid may appear to be distributed in a perilobar distribution on a lateral view and be mistaken for lower lobe consolidation. The zone of opacity is sharply marginated anteriorly by a pseudo-major interlobar fissure, which usually reaches the hemidiaphragm more anteriorly than one would expect for lower lobe consolidation. On the PA view the appearance is inconsistent with that expected in cases of lower lobe consolidation (Figs. 3-4C and D, 3-5A and B). When you see these discordant images—an appearance of lower lobe consolidation on the lateral view but a

totally inappropriate appearance for lower lobe consolidation on the PA view—think of perilobar distribution of pleural fluid as the cause.

At times fluid may also accumulate along the mediastinal aspects of the pleural space adjacent to the right atrium and simulate cardiac enlargement or pericardial effusion on the PA view (Figs. 3-4G and 3-5A). A lateral decubitus view of the abnormal side will make the true situation apparent (Fig. 3-5C).

Likewise, fluid accumulating posteromedially in the left retrocardiac position can be mistaken for left lower lobe atelectasis (Fig. 3-6).

What can you say about that portion of lung obscured by pleural fluid? When pleural effusion is large in volume and obscures subjacent lung, you can reasonably infer that there is some degree of reduced volume of that lung, but you can make no objective or accurate prediction as to whether there is also pneumonia, neoplasm, or infarction within the obscured portions of lung parenchyma. Evaluation of this obscured parenchyma can be made only if films exposed with the patient in varying positions (e.g., decubitus and prone) cause enough fluid displacement to allow this portion of the lung to become visible. Sometimes, evaluation of the lung can be done only after thoracentesis. The cross-sectional format of CT scans permits better assessment of displaced lung, and the increased density discrimination permits recognition of pulmonary or pleural masses that are not distinguishable on plain films in the face of large pleural effusions (Fig. 3-7).

Pleural Fluid on Films Made With the Patient Supine

When patients are quite ill, films usually are obtained with portable equipment with the patient in bed. Modern equipment, in conjunction with meticulous attention to the details of radiographic technique, still permits these to be films of good quality. When anteroposterior (AP) chest films are exposed with the patient supine, pleural fluid in small amounts is not discernible. However, several hundred milliliters of fluid layered out along the posterior chest wall can under these circumstances be predicted by noting that there is a lighter gray tone on the affected side than on the unaffected side, as though a filter had been placed in the beam (Fig. 3-8). The pulmonary vessels can still be clearly identified as long as they are surrounded by air-containing lung. Larger amounts of fluid may also become apparent laterally by separating lung from chest wall, and medially by causing apparent widening of the paraspinal soft tissue shadow.

Anatomic Displacements With Large Effusions

Large amounts of pleural fluid may actually cause inversion of the left hemidiaphragm (see Fig. 3-4C), so that upright views may lead you to grossly underestimate the extent of the effusion from the location of its upper limits. Furthermore, after thoracentesis you might not appreciate the magnitude of the change from prethoracentesis films, unless you see that the stomach bubble is higher in the abdomen on the postthoracentesis film, indicating that the left hemidiaphragm has changed to a more normal configuration and position.

When large quantities of fluid are present there may be a shift of mediastinal structures to the opposite side. Large volumes of fluid may cause a tension hydrothorax analogous to a tension pneumothorax.

In addition, when large quantities of fluid are present, the involved pleural space may bulge across in front of the lower thoracic spine and present an edge on the opposite side, simulating a mass (Fig. 3-9A – C).

Distinguishing Free Fluid From Loculated Fluid or Chronic Pleural Thickening

In some patients, chronic pleural thickening extends high along the chest wall. From PA and lateral views alone you often cannot tell whether there is chronic thickening alone or whether there is also a free-flowing fluid component. Previous films for comparison are very helpful but often not available. A lateral decubitus view with the abnormal side down will serve to solve the problem. When the upright PA view and the lateral decubitus view are compared and show no change in the appearance of the pleural abnormality, the process is indicative of a fixed fibrous pleuritis or a loculated fluid pocket. A change in configuration indicates the presence of a free-flowing pleural fluid component. A free-flowing component and a fixed component may be present at the same time in some patients (Fig. 3-2D and E).

CT Scans for Pleural Fluid

CT scans of the chest are ordinarily obtained with the patient supine, and very small amounts of fluid can be detected layered against the posterior chest wall. Even small loculated pockets around the periphery of the chest can be seen because of the superb contrast afforded by the adjacent lung. Although CT scans frequently show significant amounts of pleural fluid that go undetected on upright PA and lateral films of the chest, it is doubtful that a discrepancy would persist if comparisons were made with proper decubitus views. It should not be necessary to obtain CT scans solely to detect pleural fluid if you utilize decubitus views in clinically suspected cases. The surprises then will be limited to those patients in whom you did not suspect pleural fluid at all but who had chest CT scans for other reasons.

CT scans also may not permit distinction among chronic pleural thickening, loculated pockets, and small free-flowing effusion, unless the scans are repeated after a change in body position to demonstrate changes in location of the free-flowing component. Ultrasound studies also may be useful in making these distinctions.

In cases of acute chest trauma, CT scans can distinguish relatively fresh blood in the pleural space (because of high CT numbers, on the order of 50 to 60 Hounsfield units) if the examination is done shortly after the bleeding occurred. CT is not sensitive enough to distinguish between transudates and exudates, old blood, or chyle.

Sometimes it is challenging to determine from CT scans on which side of the diaphragm a fluid collection is located. That is, does the patient have subpulmonic fluid in the pleural space or fluid in the abdomen, or both? Usually these distinctions can be made with careful image analysis. However, when there are combinations of consolidation and atelectasis of the lower lobe, subpulmonic fluid, parietal pleural thickening, and/or inversion of the diaphragm, great care and critical analyses are required to properly locate supra- and infradiaphragmatic fluid collections on CT. These distinctions are especially important in distinguishing pleural effusion from ascites, and empyema from subphrenic abscess. Useful image details have been elucidated that facilitate correct analyses (Fig. 3-8B to E).[4,14]

THE OPAQUE HEMITHORAX

Occasionally you will encounter a patient who presents with a radiographically opaque or near-opaque hemithorax. It is helpful to first decide whether or not there is evidence of increased or decreased volume on the involved side by evaluating the position of the mediastinum and other signs of volume change (see Ch. 4).

Increased Volume

If the opaque hemithorax shows signs of increased volume, you know that lung atelectasis alone cannot account for the abnormality, and you can deduce the presence of either concomitant pleural effusion, a mass lesion, or both (Fig. 3-9A). Even when obstruction of a main bronchus results in opacification due to massive accumulation of mucus and fluid in the lung — the so-called "drowned lung" — there is almost never an actual increase in lung volume.

Occasionally, however, you will encounter a thoracic mass that is so large than even with atelectasis of the lung there is a net increase in volume of the hemithorax. Under these circumstances, repeated thoracentesis to remove suspected pleural fluid would be futile.

In practice, the majority of patients who first present with an opaque hemithorax with increased volume on the abnormal side will have a malignant neoplasm of the lung (rarely of the pleura), with associated pleural fluid (Fig. 3-9A and B); massive fluid alone, from inflammation (Fig. 3-9C), infection, or hemothorax after trauma, could not be distinguished radiographically with routine films.

Patients with hepatic cirrhosis may have massive right-sided pleural effusions, usually with ascites. Repeated thoracenteses in an attempt to control rapid reaccumulation of fluid can lead to severe protein loss. Chemical pleurodesis in a few cases has been reported to be effective. Pleural effusions in patients with cirrhosis are most often on the right but can be bilateral or on the left.[6]

Occasionally a patient with chronic pancreatitis may present with massive left pleural effusion accompanied by chest pain and shortness of breath. Determination of the pleural fluid amylase (Table 3-4) permits the correct diagnosis, which otherwise might be missed (Fig. 3-9C). Patients with acute pancreatitis have left-sided effusions more often than right, but bilateral effusions also occur in these patients.[6]

Decreased Volume

If the opaque hemithorax is accompanied by signs of ipsilateral decreased volume, pleural fluid alone cannot account for the findings. There may be an absence of lung tissue (most commonly surgical, rarely congenital), or there may be massive atelectasis of lung, with or without any associated mass or pleural fluid.

As long as the hemithorax remains opaque, you can make only limited deductions as to the cause. Signs of previous thoracic surgery are readily apparent on physical examination or roentgenographic study, but the extent of the lung resection cannot be reliably deduced from chest films alone. In fact, however, the majority of asymptomatic patients who present with clear signs of previous thoracic surgery and an opaque hemithorax with diminished volume will have had pneumonectomy (Fig. 3-9D and E).

Detection of recurrent neoplasm, or even empyema, in a postpneumonectomy opaque hemithorax is usually not possible with chest film studies. When comparison films are available, however, and there is clear evidence that the mediastinal structures are shifting away from or out of the opaque side, one can deduce that some new abnormality is increasing the volume of the opaque side. Empyema and recurrent neoplasm are the most common causes of this type of shift. You might reach the same conclusion without prior comparison films if the heart and mediastinum on the current film are not shifted to the postpneumonectomy side, but the conclusion would be less reliable.

Uncommonly, there is atelectasis of lung (e.g., due to obstruction of a major bronchus) plus a large volume of pleural fluid in spite of a net appearance of reduced volume on the opaque side. Thoracentesis in these patients can produce high negative pleural pressures and consequently pulmonary edema. Relief of the bronchial obstruction prior to pleural drainage by tube thoracostomy is therefore important.[6]

Computed Tomography in Evaluation of the Opaque Hemithorax

CT scans have been extremely useful in the examination of the opaque or near-opaque hemithorax. What appears to be a uniform appearance on chest films may be readily separated into fluid (either loculated or free), mass, and/or atelectatic lung components. Even the small amount of air remaining in the bronchi of an atelectatic lung can be detected on CT scans. The use of intravenous contrast agents is very helpful, since there will be density enhancement of atelectatic lung, whereas pleural fluid will not show such enhancement (Fig. 3-7B and C).

Furthermore, continuing the CT study into the abdomen permits assessment of the liver and the pancreas; disease in either of these organs can cause massive pleural effusion. The possibility that disease in these organs is responsible for the effusion may escape initial clinical evaluation.

LOCULATED PLEURAL FLUID, EMPYEMA, AND BRONCHOPLEURAL FISTULA

Adhesions between the visceral and parietal pleura in some patients bind the surfaces one to the other over areas of inflammation yet leave portions of the pleural space intact. When fluid collects in the pleural space of these patients, it may form loculated pockets. When these loculations occur in fissures, they appear with biconvex contours in at least one radiographic projection (Figs. 3-9D and E, 3-10A and B). When loculated pockets occur adjacent to the noncompliant chest wall, only that edge that has an interface with the lung will have a convex contour when viewed tangentially. When viewed en face, these fluid collections may be difficult to recognize, since they may show no effect other than that of additional absorber in the beam; rarely, however, they may simulate lung masses. In addition, loculated effusion in the minor interlobar fissure has been mistaken for right middle lobe atelectasis and vice versa.

When the character of these lesions is obscure on routine films, it is helpful to perform fluoroscopy of the patient and obtain spot films at angles of rotation that best show the tangent of the lung-pleural loculation interface. A change in shape with respiration may be seen with loculated effusion, but other soft solid tumors such as benign fibrous mesotheliomas may do the same, and thus this feature is not distinguishing.

Most of the interlobar loculated effusions (those occurring in the minor or major fissures), that I have seen, occurred in patients with congestive heart failure or following thoracic surgery or repeated thoracenteses, and rarely have these been infected. Bland loculated effusion should resolve with time when its underlying cause is relieved. From their radiographic appearance alone, one cannot distinguish noninfected pleural pockets from empyema pockets. Further study in any given patient is dictated by the clinical signs, symptoms, and suspicions.

Unfortunately, lung carcinoma in rare cases may abut on a fissure and mimic an interlobar loculated effusion. This confusion can occur when the patient presents with the abnormality on the first radiographic study and there are no previous films to show the evolution of the lesion.

When there are no clinical findings to explain why a patient should have a loculated effusion, further study is needed. CT scans made through the lesion both before and after intravenous contrast injection would show whether or not the lesion has a blood supply, and thus distinguish a tumor mass from loculated fluid. A CT scan without intravenous contrast might suffice if the lesion showed a uniformly low density such as would be expected for fluid, but if the fluid were an exudate or contained blood, the Hounsfield numbers could be high enough that the distinction between liquid and a cellular mass could not be made reliably. An MRI study could also be used to distinguish loculated fluid from a neoplasm.

A fluoroscopically controlled needle aspiration would be effective for obtaining specimens for cytologic or bacteriologic study when indicated.

Gas in a Pleural Pocket

When gas is found mixed with fluid in a loculated pocket, one can consider four possibilities:

1. The gas has been introduced as a result of thoracentesis, surgical manipulation, or trauma.
2. The patient has developed a bronchopleural fistula or, rarely, a fistula between the pocket and the esophagus.
3. The patient has a gas-forming organism in the pocket.
4. Any combination of 1, 2, and 3.

In the absence of surgery, trauma, or attempts at needle aspiration, the appearance of gas in a pleural pocket is presumptive of a bronchopleural fistula (Fig. 3-11). Usually it is not necessary to resort to contrast injection studies for diagnostic purposes.

Bronchopleural fistulas, however, can be demonstrated with bronchographic contrast material. The contrast medium can be instilled via the tracheobronchial tree or injected into the pocket, preferably under fluoroscopic guidance; the patient is then placed in various positions to see if any drainage occurs into bronchi (Fig. 3-11F). Such an examination is not necessary for diagnosis but may be reserved for those patients for whom surgery is contemplated, if the thoracic surgeon feels the information is necessary to plan a surgical approach.

Distinguishing Gas-Fluid Pockets in Pleura From Those in Lung

Gas-fluid pockets occurring in the pleural space can be distinguished from gas-fluid pockets in lung substance when there is a significant discrepancy in the length of the contained fluid level between films made in PA and lateral projections[3] or between films made with the patient upright and those made in the lateral decubitus position. If you think about the conformation of the pleural space and its fissures, you can see why such discrepancies in fluid level lengths would be readily expected. Pleural pockets along the anterior or posterior chest wall will be wider in the coronal plane than they are deep in the sagittal plane, and pockets along the lateral chest wall will be wider in the sagittal plane than in the coronal (Fig. 3-11A to E). If you think of the pockets as comparable to hot water bottles with slanted rather than rounded shoulders, you can see that the closer the fluid level is to the top of the pocket, the smaller will be the discrepancy in the lengths of the air-fluid levels seen on these two views (Fig. 3-11G).

In the lung substance, cavities, infected cysts, or infected bullae will usually be rounded or oval, and if they contain gas-fluid levels, the lengths will be of more nearly equal dimension in the two planes under study. Unfortunately, some pleural pockets may also show similar fluid level lengths in the two projections, thus mimicking intraparenchymal disease. When positive, however, the discrepant fluid level length sign is extremely helpful in distinguishing gas-fluid levels in pleural pockets from air-fluid pockets in pulmonary cavities.

Empyema Without Bronchopleural Fistula

Distinction between infected and noninfected pleural fluid collections cannot be made on radiographic findings alone. The diagnosis will depend on retrieval of pleural fluid samples for determination of pH, lactate dehydrogenase, glucose, protein concentration, culture, and microscopic study. The possibility of empyema should be considered whenever a pneumonia is accompanied by significant pleural fluid, especially if there is a rapid change in the quantity of pleural fluid or if there is evidence that the fluid is viscid or has spontaneously loculated along the chest wall (Fig. 3-12). Pleural effusion in association with pneumonia, however, is not in itself indicative of empyema. It is important to determine whether or not microorganisms are present. Parapneumonic pleural effusions are frequently sterile.

Computed Tomography in the Evaluation of Pleural Pockets

CT scans may be of great help in distinguishing a pleural pocket and bronchopleural fistula from a lung abscess (Figs. 3-11C and 3-13). The CT format permits clear localization of a fluid collection in reference to the inner chest wall and a better appreciation of the shape of the lesion in three dimensions when sequential scans are obtained through the entire cephalocaudad length of the lesion. In addition, it is possible to recognize gas collections that defy recognition on chest films. Similarly, small amounts of air remaining in bronchi (i.e., air bronchograms) are recognizable on CT scans with greater ease than on chest films.

In general, a pleural pocket has thinner walls than a lung abscess, but this difference is often not apparent when a thick border of atelectatic lung forms about an empyema pocket. The atelectatic lung, however, is usually recognized because the CT format permits identification of remnants of air bronchograms within it. When gas is present within an empyema pocket, the inner wall-gas interface is much sharper and smoother than it is in a lung abscess; this is a most reliable sign (Fig. 3-11C).

CT scans augmented by intravenous contrast injection are very helpful. Empyema contents will not opacify but frequently will be sharply delimited by an enhancing wall of pleura a few millimeters thick, with or without an adjacent mantle of enhancing atelectatic lung. Chronic empyema pockets may appear as crescentic low-density

fluid collections between thickened layers of visceral and parietal pleura. Pulmonary margins about lung abscess cavities enhance up to the necrotic zones (Fig. 3-14A–C).

Ordinarily on CT, the angles at the junctions between the chest wall and an empyema pocket are obtuse, whereas when an abscess pocket is located in lung adjacent to the chest wall the angle at the junction is acute. However, these configurations are not invariable and are unreliable signs.

There are times when reliable distinctions cannot be made. Empyema pockets loculated in fissures may mimic lung abscesses, and complex abnormalities consisting of an empyema pocket with adjacent pulmonary abscess and cavity formation occur often enough to thoroughly test one's abilities (Fig. 3-14D and E).

Sometimes bubbles of gas are seen within the fluid components of a pleural pocket rather than rising to the top, suggesting that the fluid components are very viscid. Care is required to avoid mistaking the trapped bubbles for air in distorted bronchi.

Most often, the attempt to distinguish empyema from lung abscess is dictated by anticipation of different treatment strategies. Lung abscesses may be treated by appropriate antibiotics or chemotherapy when the organisms responsible are known. In addition to antibiotics or chemotherapy, empyema usually requires treatment by tube drainage, and in a minority of patients rib resection also may be necessary.

Pleural Thickening

Obliteration or blunting of a lateral costophrenic angle or a posterior gutter is a common radiographic manifestation of pleural thickening due to laying down of collagen within the pleura. In any single individual, it is not possible to distinguish accurately such pleural thickening from a small effusion without decubitus views or old films for comparison. However, pleural effusions rarely maintain a monotonous similarity from film to film in any patient, whereas pleural thickening invariably does so if the projections to be compared are similar. What appear to be changes in the extent of pleural thickening are more often in my experience due to changes produced by differences in projection (this is particularly true for blunted posterior gutters seen on a lateral view) rather than any real change in the abnormality itself. Even differences in the position of the diaphragm at the time of filming may account for spurious changes from film to film.

Since pleural thickening alone may be a residual of remote infection, inflammation, chest surgery, or trauma, its etiology is seldom pursued when older films for comparison show stability over a long period of time. However, even apparently minor degrees of pleural thickening may alter regional ventilation and perfusion, and may also alter local anatomic structures such as bronchi and blood vessels. Recognition of these facts may prevent misinterpretation of perfusion lung scans.

Pleural thickening may be seen extending along the lateral, posterior, or anterior chest wall. Radiographs made in oblique projection often indicate that there is more extensive circumferential pleural thickening than one might deduce from analysis of PA and lateral views alone. Spot films made in varying degrees of obliquity serve the same purpose. Correlation of radiographs and autopsy examinations convinced me that radiographs almost always underestimate the degree of chronic pleural thickening when it is present.

Pleural thickening as a remnant of past disease is common not only at lung bases but also over the apices. However, histopathologic study of so-called apical pleural thickening usually demonstrates a combination of pleural fibrosis juxtaposed with a more conspicuous rind of atelectatic, scarred lung constituting an "apical cap." The individual components are often not distinguished radiologically. In the past, apical caps were considered to be residuals of tuberculous infection. Studies based on gross and histopathologic tissue analyses cast doubt on this supposition.[16] However, any study that does not include culture of these specimens or injection of tissue extracts into guinea pigs does not really resolve the issue, because tubercle bacilli have been cultured from lung specimens that showed no characteristic histopathologic changes of tuberculosis.

A thickened apical cap is so common that it is hard to conceive of tuberculosis as the sole cause in so many patients today. However, the presence of small nodules in the lung apex is still suspicious for residuals of tuberculous infection (see Ch. 5), regardless of the presence or absence of an apical cap.

Significance of Changes in the Degree of Pleural Thickening

Whenever the degree of pleural thickening, whether focal or diffuse, is seen to change from examination to examination, activity of the responsible disease process is considered likely. For example, many pulmonary infections may manifest first by changes in the pleura. The organisms responsible can be recovered from pleural fluid or biopsy specimens. The infectious granulomatous diseases (most commonly tuberculosis) may first present as pleural effusion adjacent to a peripheral parenchymal focus of infection. The parenchymal focus may not be apparent roentgenographically. Other infec-

tious agents, such as *Aspergillus, Nocardia, Blastomyces,* and *Actinomyces,* may cause similar phenomena. Indeed, some of the extrapulmonary manifestations of these infections may be so aggressive as to actually penetrate the chest wall and result in sinus tract formation, with or without evidence of involvement of adjacent ribs (see Ch. 5).

Diffuse mesothelioma, extensive metastases to the pleura, and fibrothorax from past infection may be indistinguishable entities on any given radiograph. Obtaining old films for comparison is the least expensive and often clinically the most useful service you can perform for the patient. Postinflammatory fibrothorax is characterized by its stable appearance over a long time, whereas pleural lesions due to neoplasm or infection show fluctuations, which may be gross or subtle. Careful correlation of history, physical findings, and laboratory data is helpful in defining probabilities, but cytologic, histologic, or bacteriologic study of pleural specimens may be needed for definitive diagnosis.

Rarely, a primary peripheral lung cancer can infiltrate juxtapleural lung in a fashion that radiographically mimics focal pleural thickening, leading to an erroneous diagnosis. Also, Pancoast tumors occur in the pulmonary apices, and the combined effects of the pulmonary neoplasm and its adjacent pleural reaction can produce radiographic appearances that are indistinguishable from postinflammatory pleural thickening. Focal convexity of the lesion toward the lung makes one suspect neoplasm rather than quiescent postinflammatory reaction, but there are those cases where distinction is nearly impossible prior to manifest destruction of overlying rib or adjacent vertebrae. Careful attention to correlation of clinical findings—primarily pain—and careful comparison with prior films can sometimes prevent this error (See Ch. 6). However, there are also active inflammatory lesions, such as the "tumoral" forms of actinomycosis or blastomycosis, which may produce indistinguishable destructive lesions in adjacent bone; fortunately these conditions are rare.

CALCIFICATION, PLEURAL PLAQUES, AND ASBESTOS-RELATED PLEURAL DISEASE

Plaques Due to Prior Inflammation

Calcification may be laid down in the pleura; small or large sheets are usually consequent to pleural thickening attendant on an old healed empyema, chronic tuberculous pleuritis (especially in those patients who had pneumothorax therapy), and perhaps previous hemothorax from trauma. These calcifications often have a distinctive appearance that is easier to recognize than to describe. It may or may not be obvious that the material in these plaques absorbs the beam as you would expect calcium to do. Modern high-kilovoltage films decrease the contrast between calcified and noncalcified tissue, so that you must take exposure factors into consideration in your interpretation. When viewed en face, these plaques are characterized by nonhomogeneity of the calcific foci, which appear to be laid down in rather sharply defined, small, irregularly shaped or stippled clusters. When these plaques are projected tangentially, you can recognize that the calcific components are separated from the adjacent ribs by a noncalcified layer of thickened pleura about the thickness of shoe leather (Fig. 3-15). The thickened pleura and calcific plaques produced by postinfectious lesions almost always result in symphysis of the pleural surfaces and at least focal obliteration of the pleural space.

Asbestos-Related Pleural Disease

Plaques due to asbestos[17] (Figs. 3-16 and 3-17) occur mostly in the parietal pleura, but some occur in the fissures. When viewed tangentially with respect to the chest wall, the calcific components do not appear as far from the inner rib margin as do calcific plaques in postinflammatory pleural lesions from other causes. In fact, the pleural plaques of asbestos usually do not cause even a local obliteration of the pleural space, so that induced pneumothorax will demonstrate them to be localized in the parietal pleura, and fluoroscopy will show that the plaques move synchronously with the chest wall and not with adjacent pulmonary structures. At present it is felt that most benign hyaline pleural plaques are the result of exposure to asbestos-laden dust. All types of asbestos fibers have been implicated, some more commonly than others. Even so, there is an incompletely understood association, since the incidence of pleural plaque formation in workers and inhabitants of various mining communities shows considerable variation. Asbestos fibers can be identified in the pleural plaques by means of electron microscopy.

Radiographically, these plaques become visible when there has been sufficient focal thickening of the pleura (about 3 to 10 mm) to produce an edge that has an interface with adjacent lung and thus, when seen in profile, produces a focal convexity of varying length, which deforms the normal interface between lung and adjacent chest wall. When seen en face, noncalcified plaques may easily escape detection; since they have an interface with lung on only one surface, they appear as very low density shadows with poorly defined edges.

Multiple projections of the chest and fluoroscopic examinations enhance the detection of pleural plaques.

These techniques afford the opportunity to project the plaques tangential to the beam, thus increasing the length of the absorber in the beam and projecting the interface of the plaque with adjacent lung so that a sharper contrast gradient is seen.

Pleural plaques due to asbestos are usually bilateral and may be symmetric. However, sometimes only a single plaque may be identified in any given projection. These plaques have been most commonly recognized adjacent to the fifth, sixth, seventh, and eighth ribs and interspaces, and they may also be found over the diaphragm in the vicinity of the central tendon and rarely on the pericardial surface. Asbestos pleural plaques are rarely found over the apices or costophrenic angles—a fortunate circumstance, since pleural thickening from other causes is so common at these sites. Only a minority of patients with asbestos plaques also have interstitial lung disease. Ordinarily the term "asbestosis" implies parenchymal disease and is not meant to designate the condition in which pleural plaques are unassociated with pulmonary lesions.

Asbestos contamination of the air is and has been common in industrialized communities and in certain mining communities. To complicate matters, the individual's exposure to asbestos may be relatively brief, and the time interval from exposure to manifest clinical symptoms or radiographic signs may be a matter of many years. It is estimated that radiographically visible pleural plaque calcification takes about 20 years to evolve. Hence, very careful history taking is often necessary to uncover the exposure episode. Most asbestos-induced pleural plaques are not calcified enough for radiographic detection by routine techniques, but those that are calcified are more easily seen. Calcification within pleural plaques, as within malignant lung tumors, is frequently detectable on histopathologic specimens, although not present in sufficient quantity to be radiographically evident on routine films. CT examination greatly simplifies the task of identifying and localizing pleural plaques as distinguished from pulmonary lesions (Fig. 3-17A and B).

Pleural effusions, usually small and either unilateral or bilateral, may occur in persons exposed to asbestos. A survey of a large group of workers exposed to asbestos[2] found that pleural effusion was of low overall prevalence (less than 5 percent), but was of higher prevalence (about 7 percent) in those more heavily exposed. In the 10 years following initial asbestos exposure, effusion was the only manifestation of disease. Even in the first 20 years, small effusions were more common than either pleural plaques or parenchymal asbestosis. Some patients had recurrent effusions, and half went on to develop a diffuse pleural thickening indistinguishable from any other postinflammatory pleural thickening. Half had only residual blunting of gutters. Most had no symptoms. It is important to elicit a history of possible asbestos exposure in patients who present with small effusions of unknown etiology. Some patients may develop mesotheliomas many years after asbestos exposure, but there is no evidence that a pleural plaque per se becomes a mesothelioma.

INVOLVEMENT OF THE PLEURA BY NEOPLASM

Metastases and Malignant Lymphoma

Involvement of the pleura by neoplasm is common, and some type of effusion, whether hemorrhagic, chylous, or exudative, is the usual radiographic presentation. Pain may or may not be associated, and the clinical evidence of respiratory impairment is related to the quantity of fluid present and the condition of the lung. When fluid alone is the sole recognized manifestation of pleural disease, there are no radiographic criteria to permit distinction between benign and malignant pleural effusions. When pleural fluid specimens are positive cytologically for neoplasm, that is a reliable indication of pleural metastases, but even multiple thoracenteses may be unsuccessful in retrieving positive specimens in patients who have pleural metastases subsequently proven by biopsy. The problem is complicated by the fact that not all pleural effusions in patients with known malignant tumors are due to pleural metastases.[6] Some are due to obstruction of lymphatic or venous pathways centrally (e.g., mediastinal lymphadenopathy) or to concurrent inflammatory processes in the lung (see Fig. 3-9D and E).

Pleural metastases may also present radiographically as focal soft tissue masses that appear to have only one edge — the edge that has an interface with adjacent lung (Fig. 3-18). When projecting en face to the beam, the lesions may go undetected or may project as areas of increased soft tissue density with no distinct edges. Small pleural metastases may be indistinguishable from asbestos-related noncalcified pleural plaques.

A large variety of primary tumors are known to metastasize to the pleura, and none has distinguishing features. The fact that the patient has or had a primary cancer at some site is usually known from previous studies, including the results of surgery or biopsy. In other cases the patient presents with compelling signs or symptoms referable to an organ or organ system and warranting strong suspicion of the presence of a primary neoplasm. Pleural lesions occasionally may appear as a first sign of recurrent disease in patients with known previously treated Hodgkin's disease and non-Hodgkin's malignant lymphoma (Figs. 3-19 and 3-20), yet at the time of initial diagnosis, pleural lesions are rarely seen as the only sign of malignant lymphoma.

It is quite possible that the extrapleural lesions of the malignant lymphomas — and of metastases from other primary sites for that matter — may originate as metastatic neoplastic foci in the parietal intrathoracic nodes located along the course of the ribs and intercostal spaces. By the time these lesions are large enough to produce radiographic signs, they may no longer be recognized, even histologically, as having originated in lymph nodes.

The absence of effusion cannot be considered as ruling out the likelihood of metastasis as an explanation for a pleural mass.

Malignant thymoma may propagate or metastasize to the pleura, so as to cause solitary or multiple, discrete or seemingly continuous pleural masses. The time lapse between treatment or removal of the thymoma and evidence of pleural recurrence may be several years, so that a careful history is required if error is to be avoided. The patient may have few symptoms, and the complex may mimic diffuse mesothelioma (Fig. 3-21).

Primary Chest Wall Neoplasms

A small proportion of pleural neoplasms are primary, and of these mesothelioma, benign or malignant, is the most common. If we modify our concept to include all chest wall neoplasms other than skin, and if we recall the tissues that make up the chest wall, sooner or later we will encounter neoplasms originating from those tissues and presenting as extrapleural masses, such as lipomas, fibromas, neurogenic tumors, sarcomas, and tumors of vascular origin such as hemangiomas and lymphangiomas. We eliminate skin from consideration since we do not need radiographic studies to identify skin tumors.

Chest wall tumors of bone tissue origin sometimes have bulky extraosseous components so that it is difficult to know whether the neoplasm involves bone by extension or whether it originates from bone.

Mesothelioma

Mesotheliomas may be localized or diffuse. The localized benign form may be pedunculated and simulate a pulmonary nodule or mass or even a loculated effusion if located in a fissure (Fig. 3-22). When mesothelioma presents as a focal pleural mass along the chest wall, its benign or malignant nature cannot be predicted with enough assurance to warrant a diagnosis without histologic proof. Even accompanying effusion is not always reliable evidence that the lesion is malignant.

A variety of extrathoracic signs and symptoms have been associated with benign fibrous mesotheliomas. These include hypertrophic osteoarthropathy, uncommonly hypoglycemia, chills and fever, and rarely dyspnea even in the absence of associated effusion. Of these, the hypertrophic osteoarthropathy is the most common, and the symptoms regress when the benign mesothelioma is resected.[6] Many patients have no symptoms or signs. Mesotheliomas located along mediastinal pleural reflections may produce mass lesions indistinguishable from those of thymoma, and rarely even from ventricular aneurysm.

Diffuse mesotheliomas of the pleura are almost all malignant. They may present as an extensive series of pleural-based masses or as a diffuse increase in the thickness of the pleura about much of a hemithorax (Fig. 3-23). Either form may be encountered with or without associated effusion. When massive effusion is present, the pleural mass components may be inconspicuous and can be masked until postthoracentesis films are obtained (see Fig. 3-9). There is virtually no way to distinguish diffuse mesothelioma from pleural metastases radiographically, and even histologically the distinction may not always be possible. Histochemical and electron microscopic study offer additional useful information, but still a clear distinction may not be reached.

Although there is a high correlation between a history of asbestos exposure and the occurrence of malignant mesothelioma, there is no direct evidence that asbestos-induced pleural plaques evolve into mesotheliomas. The history of asbestos exposure is often brief and remote. The number of malignant mesotheliomas that are not associated with a history of asbestos exposure varies considerably in different series. Evidence indicates that not all malignant mesotheliomas are due to asbestos exposure.

Computed Tomography for Pleural Neoplasm and Neoplasm of the Chest Wall

The sharp density discrimination between the lung and its pleural-chest wall boundary permits recognition of minor contour variations using the axial format of CT scans. Small pleural and extrapleural masses around the perimeter of the chest, whether due to benign plaques or malignant neoplasm, produce encroachment on adjacent lung, and they are recognized much more easily on CT scan than on chest films. The normal structures of the chest wall are also more easily distinguished from abnormalities with CT. The CT format also permits recognition of smaller quantities and smaller concentrations of calcium, so that calcification insufficient to be recognized by means of chest film technique can be identified on CT scans (see Fig. 3-17).

Small, uncalcified pleural lesions in the apices or over the diaphragm may escape recognition when the usual axial cross-section format is used, because one does not see their interface with adjacent lung tangentially. Use of coronal or sagittal reconstructions may be required to correct that error. This requires forewarning, since use of those options is not routine. MRI studies in the coronal plane should also be effective in detecting these lesions.

The plain-film features of a pleural or extrapleural mass are similar to those of a loculated pleural fluid pocket. CT makes it possible to distinguish between lesions of high fat content (such as lipomas) and those due to fluids or to solid, nonfatty tissue. In addition, use of intravenous contrast during the CT scan can enable you to demonstrate that a pleural mass lesion has a blood supply, as would be expected with neoplasm but not with loculated fluid (Fig. 3-23). However, a large, relatively avascular neoplasm might not show expected vascular enhancement until delayed sections (minutes after the beginning of contrast injection) are obtained.

Small rib lesions can be difficult to recognize on CT because different segments of any given rib are displayed on successive stacked CT scans, and only small portions of the lesion may be seen on any single scan. It is also difficult to count ribs accurately on CT scans.

Bone Lesions May Produce Extrapleural Masses

Metastases or myeloma involving rib, sternum, or vertebra may have soft tissue components that present characteristic signs of extrapleural lesions. Invariably, careful radiographic study will show underlying bone destruction. Similarly, primary malignant bone tumors such as Ewing's sarcoma or osteogenic sarcoma, which may occur in bones of the thoracic cage, can present with large, extrapleural soft tissue components.

Hematoma accompanying rib fracture or fracture of the sternum may account for an extrapleural mass. When the fracture is nondisplaced and the fracture line not visible, diagnosis is difficult. Study of the lesion in multiple projections will usually solve the problem. If not, short-interval follow-up films can be obtained to show developing callus about the suspect fracture site or demineralization of the bone about the fracture, allowing it to be recognized more easily.

Certain infections, particularly those of actinomycosis, blastomycosis, and even tuberculosis, may cause rib lesions and associated extrapleural pockets of infection that may mimic neoplasm.

Eosinophilic granuloma involving a rib may be misleading because of its destructive and malignant radiographic appearance. Neurogenic tumors may present as extrapleural masses in the apex of the thorax, paraspinally, or much less commonly in other regions of the chest wall or mediastinum.

When malignant tumors infiltrate adjacent lung and pleura, the lung-pleura interface will not be sharp, but rather irregular and poorly defined. Similarly, when pulmonary infection involves contiguous lung and pleura, the pleural involvement may be inseparable radiographically from the parenchymal components.

Normal Anatomic Structures That May Be Mistaken for Pleural Lesions

The pleural membranes normally are not seen except where they border on fissures. However, there are chest wall muscles, as well as muscular slips of origin of the serratus anterior and external oblique muscles, areolar tissue of the endothoracic fascia, and accumulations of fat located at various sites along the inner chest wall that interface with pleural surfaces and adjacent lung. These produce so-called companion shadows, which have been discussed and illustrated in Chapter 1.

Extrapleural deposits of fat produce a wavy margin that is most prominent on the posterolateral surfaces of ribs and usually spares anterior and paravertebral areas. They are best seen on oblique projections and may become quite prominent in patients who are receiving long-term, high-dose steroid therapy. They can mimic pleural plaques but are readily distinguished from them on CT scans.

PNEUMOTHORAX, HYDROPNEUMOTHORAX, AND PNEUMOMEDIASTINUM

Pneumothorax

Air may enter the pleural space from outside the chest, for example from penetrating chest trauma or as a complication of thoracentesis, thoracoscopy, or thoracotomy, but often there is also a tear of lung. Air may enter the intact pleural space from the lung as a result of rupture of apical bullae; this is the most common explanation for spontaneous pneumothorax occurring in otherwise healthy young males. In patients with acute or chronic obstructive airway disease, zones of high pressure occur in the lung as a result of air trapping. Air may leak into perivascular sheaths from rupture of adjacent alveoli and break through the visceral pleura into the pleural space. Interstitial perivascular air may also dissect into the mediastinum to produce pneumomediastinum.[9,10] Rupture of peripheral bullae may occur in patients with emphysema or in those with bullous disease without diffuse airway obstruction. In addition, in the late phases of diseases causing chronic interstitial

fibrosis or interstitial lung disease such as eosinophilic granuloma, "cystic" changes in lung also occur. These may rupture to produce pneumothoraces.

Barotrauma from the high-pressure mechanical respirators required to treat some patients is another common cause of pneumothorax. It is especially common in infants with respiratory distress syndrome in whom an antecedent phase of interstitial air may be seen on chest films. Adults with adult respiratory distress syndrome who are subjected to respirator-induced barotrauma are also at high risk for pneumothorax. Ruptures or tears of the trachea and major bronchi or of the esophagus may also produce pneumothoraces or combined pneumothorax and pneumomediastinum.

Pneumothorax may also be associated with a diverse group of conditions for which the pathogenesis is conjectural. These include metastases to the lungs from many different types of primary malignant neoplasms, but especially osteogenic sarcoma. A small number of women suffer recurrent pneumothoraces with their menstrual periods (catamenial pneumothorax), and there is an uncommon condition of pneumothorax associated with renal malformation of the newborn. Women with lymphangioleiomyomatosis or tuberous sclerosis may present with pneumothorax at the time of initial diagnosis and suffer recurrent pneumothoraces as well.

Finally, any process that can result in necrosis and cavitation of the lung can break through to the pleural space and cause pneumothorax, pyopneumothorax, or hemopneumothorax. Rapid evacuation of a large pneumothorax has been implicated as a cause of pulmonary edema.

Imaging of Pneumothorax

The radiographic hallmark for the presence of pneumothorax is the demonstration of a pleural line or lung edge. A pleural line is a fine white line, produced by the tangential view of a segment of visceral pleura, which becomes visible about the margins of lung separated from adjacent chest wall by air in the pleural space. The linear shadow of the visceral pleura becomes visible only when there are different absorbers on either side of it. Thus, under conditions of pneumothorax, this thin layer becomes visible by virtue of there being air-containing lung on one side of it and air in the pleural space on the other (Fig. 3-24A). The normal visceral pleura is roughly the thickness of a fine pencil line, but when the pleura over the region of pneumothorax is abnormal, or associated with adjacent lung consolidation or atelectasis, this line may be thick and irregular.

When you suspect the presence of a small pneumothorax but do not feel entirely confident of your diagnosis, it is almost always possible to resolve the doubt by obtaining films exposed during the expiratory phase of respiration. Under these conditions, the lung volume decreases, the pleural edge is further displaced from the chest wall, and the intrapulmonary air-water ratio decreases so that the lung appears lighter gray. Thus, the film density gradient across the lung-pneumothorax interface increases and is easier to detect (Fig. 3-24B). The increased tissue density of the adjacent lung in expiration often converts the pleural line to a lung edge.

Along the apical and subapical convexities of a lung that is partially collapsed by pneumothorax, one will not expect to see vessel shadows protruding beyond the pleural boundary. Attention to this detail will prevent us from mistaking fine linear shadows produced by adhesive tape, dressings, skin folds (Fig. 3-25), rib margins, or folds in dressing gowns for the pleural line or lung edge seen consequent to pneumothorax. However, it is important not to rely on the absence of apical vascular shadows by itself as a sign of pneumothorax. Such an assumption can lead to the error of mistaking an area of emphysema or bulla formation for a pneumothorax, and run the very real risk of creating a truly large pneumothorax if you attempt to aspirate such regions.

There are rare occasions when a segment of the wall of a large bulla may simulate a pleural line, and thus a pneumothorax. The distinction between a loculated pneumothorax and a bulla may rarely be impossible on routine films. Usually the distinction is not that difficult, because the walls of bullae are shorter in length and their radius of curvature is smaller than the arc of a pleural line or a lung edge due to pneumothorax. Giant bullae, however, may present a problem in distinction.

Appearance of Pneumothorax on Films Made With the Patient Supine

When films are obtained with the patient supine, which is often the case after trauma or in the very ill, pneumothorax can accumulate under the middle lobe or the lingula. You can then see a very distinct line of pleura (provided you look for it), but, in addition, you will see lung vessel shadows extending caudally beyond the pleural line. Reflection about the shape of the lung will make it clear that vessels coursing into the tongue of the lower lobe that occupies the posterior sulcus can be expected to project caudal to the more anteriorly located middle lobe or lingula, whose inferior edge is made visible by the pneumothorax (Fig. 3-26A). Ordinarily, pneumothorax air seen under the lung on supine films will move to the apex when the patient is erect, but some can still remain briefly under the lung (Fig. 3-24B).

Fairly large collections of air also can accumulate in the caudal recesses of the pleural space when the patient is supine. These pneumothoraces present as zones of lucency projected over the lung bases and the upper abdomen (Fig. 3-26B–D) on supine AP chest films.

Occasionally it is possible to mistake these collections for air under the diaphragm rather than under the lung. That could be a serious error, since the implications in terms of treatment planning are so critical. This dilemma is infrequent but could be resolved by obtaining a decubitus film with the suspect side up. In the case of pneumothorax, the air should move from under the lung to a position between the lung and the chest wall on the high side, whereas subdiaphragmatic air will remain subdiaphragmatic, even though it shifts to the high flank. A word of caution about ordering the films, however: The patient must remain in the decubitus position long enough to allow the air to move (about 20 minutes); and remember, *extrapleural* air over the diaphragm is unlikely to shift significantly (see Fig. 3-30A).

In most cases, when you order a right lateral decubitus view of the chest, the technologist will assume you are looking for free-flowing fluid and will center the film to give you optimum viewing of the dependent side. In those rare cases when you order a right lateral decubitus view in order to evaluate the presence of a pneumothorax on the left — the high side — you should make that fact clear to the technologist, so that you do not waste the patient's time or cause the patient unnecessary discomfort or x-ray exposure. Obviously, the same holds true for examining the opposite side.

On supine chest films small pneumothoraces are likely to go undetected when the pleural air accumulates centrally under the anterior chest wall. Experience with CT substantiates that contention. On CT even very small pneumothoraces can be seen in supine patients. A small pneumothorax in a patient with healthy lungs causes little physiologic deficit. However, it is important to obtain short-interval follow-up studies to be sure the pneumothorax does not increase. A moderate pneumothorax may be life-threatening in a patient with severe underlying obstructive or restrictive lung disease from any cause.

Detection of even a small pneumothorax is critical in a patient who requires positive-pressure ventilatory assistance, which can rapidly convert a small pneumothorax into a large pneumothorax.

Tension Pneumothorax

Large amounts of air in the pleural space, as a result either of an initial event or of continuous one-way leakage from the lung, will result in tension pneumothorax. If the underlying lung is normal, it will completely collapse and retract toward its hilum, and there may be signs of increased volume of the hemithorax as well (Fig. 3-27). However, the *absence* of total lung collapse cannot be invoked as a sign eliminating tension pneumothorax from consideration. Diseased lungs with decreased compliance often do not collapse completely, even in the face of high pressure in the pleural space (Fig. 3-28). Therefore, in these patients the signs of increased volume of the hemithorax (e.g., fixed mediastinal shift during inspiration and expiration, or a depressed diaphragm) become quite important in indicating tension pneumothorax.

Hydropneumothorax

The designation of a combination of air (or gas) and fluid in the pleural space as "hydropneumothorax" is convenient but not accurate. The prefix "hydro" does not fit all situations, since the fluid component may be a transudate, an exudate, blood, pus, or chyle (or soup for that matter, if there is leakage from a perforated esophagus). The radiographic appearance of the fluid permits no distinctions.

Liquid in the pleural space, usually in small amounts, may be found in cases of spontaneous pneumothorax, probably due to bleeding from the site of lung rupture or tearing of pleural adhesions, or alterations in the physiology of pleural fluid formation and transport. Liquid in large amounts may accompany pneumothorax consequent to trauma, usually as a result of hemorrhage, or pneumothorax consequent to malignant neoplasm, usually metastatic, much less often primary. Pleural air and liquid may also be due to empyema associated with pneumothorax. A film made to project a tangent of an air-fluid interface (an upright or decubitus view) will show a true meniscus just as one would expect to see in a test tube (Fig. 3-28). The relatively straight edge of the liquid at the interface is almost never seen with intrathoracic fluid collections not associated with extrapulmonary air. Therefore, whenever you see such a true meniscus in the pleural space, you should find an associated pneumothorax or a loculated pocket in which both air and liquid are free.

Pneumomediastinum

Spontaneous pneumomediastinum occurs most frequently as the result of the escape of air from overdistended and ruptured alveoli generated in association with air trapping or high-pressure assisted ventilation. Various effort-related maneuvers against a closed glottis such as heavy lifting, coughing, straining, or grunting have also been implicated as causes of rupture of perivascular alveoli into the interstitium. This interstitial air then dissects along the perivascular sheaths into the mediastinum; this event is similar to one of the mechanisms for production of pneumothorax.[9,10]

Why some patients develop pneumomediastinum alone, some develop pneumothorax alone, and some develop both from the same mechanism is not always clear.

Pneumomediastinum occurs after some dental procedures and has been attributed by some to dissection of air into the submucosal planes of the alveolar ridge, then into the prevertebral fascial planes of the neck, and subsequently into the mediastinum. I wonder if it is not more likely due to straining against a closed glottis at the time of the procedure.

Pneumomediastinum may also result from entry of air consequent to esophageal rupture, tracheal or bronchial tear, surgery, or penetrating wounds.

Air in the mediastinum is recognized on chest films by streaks of gray-black density separating portions of mediastinal pleura from mediastinal contents in PA or lateral views (Fig. 3-29). Frequently, streaks of air density are also visible in the soft tissues of the neck and chest wall. Remnants of the thymus may be seen on lateral view — even in adults — when outlined by pneumomediastinum, and more commonly outlined in both PA and lateral views in infants. Air in the mediastinum may also dissect extrapleurally over the diaphragm (Fig. 3-30) or into the retroperitoneal space. The air may dissect into the mesentery and gut wall, producing pneumatosis cystoides intestinalis, and may even break through the peritoneum or mesocolon to produce free intra-abdominal air, simulating a perforated viscus. Likewise, retroperitoneal air originating from abdominal procedures or abdominal catastrophe may dissect into the mediastinum.

As an event, pneumomediastinum alone probably accounts for few serious physiologic disturbances. However, air in the pulmonary interstitium, which leads to pneumomediastinum, is often due to ruptured alveoli associated with severe underlying lung disease. Furthermore, bilateral pneumothoraces may be associated and cause severe physiologic deficits.

Tension pneumomediastinum is rare but may result in impaired venous return to the heart and in airway distortion, impeding air flow. Decompression may thus be required.

A more important problem, however, is that pneumomediastinum consequent to a catastrophe such as esophageal tear cannot be distinguished on plain films from the far more common spontaneous pneumomediastinum. Untreated esophageal tears, both iatrogenic and spontaneous, have a poor prognosis. It is necessary to consider this potential disaster in patients with pneumomediastinum, and use water-soluble contrast agents to examine the esophagus under fluoroscopic guidance in those patients whose antecedent history (retching or vomiting followed by pain) or clinical signs and symptoms suggest the possibility of esophageal tear. The detection of salivary amylase and low pH in pleural fluid specimens is a strong indication of esophageal perforation.[6,7]

Air in a distended esophagus or in a portion of gut brought up to replace the esophagus may occasionally mimic pneumomediastinum, but these conditions usually can be distinguished by careful analysis.

Pneumopericardium may occur alone or in patients who also have pneumomediastinum. At times it is not clear as to whether there is a pneumomediastinum or a pneumopericardium, or both. When the distinction is felt to be important clinically, lateral decubitus views can be obtained. Air in the pericardium usually shows significant redistribution on lateral decubitus views whereas air in the mediastinal pleura does not. Air in the pericardium extends only as high as the pericardial attachments to the ascending aorta. Air in the mediastinum usually extends into the soft tissue planes of the superior mediastinum above the aorta and frequently (except in infants) into the neck.

Computed Tomography in Detection of Pneumothorax and Pneumomediastinum

CT allows us to recognize small amounts of air in the pleural space and in the mediastinum even when plain films raise no suspicion of either pneumothorax or pneumomediastinum. Usually, however, the plain films have been made only in the AP projection, often with the patient supine, because the patient is quite ill or on a respirator, or is early in the postoperative period. It is easy to see how small pneumothoraces may go undetected on these films.

Very rarely, in my experience, have CT scans been requested primarily to rule in or out a pneumothorax or pneumomediastinum. However, in trauma patients who are being examined by CT to assess intra-abdominal injury, it is worthwhile to obtain at least a few scans through the lower chest to assess the possibility of pneumothorax. A positive finding may warrant insertion of a chest tube for drainage if the patient is to be placed on positive-pressure ventilation for any reason (see Ch. 11).

SUMMARY

1. Imaging studies are important in detecting and defining pleural abnormalities, which are often clinically occult and yet significantly influence diagnosis, staging of disease, treatment and prognosis.
2. Imaging studies can be used to distinguish free-flowing pleural effusions from fixed pleuritis, loculated pockets, noncalcified or calcified pleural plaques, and pleural masses.
3. Pleural effusions may occur as a consequence of conditions that increase systemic or pulmonary capillary pressure, decrease colloid osmotic pressure, markedly decrease pleural pressure, or alter pleural capillary or lymphatic permeability.
4. Pleural fluid may be a transudate or an exudate; it may be serous, purulent, hemorrhagic, chylous, or pseudochylous. These distinctions cannot be made reliably from imaging studies; they should be based on analysis of pleural fluid samples. The determinations are important for diagnosis and management.
5. Radiographically, pleural fluid presents a variety of configurations that depend on its quantity, physical characteristics, compliance of adjacent lung or soft tissues, patient position and radiographic projections, and the presence or absence of pleural adhesions. Understanding the variety of these configurations is important for correct interpretation.
6. For practical purposes, empyema (pus in the pleural space) associated with pneumonia is diagnosed when microorganisms are determined to be present in pleural exudates. Noninfected pleural exudates may also be associated with bacterial or viral pneumonias (parapneumonic effusion), and the distinctions cannot be made from radiographic appearances alone. However, large or rapidly increasing effusion, or loculated effusion associated with pneumonia, is highly suspect for empyema.
7. Benign loculated effusions may occur in interlobar fissures and completely resolve when the underlying cause is remedied.
8. Loculated pleural pockets in association with pneumonia or in patients who have clinical signs and symptoms of infection are highly suspect as empyema pockets. Correct diagnosis is important, as some form of drainage procedure is usually required in addition to appropriate antibiotic therapy.
9. The spontaneous occurrence of gas in a pleural pocket raises the likelihood of an associated bronchopleural fistula or, less commonly, the presence of gas-forming organisms. CT scans are very useful for distinguishing between lung abscess and empyema with gas.
10. Calcific pleural plaques are most commonly due to asbestos exposure when they are present bilaterally. Extensive pleural calcification may also be the result of old empyema, old tuberculous pleuritis, or possibly an old hemothorax.
11. Neoplastic disease of the pleura often is seen as a nonspecific pleural effusion on chest films. Solitary or multiple pleural masses with or without effusion are less common. Metastases from intrathoracic or

extrathoracic malignancies are more common than mesotheliomas, but the distinction may be difficult even after biopsy in some cases of diffuse disease. There are a variety of other primary pleural neoplasms, but they are rare.

12. Pneumothorax has diverse causes. The radiographic diagnosis is seldom difficult when films are interpreted with care. However, small pneumothoraces are easily overlooked even by the most conscientious observers when they are unaware of the presence of a clinical suspicion. A visible line of visceral pleura separating the lung from the pneumothorax space is a most reliable radiographic sign. Small pneumothoraces are probably not visible frequently on supine films. Tension pneumothoraces are life threatening.

13. Pneumomediastinum is usually seen as streaks of air in the mediastinum, with frequent extension of air into the soft tissues of the neck in adults.

14. Pneumomediastinum is frequently related to rupture of peripheral air spaces and dissection of air along perivascular sheaths to the mediastinum. The basic cause of the pneumomediastinum may be a single, self-limited event requiring no specific treatment, or may be related to underlying chronic lung disease whose management is critical to the cause and amelioration of the pneumomediastinum. Less commonly, pneumomediastinum is caused by a catastrophic event such as rupture of the esophagus or tears of major airways.

15. CT examinations are very effective in detecting:
   a. Minimal quantities of air or fluid in the pleural space and mediastinum
   b. Differences between empyema with bronchopleural fistula and lung abscesses
   c. Pleural plaques and pleural or extrapleural masses
   d. The nature of the structural abnormalities within an opaque hemithorax
   e. Pleural or pulmonary masses hidden on chest films by large pleural effusions.

BIBLIOGRAPHY

1. Bower GC: Chylothorax: observations in 20 cases. Dis Chest 46:464, 1964

2. Epler GR, McLoud TC, Gaensler EA: Prevalence and incidence of benign asbestos pleural effusion in a working population. JAMA 247:617, 1982

3. Friedman PJ, Hellekant CAG: Radiologic recognition of bronchopleural fistula. Radiology 124:289, 1977

4. Halverson RA, Fedyshin PJ, Korobkin M: Ascites or pleural effusion? CT differentiation: Four useful criteria. Radiographics 6:135, 1986

5. Hessen I: Roentgen examination of pleural fluid: A study of the localization of free effusion, the potentialities of diagnosing minimal quantities of fluid and its existence under physiological conditions. Acta Radiol Suppl 86, 1951

6. Light RW: Pleural Diseases. Lea & Febiger, Philadelphia, 1983

7. Light RW, Ball WC: Glucose and amylase in pleural effusions. JAMA 225:257, 1973

8. Light RW, MacGregor MI, Luchsinger PC, Ball WC: The diagnostic separation of transudates and exudates. Ann Intern Med 77:507, 1972

9. Macklin CC: Transport of air along sheaths of pulmonary blood vessels from alveoli to mediastinum. Arch Intern Med 64:913, 1939

10. Macklin CC: Pneumothorax with massive collapse from experimental local over-inflation of the lung substance. Can Med Assoc J 36:414, 1937

11. Meigs JV: Pelvic tumors other than fibromas of the ovary with ascites and hydrothorax. Obstet Gynecol 3:471, 1954

12. Meigs JV, Cass JW: Fibroma of the ovary with ascites and hydrothorax. Am J Obstet Gynecol 33:249, 1937

13. Proto AV, Ball JB: The superolateral major fissures. AJR 140:4311, 1983

14. Proto AV, Rost RC: CT of the thorax: pitfalls in interpretation. Radiographics 5:693, 1985

15. Raasch BN, Carsley EW, Lane EJ, et al: Pleural effusion: explanation of some typical appearances. AJR 139:899, 1982

16. Renner RR, Markarian B, Pernice NJ, Heitzman ER: The apical cap. Radiology 110:569, 1974

17. Sargent EN, Jacobson G, Gordonson JS: Pleural plaques: a signpost of asbestos dust inhalation. Semin Roentgenol 12:287, 1977

Atlas

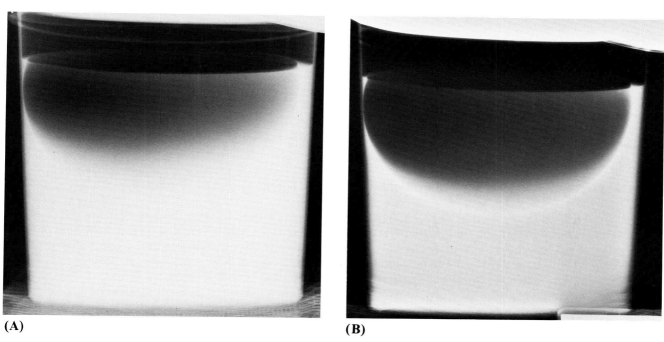

(A)

(B)

Fig. 3-1.   Balloon-in-a-Bucket Model

Two radiographs of a balloon partially submerged in water in a plastic bucket. The interface of fluid with the bottom and sides of the balloon creates an easily recognized meniscoid image. Actually, however, the only true meniscus is seen at the very top of the fluid column where it interfaces with the air above it.

The arclike (meniscoid) projections of fluid along the lateral margins of the balloon are analogous to images commonly seen on chest films where pleural fluid interfaces with adjacent lung. Very often this "balloon-in-a-bucket" effect is only seen laterally at the interface between pleural fluid and lung on the PA view, whereas its comparable image along the medial aspect is obscured.

The thin fluid columns in front of and behind the balloon present very subtle images in contrast to the large volume of air in the balloon, but it is important to understand that the fluid does *surround* the balloon.

In the more heavily exposed film (Fig. B), one can see the sharp interface of the bottom of the balloon and the water, and above it a mantle of lighter gray that merges gradually into the blackness of the air-filled balloon. You can relate this appearance to the relative thickness of the fluid mantle as judged by its projection along the sides of the balloon. On the less heavily exposed film (Fig. A), the sharp interface of the bottom of the balloon and the water is lost, and the contrast gradient is similar to that usually seen at the lower aspects of lung-fluid interfaces on chest films.

Fig. 3-2. (A,B) Large Left Effusion Showing the "Balloon-in-the Bucket" Effect on PA View

(A) A large pleural effusion occupies the lower left hemithorax. A slight mediastinal shift to the right attests to the increased volume on the left. An interface between lung and pleural fluid extends from the level of the posterior sixth interspace up to the apex in the shape of an arc that is concave toward the lung on this PA view, analogous to the balloon-in-the-bucket effect. This is not a true meniscus but rather a property of the projection. There is actually a layer of fluid surrounding the lung to the height of the apex, but it is not recognized because of its thinness relative to the lung it surrounds. (Cover the top of the fluid level surrounding the submerged balloon in Fig. 3-1A and you will obtain an effect similar to that seen here.)

(B) Lateral view shows the lighter gray tones of a fluid-filter effect, with an undulant sloping upper margin from front to back but no balloon-in-the-bucket effect. It does not clarify the true shape of the effusion surrounding the lung because the thin fluid components about the upper third do not register recognizable images in this view; thus, the balloon-in-the-bucket effect is lost.

If you had this lateral view and no PA view, could you deduce that the effusion is on the left and not the right?

1. A large pleural effusion effaces the image of the ipsilateral diaphragm, since the lung-diaphragm interface, which permits the diaphragm to be seen, is no longer present. Thus, in this case you see only one hemidiaphragm image. It is seen sharply along its entire course from front to back. This favors its being on the right.
2. You can identify the posterior edge of the inferior vena cava, which interfaces with the right lower lobe. This indicates that the aerated right lower lobe has not been displaced from this interface.
3. You cannot identify the posterior wall of the left ventricle, which normally interfaces with the left lower lobe. This indicates that some unit-density absorber has been substituted for normal lung at this interface.

All the visible data therefore indicate that the pleural effusion is on the left. Of course, you would never obtain a lateral view of the chest without a PA view, so what is the point of the exercise? If you practice analyzing every lateral view of the chest as though there were no PA view, you can use that skill when presented with a case in which a significant lesion is seen well only on the lateral view, or when there is a visible lesion on the PA view and one on the lateral view that superficially appear to be the same lesion, but on more critical analysis the two lesions are clearly localized to different sides of the chest.

When you cannot lateralize a lesion seen only on the lateral view, you can fluoroscope that patient and obtain spot films in appropriate degrees of obliquity to document the correct location.

(C) Large Pleural Effusion Due to Tuberculosis

Same woman as in Fig. A. There has been further opacification of the left hemithorax by increasing pleural effusion. There is an area of lung faintly visible inferior to the medial half of the left clavicle and adjacent to the left side of the mediastinum. Think about the configuration of lung and pleural effusion that might explain this appearance, and recall of the analogy of a balloon completely submerged in a bucket of water.

This woman had a sudden onset of left shoulder pain made worse by breathing; pain was also present in the left lower chest. Initially, on physical examination she had percussion dullness, decreased breath sounds, bronchiolar breath sounds, and pectoriloquy at the left base along with a few rales. She was febrile. Her tuberculin was positive at 1/10,000, whereas 4½ years before it was negative. Treatment for tuberculous effusion resulted in a rapid clinical response and near-complete clearing of the effusion in 1 month, except for residual blunting of the left costophrenic angle.

Tuberculous pleural effusions may be small or large in quantity. They are more commonly unilateral but may be bilateral. The parenchymal component of tuberculosis may or may not be detectable. *(Figure continues.)*

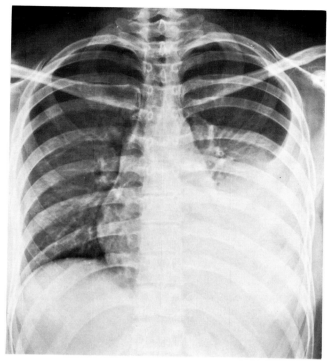

(A)

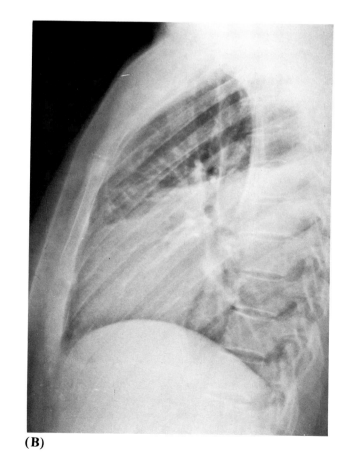

(B)

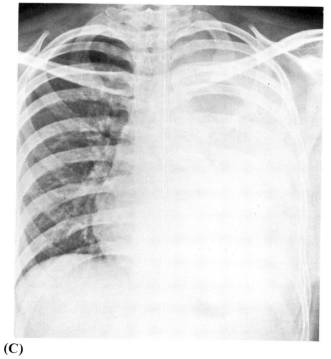

(C)

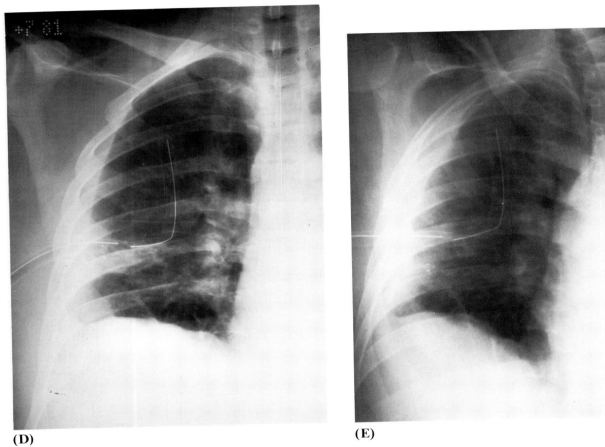

(D) **(E)**

Fig. 3-2. *(Continued).* **(D,E) Free Fluid and Fixed Components of Pleural Reaction**

Coned views of the right chest in the semi-upright (Fig. D) and right lateral decubitus (Fig. E) positions. The decubitus view is placed on the viewer as though it were also made with the patient upright in order to facilitate comparison. The decubitus view is made at a shorter target-to-film distance so that there is greater magnification. The film is behind the patient and the x-ray tube is in front. The head of the table is lower than the foot so that the patient is not only side-down but also slightly head-down.

Semi-upright film shows easily recognized pleural reaction along the right chest wall and effacement of the right costophrenic angle. A chest tube is in place.

(E) Right lateral decubitus film shows little change in the configuration of the right costophrenic angle and the pleural thickening along the chest wall. However, there is a larger amount of water absorber separating the aerated lung from the ribs than in Fig. D. We conclude therefore that:

1. The bulk of the pleural abnormality on the right is not free-flowing and is either loculated fluid, viscid fluid, pus, or a fibrous peel.

2. There is also a smaller free-flowing fluid component, which accounts for the change in configuration of the pleural reaction along the inner aspect of the ribs.

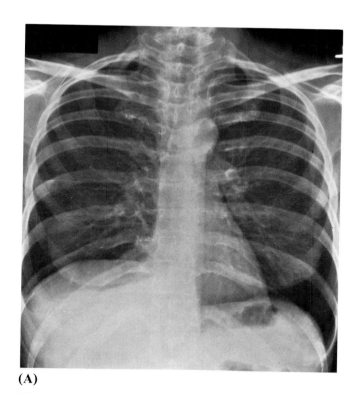

(A)

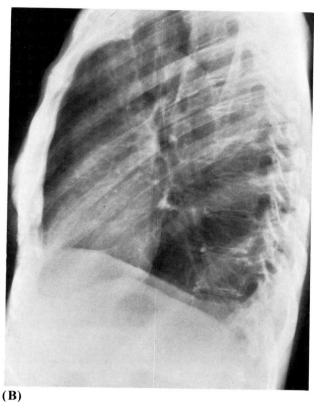

(B)

Fig. 3-3. Pleural Effusion Mimicking a High Hemidiaphragm

(A) The right hemidiaphragm is higher than the left. This is the usual relationship, but is the discrepancy greater than usual? On this PA view, the right costophrenic sulcus is relatively sharp. (This reproduction does not permit adequate evaluation of the lungs).

(B) On lateral view, the higher hemidiaphragm anteriorly is the right. You cannot follow the sharp interface of this hemidiaphragm all the way back to a set of ribs. The diaphragm becomes unsharp posteriorly and actually appears to arc cephalad, so that the right posterior gutter is rounded or blunted.

Pleural effusion layered over the true diaphragm and filling the posterior gutter is a likely explanation for this appearance. A decubitus view on the involved side would be confirmatory.

Blunting of a costophrenic recess (gutter) either laterally or posteriorly is often due to an old, stable, chronic fibrous pleuritis. When there are no old films for comparison to confirm the stability of the finding, a small effusion cannot be excluded without decubitus views. *(Figure continues.)*

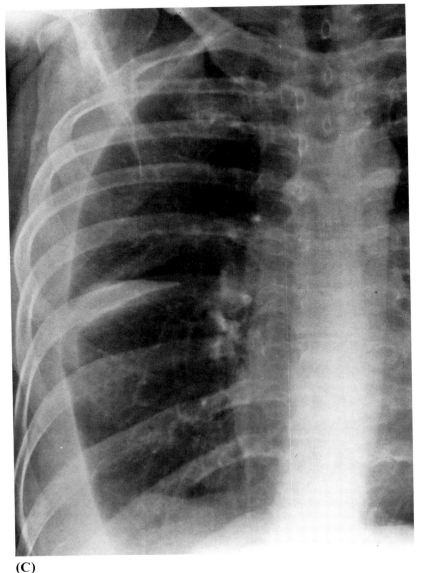

(C)

Fig. 3-3. *(Continued).* **(C)** This decubitus view is made with the patient lying on the right side with the head of the table a few degrees lower than the foot. It is viewed as though the patient were upright in order to facilitate comparison with the PA film.

A moderately large, free-flowing pleural effusion is layered on the dependent right side. The extension of the fluid into the minor interlobar fissure helps to identify the true width of the fluid mantle.

You can estimate the volume of the effusion as follows:

1. Measure the length in centimeters of the meniscoid interface from apex to base.
2. Measure the width in centimeters of the meniscoid interface of lung and fluid mantle from the inner chest wall (you can measure at three sites and average them if you prefer). This is not the true width of the fluid mantle any more than it is when a meniscoid interface is seen on a PA view, and therefore it presents one source of error in the calculation. However, it probably introduces less error than does a guess at the volume of the mantle anterior and posterior to the lung.
3. Estimate the third dimension: the depth of the fluid mantle from anterior to posterior. I use 12 cm as an average, or you can use the lateral view and measure from the estimated anterior axillary line to the estimated posterior axillary line.
4. Multiply dimensions 1 × 2 × 3 to find the volume in cubic centimeters; expect an error of ±25 percent.

An interesting question remains: How much of the apparent diaphragm seen in Figs. A and B is actually a pseudodiaphragm image produced by layered pleural effusion?

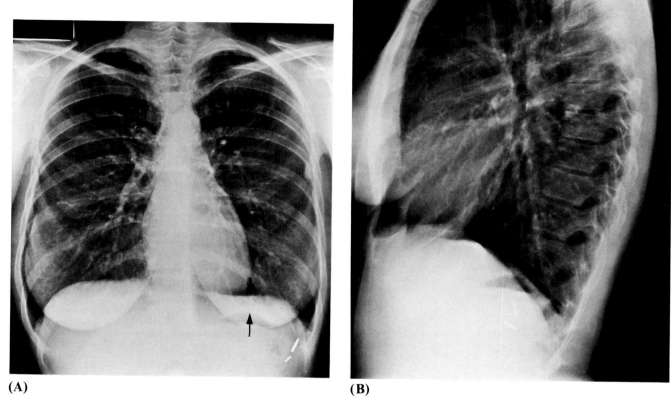

(A)　　　　　　　　　　　　　　　　　　　　**(B)**

Fig. 3-4.　(A,B) Pseudodisplacement of the Gastric Fundus From the Diaphragm After Splenectomy

PA and left lateral views, respectively, of the chest of a young woman with acute leukemia to serve as a base line for Figs. C through G.

(A) Notice the clips in the left upper quadrant from a previous splenectomy. There is a distinct separation between the dome of the left hemidiaphragm and the top of the air in the gastric fundus. (This separation is variable normally but becomes worrisome at approximately 2.0 cm). This may raise the possibility of a subpulmonic pleural effusion.

(B) On lateral view, the gastric fundus is seen well up under the posterior third of the left hemidiaphragm. One can visualize how the beam traversing from posterior to anterior would project the high tangent of the diaphragm so far above the fundus on the PA view, giving the spurious appearance of separation of these structures (see Fig. 2-7A and B).

The PA view, incidentally, also shows a deformity of the left seventh rib in the posterior axillary line, which is due to exuberant callus about an old, healed fracture. *(Figure continues.)*

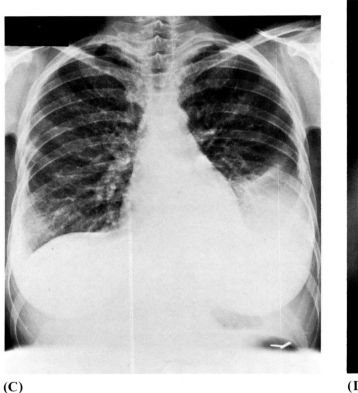

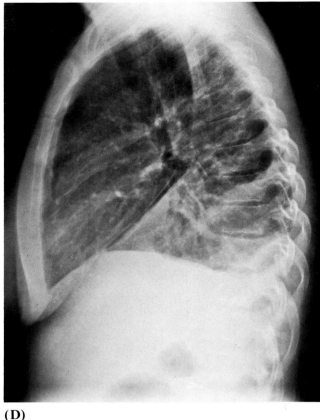

(C)   **(D)**

Fig. 3-4. *(Continued).* **(C,D) Bilateral Effusions of Different Volume: Perilobar Effusion and Inversion of Left Diaphragm**

(C) PA view of the same young woman as in Figs. A and B. Now, 5 weeks later, there is a diffuse increase in water-density absorber over the lower half of the left hemithorax, with an upper edge that appears to arc upward and laterally (one side of the balloon in the bucket). The location of the gastric fundus air and the left upper quadrant clips, in comparison with Fig. A, indicate that the left diaphragm is low.

(D) On lateral view one can only identify one hemidiaphragm. There is a sharp density gradient in the form of an edge shadow corresponding to the location of the left major fissure. This is due to a left lower lobe perilobar effusion. On the lateral view it mimics left lower lobe consolidation. The left hemidiaphragm is obscured by the pleural effusion and cannot be recognized.

Are we looking at a high right hemidiaphragm or fluid layered over the right diaphragm? On the PA view (Fig. C) the right costophrenic angle is obliterated. Laterally, the lung is separated from the ribs by a band of water density, which arcs medially at the level of the posterior right fifth and sixth interspaces corresponding to the location of the lateral aspects of the right major fissure (compare with Fig. A). The superimposed breast shadow is distracting and might cause you to overlook or explain away the abnormalities along the right lower lateral pleural space.

On the lateral view (Fig. D), the right major fissure is seen as a slightly thickened *line* shadow just anterior to the *edge* shadow of the left major fissure. We have deduced that the hemidiaphragm seen on the lateral view must be the right. Posteriorly it is totally effaced, and the posterior sulcus is filled in. Now look at the sharp slope of the right hemidiaphragm just anterior to the intersection of the right major fissure. Compare this appearance with its nearly flat configuration anteriorly in Fig. B. This *change* in configuration supports the diagnosis of a right pleural effusion with a significant subpulmonic component. Thus, the patient has developed bilateral pleural effusions with a larger volume of fluid on the left. *(Figure continues.)*

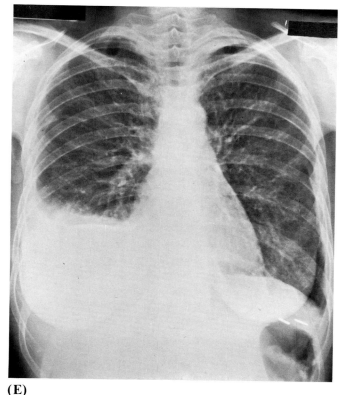

(E)

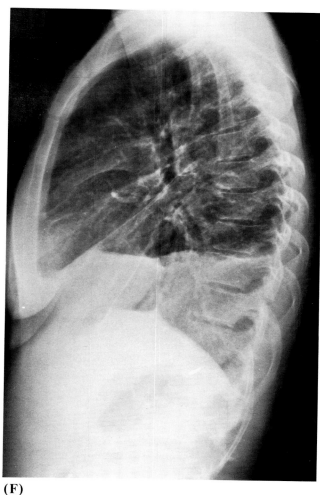

(F)

Fig. 3-4. *(Continued).* **(E,F) Sharp Caudal Inclination of the Anterior Pseudodiaphragm Image of Subpulmonic Component of Pleural Effusion**

(E) PA view of the same woman as in Figs. A to D, 11 days later. The left pleural effusion is markedly reduced as a result of thoracentesis but not entirely gone. There is still evidence of pleural fluid (or pleural thickening) along the lateral aspects of the left major fissure adjacent to the chest wall (compare to Fig. A).

(F) On lateral view there is a sharp slope immediately anterior to the lower end of the left major fissure. A few centimeters behind the left major fissure-diaphragm intersect there is a short, tentlike elevation. This probably represents the intersection of the left inferior pulmonary ligament with the diaphragm.

The amount of pleural fluid on the right side has increased considerably (compare with Figs. A and C). The right hemidiaphragm image is effaced, and a meniscoid image is present laterally. On the lateral view (Fig. F) there is an undulating lung-fluid interface extending over the diaphragm from the obliterated posterior gutter up to the intersect of the right major fissure, which is forward. Anteriorly from here the slope is sharply downward. Thus, there is evidence of bilateral pleural effusions, greater on the right than on the left. What appear to be diaphragm shadows are really pseudodiaphragm shadows. *(Figure continues.)*

Fig. 3-4. *(Continued).* **(G) Pseudodiaphragm Image of Subpulmonic Effusion**

The same woman 10 days later. There is recurrent effusion bilaterally. Compare the contour of the right hemidiaphragm to that seen in Fig. A. The high tangent is located considerably more laterally. This seeming lateral shift of the high point of a hemidiaphragm is a sign that correlates well with the appearance of a pseudodiaphragm due to a subpulmonic effusion. Here there are many other confirmatory signs: loss of the lateral gutter, extension of fluid into fissures, and loss of the right heart border due to fluid displacing the right middle lobe (compare with Fig. A).

Occasionally this appearance of lateral shift of the high point of a hemidiaphragm, with a sharp slope laterally to its costophrenic angle, may be the only sign or the more easily recognized sign of subpulmonic fluid. In such cases, confirmation by means of decubitus views is recommended. (Notice that now there are patchy foci of consolidation in both lungs).

(H,I) Subpulmonic Effusion Before and After Thoracentesis

(H) Coned upright PA film of the right chest of a young man who has had radiation therapy to the mediastinum for a known malignant lymphoma. There is a subtle but definite change in the contour of the right hemidiaphragm from Fig. H to Fig. I. In Fig. H the high point of the dome of the diaphragm is situated more laterally than in Fig. I. In addition, the diaphragm appears considerably higher in Fig. H than it does in Fig. I.

Fig. H is a rather classic example of subpulmonic effusion producing a pseudodiaphragm appearance. The fluid is layered over the right hemidiaphragm under the right lung. The right costophrenic angle appears to be sharp, but it does not extend all the way to the inner aspects of the lower lateral right ribs. It is not a true costophrenic angle, but rather a distortion produced by the subpulmonic effusion.

On the corresponding lateral view of the chest (not shown) there was definite blunting of the posterior gutter on the right side. A right lateral decubitus view of the chest would serve to estimate the amount of fluid present in the right hemithorax, but is not essential to predict that the pleural effusion is present.

(I) Appearance of the hemidiaphragm after a thoracentesis on the same day as Fig. H. The dome of the diaphragm now has its high point in approximately the midclavicular line, a more medial location than in Fig. H. In addition, the diaphragm now is projected in its usual location: lower in position than the pseudodiaphragm seen in Fig. H. Additionally, vessels extending into the posterior portions of the right lower lobe can be seen projected below the dome of the right hemidiaphragm in Fig I; in Fig. H no vessels are seen below the dome of the pseudodiaphragm because the lung has been floated out of this space.

In Fig. I the lateral margin of the right hemidiaphragm is projected all the way to the medial edge of the lower right ribs as is normal.

On both Figs. H and I one can see the arclike edge of the major interlobar fissure (arrows in Fig. H) contrasted against the aerated lung of the lower lobe, because there is thickening of the pleura extending into the major interlobar fissure. There is also thickening of the pleura along the upper lateral chest wall as well as over the right apex. These are common findings in patients who have received mantle irradiation therapy. There is also distortion of the mediastinum and the right hilum, but those components of postirradiation reaction are not shown well on these reproductions.

In some patients the major interlobar fissure may be seen on the PA view even when normal, because there is a lateral interface with fat in the pleural boundaries of the major fissure.[13] *(Figure continues.)*

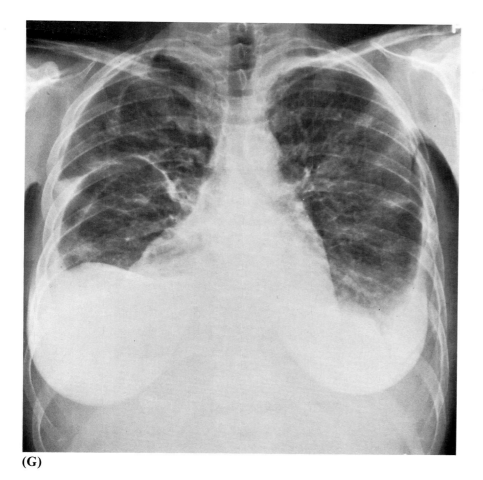

(G)

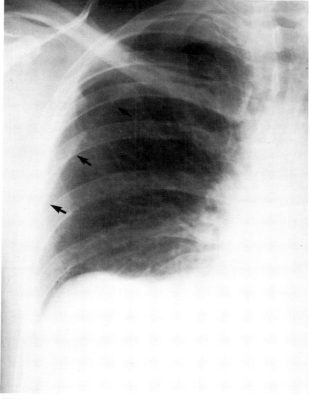

(H)

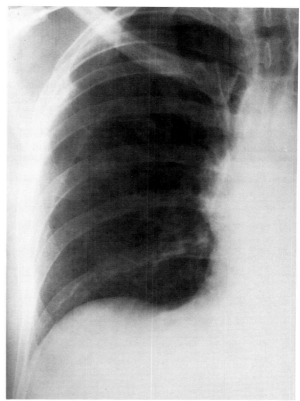

(I)

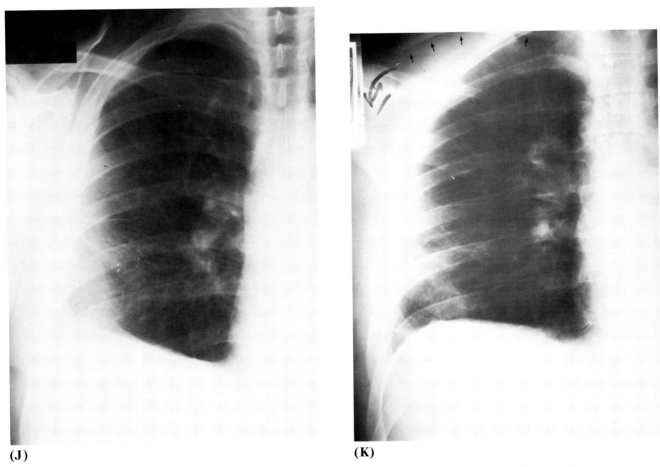

(J)   (K)

Fig. 3-4. *(Continued).* **(J,K) Effects of Lordotic Projection on Diaphragm and Pleural Abnormalities**

(J) Coned PA view of the right chest of a man who has undergone drainage of a right hemothorax following a gunshot wound. There is lateral tenting of the diaphragm on the right due to pleural adhesions. Superficially this resembles the contour of the pseudodiaphragm due to layering of subpulmonic fluid (Fig. H), but it can be distinguished by the sharp lateral peak and the short, thick linear strands (adhesions) coursing to the thickened pleura along the chest wall. These adhesions may remain fixed for life in some patients, but in others the fibrin components resolve, the adhesions decrease, and the diaphragm resumes a near-normal configuration.

(K) Coned AP view of the same hemithorax. The x-ray tube is centered so that the divergent beam produces a marked lordotic projection. Notice that the clavicle, which is seen at the extreme upper edge of the film, is projected high above the apex (arrows) compared to its position in Fig. J. The contour of the right diaphragm is more rounded, the pleural adhesions are less conspicuous, and the right costophrenic angle appears sharper. These changes are due not to resolution of the pleural reaction but to differences in projection and patient position. One cannot use films made in these different projections (AP versus PA or upright versus supine) to compare and interpret changes in the volume of pleural fluid or pleural thickening.

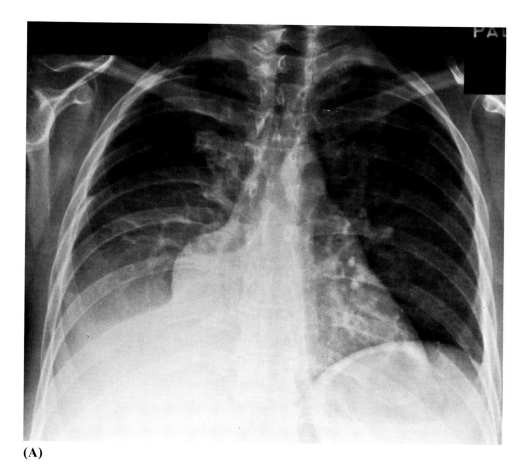

(A)

Fig. 3-5. Perilobar Effusion

(A) PA view shows an overall increase of water-density absorber in the lower half of the right hemithorax with complete loss of the image of the right diaphragm. There is no recognizable edge to the upper limits of the abnormality, but rather the gray tones change gradually so that above the level of the posterior sixth rib the right and left sides of the chest are comparable, except for a small region adjacent to the right side of the mediastinum. Just medial to the axillary portion of the right fifth rib and partly superimposed on the sixth, there is a subtle but definite water-density edge concave to the adjacent lung. It comes to a point at the level of the lateral aspect of the minor fissure, which is in its normal position. The right heart border has an unusual bumplike configuration. *(Figure continues.)*

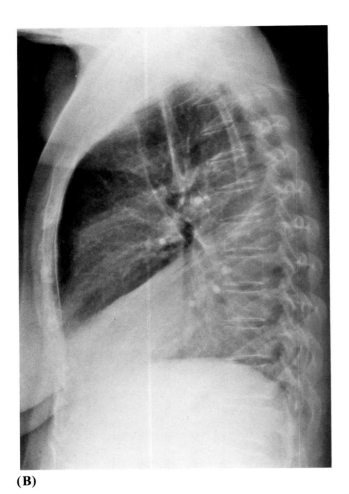

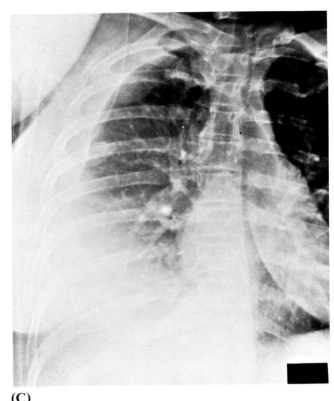

(B)   **(C)**

Fig. 3-5. *(Continued).* **(B)** On lateral view, only the left hemidiaphragm is seen. The right is not visible along any portion of its surface. There is a uniform filter effect over the lower two-thirds of the posterior portion of the chest, with anterior limits that slope rather sharply inferiorly until they reach the lower anterior chest wall. This appearance can be mistaken for a consolidation of the right lower lobe delimited anteriorly by the major fissure. Why is that unlikely? Consolidation of a lobe, even when due to an obstructed bronchus, rarely results in an increase in volume of that lobe. Since we can identify the minor fissure in its normal position, we can eliminate consolidation and reduction in volume of both the right middle and lower lobes as an alternative explanation. What is left to consider? Perilobar pleural effusion.

(C) The right lateral decubitus view is shown as though upright to facilitate comparison with the PA view. There is layering of a moderately large pleural effusion between the rib cage and the lung. The "bump" along the right heart border is gone (compare to Fig. A). You can clearly see vessel shadows in the medial half of the lower right lung now, even though you still cannot see the right hemidiaphragm. The position of the right hilar vessels is normal.

This is an example of perilobar effusion, which can simulate consolidation of lung in the lateral view. The disappearing bump along the right heart border is also due to fluid in the pleural space adjacent to the mediastinum — it moves away in the decubitus position.

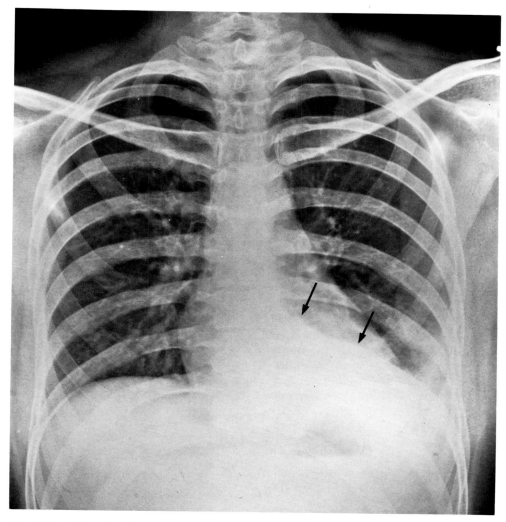

Fig. 3-6. Pleural Effusion Resembling Left Lower Lobe Atelectasis

PA view showing a wedge of increased water density inferomedially in the left retrocardiac area plus effacement of the left hemidiaphragm image. This configuration is frequent in small to moderate-sized left pleural effusions.

Superficially, this increased density resembles atelectasis and consolidation of the basilar segments of the left lower lobe, but the hilum is not depressed, nor is the left lower lobe bronchus displaced medially (see Ch. 4). A left lateral decubitus view would be useful for estimating fluid volume. It can also be used when you do not feel confident as to whether there is left lower lobe atelectasis or pleural effusion. The fluid will shift to the dependent left lateral chest wall whereas the atelectatic lung will not.

Fig. 3-7. Value of CT in the Study of Patients With Large Effusions

(A) PA view of the chest of a middle-aged man shows a large right pleural effusion that effaces detail of the lower half of the right hemithorax. A mass in the right side of the superior mediastinum is abnormal and highly suspect for lymphadenopathy. This constellation is presumptive evidence of a malignant neoplasm involving lung and/or pleura, with metastases to the mediastinal nodes. Alternatively, metastases from an extrathoracic malignant neoplasm (e.g., from the breast or the gastrointestinal or genitourinary tract) could produce the same findings. Primary tuberculosis or other infectious granulomatous disease could theoretically produce this constellation but would be unusual.

(B) CT scan shows a large right hilar and subcarinal mass that is obscured on the chest film. The mass is easily seen on CT because the patient is supine and the pleural fluid is layered posteriorly. However, even if the fluid surrounded the mass, distinction would be possible because of differences in tissue density. The mass also changes in radiodensity after intravenous contrast administration whereas the pleural fluid does not.

The mass impinges on a left pulmonary vein and on the left atrium (small arrows). A markedly distorted lower lobe bronchus is seen as a small, black, round image (long arrow) within the right hilar mass.

The patient underwent bronchoscopy, and a diagnosis of oat cell carcinoma was made from a biopsy. It is not possible to know how much of the mass component seen on the CT scan is due to the primary neoplasm and how much to extension into adjacent lymph nodes. The patient had a favorable response to chemotherapy.

(C) CT scan at a more caudal level than Fig. B. The pleural fluid floats the consolidated right middle and lower lobes away from the chest wall, but a tongue of the right upper lobe remains aerated. This scan was filmed at window and level settings such that aerated lung appears black. Compare the black, aerated right upper lobe seen anteriorly (single arrow) with the blackness of the aerated left lung. The right lower and middle lobes are reduced in volume and consolidated as a result of obstruction of the bronchus intermedius. These partly collapsed lobes can still be opacified by iodinated contrast material via bronchial artery supply if the pulmonary arterial flow is compromised. Faint air bronchograms are present in the otherwise opaque right lower lobe.

Notice that there is also a pericardial effusion accumulated laterally and posteriorly about the heart (small arrows). The heart and thoracic aorta contain intensely opacified blood.

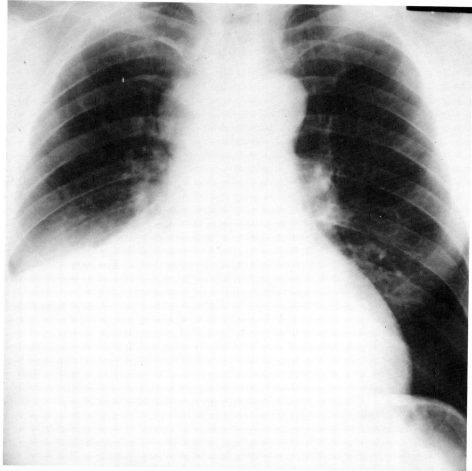

(A)

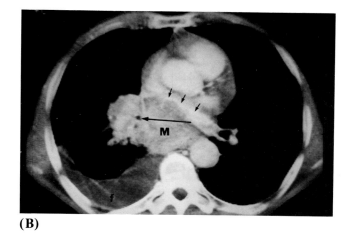

(B)

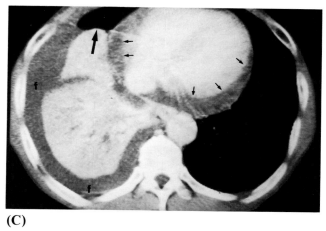

(C)

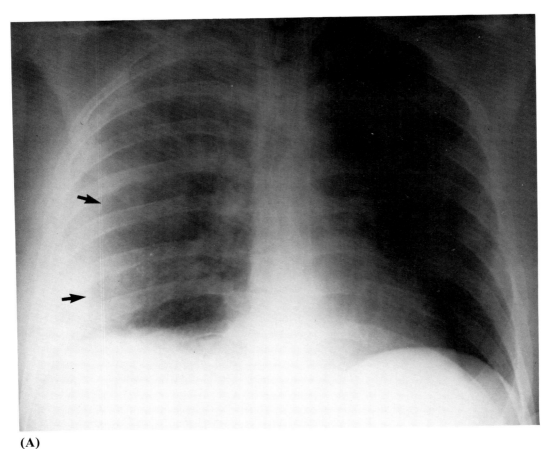

(A)

Fig. 3-8. Pleural Fluid Appearance on AP Supine View

(A) This man had a bullet enter his left upper quadrant and exit through his right chest. The film was made with the patient supine. There is a marked density difference between the two sides of the chest, more than can be accounted for by off-centering of the x-ray tube, which is also present (notice the lighter gray tone over the right axilla and scapula compared to the left).

When a moderate to large amount of pleural fluid (blood in this case) is layered along the posterior chest wall in the supine patient, it will act as a filter that increases the radiodensity of the affected side. In this instance the quantity of fluid is large enough that you can see a mantle of fluid, extending from apex to base, separating the lung from the ribs. A wider band of fluid separating the lungs from the ribs in the caudal half of the chest shows a sharp curvilinear interface with lung (arrows). This is probably due to greater atelectasis of the right lower lobe, permitting more local accumulation of pleural fluid. However, it could also be due to accumulation of fluid in an incomplete major fissure that does not extend medially to the hilum. The original film was overexposed so that no lung details are seen on the left. (Courtesy of Dr. Martin Spellman, Fremont, California.).

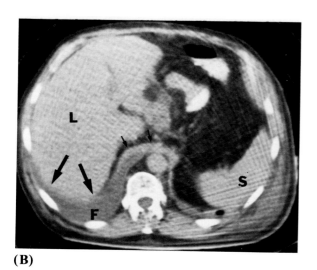

(B)

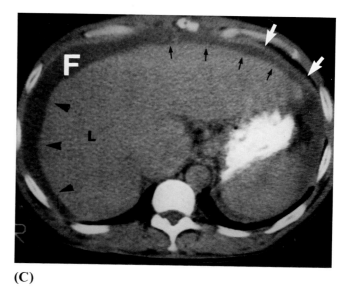

(C)

Fig. 3-8. *(Continued).* **(B-E) CT Criteria For Distinguishing Pleural Effusion And Ascites[4]**
(B) Pleural Effusion Can Accumulate In The Caudal Recess Of The Pleural Space Posterior And Medial To The Upper Aspects Of The Liver

CT cut through the caudal recesses of the pleural space. A mantle of *pleural effusion (F) displaces the right diaphragm crus (small arrows) anteriorly. The interface (large arrows) of the liver (L) with the pleural effusion is unsharp.* In part this is due to the fact the fluid is not in actual contact with the liver, but is separated from the liver by the right hemidiaphragm. The diaphragm image is not seen because it is inseparable from the curvature of the liver at this level. "S" marks the spleen. There is also a small amount of pleural fluid seen posteromedially on the left side. This demonstrates two CT criteria useful in the identification of pleural fluid. One is the *anterior displacement of the crus of the diaphragm* and two is the *unsharp or blurred interface between the margins of the liver and the pleural fluid.*

(C) Ascitic Fluid Can Accumulate About The Liver But Not Along Its Posteromedial Aspects In The Region Of The Coronary Ligaments

Example of a patient with *ascites, but no pleural effusion.* A mantle of fluid (F) surrounds the liver (L) laterally and anteriorly, but no fluid is seen posteromedially. Posteromedially, the coronary ligaments separate the bare area of the liver from the peritoneal space extending from the level of the diaphragm caudally for a variable distance. Therefore, *ascitic fluid does not have access to this aspect of the liver.* This area is occupied by lung (black) in the posterior gutter dorsal to the liver and diaphragm. Since the pleural space extends this far caudal, pleural effusion can occupy this space as in Fig. B. When the bare area of the liver enclosed within the coronary ligaments is small, either in the cephalocaudal or in the mediolateral dimension, then ascitic fluid may appear to intrude into the posteromedial region about the subdiaphragmatic portions of the liver and become confused with pleural effusion. This is uncommon.

The *interface of the liver with ascitic fluid along the right side is seen as a sharp image (arrowheads).* Anteriorly, the margin of the left lobe of the liver, which interfaces with fluid, is not as sharp (small arrows). This can be explained by the fact that the interface, anteriorly, is on a slope rather than on a vertical plane as it is along the right side of the liver. When the plane of the cut is through an interface between liver and surrounding ascitic fluid that is on a slope, the margin of the liver will be unsharp. This phenomenum is particularly deceptive when ascitic fluid accumulates over the dome of the liver. This pitfall, however, can be avoided by analyzing a series of stacked cuts through the region of interest. An arc of the diaphragm is seen anteriorly on the left (white arrows). It is distinguished from lung (black) anteriorly and the mantle of fluid (dark gray) along its inside margin. The density difference between the diaphragmatic muscle and the ascitic fluid is sufficient to be recognized by the CT technique. *(Figure continues.)*

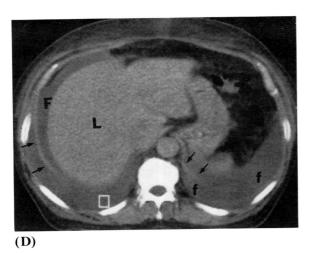

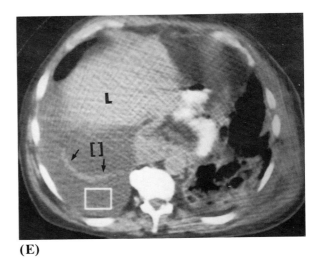

(D)   **(E)**

Fig. 3-8. *(Continued).*   **(D) CT Appearance of Pleural Effusion and Ascites in the Same Patient**

This patient has both pleural effusion and ascites. An arc-like image of the right hemidiaphragm (small arrows) is seen because a mantle of fluid (F) separates this segment of the diaphragm from the liver medially and from the lower chest wall laterally. In addition, this segment of diaphram is perpendicular to the plane of the cut.

A white square marks the pleural fluid in the posterior, inferior recess of the right pleural space behind the liver. Notice that laterally, *where the liver (L) has an interface with the ascitic fluid (F) the margin of liver appears quite sharp.* Posteriorly and medially, however, where the liver has an interface with the fluid in the inferior recess of the right pleural space, the liver margin is unsharp or blurred as in Fig. B.

On the left side a short segment of the crus of the left hemidiaphragm is seen (small arrows). It is slightly displaced from the spine by a mantle of fluid posteriorly (f). There is also a mantle of fluid seen anterior to this segment of the diaphragm. Since the diaphragm has a different tissue density then either the pleural fluid behind it or the ascitic fluid in front, it can be recognized as a distinct image. Compare the gray tone of this fluid to the much darker image of the abdominal fat lateral to the left diaphragm crus in Fig. B.

The ability to image even short segments of the diaphragm is very helpful in the analysis of fluid collections in the lower chest and upper abdomen. *Fluid which is seen outside of the perimeter provided by the image of the diaphragm can be localized to the pleural space whereas fluid which is seen inside that perimeter is usually in the abdomen due to ascites.* In a small percentage of cases when there is a large pleural effusion, the diaphragm may be inverted. In such a case, the pleural fluid will be located *inside* a peripheral ring of diaphragm image. If ascites is also present, the ascitic fluid will be located *outside* of the perimeter image of the inverted diaphragm. This pitfall is the reverse of the usual expectation, but can be recognized when stacked cuts are made at short intervals. As the cuts progress caudally, the image of the fluid located in the inverted cup of diaphragm becomes progressively smaller. This would not occur if the fluid was in the abdomen.

(E) A Band of Atelectatic Lung Surrounded By Pleural Effusion Can Mimic a Segment of Diaphragm

This patient has a large right pleural effusion. A short arc of tissue (small arrows) has a different density than the pleural fluid anteriorly (black brackets) and the pleural fluid posteriorly (white square). This image mimics a segment of the diaphragm. Therefore, one could deduce that there is both pleural effusion and ascites present. However, this patient has no ascites, and this arc represents the image of a narrow band of atlelectatic lung that is immersed in pleural effusion.

The pitfall of a band of atelectatic lung simulating an arc of the diaphragm can also be avoided by obtaining a series of stacked cuts through the region. Figure B is a CT scan of this same patient made through a plane several centimeters caudal to that of E. There is no lung left in the posterior gutter, only pleural effusion. There is no ascites. In general, careful analysis of sequential CT scans and utilization of all the criteria will allow for the correct interpretation of the vast majority of cases. (Courtesy of Dr. Marcia J. McCowin.)

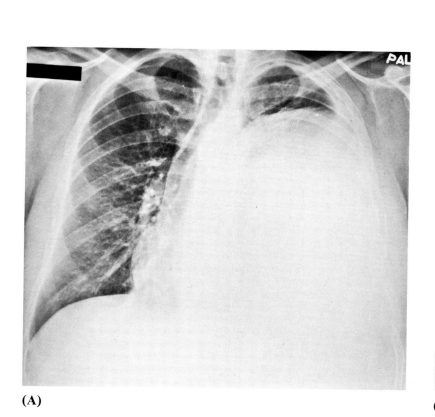

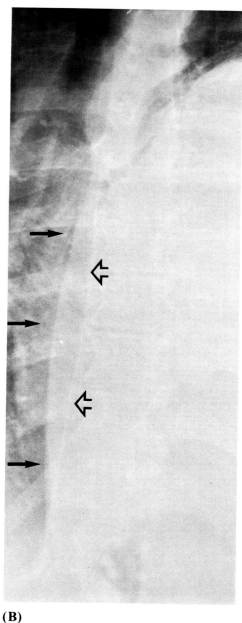

(A)

(B)

Fig. 3-9. (A,B) Opaque Hemithorax From a Large, Loculated Pleural Effusion With Herniation Across the Midline

(A) PA view. There is a large, loculated, left pleural effusion with a rounded upper edge. The left hemithorax is nearly opaque, and there is shift of the airway and the heart to the right.

  (B) Left lateral decubitus view of the chest shown as though upright; the illustration is coned to the region of the spine on the "up" side. Notice that even with the patient's left side down, there is still a herniation of the medial edge of the left pleural space (black arrows) across the midline to the right side because of the massive amount of left pleural fluid. The herniation is anterior to the spine. In cases of massive right pleural effusion the herniation occurs to the left. Notice that the paraspinal pleural reflection (open arrows) is normal.

  The cause of the large effusion was a malignant mesothelioma. *(Figure continues.)*

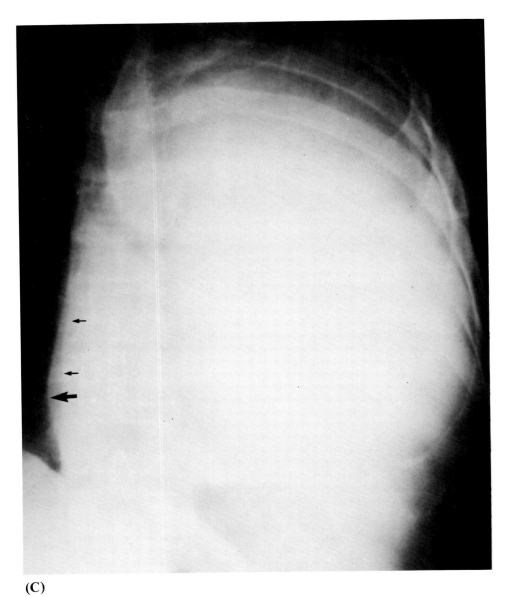

(C)

Fig. 3-9. *(Continued).* **(C) Large Left Effusion Due to Pancreatitis With Herniation Across the Midline**

This middle-aged man had a history of rapidly progressive shortness of breath. There is massive opacification of the left hemithorax, with shift of the trachea to the right. The heart is also shifted to the right, but the right heart border is shifted beyond the edge of this coned view. The curved soft tissue adjacent to the right side of the spine (larger arrow) that resembles a heart border is due to herniation of the left pleural space across to the right, similar to that seen in Fig. B. The right paraspinal stripe is normal (small arrows). A CT scan (not shown) showed a large pleural effusion with reduction in lung volume but no abnormal masses. The CT scan included the upper abdomen, however, and calcifications in the pancreas, like those commonly seen in chronic pancreatitis, were evident.

The pleural fluid was an exudate with a high amylase level.

Large pleural effusions, especially on the left side, are a known complication of chronic pancreatitis. They are probably caused by pancreaticopleural fistula. Pleural effusions also occur in association with acute pancreatitis and less commonly with pancreatic carcinoma. (Courtesy of Drs. R. Dunn and Gilbert S. Stacy.) *(Figure continues.)*

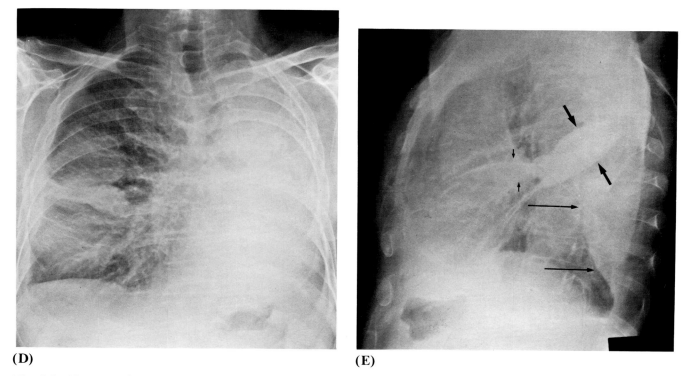

(D)   **(E)**

Fig. 3-9. *(Continued).*   **(D,E) Left Pneumonectomy and Loculated Right Pleural Effusion**

(D) PA view shows marked shift of the heart and mediastinal contents into the left hemithorax. The air column remaining in the left main bronchus terminates abruptly with a square configuration. The axillary portions of the left sixth rib are missing and have been replaced by an irregularly contoured column of bone, which is barely visible. This appearance is characteristic of regeneration of rib along the periosteal tract following partial rib resection. These findings support the conclusion that the patient has had a left pneumonectomy, which is indeed the case. He had this operation 10 months ago because of a carcinoma of the left lower lobe bronchus. He did well until 1 month before this film was taken, when he noticed increasing dyspnea.

On the right side, there is thick pleura extending along the lateral chest wall from apex to base. There is also a series of rounded and oval abnormal shadows of soft tissue density.

(E) Lateral view shows a biconvex soft tissue density in the distribution of the upper third of the major fissure. This appearance is consistent with loculated fluid. There is also a faint image of loculated fluid in the minor fissure, yet there is also a line shadow in the position of the minor fissure, indicating that a portion of the fissure is still bounded by closely applied pleural surfaces. Judging from the PA projection (Fig. D), the loculated fluid appears to be located in the middle third of the minor fissure (from side to side) and in the posterior half from front to back as judged from the lateral view. It is not uncommon to see loculated fluid in a portion of a fissure and a superimposed line or band shadow due to the presence of much less fluid in other portions of the same fissure.

In addition to the fluid loculated in the fissures, another large, loculated pocket of fluid along the posterior chest wall is clearly recognized only on the lateral view because of its long tangent with adjacent lung. It is seen on the PA view only as an area of increased tissue density with poorly defined edges.

A right pleural biopsy showed granulomatous disease consistent with tuberculosis. The patient had a moderately febrile course but improved on antituberculous chemotherapy. Within 6 months his chest cleared except for some residual pleural thickening. Seventeen months later he died of brain metastases, and at autopsy neither tumor nor residual tuberculosis was found in the chest.

This case illustrates an important point. One must resist the temptation to proceed directly to one diagnosis without formulating a differential diagnosis. For example, in a patient who carries a diagnosis of a malignant neoplasm anywhere in the body (aside from the brain), a pleural effusion might reasonably be considered to be due to metastases to the pleura. You can order that contingency as number one in the differential diagnosis, but you cannot *assume* that it is the correct diagnosis. This is especially true whenever the finding is the sole manifestation of disease activity.

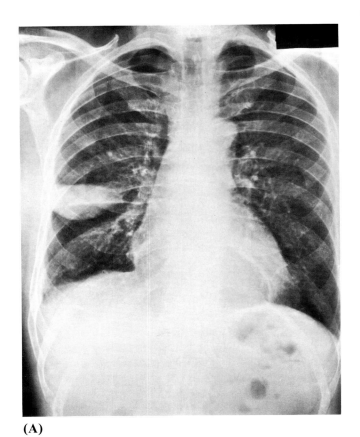

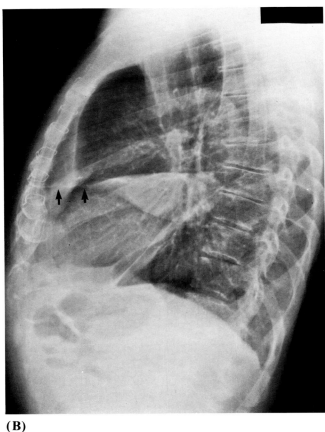

(A)   (B)

Fig. 3-10.   Loculated Pleural Fluid

(A) PA view in a postoperative male patient following aortic valve replacement. A well-defined mass is seen on both this and the lateral view (Fig. B). It has sharp, biconvex edges on the PA view, whereas on the lateral view its upper edge appears straighter while its lower edge is convex toward the lung.

The right costophrenic sulcus is blunted, and pleural thickening extends up the right chest wall laterally to the level of the mass. A thick line (or a thin band) is superimposed on the mass in the PA view.

(B) Lateral view. Arrows indicate the anterior portions of the minor interlobar fissure. This portion of the fissure, as it is projected on the PA view, accounts for the line shadow superimposed on the mass.

Follow-up films 8 days later showed the mass to be gone. The mass consisted of loculated pleural fluid, often called "vanishing tumor," "phantom tumor," or "pseudotumor."

Loculation of pleural fluid may occur between the visceral and parietal pleurae anywhere in the thorax. Loculations along the chest wall or major fissure may be difficult to distinguish from pulmonary lesions when seen en face. Retrosternal loculations may not be recognizable at all on a PA view, because the density of mediastinal structures, as well as the bone of the sternum, may not allow the relatively small increment of absorber in the beam path to be recognized. Notice that on the lateral view a relatively thin pleural loculation is seen anteriorly behind the sternum, but it is totally lost in the image of the mediastinum on the PA view.

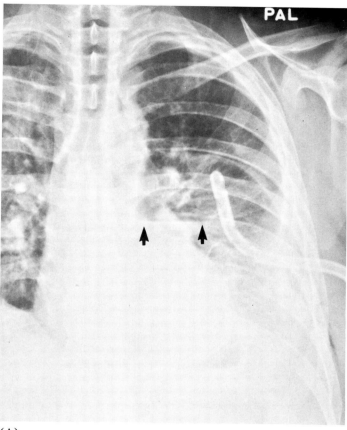

(A)

Fig. 3-11. Bronchopleural Fistula

(A) This patient had sustained a gunshot wound 17 days before these films were taken. The entry site was in the left upper quadrant of the abdomen, and the exit below the right scapula. Initially the patient had a right hemothorax drained and a laparotomy. Two holes in his stomach and a liver laceration were repaired. He later developed a left pleural effusion.

Chest tubes are now present on both sides. There is considerable pleural reaction and thickening in a mantle about the right hemithorax, a residual from the hemothorax and empyema that were drained.

The abnormalities on the left are complex. The bulk of the abnormalities are pleural. No pulmonary vessels are seen superimposed on the left heart. The left lower lobe bronchus is more lateral in position than usual, indicating that lung is being displaced. The left hemidiaphragm image is lost. There is a well-defined air-fluid level projected over the left posterior eighth rib on the PA view (Fig. A, arrows) and over the thoracic spine and intervertebral foramen on the lateral view (Fig. B, arrows). The fluid level lengths are quite different on the PA and lateral views. The chest tube is not in the loculated pocket.

The disparate lengths of the air-fluid levels favor this being a pleural pocket. Interestingly, however, on films made only the next day (not shown) the fluid level lengths were much more alike because there was more fluid in the pocket and the level was higher in the dome. *(Figure continues.)*

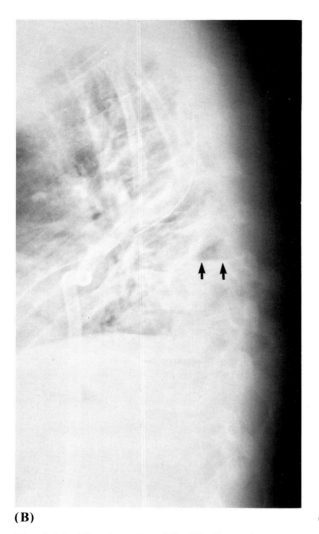

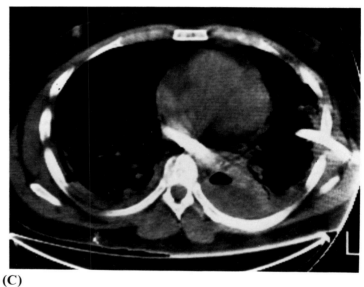

(B)   **(C)**

Fig. 3-11. *(Continued).* **(C)** CT slice 6.0 cm below the level of the carina. There is a low-density pocket with an air-fluid level in the posteromedial aspect of the left chest. The inner margins of the pocket are very sharp and smooth. Air bronchograms in atelectatic lung are seen along the anterior margins of the pocket. Pleural reaction extends laterally for a short distance beyond the pocket. A portion of a chest tube (white) is seen traversing the left lateral chest wall.

This is an empyema pocket. The air in the pocket is due to a bronchopleural fistula. The very bright band seen in front of the spine is an artifact.

Pleural abnormalities associated with empyema may involve much more of the pleural surface than would be estimated from the size of a loculated pocket alone. These may produce nodular excrescences along the pleura away from the main pocket, which mimic nodules due to neoplasm.

Notice that there is also considerable pleural reaction along the right posterior chest wall. Recall that the patient recently had a right hemothorax and empyema drained. *(Figure continues.)*

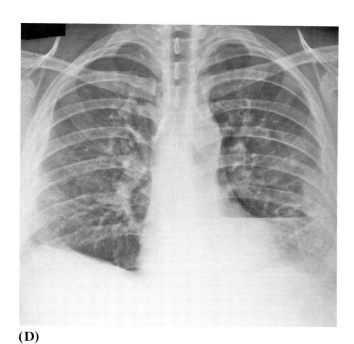

(D)

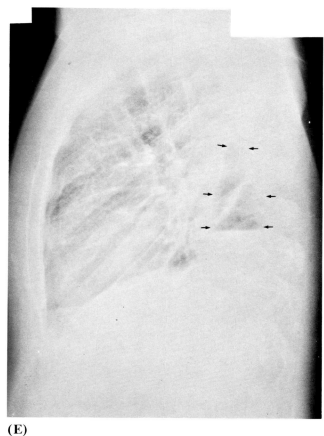

(E)

Fig. 3-11. *(Continued).* **(D,E)** PA and lateral views respectively, of the same patient at a later date. All chest tubes have been removed. A long fluid level is now projected at the posterior eighth interspace on the PA view. It is nearly twice the length of the fluid level projected on the lateral view. Arrows outline the pocket's margins on the lateral view. There is now much less fluid in the pocket, and the discrepancy in fluid level lengths becomes more apparent as the level moves down. *(Figure continues.)*

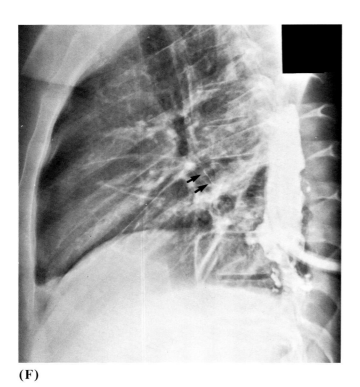

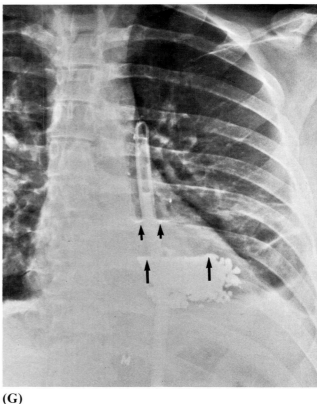

(F)   **(G)**

Fig. 3-11. *(Continued).*   **(F)** A wide-bore tube was placed into the cavity, and a variety of anaerobes were cultured from the fluid drained. After the pocket had drained for several days, contrast material was injected under fluoroscopic control. A thin rim of contrast material (arrows) can be seen outlining one wall of the left lower lobe bronchus, confirming the presence of a fistula, which was also seen at fluoroscopy. It was also noticed that the patient coughed and complained of a salty taste in his mouth when the tube was irrigated; this alone is adequate evidence of a bronchopleural fistula but does not identify the bronchus involved. The bronchus involved does not have to be known unless a surgical correction is planned.

Notice the relatively uniform depth of the cavity from front to back. The considerable cephalocaudad length of the pocket in comparison to its relatively narrow AP dimension is also a discrepancy seen in patients with pleural pockets rather than lung abscesses.

(G) This view permits appreciation of the shape of the pocket with the patient erect. It shows how fluid level lengths can vary depending on how much fluid is present. The heavy contrast material sinks to the bottom of the pocket and creates a fluid-fluid interface (long arrows) with the immiscible lighter liquid in the pleural pocket. This liquid then shows an air-fluid level (with a thin layer of floating contrast) at a higher, narrower level in the pocket (short arrows). Do not mistake the left heart border for part of the pocket's margins.

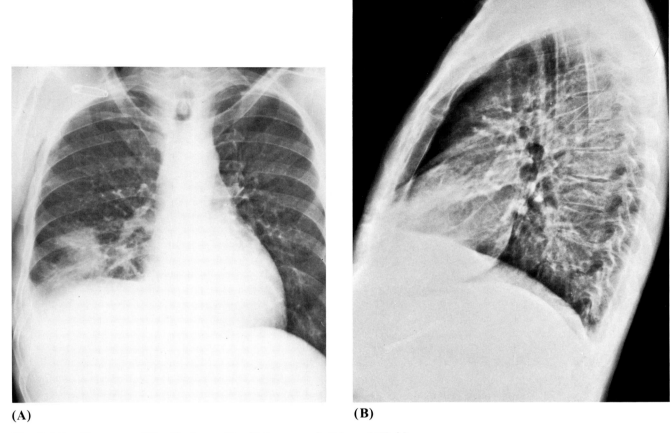

(A)   (B)

Fig. 3-12.   Empyema Manifest as a Rapid Increase in Pleural Fluid

This man developed a slowly progressive right middle lobe pneumonia following laryngectomy for carcinoma of the larynx.

(A) PA chest film showing an area of consolidation with ill-defined margins. Laterally a small pleural effusion fills in the right costophrenic angle and accounts for the loss of the sharp margin of the lateral aspect of the right hemidiaphragm.

(B) Lateral view shows the pulmonary consolidation in the right middle lobe. The right posterior gutter is not shown well on this reproduction but was blunted on the original film *(Figure continues.)*

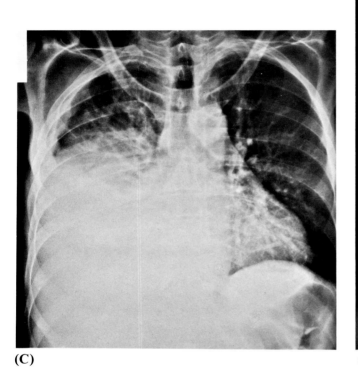

(C)

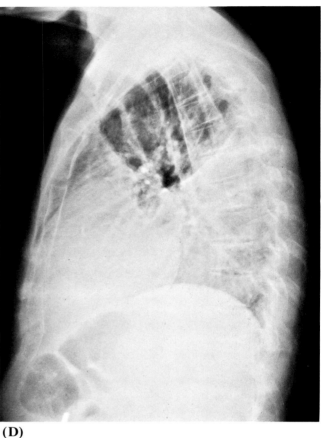

(D)

Fig. 3-12. *(Continued).* **(C,D)** PA and lateral views, respectively only one day after those shown in Figs. A and B. There has been a rapid increase in the amount of pleural fluid. On the lateral view the fluid shows a balloon-in-a-bucket effect, but this is not seen on the PA view. Discordance between PA and lateral views is not uncommon in cases of pleural effusion, but the balloon-in-a-bucket effect seen on either view is a strong indication of the presence of pleural fluid.

A right lateral decubitus view of the chest (not shown), however, showed no significant shift of fluid in comparison to the PA view. This indicates that the extensive increase in pleural fluid is either loculated or extremely viscid. Either of those conditions associated with a pneumonia prompts the diagnosis of empyema.

A large-bore tube was inserted into the pleural space, and the patient was treated with drainage and antibiotics. Anaerobic organisms were responsible for the empyema and presumably for the pneumonia as well. Anaerobic organism pneumonia can have a surprisingly indolent course, but empyema is still a serious complication.

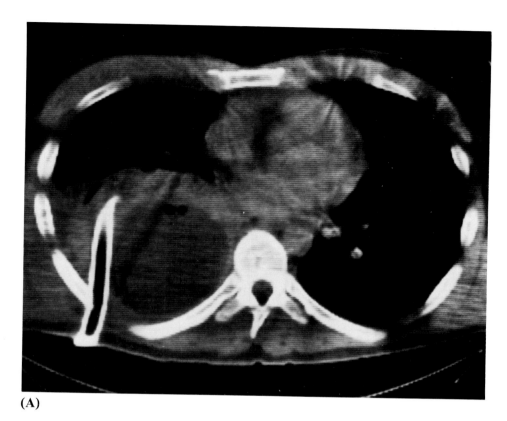

(A)

Fig. 3-13. Empyema and Bronchopleural Fistula Versus Lung Abscess

(A) CT scan of a man who developed progressive opacification of the right hemithorax in the distribution of the right lower lobe accompanied by a pleural effusion. The clinical question was whether he was developing an empyema or a lung abscess.

The scan is at a level 4 cm caudal to the tracheal carina. There is a large, round, loculated pocket posteriorly. It contains fluid and has very sharp inner margins against a higher density mantle of atelectatic, compressed lung. Part of an air bronchogram is seen on this scan as a short, black, tubular structure in the atelectatic portion of lung lateral to the chest tube. Also, a black band artifact crosses the pocket obliquely. Notice that the chest tube does enter into the fluid pocket but skirts around its lateral side. This fact was not appreciated on the PA and lateral chest films.

Within the low-density fluid collection, there are air bubbles (black holes) both anteriorly and posteriorly, consistent with the viscid nature of the fluid contents. The appearance of this pocket fits well with that of an empyema. The tube was removed since it was not really draining the pocket. *(Figure continues.)*

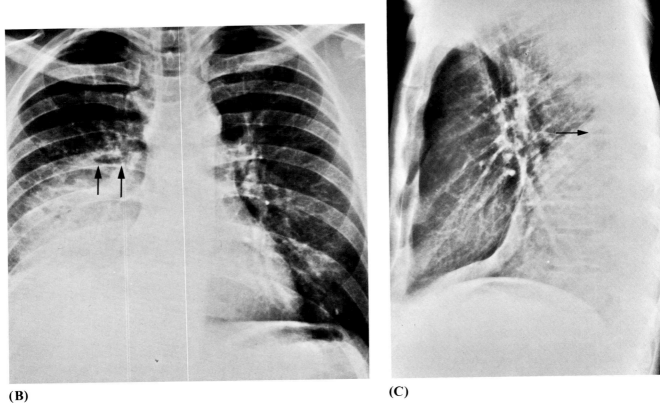

(B)   **(C)**

Fig. 3-13. *(Continued).*   **(B,C)** PA and lateral chest films, respectively, show a large zone of opacification in a distribution conforming to the right lower lobe. A well-defined margin, which bulges anteriorly, is seen on the lateral view. On the PA view a small air-fluid level is seen at the top of the opaque zone superimposed on the right seventh rib. On the lateral view it is seen at the top of the opaque zone superimposed on the spinal canal. A rib was later resected, and large-bore tube drainage of the empyema was successfully carried out. Anaerobes were the bacteria responsible. After the infection resolved, a decortication was required.

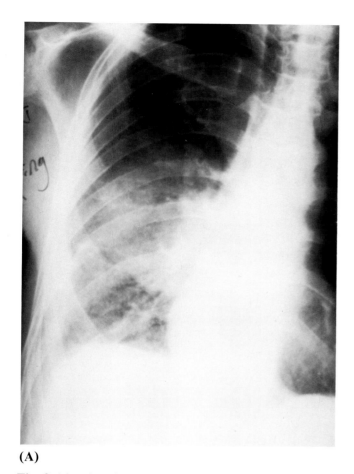

(A)

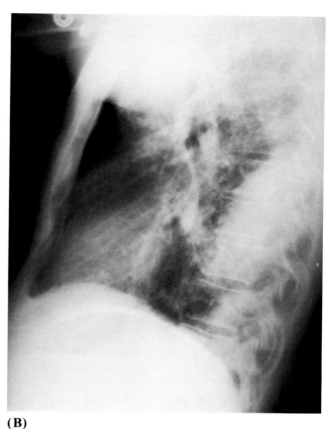

(B)

Fig. 3-14. (A–C) Lung Abscess on CT With Possible Empyema on Chest Films

(A,B) PA and lateral views, respectively, of the chest of a young man with cerebral palsy and a history of previous aspiration pneumonias. Once again he has developed clinical signs and symptoms of pulmonary infection.

(A) PA view shows increased opacity of the lower two-thirds of the right hemithorax, with a rounded, masslike zone of opacity in the right parahilar region. Its edges are unsharp except on the most caudal margin. There is also effacement of the right costophrenic angle, loss of the sharp outline of the right diaphragm, and separation of aerated lung from the lower ribs laterally.

(B) On lateral view there is a long, mass like zone of opacity behind the hilum, adjacent to the posterior chest wall. It has a fairly sharp interface anteriorly with the lung, and its location corresponds to the zone of opacity seen on the PA view. The posterior margin of the right diaphragm and the posterior gutter are effaced. (Note that only one hemidiaphragm is seen posteriorly on the lateral view).

The obliteration of the lateral and posterior gutters on the right and the loss of diaphragm image fit well with the presence of pleural thickening or fluid or both. The question, however, is whether the masslike zone of consolidation represents a necrotizing gram-negative organism pneumonia or a loculated empyema pocket. *(Figure continues.)*

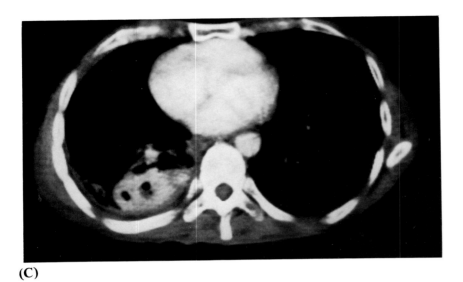

(C)

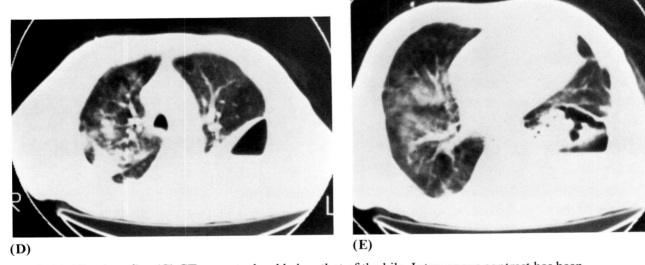

(D)   **(E)**

Fig. 3-14. *(Continued).*   **(C)** CT scan at a level below that of the hila. Intravenous contrast has been used; notice the density of the cardiac chambers and the descending aorta to the left of the spine. The zone of opacity on the right, corresponding to that seen posteriorly on the chest films, also shows marked enhancement. Compare its density to that of the adjacent rib and to the muscles dorsal to the rib. This CT scan was photographed at window and level settings at which normal lung appears black.

The rounded but irregular black foci within this enhancing, consolidated lung are small air pockets.

The CT findings support a diagnosis of necrotizing pneumonia or abscess such as may be seen in gram-negative or anaerobic organism (or mixed flora) pneumonias. Some of the pleural component — fluid or thickening — is seen as a thin rim of soft tissue paralleling the inner aspect of the rib behind and lateral to the parenchymal lesion.

(D,E) Lung Abscess Communicating With an Empyema Pocket

(D) CT scan of a man who developed bilateral pneumonia and sepsis following abdominal surgery. This cut is above the level of the carina. There is a sharply marginated empyema pocket, showing a fluid level, in the posterolateral aspects of the left hemithorax. Patchy foci of consolidation are also seen in the right lung.

(E) CT scan at a lower level, caudal to the carina. The fluid level in the empyema pocket can still be seen posterolaterally on the left. Immediately adjacent to its anteromedial aspect, however, there is a serpiginous, branching, black structure with lobulated margins, buried in consolidated lung. This is a lung abscess, which was communicating with the empyema pocket. *Escherichia coli* and *Proteus mirabilis* were cultured both pre- and postmortem, and mixed anaerobes were cultured premortem from one specimen of thoracic fluid.

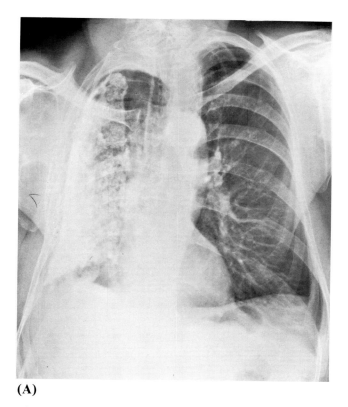

(A)

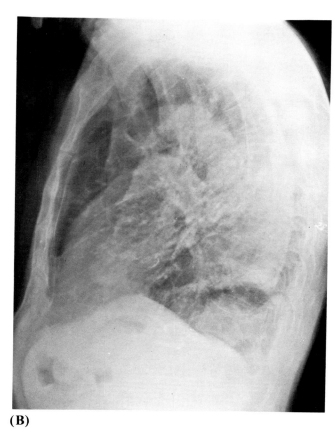

(B)

Fig. 3-15.   Extensive Pleural Calcification

(A) PA view. There is extensive calcification of the pleura about the right lung extending from the apex to the base. The calcified envelope, however, is separated from adjacent ribs on the PA and the lateral view, indicating that there is also a thick (fibrous) pleural peel layer that is not calcified. The pleural calcification is diffuse, but is nonhomogeneous and stippled in appearance. There is also contraction in volume of the right hemithorax; compare its size to that of the left.

(B) On lateral view the calcification is seen as stippled densities—which mimic parenchymal nodules—in a "wrapper" distribution, with a more intense band of increased tissue density adjacent to the posterior ribs. What would you expect a ventilation-perfusion scan to tell you about the right lung?

This is the type of extensive pleural calcification that may occur following empyema, especially tuberculous, or after pneumothorax inductions for treatment of tuberculosis. Theoretically, extensive pleural calcification may occur following hemothorax, usually one that has been inadequately drained following trauma. It is unlikely that you will see calcific plaques this extensive in younger patients, because of improved methods of treatment.

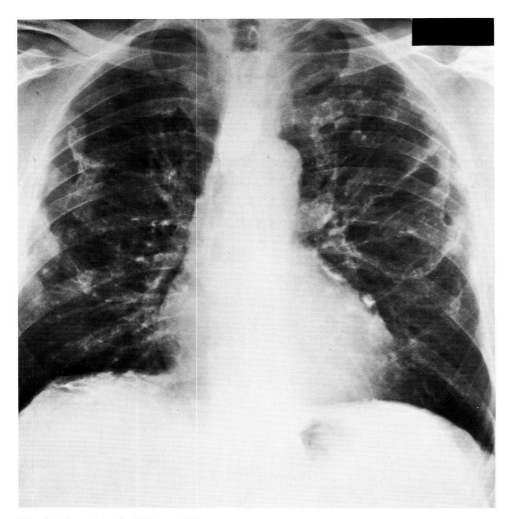

Fig. 3-16. Calcified Pleural Plaques

There are large, bilateral, relatively symmetrical, calcific pleural plaques of the type seen in persons with a remote history of exposure to asbestos. The edges of the plaques appear more heavily calcified than does the central portions; this may be a matter of projecting longer segments in tangent. Most calcified pleural plaques from asbestos exposure are not this large or obvious. Notice the plaques over the diaphragms (the right reproduces better than the left); these are common sites for asbestos pleural plaques and are often the most easily recognized.

Many pleural plaques due to asbestos exposure will not be calcified and will be more difficult to recognize on chest films. CT scans are more sensitive than chest films in detecting pleural plaques.

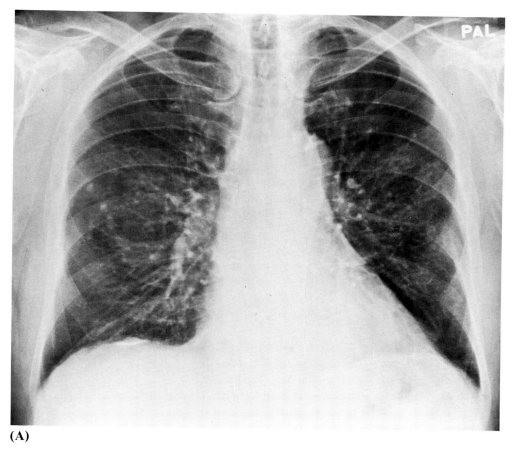

(A)

Fig. 3-17. CT of Pleural Plaques

This man had chest films and CT scans taken as part of his workup for diffuse histiocytic lymphoma. He also had a history of occupational asbestos exposure.

(A) The chest film shows a calcific plaque over the right diaphragm. In addition, there are scattered small, nodular shadows in the right midlung zone and to a lesser extent on the left. Some of them appear dense for their size, but others do not. *(Figure continues.)*

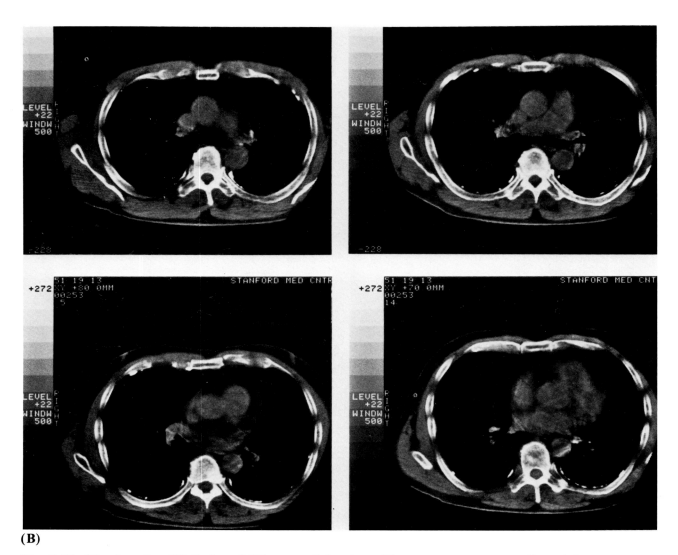

(B)

Fig. 3-17. *(Continued).* **(B)** Series of CT scans of the chest. There are numerous small, nodular, calcific pleural plaques scattered about the periphery of the chest cradled adjacent to ribs. Most of the plaques are located posteriorly and only a few anteriorly. They account for the nodular shadows seen on the chest films, but on CT they are much more easily recognized as being pleural in location as well as calcified.

CT images at lung detail settings showed no nodules in the lungs per se. This is an important distinction, since noncalcified pulmonary nodules may be a manifestation of lung involvement by diffuse histiocytic lymphoma, which this man had.

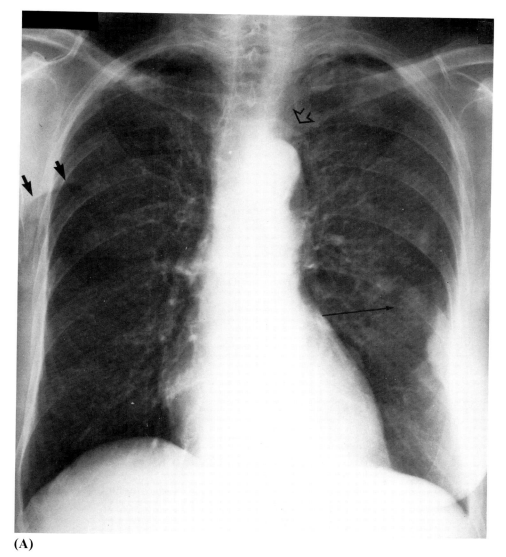

(A)

Fig. 3-18. Pleural Metastases

Nine years ago before these films were taken, this woman had a radical mastectomy for carcinoma of the right breast and has had no evidence of metastases up to this time.

(A) PA view. The lower two-thirds of the right chest appears blacker than the left because of the absence of the right breast and pectoralis muscles. The edge of a ridge of soft tissue is seen over the upper right hemithorax (short arrows). This is a telltale sign of a radical mastectomy, which produces marked change of the ipsilateral axillary soft tissues.

A prominent soft tissue mass (not marked) is seen along the inner aspects of the posterior axillary portion of the left eighth rib. It has one sharp edge (medially, adjacent to the lung), and its superior and inferior margins taper to the chest wall — an appearance characteristic of an extrapleural mass. There are other ill-defined, focal, nodular areas of increased tissue density superior and medial to the obvious mass. The largest of these also has one sharp, although faint, edge along its medial aspects (thin arrow). The smaller ones do not show any definite edges. They are all extrapleural masses.

The patient is slightly rotated, so that the edge of the manubrium is seen as a faint image above the aortic arch, adjacent to the inferomedial end of the left clavicle (open arrow). It could be mistaken for the edge of a mass, because it is a relatively thin bone in a woman with bone demineralization. The high-kilovoltage technique further contributes to its loss of contrast. Recognition of its shape and its location prevents that error. *(Figure continues.)*

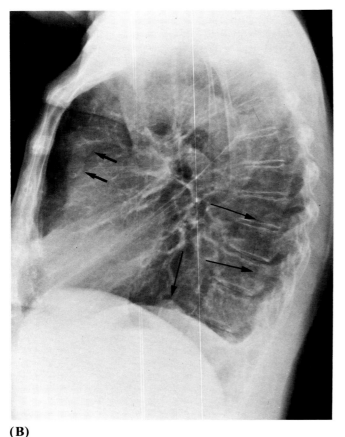

(B)

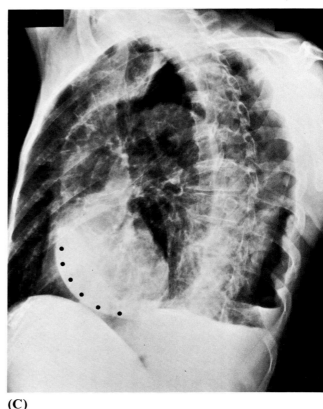

(C)

Fig. 3-18. *(Continued).* **(B)** Lateral view. One posterior gutter is obliterated by pleural reaction. Can you tell for certain whether or not there is free fluid? Which side is it on?

Very low density, one-edge shadows are seen superimposed on the spine posteriorly over a hemidiaphragm, and anteriorly partly superimposed on the ascending aorta (arrows).

(C) Left anterior oblique view, after pneumothorax. There is a series of lobulated masses adjacent to the inner aspects of the left posterior ribs. They are seen well because of air in the pneumothorax. Their images are no longer degraded by the anatomic noise of superimposed pulmonary vessels. Notice how sharp and uninvolved the visceral pleura appears where it interfaces with the pneumothorax air.

There is a true meniscus at the bottom of the pneumothorax. This indicates that some fluid is certainly present, but on the lateral view before the pneumothorax you cannot distinguish between chronic pleural thickening and a small effusion as the cause of the blunted posterior gutter. Biopsy of one of the pleural masses showed poorly differentiated adenocarcinoma consistent with breast primary tumor.

The free margin of the left breast (dots) is superimposed on the heart as a sharp, curved edge. This could be confusing if you did not understand what structure was responsible for the image.

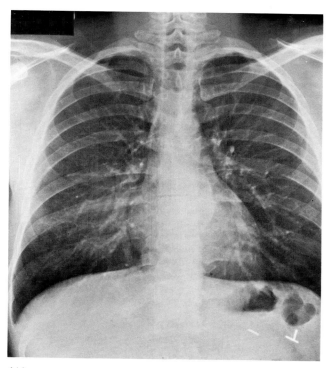

(A)

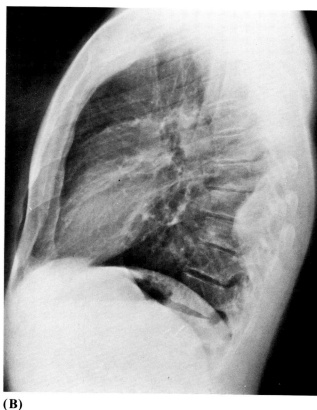

(B)

Fig. 3-19. Extrapleural Masses Due to Hodgkin's Disease

(A,B) PA and lateral views, respectively, of the chest of a young man who has received treatment for Hodgkin's disease in the past and is returning to clinic for a follow-up visit.

(A) A soft tissue mass is projected adjacent to the left side of T7, T8, and T9 on this PA view. Its lateral edge against lung is easily seen. Its medial edge is not recognizable, although the adjacent vertebral margins are.

(B) On lateral view there is a large soft tissue mass along the posterior chest wall, behind the heart. It has a relatively sharp anterior edge. Its posterior margin is not identifiable separate from the posterior chest wall.

Do you think the mass seen on the PA view on the left side accounts for the mass seen posteriorly on the lateral view? If a posterior extrapleural mass is seen well on a lateral view because it presents an anterior edge tangent to lung, would you also expect to see that tangent well on the PA view, or would you expect to see it en face, and thus indistinct? *(Figure continues.)*

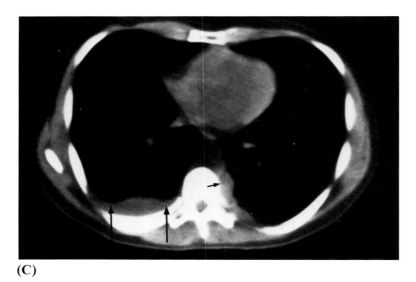

(C)

Fig. 3-19. *(Continued).* **(C)** CT scan (1.0 cm thick) through the approximate middle of the long axis of the left-sided mass seen on the PA chest film. There is a soft tissue mass along the left side of the spine behind the descending aorta, and a larger soft tissue mass is cradled adjacent to a posterior rib on the right. Both of these masses are extrapleural, and both contribute to the radiodensity of the lesion seen on the lateral chest film, but the visible edge (tangent) is produced by the lesion on the right. The lesion on the left accounts for the paraspinal mass so readily seen on the PA view.

Search the PA view from the level of the posterior right seventh rib to the ninth rib lateral to the heart. This area shows a subtle increase in soft tissue density (compare it with the density of a similar area lateral to the heart on the left). This fits the appearance of an extrapleural lesion whose tangent with lung is projected en face. This shows how a filter effect can be produced by a peripheral mass when none of its interface with lung is projected tangentially to the beam.

The CT scan findings are anatomically more graphic than the plain films and serve as a permanent record. They can be very useful in planning radiotherapy. Aside from that, they are not vital to simply proving that there are lesions on both sides. Fluoroscopy and spot films would suffice for that purpose. (CT scan courtesy of Palo Alto Medical Clinic. Reprinted from Blank M, Castellino R: The intrathoracic manifestation of the malignant lymphomas and leukemia. Semin Roent 15:227, 1980.)

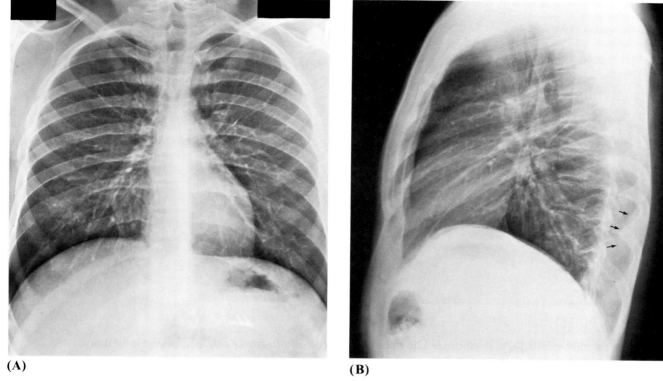

(A)   **(B)**

Fig. 3-20.   Extrapleural Recurrent Hodgkin's Disease

This young man is being followed in clinic after having received radiation treatment to the mediastinum in the past for the treatment of Hodgkin's disease.

(A) PA view. The slight medial deviation of the upper portions of the large vessels emanating from the hila is due to contraction in volume of the paramediastinal portions of both lungs, which is common after mediastinal and hilar radiation treatment. The contraction in this patient is minimal. Aside from this and a slight distortion of the mediastinum, the PA view shows no compelling abnormality.

(B) Left lateral view shows separation of the tangents of the posterior left and right ribs due to slight obliquity off of true lateral. The diaphragm images are projected so closely to one another that it is difficult to decide which is which. The right posterior gutter is the more caudal and identifies the more posterior set of ribs as those of the right side.

Scrutinize the posterior right lung-rib interfaces. You can see them well a little more than halfway up toward the apex. Further cephalad the more abundant soft tissues of the upper chest wall and shoulder girdles obscure detail. At the level of the posterior eighth rib there is an abnormal soft tissue shadow with a faint but sharp interface with lung (arrows). It is subtle but definite. If it is in close association with the posterior eighth rib on a lateral view, then we know it has to be somewhere along the distribution of that rib on the PA view.

On the PA chest film, where the posterior right eighth rib is superimposed on the image of the anterior right fifth rib, and extending inferomedially, there is a very subtle difference in film radiodensity compared to a similar area of the left side. Most observers would probably not call this an abnormality if the finding on the PA view had to stand alone. Two factors account for this: First, a low peripheral mound with tapered edges projected en face does not permit edge recognition; second, interference by the overlying ribs hinders recognition of an increase of tissue in the beam path.

This lesion was biopsied and represents recurrent Hodgkin's disease. The discovery of this lesion on routine surveillance films of this asymptomatic patient depended on the chance occurrence that the lateral view of his chest was made in the RPTL variant of the left lateral view. Had this been a true left lateral projection, the lesion would have been obscured by the superimposed images of the posterior ribs (see Fig. 2-8B).

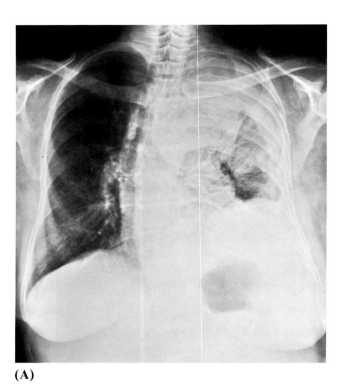

(A)

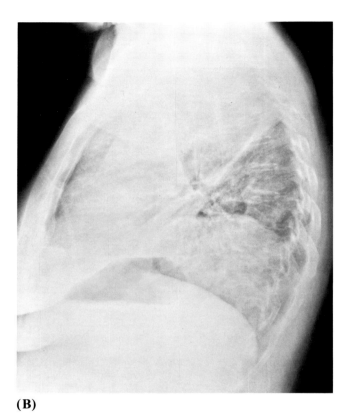

(B)

Fig. 3-23. Malignant Mesothelioma

This 67-year-old woman had a history that was questionable for tuberculosis. She also had chest pain and had lost 50 pounds over 6 months.

(A) PA view. There is extensive opacification of the periphery of the left hemithorax, with efface-ment of the images of the aortic arch, the left pulmonary artery, and the left anterior mediastinum. The trachea deviates to the right. There is marked separation of the air in the stomach from the apparent left hemidiaphragm. On the left lateral decubitus view (not shown) there was no detectable change in the appearance or position of these pleural abnormalities.

The appearance of the air-filled major bronchi indicates compression of the left upper lobe and downward displacement of the left main bronchus.

Incidentally noted are coarsely nodular foci of calcification in right paratracheal nodes just above the level of the azygos vein on the PA view.

(B) Lateral view confirms the findings on the PA view and shows that most of the remaining aerated lung on the left is in the lower lobe.

At this point there are two main diagnostic possibilities:

1. There is marked permeation of the left pleural space by lobulated masses of neoplasm, ei-ther malignant mesothelioma or metastases from an unknown primary.
2. There is extensive loculation of pleural fluid, either infected or noninfected. Loculations this extensive would be unusual, although still possible, in someone who has never had chest surgery, prior thoracentesis, or known ante-cedent pneumonia. This, then, is the less likely choice. *(Figure continues.)*

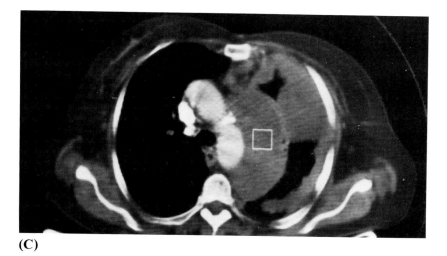

(C)

Fig. 3-23. *(Continued).* **(C)** CT scan through the level of the bottom of the aortic arch following the intravenous injection of a bolus of contrast material. The superior vena cava and the aortic arch are opacified.

The very dense, (white) wedge-shaped image along the midcourse of the aortic arch represents calcified lymph nodes in the subaortic space—the ductus nodes. Calcified right paratracheal nodes (bright white lobular mass medial to ascending aorta) are also seen. These are probably due to prior tuberculosis or histoplasmosis.

The settings used to photograph this section were such that the right lung appears black. The left should appear the same, but instead there are extensive, lobulated soft tissue masses about the periphery of the chest, with a large component (open white box) against the aortic arch. (Compare the density of these masses with that of the muscles about the scapulae.)

The CT numbers of these masses before injection of intravenous contrast were higher than those of a transudate, but fluid collections high in protein can have relatively high CT numbers. Following intravenous contrast, however, there was an inhomogeneous increase in the CT numbers such as may be seen in large neoplasms. Loculated fluid would not show an increase in CT numbers following IV contrast infusion. Under CT guidance, a needle biopsy was obtained from the anterolateral mass component seen on this scan.

The pathologic diagnosis was that of malignant tumor, favoring malignant mesothelioma, although the possibility of adenocarcinoma metastatic to the pleura could not be entirely ruled out.

On caudal CT levels (not shown), an additional bulky mass was present at the left base. Thus, what appears to be an elevated left diaphragm on the chest film is neither a diaphragm nor subpulmonic fluid, but tumor mass simulating the diaphragm.

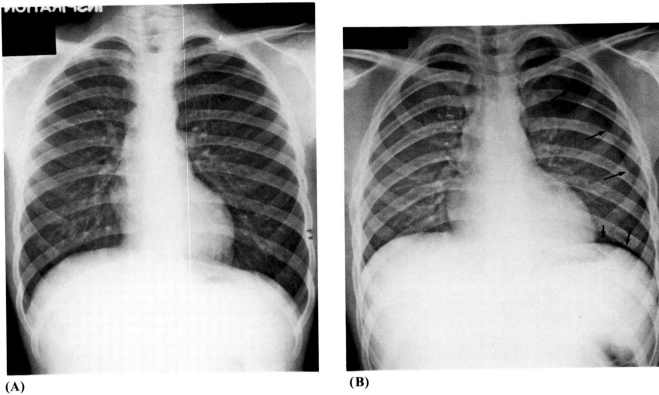

(A)

(B)

Fig. 3-24.   Influence of a Film at End-Expiration on the Visibility of a Pneumothorax

(A) PA view of the left lung of a young man who has a small left pneumothorax. A very fine line of visceral pleura could barely be seen between the very minimally collapsed lung and the surrounding mantle of pneumothorax. On the original films this pleural line could be seen not only over the convexity of the left upper lobe but also under the lingula and adjacent to the mediastinum. On this print the lines are not visible.

(B) Film of the same young man taken at the end of expiration. It is easy to detect the left pneumothorax. The film contrast gradient between the smaller, more opaque lung and the pneumothorax is increased.

Although the film is made with the patient erect (note the fluid level in the stomach), there is still a black crescent of air over the left diaphragm representing residual pneumothorax under the lung. If the patient remained erect long enough, that air should rise to the apex, since the pleural space is seen to be free of loculations.

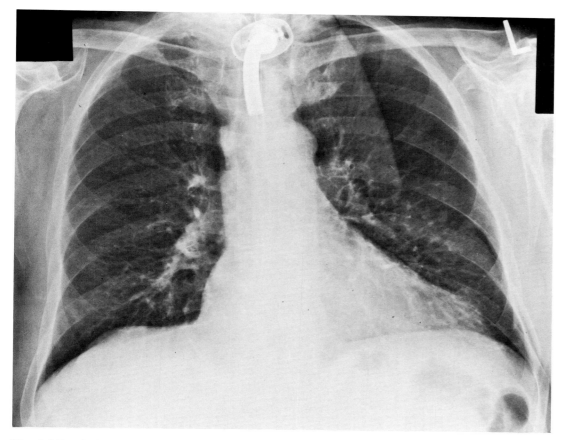

Fig. 3-25.   Skin Fold Simulating Pneumothorax

There is a well-defined edge of an arc over the upper half of the left hemithorax. Superficially it resembles a pneumothorax, but you know it is not. Why?

First, it is an edge, not a line. It would be unlikely for the margins of a pneumothorax about the convexities of the lung to present as an edge rather than a pleural line unless the film was made in maximum expiration, which would permit the adjacent lung to empty of air, or unless there was consolidation of adjacent lung. Neither of these conditions is present, as you can see from the overall appearance of the chest.

Second, vessel shadows are present lateral to the edge. The only way that could occur with a pneumothorax over the convexity of the lung would be if the pneumothorax were loculated so that part of the lung was collapsed and part expanded. Loculated pneumothoraces can and do occur, but they are rare in patients who have not had surgery on the ipsilateral side, multiple thoracenteses, or prior chronic infection. Occasionally, pleural adhesions may prevent a portion of lung adjacent to a pneumothorax from collapsing away from the chest wall, but the point of fixation causes the free portions of adjacent lung to assume an obvious tentlike configuration.

Infrequently the margin of a lobe partially collapsed from pneumothorax is superimposed on an adjacent, less collapsed lobe so that vessel shadows pass beyond its pleural line. This situation rarely presents a difficult recognition problem.

This image is due to a deltopectoral flap that has been raised in order, eventually, to be brought up to cover the defects from extensive prior surgery for carcinoma of the floor of the mouth. The thickness of the flap itself accounts for the lighter gray tone medial to the free edge.

Skin folds in both infants and adults can be confused with manifestations of pneumothorax unless one analyzes the image correctly. Even adhesive tape or projections of intravenous tubing can trap the unwary.

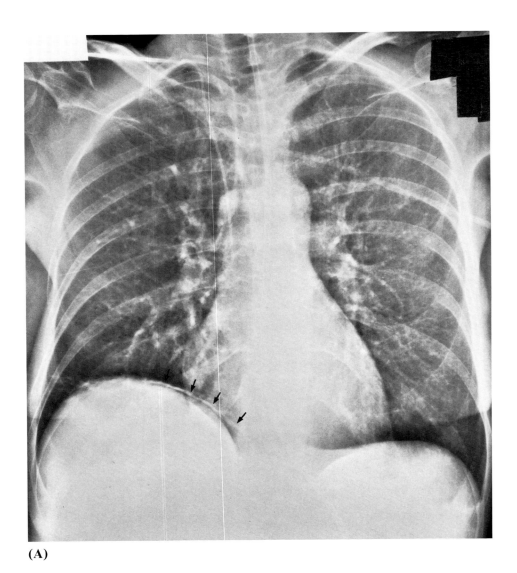

(A)

Fig. 3-26.   (A) Pneumothorax Under the Lung Base on an AP Film of a Supine Patient

Portable chest radiograph of a supine woman who had just had a right-sided central venous pressure line inserted. There is a thin rim of pneumothorax under the right lung. It can cause confusion since it simulates air under the diaphragm if the slightly thickened visceral pleural line (arrows) under the right lung is mistaken for a diaphragm. The problem was solved by repeating the film with the patient erect. The pneumothorax moved to the apex. If the patient had been unable to assume the erect position, a left lateral decubitus position would have been an acceptable alternative.

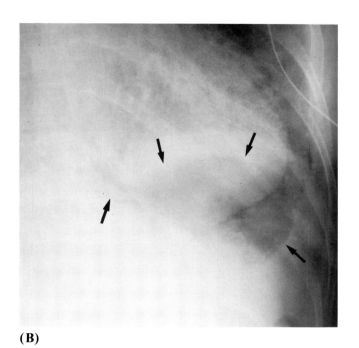

(B)

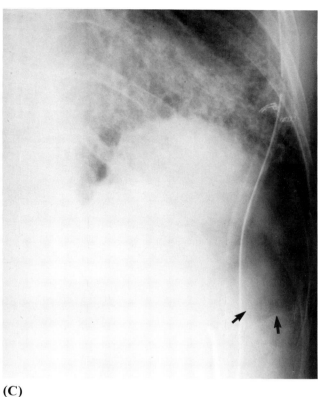

(C)

Fig. 3-26.   (B – D) Large Pneumothorax in the Caudal Pleural Space of a Patient on Positive-Pressure Ventilation

Series of coned views of the left upper quadrant of a young woman who was being treated with positive-pressure ventilation. Each view is taken from a chest film made in the AP projection with the patient supine.

   (B) An oval collection of gas is seen in the left upper quadrant. It is quite characteristic of air in the fundus of the stomach (arrows). Some air can be seen in the cardia of the stomach and the distal esophagus (medial arrow).

   (C) Film taken at a later date shows an oval zone of radiolucency (dark gray) projected over the left lower ribs laterally. It could be mistaken for a collection of gas in a high splenic flexure of the colon. However, it is a pneumothorax with air extending caudally as far as the limits of the lateral aspects of the pleural space permit (arrows). The patient had recently undergone lung biopsy, and a string of metallic staples is seen above the diaphragm at the biopsy site. A chest tube is present with its tip at the left base. *(Figure continues.)*

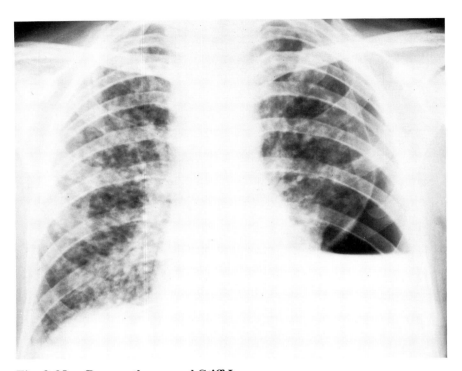

Fig. 3-28. Pneumothorax and Stiff Lungs

PA view of a patient with markedly abnormal lungs and a moderately large pneumothorax. The opaque area at the left base has a horizontal upper edge. This is a true meniscus in a hydropneumothorax.

The pleural line about the lateral aspects of the partially collapsed left lung is abnormally thick. The medial edge of the left scapula is projected over the partially collapsed lung.

Abnormal lungs may have markedly reduced compliance, and therefore one cannot use the absence of complete collapse as a sign indicating that a tension pneumothorax is not present. The recognition of tension pneumothorax in these cases may be delayed until there is a recognizable, fixed mediastinal shift, which is not present in this case.

The size of a pneumothorax often dictates treatment, and various methods of estimating quantity as a percentage of thoracic volume have been proposed. We ordinarily find subjective estimation (small, moderate, and large) adequate because most pneumothoraces that are easily detected (moderate and large) receive some type of tube drainage in our hospital. Most small, iatrogenic pneumothoraces (crescents of air a few millimeters thick) over the apex and axillary region do not receive immediate drainage. If clinical observation and 4-hour and 24-hour follow-up films show evidence of increase, then tube drainage is reconsidered. On the other hand, even small pneumothoraces may receive tube drainage if the patient is to be placed on mechanical ventilation.

R.W. Light[6] proposed the following method for determining the relative size of a pneumothorax, based upon the proposition that the volumes of the lung and the hemithorax are roughly proportional to the cube of their diameters:

1. Estimate the average diameter of the hemithorax, in centimeters, by measurement on the PA chest film.

2. Estimate the average diameter of residually expanded lung, in centimeters, from the same film.

3. Cube these diameters.
4. Then

$$\frac{(\text{Diameter of expanded lung})^3}{(\text{Diameter of hemithorax})^3} \times 100 = \% \text{ expansion present}$$

$$100 - \% \text{ expansion} = \% \text{ pneumothorax}.$$

The need to estimate variables 1 and 2 will cause the result to be imprecise; however, great precision is not required.

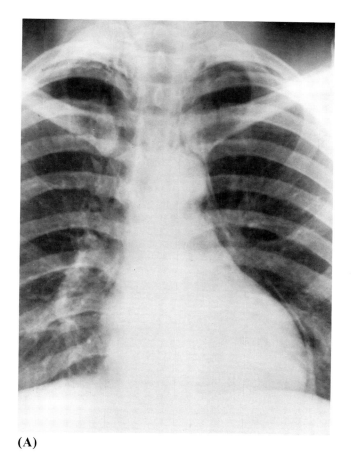

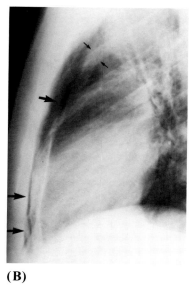

(A)

(B)

Fig. 3-29.   Pneumomediastinum

(A,B) This patient was admitted to the hosital after an episode of progressive substernal pain, which radiated into his neck following a bout of coughing. He had a history of a resolving upper respiratory infection over the preceding 7 days.

(A) On the PA film you can see the mediastinal pleura lifted off of the left side of the heart and extending above the aortic arch, where it is superimposed on the medial aspects of the left clavicle. In addition, you can see gray streaks radiating into the soft tissues of the neck.

(B) On lateral view you can see the air in the retrosternal portions of the mediastinum (arrows). An elliptical tongue of soft tissue, which probably represents residual thymus, is projected in front of the ascending aorta. These radiographic findings are characteristic of pneumomediastinum. Other than the bout of coughing, no precipitating event was uncovered. The patient was treated with codeine for control of pain and coughing and sent home the following day. (Courtesy of Drs. James J. McCort and Robert E. Mindelzun, San Jose, California.) *(Figure continues.)*

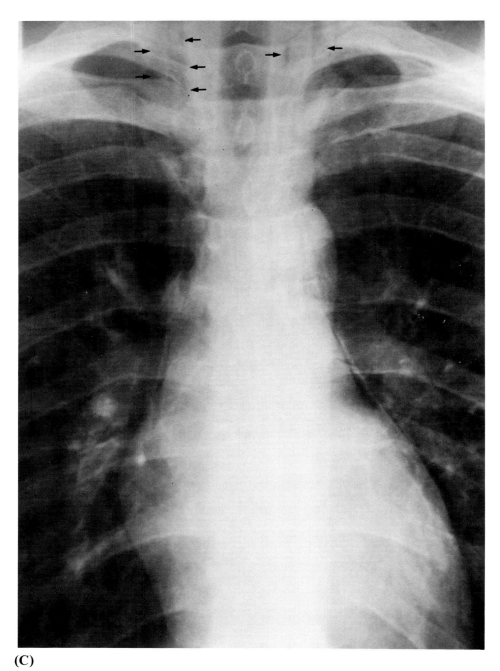

(C)

Fig. 3-29. *(Continued).* **(C) Pneumomediastinum**

This patient is a 20-year-old man who suffered from recurrent bouts of nausea and vomiting before developing severe substernal chest pain with breathing or with coughing. He also complained of dysphagia. There was a positive Hamman's sign on physical examination.

A linear opacity is seen extending from the upper portions of the left heart border, bridging the area of the main pulmonary artery, and extending up to and superimposing on the aortic arch. It is less than 2 mm thick. A similar linear opacity is seen on the right side, extending from the level of the upper aspect of the right atrium cephalad to at least the level of the upper aspect of the posterior fifth rib. In addition, however, there are gray streaks present within the soft tissues of the neck, indicating dissection of air into the soft tissues (arrows). The patient had an esophagram to rule out a perforated esophagus, and no perforation was found. The patient's signs and symptoms resolved spontaneously with conservative management. (Courtesy of Dr. James Vaudagna, Los Gatos, California.)

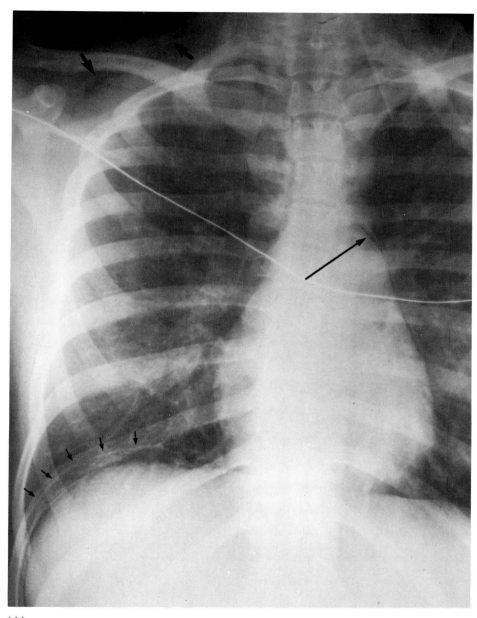

(A)

Fig. 3-30. Pneumomediastinum

There are streaks of air in the soft tissues of the neck and in the soft tissues projected above and below the right clavicle (short arrows). In addition, a very small crescent of air is seen separating a linear opacity from the pulmonary artery on the left side (long arrow). These findings are all consistent with pneumomediastinum. There is a curvilinear shadow that parallels the right hemidiaphragm (small arrows). This could be due to a small pneumothorax under the right middle lobe or to extrapleural dissection of air over the diaphragm in association with the pneumomediastinum. If the finding persisted in this location on films made with the patient erect or in the left lateral decubitus position, that would favor an extrapleural dissection. On the other hand, if the air moved with the change in the patient's position, that would indicate that it was air in a pneumothorax. (Courtesy of Drs. James J. McCort and Robert E. Mindelzun, San Jose, California.) *(Figure continues.)*

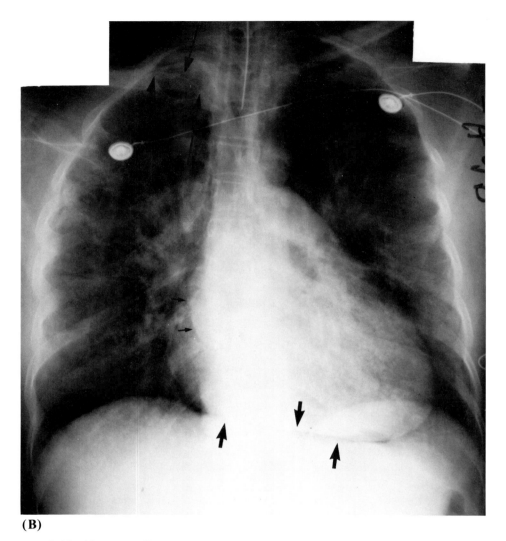

(B)

Fig. 3-30. *(Continued).* **(B) Pneumothorax and Pneumomediastinum**

Portable chest film of a woman who has developed a small right pneumothorax. The visceral pleura is seen as an arc bridging the posterior right second interspace (long arrows). She has also developed a pneumomediastinum, which is difficult to see on this reproduction except for a rather thick band of radiolucency that follows the contour of the inferior aspects of the heart (short arrows). This is a sign of pneumomediastinum, especially on films made with the patient supine. However, crescents of air projected along the inferior margins of the heart may also be present in patients who have pneumo-pericardium.

Incidentally the confluence of right pulmonary veins (small arrows) is frequently seen better on supine films than on upright views. *(Figure continues.)*

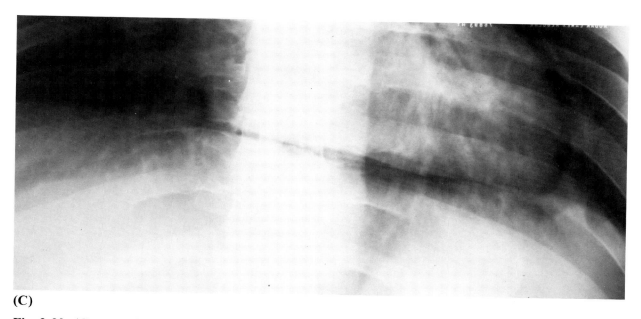

(C)

Fig. 3-30. *(Continued).*   **(C) Pneumomediastinum and Pneumopericardium**

Coned view of the lower chest and upper abdomen of a young man who had both a pneumopericardium and a pneumomediastinum. There is a striking dark gray streak produced by air between the diaphragm and the diaphragmatic surface of the heart. This may be seen in patients with pneumomediastinum or with pneumopericardium or in patients such as this one who have both (as confirmed by CT scan).

Air under the central tendon of the diaphragm from a pneumoperitoneum can produce a similar but not identical appearance. Nevertheless, if clinical doubt exists, a film in a left lateral decubitus position would serve to distinguish between these possibilities. (Courtesy of Drs. James J. McCort and Robert E. Mindelzun, San Jose, California.)

4

Localizing Pulmonary Lesions and Analyzing Pulmonary Collapse

LOBAR AND SEGMENTAL ANATOMY

Fissures Define Lobar Boundaries

Visualization of the three-dimensional relationships of the interlobar fissures is handicapped by the fact that, radiographically, we cannot actually see the fissures in their entirety. Therefore, it is difficult to appreciate their curved and undulating character. Reconstructing their course by integrating the images seen on PA and lateral chest films and CT cross sections greatly assists our understanding, however.

The pleural boundaries of the interlobar fissures frequently are projected as thin line shadows on chest films. For the sake of brevity we have simply referred to these pleural boundaries as the fissures themselves. More often than not the entire length of a fissure is not seen since only those portions that present tangentially to the x-ray beam produce a linear image. Even total absence of the image of any fissure can be normal.

Minor (Horizontal) Fissure

Anatomically, the minor (horizontal) interlobar fissure marks the boundary between the anterior portions of the right upper lobe and the lateral and medial segments of the right middle lobe.

On a PA chest film the minor interlobar fissure can be seen as a single line or occasionally a double line shadow extending laterally from about the level of the middle of the right hilum to the lateral chest wall. Its course may be parallel to the floor, or it may deviate a few degrees from the horizontal. It commonly has a caudal slope laterally. Deviations from the horizontal, however, may indeed be abnormal if they are departures from positions seen on previous films. Therefore, old films can be valuable for comparison in doubtful cases.

In the lateral view the minor interlobar fissure extends anteriorly from the level of the hilum to the anterior chest wall; modest bowing and caudal deviations from the horizontal course are common. When the right major (oblique) fissure is also visible on the lateral view, the minor fissure intersects it in the region of the hilum. The lateral end of the minor fissure extends behind the hilum and behind the medial intersect with the major fissure, although this portion is not always visible. When the lateral segment of the right middle lobe is large, the minor fissure may extend posteriorly as far as the spine.

It is common for the minor fissure to be incomplete, and it is common for it not to be seen on chest films whether complete or not.

Major (Oblique) Fissure

The right major fissure separates the right lower lobe from the right upper and middle lobes; the left major fissure separates the left lower lobe from the left upper lobe.

The major interlobar fissures may present as line shadows on the lateral view of the chest. From a high position posteriorly (approximately the level of the fifth rib on the right and the fourth rib on the left), their course is obliquely inferior. Each passes through or below the region of the hilum and reaches its respective hemidiaphragm along its anterior third. Although variations occur with respect to both the highest point of origin and the exact point of intersection of either major fissure with its corresponding hemidiaphragm, neither the right nor the left major fissure reaches the anterior chest wall normally. Unless you can clearly identify the intersection of the major fissure with a specific hemidiaphragm on the lateral view, you will not be able to tell the right from the left with accuracy. In general, however, the right major interlobar fissure reaches the diaphragm anterior to the position of the left major interlobar fissure. The major fissures may be projected as relatively straight lines or may be slightly bowed. Anatomically these fissures are not flat sheets from medial to lateral, but have a slightly undulating course, with segments showing convex arcs anteriorly or posteriorly.

It is common for the major fissures to be incomplete.[17] Much less frequently they are totally absent. The fact that fissures are not seen radiographically, however, cannot be taken as evidence of their anatomic absence. When they are oriented so that they do not present an adequate segment tangential to the x-ray beam, they will not produce a linear image. Occasionally, pleural fat or pleural thickening adjacent to the major fissure may present a sufficient tangent to the x-ray beam to allow superolateral portions of the fissure to be seen as a curved edge image on a PA view of the chest (see Fig. 4-28). Less commonly, a lateral arc may be seen as a line even in the normal individual.[16]

Major fissures or segments thereof may also be seen on the PA view when they have changed their orientation to the beam as a consequence of reduction in volume of adjacent lobes.

Anomalous Fissures

A variety of anomalous fissures may be found both radiographically and in lung specimens. Among the more common are the inferior accessory fissures, which separate the medial basal segment of the lower lobe from the remainder of the basilar segments; the superior acces-

sory fissure, which separates the superior segment of the lower lobes from the basilar segments; and the azygos lobe fissure, which has been previously described. In addition, there are a variety of short fissures, which may occur in apparently random fashion in individual lung specimens.

In infants and young children a near-vertical fissure line may be seen far laterally in the lower chest. It usually represents the lower segment of the major fissure rather than a true anomaly.

The line shadows of the fissures are important chest film images because they are helpful in localizing focal pulmonary lesions, in evaluating changes of lobar volumes, and in evaluating the extent of pleural abnormalities.

Appearance of Fissures on Computed Tomography

On CT scans the minor and major interlobar fissures can be recognized, in all but a small percentage of people, if the interval between scan levels is no more than 1.0 cm. The position of the minor interlobar fissure is inferred to be within a roughly triangular zone of marked diminution in peripheral vessels in the anterior portion of the right lung slightly above the level of origin of the right middle lobe bronchus[9] (Fig. 4-2).

The major fissure is also usually marked by a thin zone of diminished vascularity, and occasionally as a line or thin band of soft tissue density over at least part of its course.[12] At its cephalad level (higher on the left than on the right) it intersects with a vertebra medially and passes obliquely laterally and posteriorly to reach the chest wall. At successive caudal levels the image of the fissure or the zone of hypovascularity moves anteriorly, with its lateral edge moving more anteriorly than its medial margin (Figs. 4-1 and 4-3). Thus, at its caudal end it is often seen to have an obliquity opposite that seen cephalad, that is, with its lateral margin more anteriorly positioned than its medial margin. On the right side, however, the lateral aspect of the major fissure may remain slightly posterior to its medial end even caudally. When thin (e.g., 1.5 mm) slices are obtained, the fissures can be seen as actual linear images more often than is the case when 1.0-cm-thick slices are obtained (Fig. 4-2).

The azygos fissure presents a prominent and easily recognized image on the CT scan. Because of its more vertical orientation it projects as a line or thin soft tissue band. Its course may also be variable depending on how far laterally it begins its descent through the lung (see Ch. 3).

The inferior pulmonary ligaments may also appear as lines or bands along their supradiaphragmatic course.

TABLE 4-1. Bronchial Segments

Nomenclature[a]	Boyden's Numbering
Right upper lobe	
Apical segment	B_1
Anterior segment	B_2
Posterior segment	B_3
Middle lobe	
Lateral segment	B_4
Medial segment	B_5
Right lower lobe	
Superior segment	B_6
Medical basal segment	B_7
Anterior basal segment	B_8
Lateral basal segment	B_9
Posterior basal segment	B_{10}
Left upper lobe	
Apicoposterior segment	B_{1-3}
Anterior segment	B_2
Lingula	
Superior segment	B_4
Inferior segment	B_5
Left lower lobe	
Superior segment	B_6
Anteromedial basal	B_{7-8}
Lateral basal	B_9
Posterior basal	B_{10}

[a] Nomenclature of the 1955 International Anatomy Congress.

PULMONARY SEGMENTS

The modest effort required to learn the segmental anatomy of the lungs is worthwhile, since understanding the location of pulmonary lesions is useful in rank-ordering differential diagnoses and in communicating radiographic findings to others involved in the patient's care. Tedious, deliberate memorization can be avoided by repeated reference to anatomic guides when attempting to localize all focal lesions encountered in your work. Gradually, the learning task will thus be accomplished in a more challenging manner.

Table 4-1 is a listing of a common nomenclature of the pulmonary segments. In general, the names indicate the position of the segments in the hemithorax. In addition, a numbering system devised by Boyden and associates[2] is shown.

Understanding of pulmonary anatomy will be enhanced by visits to the anatomy and pathology laboratories and the surgical suites to examine specimens in three dimensions. To quote from Boyden:[2]

Whoever wishes to understand the structure of the lung—be he surgeon, radiologist, bronchoscopist, internist, or medical student—must first dissect the lungs. Then he may carry this knowledge to other disciplines and use other techniques. Without this first-hand acquaintance with the specimen, he flounders in a one dimensional field of x-rays and diagrams.

The segments and lobes of the lung have complex shapes, multiple surfaces, and significant interindividual variability.[1,2] Again quoting from Boyden:

In order to analyze the structure of organs that are as complicated as the lungs, it is necessary to establish criteria by which one may judge variations. For any given segmental or subsegmental bronchus, two such criteria are available: first, the usual point of its origin on the bronchial tree: second, the territory usually ventilated by it. These facts establish the prevailing pattern. The latter is not a matter of opinion, but a matter of statistics—the result of examining large numbers of specimens.

Further on he says:

Curiously enough, lungs that are made up wholly of prevailing patterns are seldom encountered for a variation in even one zone necessarily modifies the development of adjacent segments. . . . For purposes of instruction, therefore, it has become necessary to create a hypothetical pair of lungs that will combine the prevailing patterns of all the principal bronchi.[2]

Although segmental anatomy is relatively constant, subsegmental anatomy is awesomely variable, and it is largely the subsegmental variations that determine the size of a given segment. Go to your medical library and pick out three or four anatomy texts that show the segmental anatomy of the lungs. Commonly they show fixed inflated specimens whose segments have been selectively injected with colored gelatin so that each segment is dyed a different color. Line these books up on a counter and note the definite differences in the size of the segments from specimen to specimen, and how variable are the surface distributions of the segments anteriorly, posteriorly, laterally, and medially. The anatomy is complicated by the fact that segments are irregular, and therefore may be larger medially than laterally or vice versa.

In spite of these variations, however, radiographically you can locate a lesion within a specific segment much of the time if you can see the lesion in at least two different planes. However, at times small nodular lesions may be located in positions that do not permit a realistic or reliable choice between two adjacent segments, and occasionally even between two lobes.

Frequently neither diagnosis nor treatment depends on precise localization of a lesion; in such cases inordinate or expensive studies in an attempt to achieve precision are unwarranted. Even when considering needle aspiration of a focal lesion it is far more important to be able to localize the lesion fluoroscopically than to name the segment in which it is located. However, when a surgeon is willing to resect a segment or lobe for a lesion that cannot be palpated at thoracotomy (an uncommon event in my experience), precise, reliable preoperative localization is mandatory and warrants maximum effort. The same is true for those situations where determining the presence of disease in more than one lobe, or a lesion that extends across a fissure, would materially alter treatment planning. Judicious use of fluoroscopy and oblique projections can solve localization problems in cases that appear equivocal on the routine views. Tomograms or CT scans may also be used for accurate localization of focal lesions. Bronchography, on the other hand, is rarely necessary for this purpose alone, but would also allow for precise localization in most patients.

Figs. 4-4 through 4-10 present a series of illustrations in which pulmonary lesions are localized to specific lobar and segmental distributions.

AXILLARY SEGMENTAL DISTRIBUTION

Occasionally on a PA view you will see a wedge-shaped zone of consolidation extending from the hilum toward the axilla. On the lateral view the consolidation extends anteriorly from the hilum, just above the level of the minor interlobar fissure, or posterosuperiorly in a distribution superior to the upper portion of the major interlobar fissure, but may not reach the chest wall and may appear more dense centrally. These represent so-called axillary segmental distributions (Figs. 4-5 and 4-6). In most people the axillary portions of an upper lobe are supplied by a subsegmental branch of the anterior segment or of the posterior segment, or both.

THE SILHOUETTE SIGN

Certain zones of consolidation or atelectasis, even when seen only in one plane, can be localized to lobes or segments by virtue of the fact that they obscure marginal contours of portions of the cardiomediastinal silhouette. This concept has been popularized by Felson, who called it "the silhouette sign." [5] It is commonly applied to loss of sharp definition of the right heart border from consolidation or atelectasis in the adjacent right middle lobe (Fig. 4-7). It is also commonly used to infer the presence of such abnormalities in the lingula of the left upper lobe due to loss of definition of part of the left heart border. As Felson has pointed out, the silhouette sign can also be used to infer the presence of disease in other pulmonary segments, such as in the anterior segment of the right upper lobe when an area of consolidation obliterates the

mediastinal pleura-lung interface in the region of the superior vena cava, or in the posterior subsegment of the apical posterior segment of the left upper lobe when a zone of consolidation obliterates the descending limb of the aortic arch. You can think of other examples.

This concept has been enormously useful, and yet, like other good concepts, can be abused when applied without thought. For example, if the right middle lobe becomes severely collapsed and the adjacent portions of either the upper or lower lobe overexpand to fill the space, an air-water interface can be reestablished between the lung and the right heart border sufficient to produce a sharply defined image on film. When there is consolidation of the lateral segment of the middle lobe but sparing of the medial segment, the right heart border interface with lung can also be preserved (Fig. 4-8). As Felson has also pointed out, in a small (approximately 4 percent) but significant number of cases portions of the right heart border may be obscured even in the absence of a lung lesion or thoracic deformity. This is in addition to those cases of demonstrable pectus excavatum where the thoracic deformity distorts the lung-mediastinum relationship so that the right heart border is not seen sharply (Fig. 4-9).

Fortunately, problems in evaluating the significance of loss of portions of the heart borders can be resolved by obtaining an AP film of the chest with the subject in the lordotic position, or with the tube tilted off the horizontal toward the head and the film appropriately positioned vertically to intercept the beam. Atelectasis in the right middle lobe or in the lingula that is extraordinarily difficult to confirm on PA views, and occasionally even on lateral views, may be rendered obvious by lordotic positioning (Fig. 4-10). The effect of this change in position essentially is to increase the length of the water absorber (the collapsed portion of lung) traversed by the beam. It can be thought of as analogous to seeing a vessel end-on. In addition, this positioning aligns portions of either the minor or the major fissure, or both, tangential to the beam so that the zone of atelectasis has sharp margins.

OBFUSCATING FACTORS

All of the above points concerning localization assume that one is dealing with a "nonviolated" chest—one that has not been operated on, therapeutically irradiated, or scarred from chronic cicatrizing pulmonary disease or previous trauma. Under these circumstances significant spatial rearrangements of segments and lobes can occur, so that the usual anatomic configurations no longer apply. Localization of lesions in lungs with distorted architecture is most demanding, and frequently segmental localization in these lungs is not feasible.

Lobar localization is usually still possible when the inter-lobar fissures are visible, and obviously lobar localization is no problem when only one lobe of a lung remains in place.

Fortunately, the presence of these obfuscating factors can almost always be revealed by close study of the film, even though the precise anatomic distortion cannot be accurately predicted (Fig. 4-11).

When lesions are situated in the region of the junction between two segments, in one view or the other, both segments have to be considered as possible locations. Furthermore, since pulmonary segments vary in size from person to person, you may be left with a choice between two adjacent segments that cannot be resolved from radiographs.

When your analysis is limited to a single PA projection, it may not be possible to accurately place focal lesions in even a lobar distribution. Significant portions of the upper and lower lobes may be superimposed on one another on both the right and left, and the right middle lobe is totally superimposed on the right lower lobe on a PA view. Even when both PA and lateral views are available for analysis, the lesion in question may only be clearly identified on one of the two views. Again under these circumstances, accurate segmental localization may not be possible without using the other techniques mentioned.

CONSOLIDATION (OPACIFICATION) VERSUS ATELECTASIS (COLLAPSE)

Consolidation

The terms "consolidation" and "opacification" will be used to refer to portions of lung that appear opaque. Modifiers such as "homogeneous" or "inhomogeneous" may be used to indicate that the opacification is fairly uniform and complete in the involved zone (homogeneous) or that there are interspersed areas of radiolucency due to relatively uninvolved acini, to bronchiolectasis, or even to bronchiectasis or emphysema or cavitation (inhomogeneous). As noted in Chapter 2, the term "consolidation," as used here, does not imply a specific pathology.

Atelectasis

The term "atelectasis," when applied to the lung, implies loss of volume. Loss of volume can occur without associated consolidation and then is often difficult to recognize. Hilar displacement, shift in the position of interlobar fissures or shift of the mediastinum, crowding of vessels in the involved area, elevation of the diaphragm, and other signs of volume compensation must be recognized before the situation can be appreciated. When fissures are not visible, the atelectasis often goes unrecognized unless large amounts of lung are involved. "Collapse" indicates maximum volume loss in a segment, lobe, or entire lung.

Atelectasis and Consolidation

Fortunately, in most instances of segmental and lobar atelectasis there is an element of consolidation. This produces a more easily recognized signal by increasing the tissue density of the involved lung to a much greater degree than does atelectasis alone. Atelectasis, however, is also relative in that the loss of volume may be minimal, moderate, or marked. For example, in many cases of lobar pneumonia there is some loss of volume of the involved lobe, but it is minor in comparison to the magnitude of consolidation (Fig. 4-7).

In some cases of bronchial obstruction the degree of atelectasis is marked, and the volume opacified therefore small; in others, the main finding is opacification, with little or no reduction in volume. You cannot determine from its radiographic appearance whether a zone of atelectasis and consolidation is infected or not (see Fig. 4-20C to E). Chronic infection or inflammation often causes collapse and consolidation,[19] but there are many other causes.

Conversion of Line Shadows of Fissures to Edge Shadows

When zones of consolidation or atelectasis extend to a pulmonary fissure, the pleural boundaries of the fissure are often converted from line shadows to edge shadows (Fig. 4-12). Therefore, a working rule is: Whenever you see a long, relatively sharp edge, think of the possibility of atelectatic or consolidated lung against an interlobar fissure. Extrapleural masses or fluid loculated against the chest wall or in fissures may also cause long edges to become visible at the pleural interface between the mass or fluid collection and the adjacent lung. Hence we can modify the working rule to read: Whenever you see long, relatively sharp edges, think of pleural surfaces. In addition, skin folds or deformities of soft tissues on the surface of the chest wall interface with the air in the room; when projected in tangent they cast relatively sharp edge shadows on the chest films (see Fig. 4-6B). Thus, we can modify the rule again: Whenever you see long, relatively sharp edges, think of pleural surfaces or skin folds or superficial masses on the chest wall.

Movements of Lung Associated With Reduction in Volume

The lung is normally free in the thorax except where it is tethered to the mediastinum by vessels and bronchi that pass from the mediastinum into the lung through the anatomic hilum. In addition, there is a variable degree of tethering to the mediastinum and the diaphragm by the inferior pulmonary ligaments.

The radiology of lobar and segmental atelectasis has been studied extensively.[11,13,14,15] When lobes of the lung collapse acutely or subacutely, they move in a complex fashion that can be broken down into three main vectors. One vector is toward the tether (i.e., medially). Another can be likened to the closing of a fan with the fulcrum at the hilum. A third consists of a shift posteroinferiorly for lower lobe collapse (Fig. 4-13) and anterosuperiorly for upper lobe collapse on either side. Because the lingula is an intrinsic part of the left upper lobe there is a longer retrosternal image of atelectasis and consolidation for the left upper lobe than for the right (Figs. 4-14 and 4-15). The middle lobe collapses in a manner that might be expected from its location between the upper and lower lobes. Frequently, its volume loss on lateral view is best described as a closing of a fan with the fulcrum at the hilum (Figs. 4-7, 4-8, 4-10, and 4-16). The position and visibility of hilar vessels and the position of major bronchi can also be seen to change in a predictable fashion when there is lobar atelectasis (Figs. 4-17 and 4-18).

So long as the pleural space remains intact — that is, there is no concurrent pneumothorax or hydrothorax — the collapsing lobes or segments continue to occupy some portion of the inner aspects of the chest wall. They simply come to occupy smaller and smaller areas of the chest wall as the reduction in volume becomes more pronounced. Occasionally when the right middle lobe is severely collapsed, it may retract from the lateral chest wall, and the upper and lower lobes come into contact around the margins of the retracted middle lobe (Fig. 4.15-D). When there is also pneumothorax or hydrothorax, the atelectatic lung may retract toward its hilum and leave the chest wall entirely.

Compensating Adjustments

Variations in the radiographic appearance of collapsed lobes are greatly influenced by the degree of volume loss and the magnitude of hyperexpansion (compensatory emphysema) in the adjacent lung. The latter also depends on the compliance of the expanding portions of the lung. As part of a lung becomes reduced in volume, the adjacent hyperexpanded portions influence the shape and position of the collapsed lobes or segments.

The mobility of collapsed lobes depends in part on the completeness of interlobar fissures. Other volume-compensating mechanisms such as mediastinal shift, diaphragm elevation, and rib approximation are quite variable and depend on the relative compliance of these compensating structures, which in turn seems to depend in part on the age of the patient (Figs. 4-19 and 4-20).

Compensatory overexpansion of lung is seen as an increase in film density (increased darkness on the gray-black spectrum) accompanied by a decrease in the number of small vessels per square centimeter of film in comparison to areas of normal lung (Figs. 4-13, 4-19, and 4-20). The normal complement of vessels is simply distributed over the greater volume of the hyperexpanding lobe or lobes.

Compensatory overexpansion of lung usually can be distinguished from a similar radiographic appearance consequent to air trapping by obtaining a film of the patient during expiration. Air can be expelled from the compensating lobe, since its bronchus is open. Hence the air-water ratio will be decreased, and that portion of lung will be lighter gray on the expiratory film than on the inspiratory film. In cases of air trapping, however, the supplying bronchus is not normal, and air is not rapidly expelled on expiration. The obstructed lung will appear darker, in comparison to normally functioning lung, on end-expiratory films.

The radiographic signs of compensatory overexpansion and of air trapping are often subtle but can be recognized more easily by increasing your viewing distance from the film to about 6 feet or by using a minifying lens, which accomplishes the same effect.

Rarely, torsion of the collapsed lobe may occur and produce unusual radiographic appearances. These have been described by Felson.[6]

When portions of lung have become scarred from previous infection such as chronic tuberculosis, or from radiation treatment or other cause of inflammatory scarring or neoplastic infiltration, they become less compliant. Should collapsing forces later develop in these abnormal portions of the lung, the usual patterns of lobar and segmental collapse are often altered (see Fig. 4-11). This will also be true when pleural adhesions cause portions of the lungs to remain fixed adjacent to the chest wall, so that the usual movements accompanying the reduction in volume are modified.

Collapse Around a Mass

Whenever there is a relatively noncompliant mass — most commonly neoplasm, uncommonly an inflammatory mass — within an atelectatic lobe, the shape of the edge adjacent to the mass may remain as a bulge convex toward adjacent aerated lung. This concept has been popularized as the "S" sign of Golden[8] (see Figs. 4-14 and 4-15).

Possible Confusion With Pleural Effusion or Pleural Thickening

At times it may be challenging to distinguish lower lobe collapse from pleural effusion. Either may cause increased opacity at the base, with loss of definition of the adjacent hemidiaphragm (Figs. 4-20D and 4-21).

Usually the distinction between pleural effusion and lower lobe atelectasis can be made by careful evaluation of the position of the lower lobe bronchus. When atelectasis is the sole component of the basilar abnormality, the lower lobe bronchus moves medially in relation to its usual position and has a more vertical inclination. This also occurs when the lobar collapse is the dominant component of the basilar abnormality accompanied by a small effusion (Figs. 4-22 and 4-23). The images of larger central vessels are lost within the consolidated, collapsed lung, and often air bronchograms can be seen.

Lower Lobe Atelectasis and Pleural Effusion

Frequently, atelectasis of basilar segments and pleural effusion coexist (Fig. 4-23). When pleural effusion is layered over the diaphragm, the costophrenic angles may be deceptively lacking in the usual telltale clues that indicate its presence.

However, when the pleural effusion is a dominant component, the lower lobe bronchus does not move medially since the pleural fluid surrounds the lung base, occupies the space between the lung and the paraspinal soft tissues, and prevents the usual medial shift of the collapsing basilar segments. If there is a large mass, (e.g., primary neoplasm or adenopathy) about the proximal lower lobe bronchus, medial shift of the bronchus may be prevented even when no significant pleural effusion is present (Fig. 4-24). Whenever there is confusion as to whether atelectasis or pleural effusion is the dominant factor causing an opacity, a lateral decubitus view can be obtained for further analysis.

Rarely a severely collapsed upper lobe may be draped over the hyperexpanded superior segment of a lower lobe, simulating pleural thickening or encapsuated fluid in the apex of the involved side.[15]

MULTILOBAR COLLAPSE

Just as collapse of a single lobe can be recognized because of differences in tissue density, spatial rearrangement, fissural displacement, and loss of usual marginal anatomical contours, so can multilobar collapse. Obstruction of the bronchus intermedius, for example, can cause atelectasis of both the right middle and lower lobes

(Fig. 4-20A and B). Consolidation of adjacent lobes due to pneumonia may also be accompanied by loss of volume and mimic obstructive atelectasis (Fig. 4-20C to E). Atelectasis or consolidation of segments or lobes that do not have a common parent bronchus also may result from multiple sites of obstruction or multiple sites of intrinsic alteration of lung structure (see Figs. 4-12 and 4-15).

Atelectasis of an entire lung is accompanied by signs of reduced volume of the involved hemithorax (Fig. 4-25) except when there is also a large volume of pleural fluid or a combination of mass and pleural fluid. See Chapter 3 for a discussion of the opaque hemithorax.

CAUSES OF PULMONARY COLLAPSE

Recognition of lobar or segmental collapse is an important function of chest roentgenography. Once the reduction in volume is recognized, plans can be formulated for establishing its cause.

There are three basic causes of segmental, lobar, or multilobar collapse: compression-relaxation forces, bronchial obstruction, and intrinsic alteration of lung structure.

Compression-Relaxation

Whenever moderate to large volumes of pleural fluid or, much less commonly, pleural or extrapleural masses are present, adjacent lung is reduced in volume. This is so not only because no two things can occupy the same space, but also because there frequently is alteration of ventilatory function of lung adjacent to regions of pleural disease. Likewise, when moderate to large volumes of pneumothorax are present, there will be reduction in volume of adjacent lung. Some think of this association as a consequence of compression forces, whereas others feel that relaxation forces are functionally responsible. That is, the lung is free of the negative pleural pressure forces that normally keep it in close juxtaposition to the chest wall, and therefore the lung responds to its inherent elastic recoil properties by becoming smaller. Extensive cellular infiltration of the interstitium of the lung may sometimes be responsible for collapse of adjacent alveoli; this phenomenon can also be considered as a form of compression atelectasis or as an intrinsic alteration of lung structure.

Bronchial Obstruction

Bronchial obstruction is most commonly intrinsic, due to mucous plugging, neoplasm, foreign body inhalation, or inflammatory stricture. Bronchial obstruction may also be extrinsic, resulting from enlarged lymph nodes or pressure from adjacent masses or even an enlarged heart.

Even high-grade bronchial obstruction does not always lead to zones of total collapse. Collateral ventilation[3] between adjacent lung segments, through the pores of Kohn or the canals of Lambert, is sufficient to prevent collapse. Where interlobar fissures are incomplete, this collateral air flow may also occur between adjacent segments of different lobes.

Collateral ventilation associated with bronchial obstruction results in air trapping and is often more easily detected on films made in expiration, just as in patients with the "ball-valve" type bronchial obstruction. In fact, when segmental or lobar bronchi are obstructed, collateral ventilation of the obstructed segments may mask the effects of the bronchial obstruction on inspiratory films.

When edema, inflammatory exudate, or retained secretions fill the bronchi and alveoli and prevent collateral ventilation, the obstructed zone becomes opaque and more easily recognized. The term "obstructive pneumonitis" could be applied but should not be taken to imply that microorganisms also have to be present. In some cases microorganisms are present, and the patient also may have clinical signs and symptoms of infection. In other cases, radiographically indistinguishable from these, there are neither microorganisms present nor any clinical signs of concomitant infection. There may be an infiltrate of lipid-laden macrophages and cholesterol, which produces a "golden pneumonia," so-called because of its appearance on gross examination.

Mucous Plugging

Although mucous plugging per se may be the cause of atelectasis in patients with asthma or cystic fibrosis, in the more common case of the postoperative patient with atelectasis, invoking mucous plugging as the cause is probably an oversimplification. It is likely that such an explanation does not properly take into account the role of surfactant function and replenishment in the patient who will not or cannot breathe deeply.

Neoplasm

Either benign or malignant neoplasms may cause bronchial obstruction (see Ch. 6); the latter are by far the more common cause. An endobronchial neoplasm does not have to obstruct the lumen to cause atelectasis. There need be only a sufficient interruption of mucosal ciliary action due to mucosal or submucosal spread of tumor to interfere with the drainage function of the involved bronchus. The presence of visible air bronchograms

within a collapsed lobe or segment does not eliminate obstructing neoplasm from consideration as cause of the collapse.

Often, bronchial obstruction by neoplasm is due to primary carcinoma of the lung involving a major bronchus. All histopathologic varieties of carcinoma may do so, although squamous cell carcinoma is the most common. Metastases to major bronchi from extrathoracic primary tumors may cause radiographic appearances indistinguishable from those of primary bronchogenic carcinoma. Hodgkin's disease and non-Hodgkin's lymphomas may also cause endobronchial lesions and obstruction (see Ch. 6). Patients with bronchial adenomas frequently present clinically with an obstructive pneumonitis.

Benign neoplasms composed of any tissue found in the lungs (fibroma, lipoma, chondroma, etc.) and their sarcomatous counterparts rarely may cause bronchial obstruction. Rarely, endobronchial sarcoid lesions achieve sufficient size to behave like neoplasms and obstruct major bronchi.

Foreign Bodies

Aspirated foreign bodies of many types may cause obstruction of main, lobar, segmental, or subsegmental bronchi. Infants, children, and adults with impaired sensorium or impaired mentation are most commonly afflicted. Aspiration of peanuts or other nut fragments is a serious cause of atelectasis or obstructive air trapping in very young children.

Inflammatory Stricture

Bronchial obstruction due to inflammatory stricture is now an uncommon cause of atelectasis in western societies. However, in the years when tuberculosis was prevalent, inflammatory strictures consequent to endobronchial tuberculosis were among the common causes of atelectasis. Endobronchial tuberculosis still occurs in Western societies, but it is now quite uncommon as a cause of atelectasis. Other forms of pulmonary infection cause bronchial stenosis still more rarely.

Traumatic bronchial tears may go undiagnosed and untreated. As healing occurs, variable degrees of stricture and inflammatory bronchial stenosis take place even in the absence of infection. This can cause atelectasis of lung peripheral to the involved bronchus, which can be successfully corrected long after the event (see Ch. 11). However, when chronic infection occurs in the obstructed lung, bronchiectasis follows, and lung function usually cannot be restored by correction of the bronchial stenosis.

Broncholithiasis

Uncommonly, calcified peribronchial lymph nodes may erode into adjacent major bronchi, causing coughing, expectoration of particulate matter, and frequently hemoptysis. Consolidation and varying degrees of atelectasis of the involved lobe may be seen as a result of bronchial obstruction or aspiration of blood. Rarely a metallic foreign body (e.g., shrapnel) that has been lodged in the lung for years can erode into a bronchus and cause a similar clinical event.

Extrinsic Bronchial Obstruction and Right Middle Lobe Syndrome

Right middle lobe collapse due to causes other than endobronchial obstruction has been referred to as the right middle lobe syndrome. Its pathogenesis has been ascribed to extrinsic bronchial obstruction due to pressure from enlarged, inflamed lymph nodes, usually caused by tuberculous adenopathy. However, there have been patients in whom chronic right middle lobe consolidation with varying degrees of reduced volume has been caused by neither intrinsic nor extrinsic major bronchial obstruction.[19] In these patients, resection of the involved lobe has resulted in apparent clinical relief of symptoms. Pathologic study showed changes of nonspecific chronic inflammation not associated with obstruction of the lobar bronchus.

In some patients with massive hilar and mediastinal adenopathy due to malignant lymphoma or to metastases, there is associated atelectasis due to extrinsic bronchial involvement.

Congenital Anomalies

Bronchial atresia, lobar agenesis, pulmonary sequestration[20] (Fig. 4-26), and other congenital anomalies are not always diagnosed in infancy or childhood. Even in adults these lesions may remain silent and only be discovered incidentally, or they may cause nonspecific symptoms related to infection or bronchial inflammation. They are mentioned here because part of their radiographic spectrum includes changes similar to those of lung consolidation with loss of volume.

Intrinsic Alteration of Lung Structure

The term "intrinsic alteration of lung structure" is used to pool conceptually all of those cases in which reduction of volume is due to scarring of lung from chronic infection (particularly tuberculosis; see Fig. 4-11), repeated episodes of infection such as may occur with bronchiectasis (Figs. 4-21 and 4-27), postirradiation reaction of lung that has received high doses of therapeutic x-irradiation (Fig. 4-28), or infiltration of lung by neoplasm, granulomatous tissue, or fibrous tissue from any cause. Once again, the role surfactant deficiency plays in the collapse of these structurally altered lung zones is probably underestimated.

SPECIAL TYPES OF ATELECTASIS

Trapped Lung or Rounded Atelectasis

Atelectatic, consolidated lung may assume a rounded and masslike configuration about the periphery of the lung, usually but not exclusively posteriorly in a lower lobe. Invariably there are stigmata of pleural thickening present, and theoretically the atelectasis is due to the trapping of a portion of the lung by a zone of chronic pleuritis.[10,22] The roentgenographic diagnosis depends on recognition of the rounded mass immediately adjacent to a large zone of pleural thickening and the demonstration of a curved band shadow, composed of vessels and bronchi, which converges upon and enters the rounded consolidation along its lower margins or occasionally its upper pole (Fig. 4-29). Lateral tomograms are especially helpful in identifying this typical tail of involved vessels and bronchi when they are not clearly seen on lateral chest films. CT scans also can be used to identify these lesions.

Peripheral Atelectasis (Plate Atelectasis, Subsegmental Atelectasis, Discoid Atelectasis)

Frequently, opaque bands varying in number, width, and length are seen on chest films of patients with a wide spectrum of pulmonary signs and symptoms or with no pulmonary signs or symptoms at all. Usually the bands are seen at the lung bases — in the lower lobes, the right middle lobe, or the lingula — and are more or less horizontal in course. Occasionally, however, they are oblique or near-vertical and bear no resemblance to expected anatomic segments. They may be unilateral or bilateral.[21,23,24] Frequently they are transient or may be seen repeatedly at follow-up examination in the same patient at both short and long intervals. Although seen in the same region from film to film, they often are sufficiently (although subtly) different in appearance to make one believe that they are not truly stable but rather fluctuating (Fig. 4-30). In other cases the bands are clearly in different locations on follow-up films, whereas in still others they are absent at follow-up. Therefore, the age, the stability, and frequently the clinical significance of these bands cannot be predicted from their appearance on any isolated chest roentgenogram. They have been designated "Fleischner lines" after the radiologist who described them as zones of plate atelectasis.[7]

Studies of inflated, fixed, sliced, and radiographed lungs at postmortem have shown lesions composed of sheets of peripheral atelectasis that reached the visceral pleura, which was invaginated focally.[24] Histopathologically the lesions consisted of collapsed alveoli (atelectasis) alone, or of atelectasis with edema or with pneumonia. Neither large nor small bronchi were seen to be obstructed. In the postmortem cases studied there was a high incidence of pulmonary embolism (6 of 10 cases) but no indication that the atelectatic bands themselves were due to pulmonary infarcts. Simon reported one case where a thrombosed artery surrounded by inflammation accounted for a "line shadow" seen on a chest film and proposed that line shadows were pulmonary infarcts.[21] In the study by Westcott and Cole[24] no thrombosed vessels were felt to account for the atelectatic bands, nor did the bands have the histopathologic characteristics of pulmonary infarcts.

It seems likely that bands of peripheral atelectasis occur in association with hypoventilation from many different causes, including congestive heart failure, pulmonary embolism, postoperative state (especially after upper abdominal surgery), obesity, and diaphragmatic dysfunction. In themselves the atelectatic bands are nonspecific. Their importance may be as indications that hypoventilation is, or has recently been, occurring.

Studies of hypoxemia in postoperative patients suggest that venous shunting is a principal cause of the hypoxemia.[4] Radiographically such patients may have little evidence of hypoventilation other than small-volume lungs with or without zones of peripheral atelectasis.

Linear shadows in the lungs may also be caused by fibrotic pulmonary scars associated with varying degrees of infolded pleura. These scars may be postinfectious or postinfarction.

OTHER STUDIES

Plain chest films frequently provide the first indication that there is collapse of portions of lung. When the cause can be anticipated from radiographic findings, such as atelectasis associated with a large pneumothorax, or from the clinical situation, such as postoperative atelectasis that can be expected to resolve with time and appropriate clinical management, further diagnostic studies are not needed. However, elucidating the precise cause of segmental or lobar atelectasis, unaccompanied

by any known precipitating factor, almost always requires further investigation by fluoroscopy, tomography, CT scans, bronchography, bronchoscopy, pulmonary arteriography, radioisotope scans, or surgical exploration. In asymptomatic patients a short period of observation (days to weeks) may be desired to determine whether or not spontaneous resolution will occur or whether studies of induced sputum specimens will provide a definite diagnosis.

Since the advent of fiberoptic bronchoscopy, which permits examination of airways down to the level of fifth-order bronchial orifices, bronchography is seldom required to establish the nature of obstructing bronchial lesions. Bronchography is still a useful examination for mapping the airways of patients with bronchiectasis who are being considered for pulmonary resection. Because of the relatively infrequent use of bronchography the technique will not be discussed.

SUMMARY

1. The segments of the lungs are relatively constant in number and position, but the subsegments are variable and govern the size of the segments in a given individual. These variations are significant, and only an abstract conception of "normal" can be created against which to assess an individual patient.

2. Segments of the lung have multiple surfaces and complex shapes. Appreciation of their three-dimensional distribution is necessary in order to localize focal lesions accurately.

3. If a lesion can be identified in at least two different planes, correct lobar localization is usually possible. Segmental localization is often possible as well, but frequently it cannot be determined which of two adjacent segments is involved because you do not know the precise limits of any segment in a given individual.

4. Identification of interlobar fissures on both PA and lateral views of the chest increases the accuracy of lesion localization. However, because of the undulating nature of the fissures, and the fact that only portions of their anatomic course are seen tangentially, it is possible to locate small lesions incorrectly when they are in lung close to fissures.

5. CT can aid greatly in lesion localization because it provides a third dimension, but CT should seldom be needed to serve that function alone.

6. Localization of lesions in lungs whose anatomy has been distorted by previous surgery or by scarring processes is difficult unless interlobar fissures are still visible.

7. Segmental localization of focal lesions (e.g., pulmonary nodules) is seldom critical unless surgical removal is planned.
8. Interlobar fissures, or more likely parts of interlobar fissures, present as line images on chest films. On CT scans they may be seen as line or band images or as avascular zones between areas in which vessels often appear to be taking different courses. On thin sections (1.5 mm) the fissures are more likely to be seen as lines.
9. When consolidated lung extends to one side of an interlobar fissure, the image of the fissure will be converted from a line to an edge (the interface between two different x-ray absorbers). When you see long, relatively sharp edges on chest films, think of interlobar fissures against consolidated lung as one common cause.
10. Interlobar fissures are frequently incomplete, may even be absent, and seldom are visible in their entirety whether complete or not. Anomalous fissures are common, often incomplete, and frequently not seen on radiographs.
11. Zones of consolidation may also be localized by their association with anatomic structures whose usual lung interface they efface (silhouette sign).
12. Lobes and segments that are reduced in volume and contain less air (atelectasis) may be difficult to recognize unless accompanied by consolidation or by major shifts of interlobar fissures.
13. Lobes usually collapse in predictable patterns, with major displacements having these components:
    a. Medial shift
    b. Closing of a fan with the fulcrum at the hilum
    c. Anterosuperior shift (upper lobes) or posteroinferior shift (lower lobes).
    There is a constant tether at the hilum, and the portion of the collapsed lung extending to the hilum often is not visible.
14. The magnitude of volume loss, the degree of mobility of the collapsed lobe, the hyperexpansion of adjacent lobes, and the rotation of fissures will influence the radiographic image and account for common variations.
15. The causes of segmental and lobar collapse can be divided into three main categories:
    a. Relaxation or compression forces
    b. Bronchial obstruction
    c. Intrinsic alteration of lung structure.
16. Zones of rounded atelectasis, due to trapping of lung by thickened pleura, occur and may mimic tumor masses.
17. Bands of peripheral atelectasis (plate atelectasis, subsegmental atelectasis, discoid atelectasis) are commonly seen on chest radiographs and probably are associated with hypoventilation of diverse causes.

BIBLIOGRAPHY

1. Bloomer W, Liebow A, Hales M: Surgical Anatomy of the Bronchovascular Segments. Charles C Thomas, Springfield, IL, 1960
2. Boyden EA: Segmental Anatomy of the Lungs. McGraw-Hill, New York, 1955
3. Culiner MM, Reich SB: Collateral ventilation and localized emphysema. Am J Roentgenol 85:246, 1961
4. Diament ML, Palmer KN: Venous/arterial pulmonary shunting as the principal cause of postoperative hypoxemia. Lancet 1:15, 1967
5. Felson B, Felson H: Localization of intrathoracic lesions by means of the postero-anterior roentgenogram: the silhouette sign. Radiology 55:363, 1950
6. Felson B: Lung torsion: radiographic findings in nine cases. Radiology 162:631, 1987
7. Fleischner F, Hampton AO, Castleman B: Linear shadows in the lung (interlobar pleuritis, atelectasis and healed infarction). Am J Roentgenol 46:610, 1941
8. Golden R: The effect of bronchostenosis upon the roentgen ray shadows in carcinoma of the bronchus. Am J Roentgenol 13:21, 1925
9. Goodman LR, Golkow RS, Steiner RM, et al: The right mid-lung window. Radiology 143:135, 1982
10. Hanke R, Kretzschmar R: Round atelectasis. Semin Roentgenol 15:174, 1980
11. Krause GR, Lubert M: Gross anatomico-spatial changes occurring in lobar collapse: a demonstration by means of three-dimensional plastic models. Am J Roentgenol 79:258, 1958
12. Marks BW, Kuhns LR: Identification of the pleural fissures with computed tomography. Radiology 143:139, 1982
13. Naidich DP, McCauley DJ, Khouri NF, et al: Computed tomography of lobar collapse: 1. Endobronchial obstruction. J Comput Assist Tomogr 7:745, 1983
14. Naidich DP, McCauley DJ, Khouri NF, et al: Computed tomography of lobar collapse: 2. Collapse in the absence of endobronchial obstruction. J Comput Assist Tomogr 7:758, 1983
15. Proto AV, Tocino I: Radiographic manifestations of lobar collapse. Semin Roentgenol 15:117, 1980
16. Proto AV, Ball JB: The superolateral major fissures. AJR 140:431, 1983

17. Raasch BN, Carsky CW, Lane EJ, et al: Radiographic anatomy of the interlobar fissures: a study of 100 specimens. AJR 138:1043, 1982
18. Resnick D: Degenerative diseases of the vertebral column. Radiology 156:3, 1985
19. Rosenbloom SA, Ravin CE, Putman CE, et al: Peripheral middle lobe syndrome. Radiology 149:17, 1983
20. Savis B, Birtel FC, Tholen W, et al: Lung sequestration: report of seven cases and review of 540 cases. Thorax 34:96, 1979
21. Simon G: Further observations on the long line shadows across a lower zone of the lung. Br J Radiol 43:327, 1970
22. Schneider HJ, Felson B, Gonzales LL: Rounded atelectasis. AJR 134:225, 1980
23. Trapnell DH: The differential diagnosis of linear shadows in chest radiographs. Radiol Clin North Am 11:77, 1973
24. Westcott JL, Cole S: Plate atelectasis. Radiology 155:1, 1985

Atlas

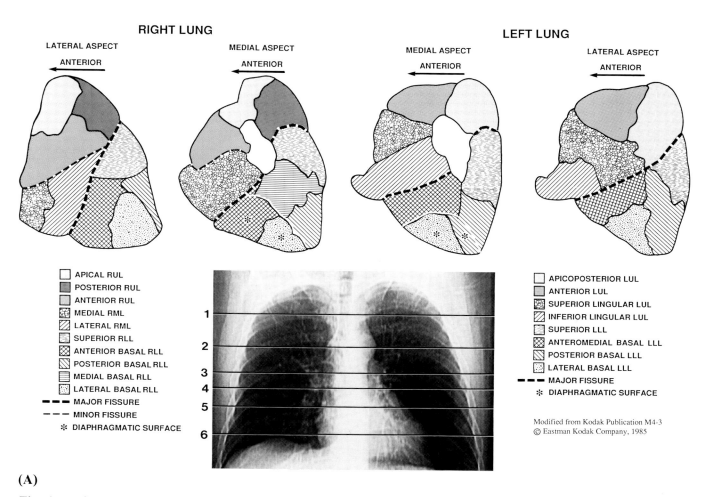

RIGHT LUNG

LATERAL ASPECT
ANTERIOR

MEDIAL ASPECT
ANTERIOR

LEFT LUNG

MEDIAL ASPECT
ANTERIOR

LATERAL ASPECT
ANTERIOR

- APICAL RUL
- POSTERIOR RUL
- ANTERIOR RUL
- MEDIAL RML
- LATERAL RML
- SUPERIOR RLL
- ANTERIOR BASAL RLL
- POSTERIOR BASAL RLL
- MEDIAL BASAL RLL
- LATERAL BASAL RLL
- ━ ━ ━ MAJOR FISSURE
- ─ ─ ─ MINOR FISSURE
- ✽ DIAPHRAGMATIC SURFACE

- APICOPOSTERIOR LUL
- ANTERIOR LUL
- SUPERIOR LINGULAR LUL
- INFERIOR LINGULAR LUL
- SUPERIOR LLL
- ANTEROMEDIAL BASAL LLL
- POSTERIOR BASAL LLL
- LATERAL BASAL LLL
- ━ ━ ━ MAJOR FISSURE
- ✽ DIAPHRAGMATIC SURFACE

Modified from Kodak Publication M4-3
© Eastman Kodak Company, 1985

(A)

Fig. 4-1. Segmental Anatomy of the Lungs

This series shows the anatomical distribution of the pulmonary segments. The whole lung specimens are oriented to face in the same direction to emphasize differences in the size and surface distributions of the pulmonary segments on the lateral and medial aspects of the lung. This can be envisioned as having the specimens on a pedestal, viewing the lateral surface, and then walking around the pedestal to view the medial surface. The view of the medial surface includes a partial view of the diaphragmatic surface due to the shape of the inflated lung and the orientation of the specimens when photographed.

The cross-sectional images of the pulmonary segments were constructed from slices of the lung specimen in the axial plane. Ramifications of each bronchial segment were identified by an injection mass of a different color before the fixed inflated lung was cut into slices.

An annotated scout view (for this CT scan of another person) shows the levels at which the correspondingly numbered CT cuts were made. *(Figure continues.)*

155

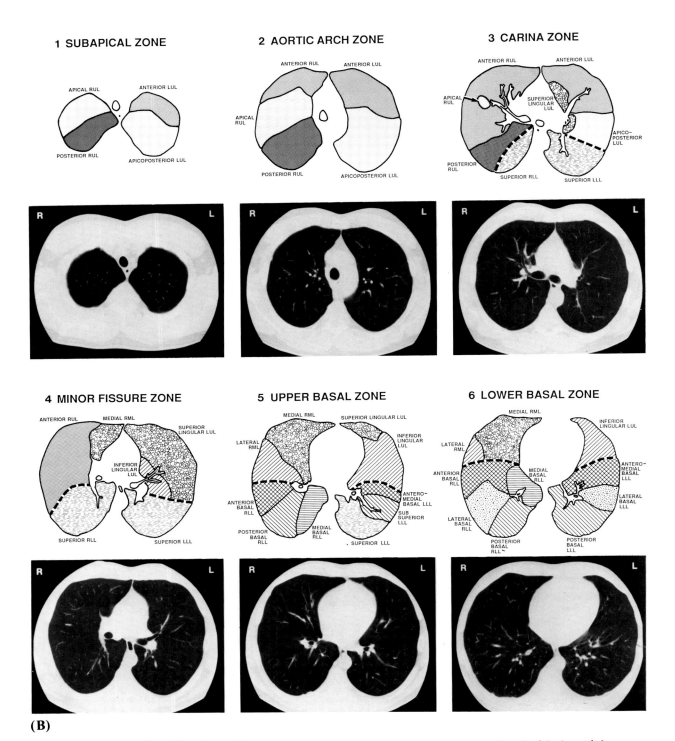

(B)

Fig. 4-1. *(Continued).* The slices of the specimen at comparable levels were correlated with the axial CT scans and slight modifications were made to fit the anatomical slices to the CT scans.

This format gives a much better appreciation of segmental shape and distribution than is given by estimated segmental boundaries drawn onto PA and lateral views of the chest because the latter make it extremely difficult to appreciate the change of a pulmonary segment from its lateral to its medial surface or from its anterior to its posterior surface. (Modified and reprinted from Kodak Publication M4-3 © Eastman Kodak Company, 1985, with permission of the company and the authors Dr. N.R. Bechai and Dr. D.J. Wise.)

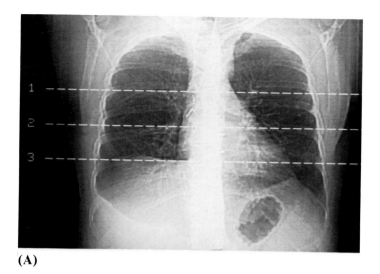

(A)

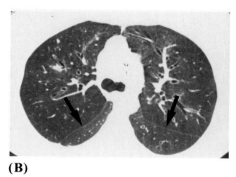

(B)

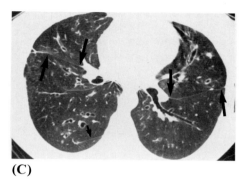

(C)

Fig. 4-2. Linear Images of the Major Interlobar Fissures

(A) Scout view of a woman who has had a heart and lung transplant and is undergoing CT of the chest using thin-section (1.5 mm) technique. The examination tabletop is calibrated so that the position of the patient in the CT gantry can be sharply defined and correlated with the level of the CT scan. The dashed lines on the scout view indicate the levels at which CT scans were obtained.

(B) CT scan made at level 1 on the scout film. It is located just above the tracheal carina at the site of the anastomosis of the donor trachea and the recipient's trachea.

The major interlobar fissures are shown as linear images (arrows) separating the superior portions of the lower lobes, which are located posteromedial to the upper lobes at this level. The vessels, in the superior segments of the lower lobes are oriented primarily perpendicularly to the plane of the scan and are seen as small white, round, or oval opacities. The vessels in the upper lobes are oriented in the scan plane as well as perpendicular to it. Therefore, some of the vessels are seen as branching tubular structures that taper as they reach the periphery, whereas others are seen as round or oval opacities representing vessels cut more or less in cross section.

At this level the major interlobar fissures have an oblique orientation, with the medial end located anterior to the lateral end. This is true on both the right and the left.

(C) CT scan at level 2 on the scout film. The major fissure on the right side (arrows) is seen in the anterior third of the slice as a linear image that has its medial end posterior to its lateral end (just the opposite of its orientation superiorly); it has a very slight bow, convex anteriorly, along its lateral third. This is a common but not invariable position of the major interlobar fissure at this level. In some patients the lateral end of the fissure may remain posterior to the medial end of the fissure.

On the left side, the major interlobar fissure has its medial end slightly posterior to its lateral end (arrows), which is its usual orientation at this level.

Incidentally noted is a short, incomplete, anomalous fissure extending into the posteromedial aspects of the right lower lobe (short arrow).

On both Fig. B and Fig. C there are numerous round and oval rings with black centers. These represent dilated, thick-walled bronchi, the result of bronchiectasis proximal to areas of bronchiolitis obliterans. Bronchiolitis obliterans is one of the serious late pulmonary complications seen in heart-lung transplant recipients.

Fig. 4-3. Location of Interlobar Fissures is Marked by Hypovascular Lung Zones on Relatively Thick (10-mm) CT Cuts

Series of sequential CT scans extending caudally towards the diaphragm from the level of the trachial carina. These sections were photographed at window and level settings which show pulmonary vessels to advantage. At these settings, however, the heart and mediastinal contents, the soft tissues of the chest wall, and even the vertebral column are shown on the same near-white gray scale.

CT scan made at level 1 is immediately caudal to the tracheal carina. The proximal portions of each main bronchus appear as black ovals. The pulmonary vessels are seen fanning out into the lungs from both hila. The top of the right major interlobar fissure has not appeared yet, but a zone lacking in pulmonary blood vessels marks the location of the top left of the major fissure (between the black arrows). The pulmonary vessels posteromedial to this zone have a different configuration than those vessels which are seen anterior to this plane of the left major fissure. At this level, the major fissure separates the superior segment of the LLL from the left upper lobe.

At level 2 the location of the right major interlobar fissure is marked by a hypovascular zone extending between the large black arrows. Pulmonary vessels of the superior segment of the right lower lobe posteromedial to the plane of the major interlobar fissure have a different pattern and course than those right upper lobe vessels which are seen anterolateral to the major interlobar fissure.

Anterior to the plane of the right major interlobar fissure there is a peripheral semicircle of small arrows which point to a fan-shaped hypovascular zone surrounding the right hilum. This is the plane of the minor interlobar fissure. Interspersed among the small arrows, however, there are images of small vessels about the periphery of the lung. This mantle of small vessels is not seen on image 3. From this pattern we deduce that the minor interlobar fissure has a slight dome-shape and that the peripheral vessels seen at level 2 are in the outer perimeter of the right upper lobe above the lateral and anterior slope of the minor interlobar fissure.

On the left, the major interlobar fissure (the zone between the black arows) has moved slightly forward from its position at level 1, but maintains a similar oblique orientation.

Image 3 shows that both the right and the left major interlobar fissures have moved slightly forward from their relative positions on the cut above. Anterior to the right major interlobar fissure there is still a relative paucity of pulmonary vessels. This is the superior peripheral portion of the middle lobe.

Vessels in the periphery of the lung are much smaller than those more centrally located within each lobe. It is helpful to recognize that the periphery of the lung is not only that mantle against the chest wall and the mediastinum, but also includes that zone of each lobe which is adjacent to a fissure. That is one of the reasons that the location of fissures is marked by relatively avascular zones on 10-mm thick CT slices.

The small black oval seen in the right hilum is the distal portion of the bronchus intermedius. A branch of the lingular division of the LUL is seen as a gray, curved, tubular image in the left hilum.

At level 4 each of the major fissures has moved anteriorly relative to its position on the more cephalad cuts. At this level on the right, the major interlobar fissures separates the lower lobe from the middle lobe, whereas on the left side the fissure separates the lower lobe from the lingula. The small black rounded images in the hilar regions on each side are cross-sections of the upper portions of each lower lobe bronchus. Anterior to the right major fissure there are large pulmonary vesssels which supply the right middle lobe. These can be contrasted with the relatively avascular zone seen on either side of the minor interlobar fissure on scans 2 and 3.

Since there is no fissure separating the lingula from the anterior segment of the left upper lobe a comparable avascular zone is not seen on the left.

On levels 5 and 6 each major fissure has continued to move anteriorly. On the right, the major fissure has a configuration such that the lateral and medial margins are nearly opposite. However, in comparison with the plane of the fissure more cephalad, the lateral edge has moved relatively more anteriorly than has the medial end of the fissure.

The lateral end of the left major fissure has rotated relatively further anteriorly than the lateral end of the right major fissure, so that the left major fissure at level 6 has an obliquity that is opposite its obliquity as seen on levels 1 through 3.

Level 6 is still several centimeters above the diaphragm. On more caudal levels (not shown) there is

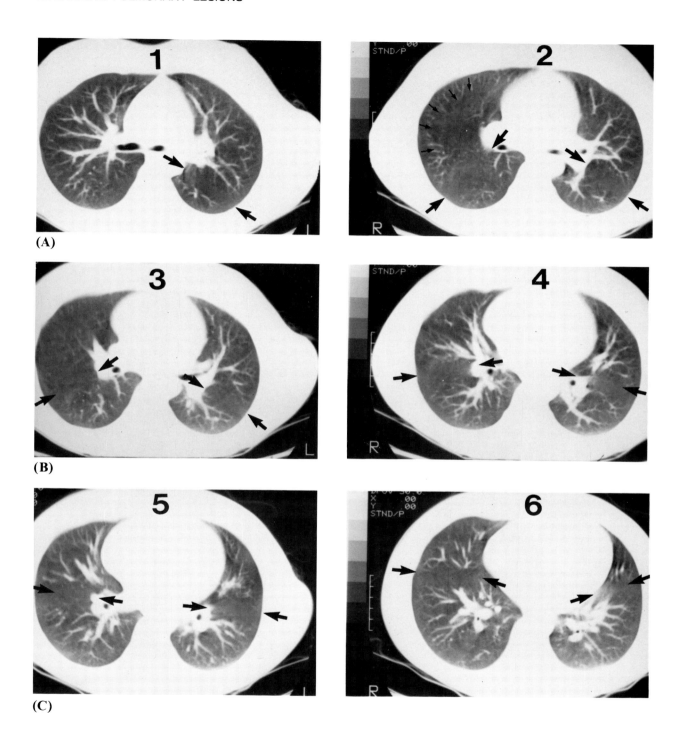

(A)

(B)

(C)

very little further change in the orientation of the fissures, but they are slightly further anterior in position. However, neither fissure reaches the anterior chest wall, even at the level of the diaphragm.

Although it is common for the left major fissure to reverse its obliquity as it passes caudally, the magnitude of this rotation is usually less for the right major fissure. Even at its caudal extremity the right major fissure may have its medial and lateral ends opposite one another or the lateral end may remain slightly posterior to the medial end. Less commonly the lateral end of the caudal aspects of the right major fissure may be significantly more anterior than the medial end, similar to the rotation seen on the left side.

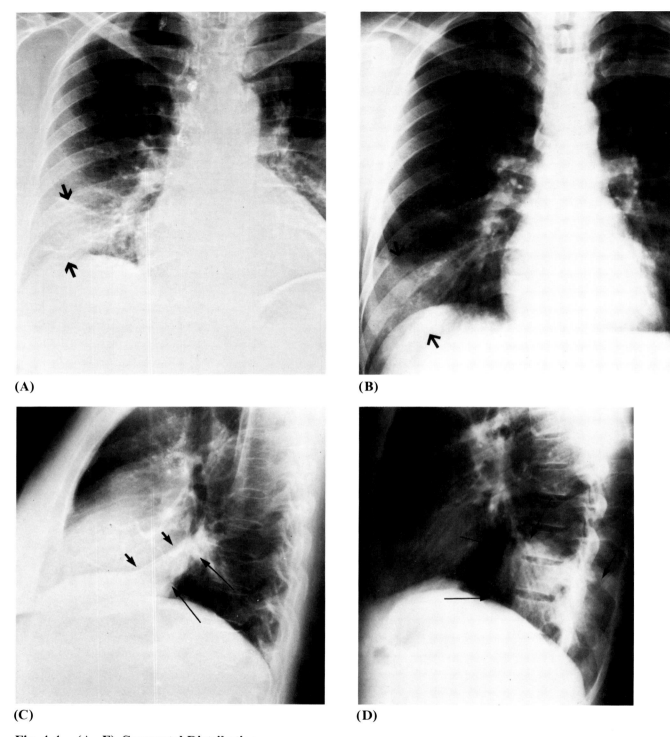

(A)

(B)

(C)

(D)

Fig. 4-4. (A – F). Segmental Distribution

(A,B) Zones of consolidation are seen laterally at the right base (arrows). The more medial vessel images are preserved whereas the lateral vessels are obscured. The consolidations appear quite similar in location. (The dense nodular opacities in the mediastinum and right supraclavicular space on Fig. A and C are lymph nodes opacified by foot lymphangiography.)

(C) Lateral view corresponding to Fig. A. The consolidation in the right lower lobe (arrows) is superimposed on the heart and is limited anteriorly by the major fissure (short arrows). From its position in Figs. A and C we conclude that the consolidation is in the anterior basal segment.

(D) Lateral view corresponding to Fig. B. The consolidation is located posteriorly on the lateral view (arrows) and is superimposed on the spine. From its position in Figs. B and D we conclude that the consolidation is in the lateral basal segment. *(Figure continues.)*

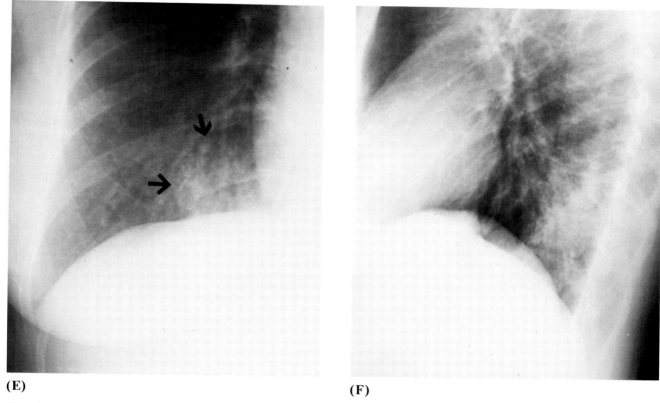

(E)   **(F)**

Fig. 4-4. *(Continued).*

(**E**) A zone of consolidation is observed medially at the right base (arrows). The medial lung vessels are obscured whereas the lateral ones are preserved — the opposite of the situation in Figs. A and B.

(**F**) Lateral view corresponding to Fig. E. The consolidation is predominantly posterior, similar to the location in Fig. D. From its position in Figs. E and F we conclude that the consolidation is in the posterior basal segment. *(Figure continues.)*

Fig. 4-4. *(Continued).*

Thus, lesions located laterally in the right lower lobe could be in either the anterior basal or the lateral basal segment. If located posteriorly on the lateral view the lesion is in the lateral basal segment; if anteriorly, but behind the major fissure, it is in the anterior basal segment.

A lesion located posteriorly in the right lower lobe could be in either the posterior basal or the lateral basal segment. If located medially on a PA view, it is in the posterior basal segment; if located laterally on a PA view, it is in the lateral base segment.

By elimination there is only one basal segment left: the medial. It is located medially on a PA view and anteriorly, but behind the major fissure, on a lateral view. Thus, a lesion located medially in the right lower lobe could be in either the posterior basal or the medial basal segment. If located posteriorly on the lateral view, it is in the posterior basal segment; if located anteriorly, but behind the major fissure, on the lateral view, it is in the medial basal segment.

(Note: In Fig. F there is a small amount of peribronchial thickening posterior to the heart and inferior vena cava that probably represents some pneumonitis in the medial basal segment as well.)

Lastly, if a lesion is anterior in the right lower lobe on a lateral view, it could be in either the anterior basal or the medial basal segment. If it is located laterally on the PA view, it is in the anterior basal segment; if it is located medially on the PA view, it is in the medial basal segment. Correlate these localizations with the segmental anatomy of the lower basal zone as shown in Fig. 4-1. *(Figure continues.)*

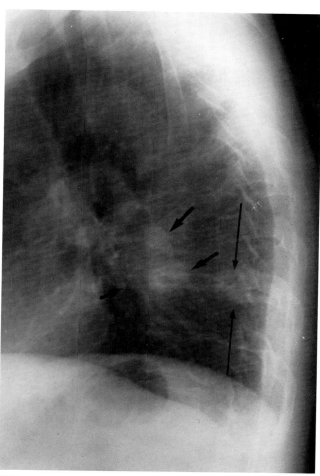

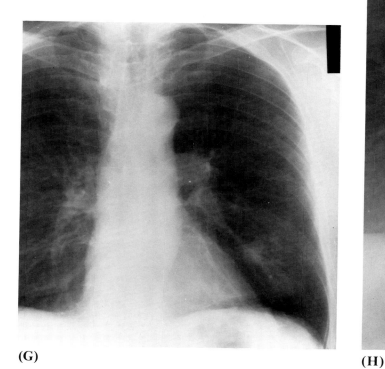

(G)

(H)

Fig. 4-4. *(Continued).* **(G,H) Location of a Nodule on Two Views**

(G) PA view. An irregular nodule is projected in approximately the midclavicular line of the left lower lobe. It could be in any of the basilar segments of that lobe, or it could be in the lingula. Since we have no way of knowing the precise size of these segments in this patient, the lesion cannot be located with greater precision from the PA view.

(H) Lateral view. The lesion is located posteriorly (long arrows). It is mostly likely in the posterior basal segment of the left lower lobe. However, the patient is rotated so that the right side is anterior and the left side posterior to true lateral. Notice the left diaphragm (identified by subjacent stomach gas) extends far posterior. Therefore, this nodule could be in the lateral basal segment of the lower lobe and projected this far posterior because of rotation, especially if the patient had a large lateral basal segment.

The clustered arrows outline opacities, which on a tomographic study were shown to be lymph nodes extending into the lung from the lower portions of the left hilum.

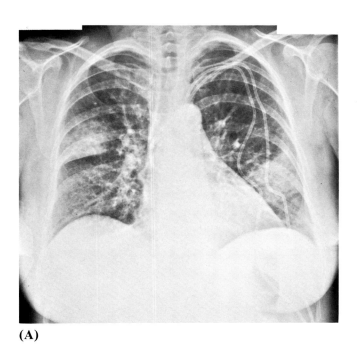

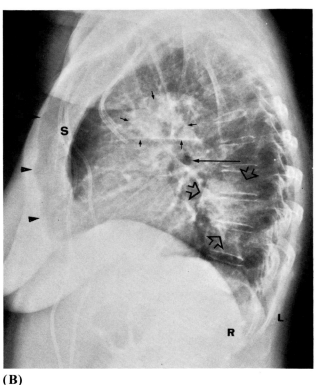

(A)   (B)

Fig. 4-5.   Consolidation in the Axillary Subsegment of the Right Upper Lobe and the Anteromedial
Basal Segment of the Left Lower Lobe Due to *Aspergillus* Infection

(A) PA view. There are two distinct zones of consolidation. That on the right is located laterally in the right upper lobe, and there is a relatively uninvolved zone of lung separating it from the hilum. Its lower margin is defined sharply by the minor fissure.

(B) Lateral view. The right upper lobe consolidation (small arrows) is neither extremely anterior nor extremely posterior, but rather more central and superimposed on the airway. Its lower margin is also well defined because it has an interface with the minor interlobar fissure (small vertical arrows).

This region is supplied by an axillary subsegmental branch of the anterior segment bronchus of the right upper lobe.

The consolidation on the left in the PA view is in the lower half of the lung. Although it extends to the image of the left heart border, the heart border remains sharply defined. The consolidation extends laterally to reach the chest wall at its low corner but not superiorly.

On the lateral view the anterior limits of the consolidation are very sharp (horizontal open arrow). This is at an interface with a portion of the major interlobar fissure. This consolidation is probably in a lateral, cephalad portion of the anteromedial basal segment of the left lower lobe. It could be in a large superior segment of that lobe, but ordinarily at this caudal level the superior segment of the left lower lobe does not reach the major fissure anteriorly. (See segmental anatomy of upper basal zone level of Fig. 4-1.)

Note incidentally that Fig. B is not a true lateral view, but rather an RATL (right shoulder anterior to true lateral) variant. Arrowheads mark the anterior limit of the right lung, which is projected more than 1.0 cm anterior to the image of the sternum (S).

There are two central venous catheters entering from the left side. Their position on the lateral view gives you a sense of the position of the left brachiocephalic vein and the superior vena cava. The black oval projection of the left upper lobe bronchus (long arrow) is clearly seen end-on.

This patient had leukemia and infection with *Aspergillus*. These pulmonary lesions are zones of infection and infarction consequent to the vascular invasion that is typical of invasive aspergillosis. Although typical, the radiographic appearance is by no means diagnostic. The consolidation in the LLL, however, went on to show the characteristic cavitation that occurs in these lesions when the patient's neutrophil count improves.

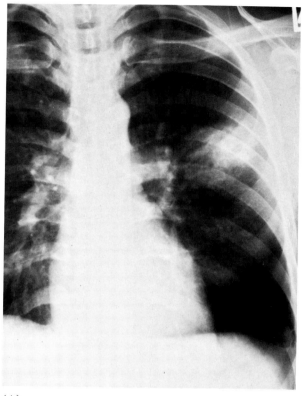

(A)

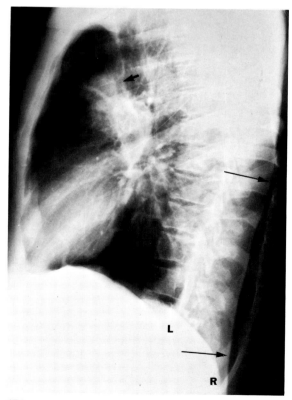

(B)

Fig. 4-6. Consolidation of the Axillary Subsegment of the Left Upper Lobe

(A) PA view. There is a poorly marginated oval zone of consolidation in the axillary region of the left midlung zone. From this projection alone you could place it either:

1. In the caudal portion of the apicoposterior segment of the left upper lobe
2. In the axillary subsegment of the anterior segment of the left upper lobe, or
3. In the lateral aspect of the superior segment of the left lower lobe. (See segmental anatomy of carina zone level of Fig. 4-1.)

(B) Lateral view. The consolidation projects anterior to the trachea. This clearly places it in the left upper lobe and eliminates the superior segment of the lower lobe from consideration. Assuming that the apicoposterior segment of the upper lobe is not unusually large, the mostly likely location for this lesion is the axillary subsegment of the anterior segment of the upper lobe. This lesion could also be in the axillary subsegment of the apicoposterior segment of the upper lobe and be projected anterior to the airway because of rotation of the patient.

Arrows in Fig. B point to a skin fold of the left side of the back that simulates a posterior pneumothorax of the right lung. The lateral view is an RPTL (right shoulder posterior to true lateral) variant. Thus, the right posterior ribs project far behind the left. You can see that the long sharp edge shadow due to the skin fold passes beyond the lowest rib visible and thus could not represent the visceral pleura of the right lung.

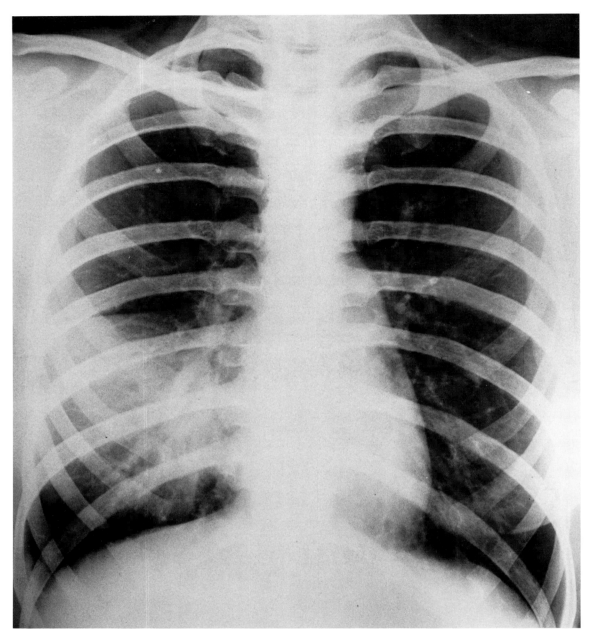

(A)

Fig. 4-7.   Right Middle Lobe Consolidation

(A) PA view shows a fan-shaped area of opacity in the lower half of the right hemithorax. The sharp upper edge of the consolidation is at the level of the minor interlobar fissure. The extreme right base is spared. The right heart border is effaced.

   (B) Lateral view shows a pie-shaped area of consolidation extending obliquely from a point just behind the right hilum to the anterior chest wall. Its upper margin is the minor fissure, which is seen as a well-defined edge. Part of the posterior margin also is a well-defined edge, representing the major fissure, which reaches the anterior chest wall just above the diaphragm. *(Figure continues.)*

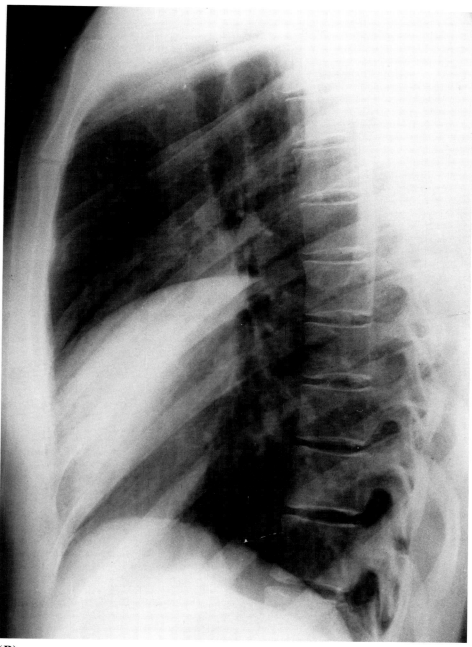

(B)

Fig. 4-7. *(Continued).* These findings are classic for right middle lobe consolidation. There is only minor reduction in volume. The fact that the major fissure intersects the anterior chest wall rather than the diaphragm testifies to the element of reduced right middle lobe volume.

Two small, dense, nodular opacities in the right upper lobe are calcified granulomata (Fig. A).

The middle lobe consolidation is easy to recognize on the PA view in this patient because the consolidated lung against the minor fissure presents a sufficient tangent to the x-ray beam to create a long, sharp edge, and the right heart border is effaced. Notice, however, that although the tangential projection of the minor fissure is seen as a nearly horizontal edge on the PA view, on the lateral view the minor fissure is clearly shown to have slight bowing and a definite caudal angulation. This serves to illustrate that the image of an interlobar fissure on any given projection only represents that portion of the fissure that is tangential to the x-ray beam and does not allow one to assess the true course of the entire fissure.

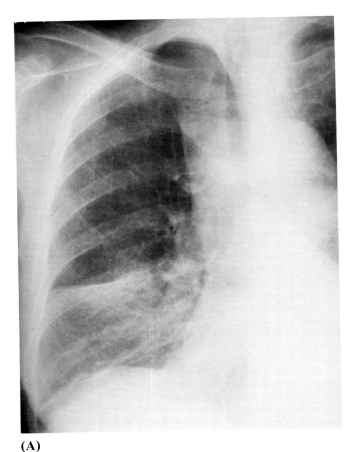

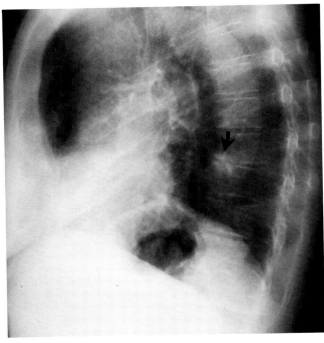

(A)

(B)

Fig. 4-8. **(A – C) Consolidation of the Lateral Segment of the Right Middle Lobe**

(A) PA view. This 73-year-old woman has stage 4 chronic lymphocytic leukemia. She developed a right middle lobe pneumonia of uncertain etiology. Increased radiopacity is seen over the lower portions of the right lung. This is sharply delimited superiorly by the minor interlobar fissure. The right heart border is still clearly visible except at the right cardiophrenic angle where there is a fat pad.

The superior mediastinum is shifted considerably to the right. This shift is due not to compensation for the consolidated right middle lobe but to the marked rotation of the patient. Relate the medial ends of the clavicles to the spine and you can see that the right clavicle is far off center.

(B) Lateral view. The middle lobe consolidation is not striking, but anteriorly, superimposed on the heart, there is a wedge-shaped zone of increased opacity within which vessel shadows are obscure (small arrows). *(Figure continues.)*

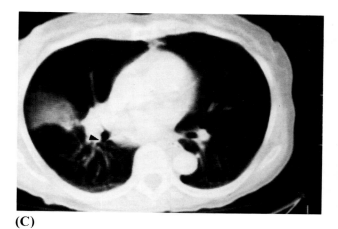

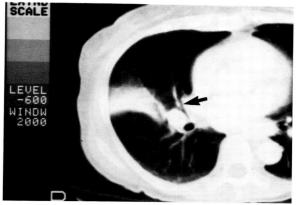

(C)

Fig. 4-8. *(Continued).* **(C)** CT scans. Scan on the left is 1 cm cephalad of that on the right. The consolidation of the lateral segment of the right middle lobe is easily recognized (light gray) and sharply demarcated from the aerated lower lobe posteriorly (black) by the major interlobar fissure. The black tubular lucency of the bronchus intermedius is seen on both scans. The takeoff of the superior segment of the right lower lobe is seen in scan on the left (arrowhead). The middle lobe bronchus is seen on both cuts, but is better defined in the scan on the right. You can see the bifurcation of the middle lobe bronchus into medial and lateral segments. The lateral segment bronchus curves toward the area of consolidation. The medial segment bronchus of the right middle lobe (arrow), however, passes into aerated (black) rather than consolidated (light gray) lung. This represents lateral segment consolidation with little reduction in volume.

The medial segment is not involved. (Correlate with anatomy of upper basal zone level of Fig. 4-1.)

Note incidentally in Fig. B:

1. How well the length of the descending aorta is seen. When the descending thoracic aorta becomes elongated and projects further into the left lung, it becomes more easily seen.
2. The nodule-like opacity that projects over the anterior aspect of a vertebral interspace in the retrocardiac position (arrow). This is a not-uncommon site for hypertrophic changes of the spine to occur. These vertebral spurs can be mistaken for pulmonary nodules. The error can be avoided by obtaining AP and lateral views of the thoracic spine when the problem arises. The hypertrophic spurs are more easily recognized as spinal abnormalities with that filming technique. *(Figure continues.)*

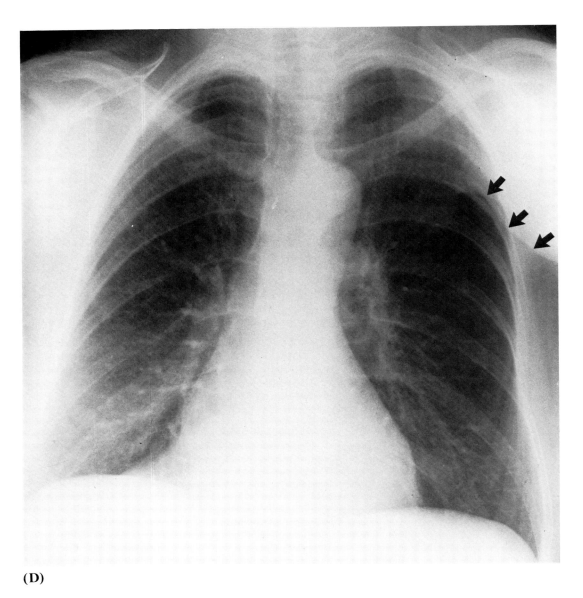

(D)

Fig. 4-8. *(Continued).* **(D–F) Right Middle Lobe Atelectasis Difficult to Recognize on a PA View**

(D) PA view of a patient who has had a left radical mastectomy. The altered axillary skin fold can be seen passing from the left arm onto the chest wall (arrows). The absence of the breast and the pectoralis muscles on the left reduces the amount of soft tissues traversed by the beam; consequently the lung appears more lucent (blacker) than corresponding areas of the right lung. (This surgical deformity is mimicked by rare unilateral congenital absence of the pectoralis muscles.)

The vessels in the lower left lung lateral to the heart are more clearly defined than the vessels in corresponding areas of the right lung. You might reason that since there is breast tissue on the right, which acts as a scatterer of photons, some relative loss of detail of these vessels would be expected. *(Figure continues.)*

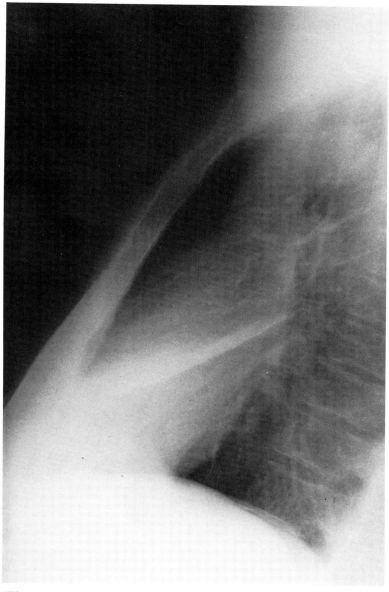

(E)

Fig. 4-8. *(Continued).* **(E)** On the lateral view, however, there is a thin wedge of opacity superimposed on the heart. Within this wedge no vessels can be seen. Its inferior boundary is sharp, as would be the case if it represented airless lung against an anteriorly displaced major interlobar fissure. Therefore, one must be concerned about atelectasis involving at least one of the segments of the right middle lobe. How, then, do we explain the fact that in Fig. A the right heart border is clear except at the cardiophrenic angle, where a fat pad obscures its lower edge?

A possible explanation is that the right middle lobe is so reduced in volume that hyperexpanded portions of the lower or upper lobes gain access to the right heart border, so that it remains visible, or that the medial segment of the middle lobe remains aerated. *(Figure continues.)*

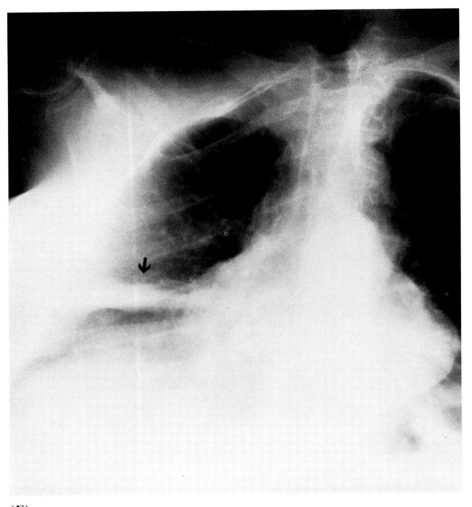

(F)

Fig. 4-8. *(Continued).* **(F)** Lordotic view graphically demonstrates the atelectasis of the right middle lobe and reinforces the findings on the lateral view. The minor fissure is faintly visible as a line shadow (arrow) separated from the atelectatic band, indicating that one segment of the middle lobe is at least partially aerated.

Since both the medial and lateral segments of the middle lobe abut segments of both the major and minor fissures, seeing or not seeing portions of these fissures is of little help in deciding which segment is involved. The medial segment does interface with the right heart border whereas the lateral segment does not. This plus the fact that the atelectatic band remains wide laterally on the lordotic view favors collapse of the lateral segment. Were it necessary to be precise, a CT scan would provide the answer.

It can be difficult to determine whether there is complete collapse or collapse of only one segment of the middle lobe. The underlying causes are the same, however, and when bronchial obstruction is a consideration in the differential diagnosis, bronchoscopy can make the distinction. Both of the middle lobe segmental orifices are within reach of modern bronchoscopes.

Right middle lobe collapse can be difficult to recognize on a PA view when the minor fissure does not present a sufficient tangent to produce an edge image as happened in Fig. A. The atelectatic wedge of lung itself simply acts as a thin filter and produces a density gradient that is difficult to recognize as abnormal, particularly when there are no prior films for comparison. An extrapleural lesion creates the same problem when seen en face.

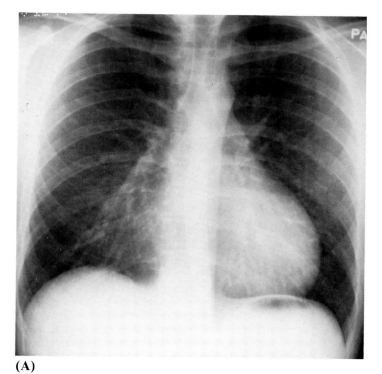

(A)

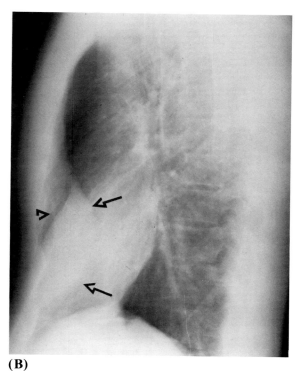

(B)

Fig. 4-9. Pectus Excavatum

(A) PA view. This young man has a pectus excavatum deformity of the anterior chest wall. The right heart border is effaced, and there is a hazy, poorly margined zone of increased opacity medially in the adjacent lung. This combination raises the question of atelectasis and consolidation in the right middle lobe.

(B) Lateral view clarifies the situation by showing the characteristic inward bowing of the lower sternum and the retrosternal soft tissues (arrows). In this case the sternum itself is difficult to see; its anterior cortex is barely visible (arrowhead), but the soft tissue components are obvious. If necessary, the sternum could be imaged better by a different technique.

In many patients with pectus excavatum, the anterior ribs show a steep downward inclination on the PA view, but that feature is not striking in this individual.

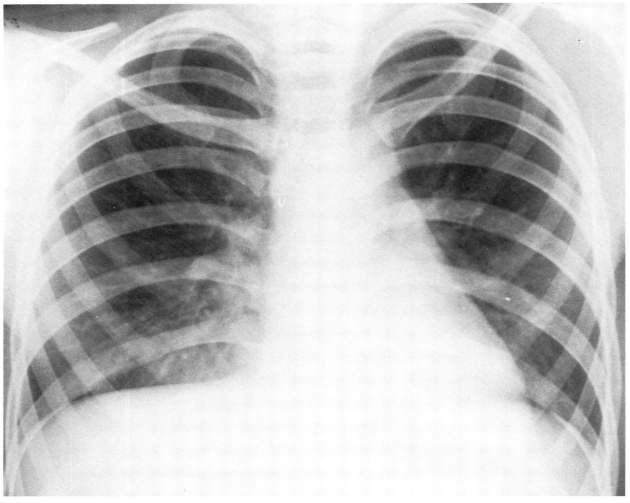

(A)

Fig. 4-10.   Right Middle Lobe Atelectasis

(A) PA view. The right heart border is not visible even in a small percentage of normal subjects, and therefore its absence here is not necessarily pathologic. There is however, right middle lobe atelectasis, which is cryptic on this view.

(B) As you scan this lateral view, you will see a wedge of increased tissue density extending anteriorly from the hilum toward the low retrosternal area (arrows). Increased density alone might be due to superimposition of ribs from both sides of the chest on one another over the intervening water-density heart shadow. Notice, however, that there is also a loss of vessel shadows in this opaque zone compared to areas of the film both superior and inferior to it. The loss of vessel images confirms that the abnormality involves lung parenchyma, and the distribution of this opacity fits very well with the right middle lobe.

(C) This lordotic view converts the very subtle finding on the PA view into a very obvious abnormality: a triangular opaque zone with its base lying medially and its apex laterally. On the original film a faint line could be seen extending laterally from the apex of the triangular zone (arrow). This represents the major interlobar fissure, which is outlined by the upper lobe above and the lower lobe below, lateral to the collapsed middle lobe, which has retracted from the lateral chest wall.

There is little mediastinal shift, diaphragm elevation, or recognizable hyperexpansion of adjacent lobes in cases of right middle lobe atelectasis. *(Figure continues.)*

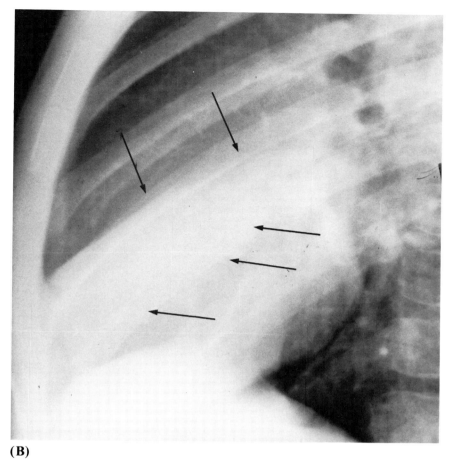

(B)

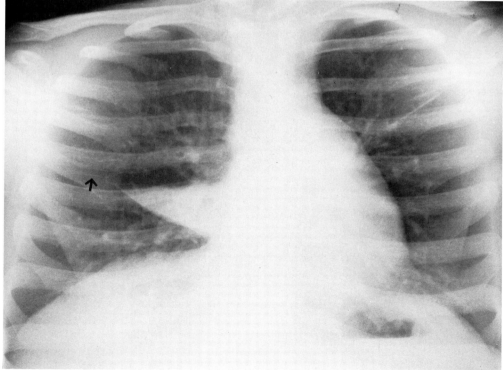

(C)
Fig. 4-10. *(Continued)*

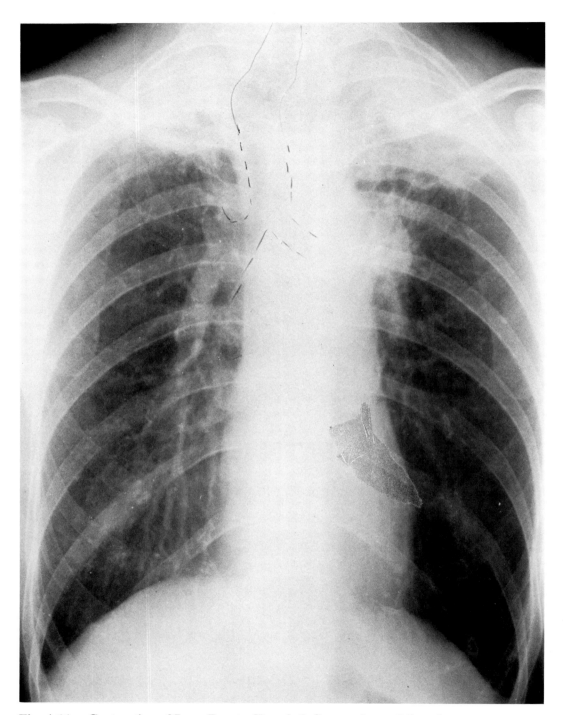

Fig. 4-11. Contraction of Lung Due to Chronic Inflammation and Scarring

There is intense opacification of the apical and subapical regions of both upper lobes, and there is buckling of the trachea to the right (retouched). There is considerable upward retraction of both hila. The vessels extending into the aerated portions of the middle and lower lung zones appear elongated and separated from one another because of the compensatory hyperexpansion of these portions of lung.

When there is such gross distortion of large volumes of lung, it is not possible to localize small lesions with accuracy unless you can identify interlobar fissures to use as landmarks.

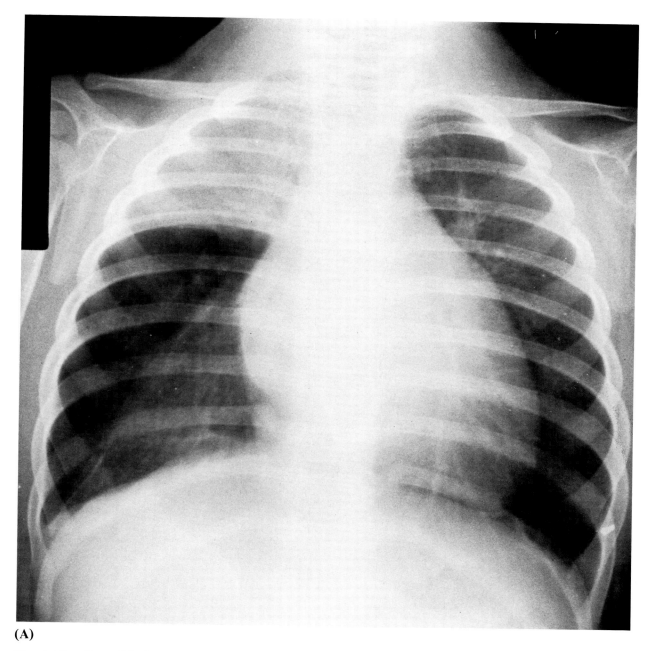

(A)

Fig. 4-12. Consolidation of the Right Upper Lobe and Atelectasis of the Right Lower Lobe

(A) PA view. There is consolidation of the right upper lobe extending down to the posterior sixth rib. Its inferior margin corresponds to the minor fissure.

Inferomedially there is a second, near-triangular zone of opacity that is much less dense than the consolidated upper lobe. A well-defined lateral edge extends obliquely inferolaterally from the hilum to the costophrenic angle. This edge represents a medially displaced and rotated major fissure and indicates that the lower lobe is reduced in volume even though not heavily consolidated. *(Figure continues.)*

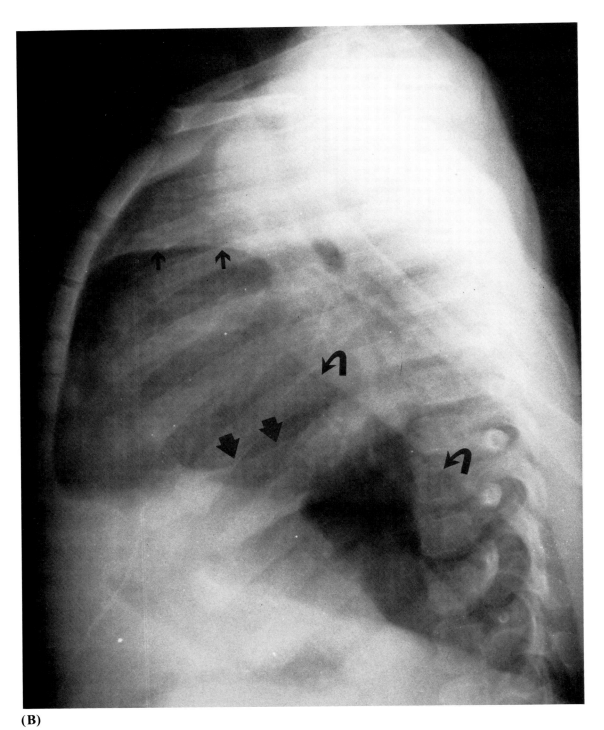

(B)

Fig. 4-12. *(Continued).* **(B)** Lateral view. The upper lobe consolidation has a well-defined lower edge at its interface with the minor fissure (paired small arrows). The manifestations of the lower lobe reduction in volume are extremely subtle. A bowed and posteriorly displaced major fissure is seen only over a short length (paired thick arrows) before it becomes lost in images of the ribs. The right upper lobe shows mainly consolidation, whereas the lower lobe shows mainly reduction in volume.

These films illustrates that reduction in volume of a lobe unaccompanied by extensive consolidation is much more difficult to recognize than is reduction in volume accompanied by consolidation.

There is a conspicuous soft tissue shadow superimposed on the lower half of the film, the result of improper positioning of the child's arms (curved arrows).

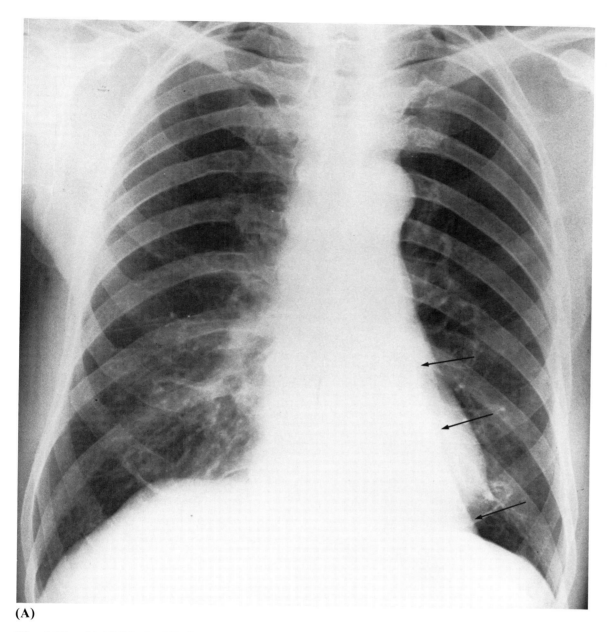

(A)

Fig. 4-13. (A,B) Marked Left Lower Lobe Atelectasis (Collapse)

(A) PA view. A fairly sharp edge image (arrows) is seen medial to the left heart border. This represents the displaced major fissure against a collapsed left lower lobe. The fissure has moved medially and rotated posteriorly; it presents a tangent to the x-ray beam in this projection, but not in the lateral view (Fig. B). (Go to the anatomical axial images of Fig. 4-1 and imagine that you are rotating the lateral end of the major fissure so far posterior in relation to its medial end that at least a portion of the fissure becomes tangential in the PA view. This can occur when the left lower lobe becomes atelectatic and shifts posteromedially.) The aerated portion of the left lung (the hyperexpanded upper lobe) is blacker than the right lung and shows fewer vessels per unit area of film. Appreciation of this finding requires careful comparison of the two sides.

The left hilum appears small because the hilar vessels entering the lower lobe cannot be seen within the collapsed lobe. The film is not adequately exposed to show the major bronchi. *(Figure continues.)*

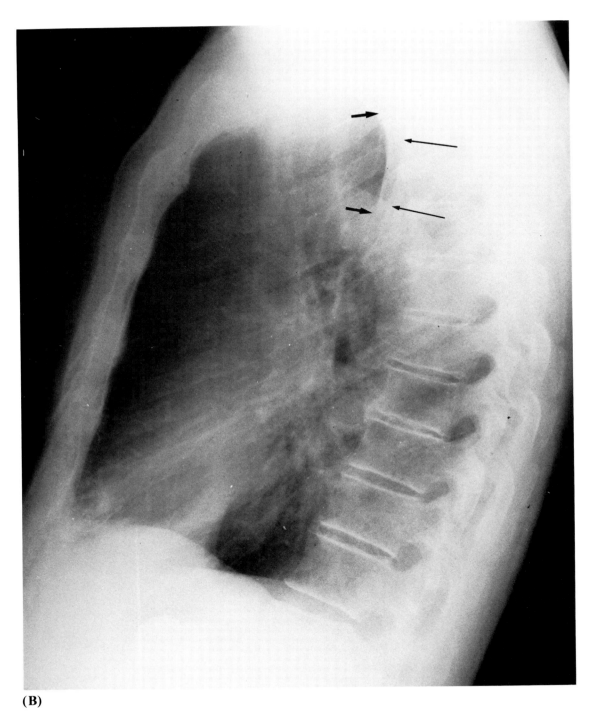

(B)

Fig. 4-13. *(Continued).* **(B)** Lateral view. The gray tones of the portion of lung superimposed on the spine are inappropriate. In the normal subject, the gray tones in this region should progress from light gray superiorly to darker gray-black inferiorly, because of the shape of the thoracic cage and increased thickness of the soft tissues relative to lung at the level of the shoulders compared to the more caudal areas. In this patient the gray tone is nearly uniform because the collapsed left lower lobe acts as an x-ray filter. Equally important, the posterior third of the left hemidiaphragm is completely effaced. It "stops" at the anterior margin of a vertebra. The displaced major fissure in this patient does not present enough of a tangent on the lateral view to be projected as a well-defined edge, but in some cases of left lower lobe atelectasis it can.

The scapulae project well-defined edges (arrows) superiorly. *(Figure continues.)*

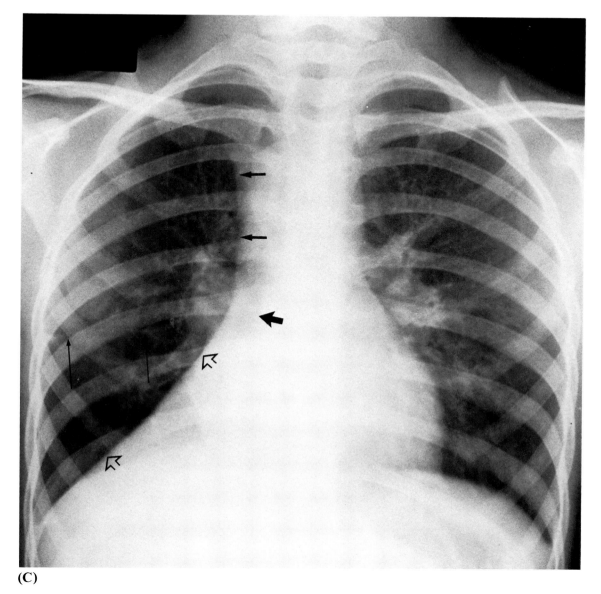

(C)

Fig. 4-13. *(Continued).* **(C,D) Right Lower Lobe Atelectasis**

(C) PA view of another patient. There is a long, sharp edge passing obliquely from the right hilum to the lateral third of the right hemidiaphragm. This edge represents the major interlobar fissure with an atelectatic right lower lobe on one side and an aerated middle lobe on the other. The major interlobar fissure has been displaced medially and inferiorly. There has also been posterior rotation so that a long tangent is seen (open arrows).

There is a shift of the upper mediastinum to the right. This is a common finding with right lower lobe atelectasis. The pleural reflection over the superior vena cava (short black arrows) appears to be in continuity with the displaced major interlobar fissure. This is a fortuitous projection since these structures are not at all in the same plane. The minor interlobar fissure can be seen in near-normal position (long arrows). The bronchus intermedius is seen faintly (thick black arrow) and has a more vertical inclination, because of the right lower lobe atelectasis, than it would have in the normal individual. *(Figure continues.)*

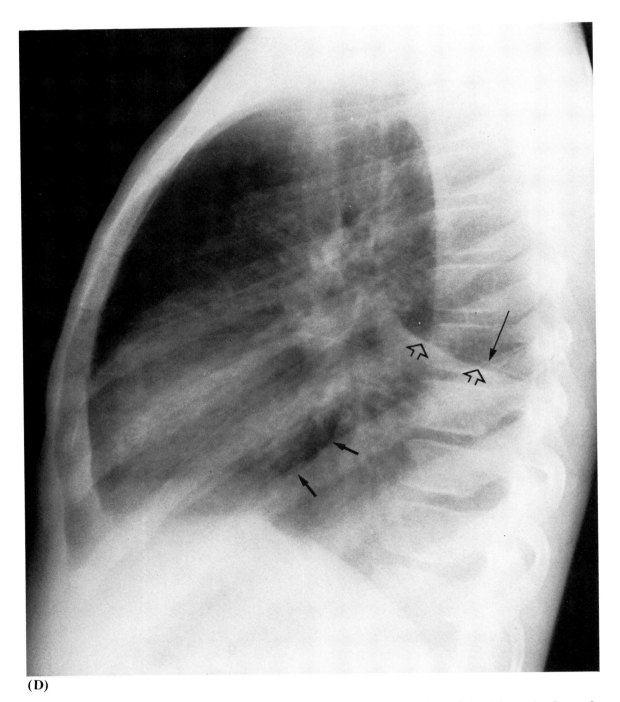

(D)

Fig. 4-13. *(Continued).* **(D)** Lateral view. Part of the edge of the lower half of the right major fissure is seen in the retrocardiac region (paired black arrows). It bows posteriorly. The edge of the upper half of the right major fissure slants posteriorly and inferiorly (open arrows) against the collapsed superior segment of the right lower lobe.

A portion of the displaced right major fissure appears as a line (long arrow). This indicates that some of the alveoli in the adjacent portion of the superior segment must still contain air.

The posterior half of the left hemidiaphragm is clearly seen, whereas that of the right hemidiaphragm is effaced because it is now in contact with the water density of the collapsed right lower lobe. The linear shadow of the right minor fissure and the lower part of the left major fissure appear as lines that cross each other, even though they are on opposite sides of the chest.

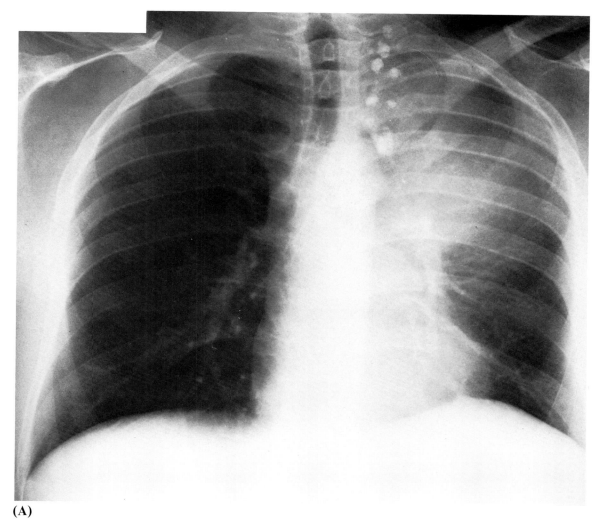

(A)

Fig. 4-14. Left Upper Lobe Atelectasis and Consolidation Around a Mass

(A) PA projection. There is a relatively homogeneous increase in tissue density in the left upper hemithorax, but there are no sharp edges to the opaque area. The apical and lateral subclavicular regions are more lucent than the perihilar portions of the lung. The upper edge of the left pulmonary artery is effaced. The left heart border is unsharp. The aortic arch is visible. The left main and lower lobe bronchi are well defined. The left upper lobe bronchus is not visible. There is slight elevation of the left hemidiaphragm but no mediastinal shift. (The lower trachea buckles around the aortic arch, but this is not a true mediastinal shift.)

The irregularly oval or rounded opacities distributed in a string along the left superior mediastinum are lymph nodes, which were opacified at the time of foot lymphangiography a few days earlier. The fact that they are opacified is not evidence that they are abnormal. *(Figure continues.)*

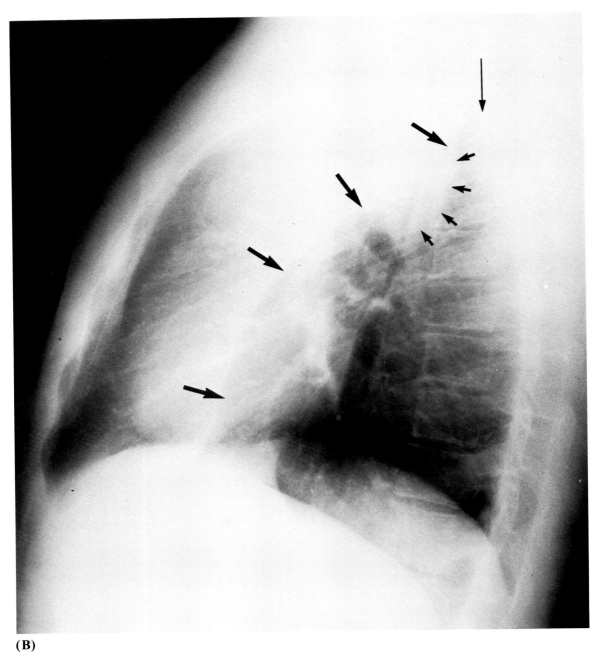

(B)

Fig. 4-14. *(Continued).* **(B)** Lateral projection. A sharp edge (large arrows) is seen extending from the posterior subapical region (long thin arrow) anteroinferiorly to the level of the diaphragm. This represents the anteriorly displaced major fissure against the atelectatic upper lobe. Since the lingula is an integral part of the left upper lobe and extends to the diaphragm, the retrosternal projection of the atelectatic lobe is quite long. In the immediate retrosternal region the film is blacker because of projection of the anterior portions of the right lung. *(Figure continues.)*

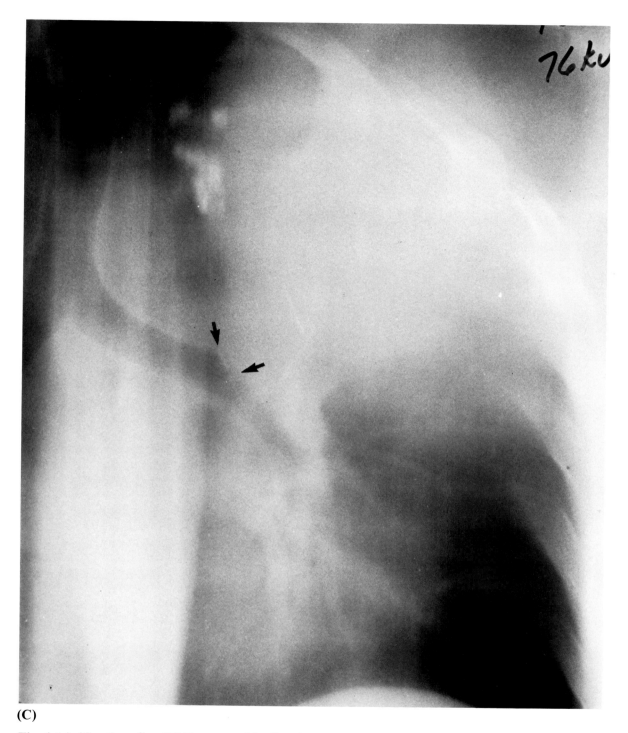

(C)

Fig. 4-14. *(Continued).* **(C)** Tomographic slice through the level of the main bronchi of the left lung shows the lower lobe bronchus to be patent, but the upper lobe bronchus contain no air. It is occluded by tumor at its origin from the left main bronchus (arrows).

If you now go back to the lateral view you can see that beginning just above the air column of the left main and lower lobe bronchi there is an edge in the form of an arc that is convex toward the aerated, hyperexpanded lower lobe (small arrows). This represents the margins of a mass, around which the atelectatic changes have occurred. Since the mass is noncompliant, the upper lobe simply wraps around it.

This is an example of left upper lobe atelectasis and consolidation in which the consolidation component is predominant.

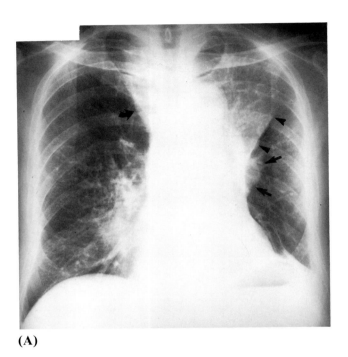

(A)

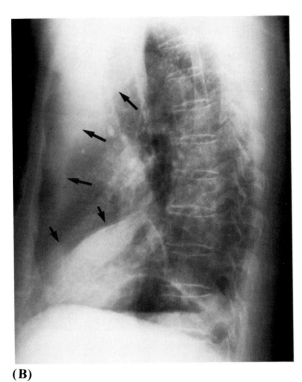

(B)

Fig. 4-15. Atelectasis of the Left Upper and Right Middle Lobes

(A) PA view of a 79-year-old man with a newly diagnosed adenocarcinoma of the left upper lobe shows a veil-like zone of increased tissue density extending from the apex to the lower portions of the left hilum. This zone has a well-defined lateral edge (arrowheads). At the level of the hilum there is a mass with an edge that is convex toward the adjacent aerated lung (short arrows). The upper portions of the left hilum are effaced. The left pulmonary artery, which can faintly be seen through the veil of increased soft tissue density, appears elevated. There is slight elevation of the left hemidiaphragm, and there is some tenting.

On the right side there is a loss of detail of the vessels just lateral to the right heart border, extending caudally but not reaching the diaphragm. The vessels in the right upper lung zone appear attenuated. There is widening of the mediastinum to the right with an abnormal, laterally oriented convexity (short curved arrow).

(B) Lateral view shows the long, relatively sharp edge of a displaced major fissure (long arrows) separating the anteriorly shifted, collapsed, consolidated left upper lobe from the overexpanded lower lobe. The lingula is markedly reduced in volume and occupies only a narrow space behind the sternum (compare with the lesser reduction in volume of the lingula in Fig. 4-14B). The darker zone immediately behind the sternum is due to projection of the right lung.

The zone of atelectatic lung that extends to the hilum (the so-called mediastinal wedge) is located between the upper two long arrows, but it does not have edges that are tangential to the beam. Therefore, this portion of the atelectatic lobe does not have a discrete image.

There is an elliptical zone of consolidation superimposed on the heart; just superior to this consolidation there is a very fine line (short arrows) that represents the major fissure on the right side. The oval zone of consolidation simulates loculated fluid in a fissure, but its anterior, caudal extremity is incomplete. This is not loculated fluid but atelectasis of the right middle lobe, which can imprecisely simulate loculated fluid. This atelectasis accounts for the increase in tissue density seen adjacent to the right heart border on the PA view.

Some very dense nodular opacities project anterior to the trachea on the lateral view. One is situated just superior to the blunt end of the middle arrow and the other between the middle and the lower arrow. These represent calcified mediastinal lymph nodes, probably from prior tuberculosis.

The radiographic findings in this case are complex. There is a classic appearance of left upper lobe atelectasis. There is also atelectasis of the right middle lobe. (If that is so, how is it that we are able to see the major interlobar fissure on the right side as a linear image?) *(Figure continues.)*

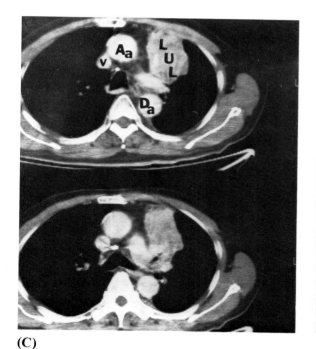 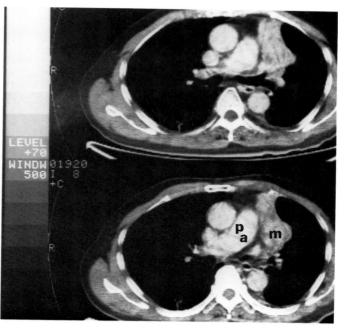

(C)

Fig. 4-15. *(Continued).* **(C)** Sequential CT scans from a level just under the aortic arch (top left) to a level 4 cm caudally (bottom right). The atelectatic left upper lobe (LUL) is seen as a broad band of soft tissue density that extends from the hilar region anteriorly to the chest wall on all of these scans. They are photographed at window and level settings such that the aerated portions of the lung appear solid black. The consolidated and atelectatic left upper lobe, however, appears as a soft tissue density and has become opacified by intravenous contrast material.

On the upper right CT scan you can see the left upper lobe bronchus disappearing into the atelectatic upper lobe. On the scan below it you can see the contour of a mass (m) around which the left upper lobe is collapsing. This corresponds to the mass that projects laterally to the displaced major interlobar fissure in the region of the lower portions of the left hilum on the PA view. It is the displaced left major interlobar fissure that accounts for the sharp interface between the collapsed consolidated left upper lobe and the aerated lower lobe on both the PA view and the CT scan. (Aa, ascending aorta; v, superior vena cava; Da, descending aorta; pa, pulmonary artery.)

Note: The bottom left scan is near the level of the carina of the trachea. Immediately anterior to the black airway there is a brilliant white, irregular nodular opacity. It is medial to the image of the superior vena cava. This represents one of the calcified mediastinal lymph nodes that is seen on the lateral view. A smaller node, or an extension of this one, is visible on the scan immediately above. *(Figure continues.)*

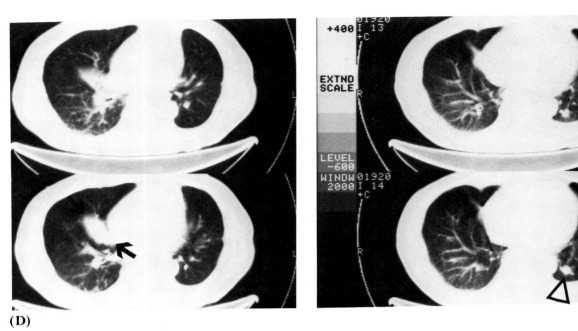

(D)

Fig. 4-15. *(Continued).* **(D)** Series of CT scans through the region of the atelectatic right middle lobe, photographed at settings such that the vessels in the lung can be seen, but the mediastinal contents and the atelectatic portions of the lingula adjacent to the left heart are inseparable and appear as a uniform white, featureless image occupying the central zone. The atelectatic middle lobe is seen as a pyramidal or oval zone of consolidation in the region of the lower portions of the right hilum (top left). It becomes a more oval image on the cut below (arrow) and becomes a thin pyramidal image on the more caudal cuts (upper and lower right). In this case the atelectatic, consolidated middle lobe reaches neither the lateral nor the anterior chest wall. The upper and lower lobes have literally surrounded the atelectatic middle lobe, and that is why we are able to see the anteriorly displaced major interlobar fissure as a line image on the lateral view.

There is a nodular opacity in the posterior portions of the left lower lobe adjacent to the edge of the descending thoracic aorta (open arrowhead). This nodule in the lung is not clearly apparent on either the PA or the lateral chest view even in retrospect. Its location conforms to that of the posterior basal segment of the left lower lobe. (See segmental anatomy of the lower basal zone in Fig. 4-1.)

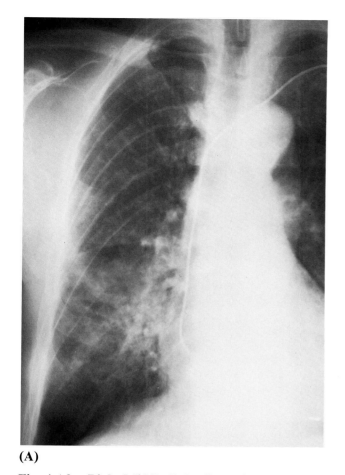

(A)

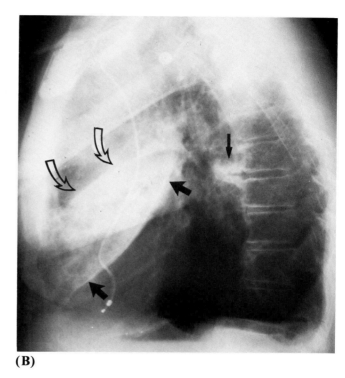

(B)

Fig. 4-16. Right Middle Lobe Consolidation Due to Pneumonia

The patient is an 81-year-old man who had a productive cough, pleuritic pain, and fever of 101 to 102 degrees F for 3 days. The cough was productive of brown and occasionally blood-tinged sputum.

(A) PA film shows increased opacity, with loss of definition of vessels, in the distribution of the right middle lobe. The diaphragm is very low in position, suggesting obstructive airway disease. A pacemaker wire is seen with its tip in the region of the right ventricle. The path of the wire marks the course of the left subclavian and left brachiocephalic veins.

(B) Lateral view. There is a sharply delimited zone of consolidation of the middle lobe outlined by the major interlobar fissure posteriorly (thick black arrows) and a depressed minor interlobar fissure (open arrows) anteriorly. The shift of the interlobar fissures indicates that there is reduction in volume. Ordinarily the major interlobar fissure does not intersect with the anterior chest wall, but rather intersects with the diaphragm.

The patient's arm (the humerus can be seen) is superimposed on the chest. The soft tissues of the patient's arm, hanging below the humerus, are projected as a very sharp edge at the soft tissue-room air interface (small arrows). This edge is partly superimposed on the consolidated middle lobe. Soft tissue-air interfaces on the chest surface can cause confusing images on chest films. Usually they can be followed beyond the confines of the lung and are thus correctly identified.

A metallic pacemaker is superimposed on the upper sternum, with metallic snaps seen as dense, small, round opacities. The thin black vertical arrow points to a large set of anterior hypertrophic spurs from adjacent vertebrae. There is also thickening and waviness of the anterior spinal ligament as it passes over the next few caudal vertebrae. This type of "flowing ossification," bridging at least four contiguous vertebrae, is part of a clinical entity known as diffuse idiopathic skeletal hyperostosis (DISH), which occurs in older people. It is of uncertain significance but may account for back pain and stiffness.[18] *(Figure continues.)*

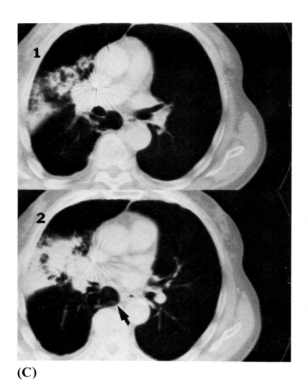
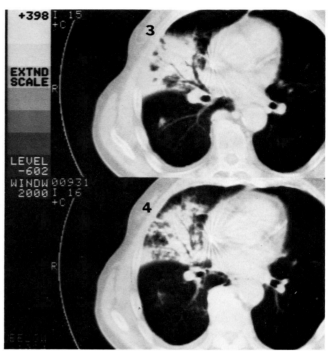

(C)

Fig. 4-16. *(Continued).* **(C)** Four consecutive CT scans, the highest of which (top left) is at a level below the tracheal carina; the right pulmonary artery is seen crossing in front of the airways. A small, dense opacity is seen just anterior to the right pulmonary artery along the posterior wall of the superior vena cava. This represents the pacemaker wire, and a starburst pattern of artifacts emanates from it. These four scans show a mottled opacification of the right middle lobe.

The major fissure provides a sharp demarcation between the opaque middle lobe anteriorly and the aerated lower lobe posteriorly. This fissure is projected more anteriorly as the cuts proceed caudally.

The anterior segment of the upper lobe (black) is interposed between the opacified middle lobe (light gray) and the anterior chest wall, as you would anticipate from the appearance on the lateral view. As the cuts move caudally, however, the middle lobe comes closer and closer to the anterior chest wall; even more caudal scans (not shown) show that the major interlobar fissure also moves anteriorly.

The top right scan (3) shows that both the medial and lateral segmental bronchi of the middle lobe extend into the zone of opacification. The consolidation of the middle lobe is mottled with rounded lucencies. These could be either emphysematous or uninvolved lung foci or a manifestation of necrosis of lung tissue.

Incidental findings are a well-defined anterior junction line and a very deep azygoesophageal recess, which is seen on all of the scans but is identified by an arrow only on the bottom left scan (2) (see Ch. 7).

CT is very helpful in understanding the three-dimensional anatomy of the lobes and segments of the lung. For example, the posterolateral extent of the lateral segment of the right middle lobe is much more easily appreciated on these CT scans than on the lateral radiograph.

Staphylococcus epidermidis was isolated from bronchial washings. This organism would ordinarily be considered a contaminant, but in this case the same species was grown from a blood culture. Therefore, this case probably represents an unusual case of pneumonia due to *Staphylococcus epidermidis.*

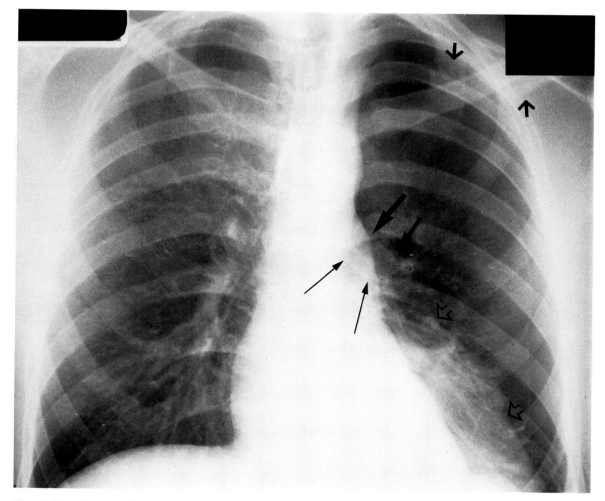

Fig. 4-17. Pneumothorax and Left Lower Lobe Atelectasis Following Blunt Chest Trauma: Effect on the Position and Appearance of the Hilum

This young man had been in an automobile accident a few days before this film was made and sustained a fracture to his left clavicle as well as the anterior left first rib (vertical arrows).

A moderately large pneumothorax is present on the left. Partially collapsed lung is outlined by a very fine line of visceral pleura. There is a short fluid level at the left costophrenic angle, probably due to a small amount of blood in the pleural space.

The left pulmonary artery, which constitutes the bulk of the left hilum, is depressed (thick arrows). There is also a downward inclination of the left main bronchus, whose upper margin (thin arrows) is outlined by the left pulmonary artery. Ordinarily the left hilum is projected at a higher level than the right.

The left retrocardiac area is totally opaque, and a zone of consolidation extends laterally beyond the left heart border. The consolidation is fairly sharply demarcated from the adjacent aerated lung by the displaced major interlobar fissure (open arrows). The fissure is displaced because of atelectasis and consolidation of the lower lobe. The depressed left hilum and the steeper inclination of the left main bronchus are useful correlative signs.

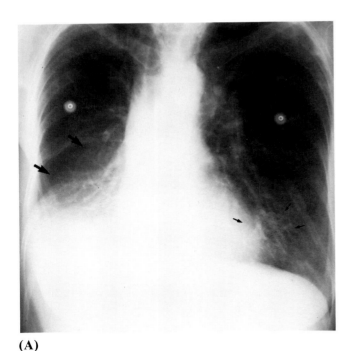

(A)

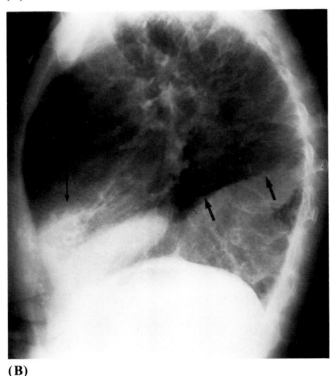

(B)

Fig. 4-18. Effect of Right Lower Lobe Atelectasis on the Position and Appearance of the Hilum

(A,B) PA and lateral views, respectively, of the chest of a woman who is being followed for known chronic lung disease.

(A) PA view. There is a large zone of increased opacity in the right lower lung, with total loss of the image of the right hemidiaphragm. There is a very faint lateral edge (arrows), across which there is a rather sharp change in gray tone. There is a marked diminution in size of the visible portions of the right hilum, and there is considerable shift of the trachea and the superior mediastinum to the right side. On the left is a rounded zone of inhomogeneous consolidation adjacent to the heart (small arrows).

(B) Lateral view shows a very sharply marginated zone of opacity in the posteroinferior portions of the hemithorax. The long, sharp edge (double arrows) represents the lateral aspect of the right major interlobar fissure, which has become displaced inferiorly and posteriorly against the atelectatic right lower lobe. Although it appears as though there is no connection between the atelectic lower lobe and the hilum, in fact a wedge of the atelectatic lobe (the "mediastinal wedge") is still tethered to the hilum. It is simply thin enough that it does not produce a discernible image on the lateral view.

The posterior half of the right hemidiaphragm is effaced. The anterior portions of the right hemidiaphragm are elevated (arrowheads) and appear to be continuous with the sloping image of the lateral aspects of the displaced major interlobar fissure (double arrows). This apparent continuity is spurious. Furthermore, anteriorly the elevated right diaphragm is superimposed on the heart shadow so that the combined image simulates consolidation of the right middle lobe. This image of superimposed structures has no connection to the right hilum, which a collapsed, consolidated right middle lobe should have on a lateral view. Open arrow identifies the posterior wall of the left ventricle.

A vertical arrow points to a rounded zone of inhomogeneous consolidation that corresponds to the abnormality seen in the left lung on the PA view. Correlation of the two views places the consolidation in the lingula. *(Figure continues.)*

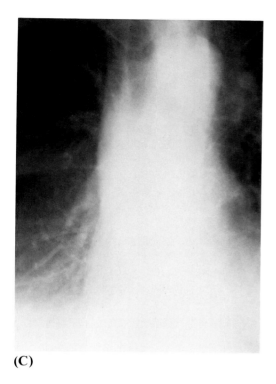

(C)

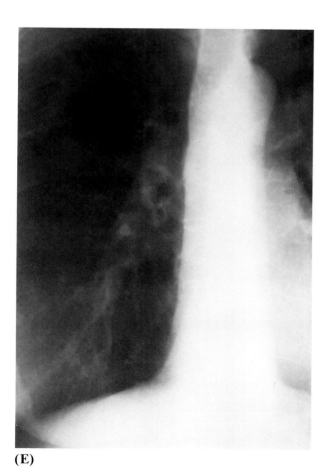

(E)

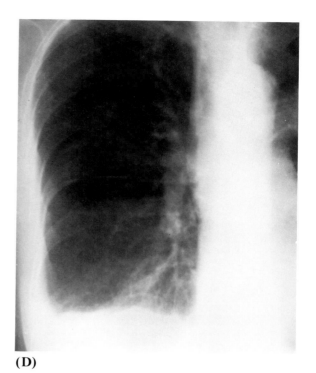

(D)

Fig. 4-18. *(Continued).* **(C–E)** Coned views of the right hemithorax show the change in the appearance of the right hilum from the time of marked lower lobe atelectasis (Fig. C), to 2 days later when it had become partially reexpanded (Fig. D), and from a time prior to the onset of atelectasis (Fig. E). There has been a progressive change in the appearance of the right hilum.

(C) Only a small portion of the vessels of the right hilum remain visible, and there is a considerable shift of the mediastinum to the right. The increase in the overall density of lung at the right base is noted, along with effacement of the right hemidiaphragm (see also A).

(D) There has been a partial reexpansion of the lower lobe; however, the descending limb of the right pulmonary artery and the adjacent bronchus still have an abnormal vertical inclination. The right hemidiaphragm is better seen than in Fig. C, but has not yet become a sharp image. There is still increased tissue density and approximation of vessels at the right base medially. Incidentally, the minor fissure is visible as an interrupted line shadow.

(E) The vascular shadows of the right hilum have their normal oblique lateral inclination as they pass caudally. The right hemidiaphragm presents a sharp image, and there is much better aeration of the right lower lobe. There is no mediastinal shift.

Careful attention to the size of the hilum and the inclination of hilar vessels and bronchi can be very helpful in detecting lobar atelectasis on either the right or the left side.

Assessment of hilar size and position can be used to detect not only lower lobe but also upper lobe atelectasis.

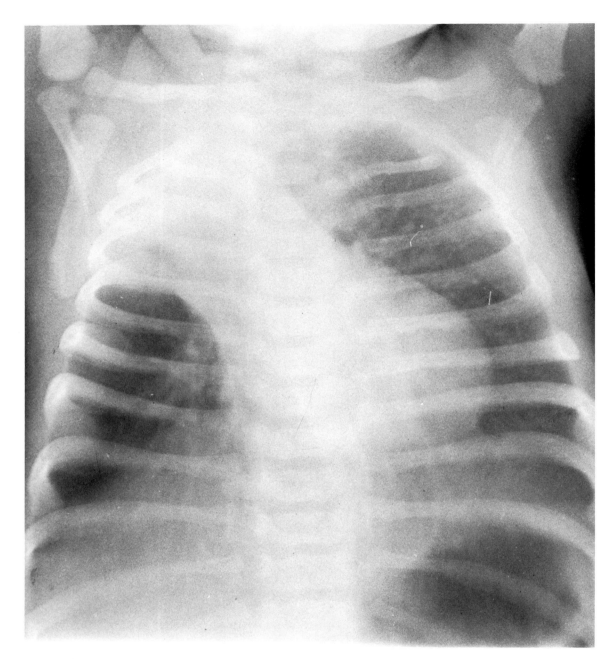

Fig. 4-19. Right Upper Lobe Consolidation and Atelectasis With Marked Mediastinal Shift

AP view shows near-homogeneous opacification of the right upper hemithorax in this infant. The opaque right upper lobe is contracted in volume and is separated from the middle lobe by a sharply defined minor interlobar fissure. There is marked shift of the superior mediastinum to the right and "herniation" of the left lung across to the right superiorly. Infants and children often demonstrate much greater shifts of mediastinal contents than do adults with comparable degrees of lobar atelectasis.

Neither hemidiaphragm is sharply outlined. The clavicles project above the pulmonary apices, telling you that the image is a lordotic projection. This projection changes the orientation of the diaphragm so that the beam sees a continuous slope without enough of a tangent to the beam to record a sharp diaphragm-lung interface.

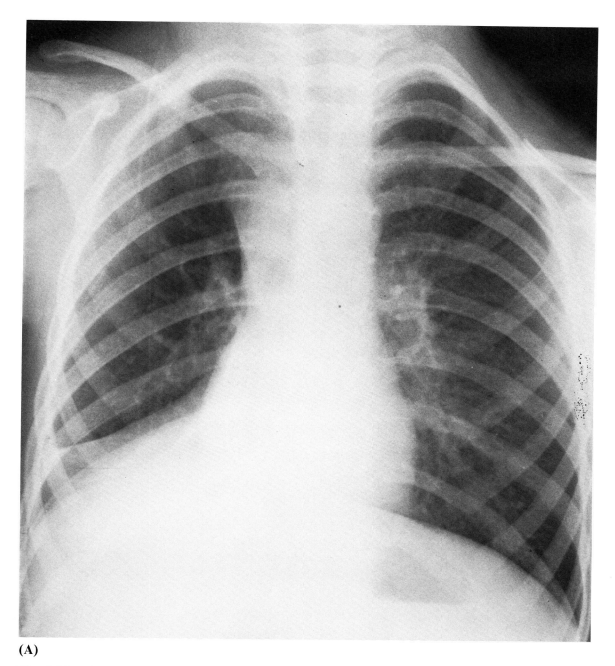

(A)

Fig. 4-20. (A,B) Atelectasis of the Right Middle and Lower Lobes With Mediastinal Shift

These are PA and lateral views of a child who has atelectasis of the right middle and lower lobes. The right hemidiaphragm shadow is effaced from front to back on both views. The hemidiaphragm seen sharply outlined on the lateral view is the left hemidiaphragm.

(A) There is a long, relatively sharp, slightly curved edge projected at the level of the posterior right eighth interspace. There is also a pronounced shift of the superior mediastinum to the right.

The film is not penetrated well enough for the right lower lobe bronchus to be seen, but the right hilum is smaller than expected. In addition, the expanded portion of the right lung—now limited to the upper lobe—is hyperlucent (darker gray) compared to the left lung. A fairly long segment of the right heart border is still sharply defined, because it now forms an interface with the aerated portions of the expanded upper lobe. *(Figure continues.)*

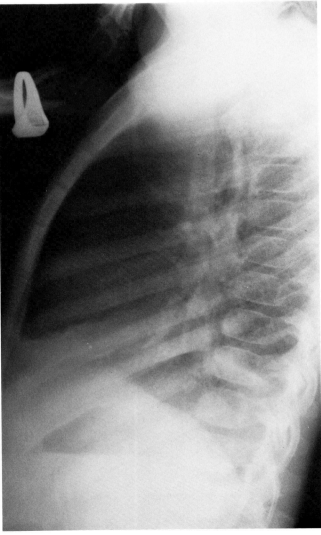

(B)

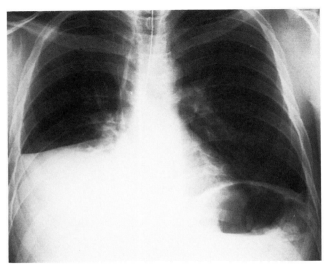

(C)

Fig. 4-20. *(Continued).* **(B)** From the appearance of the lung behind the hilum on the lateral view, it is likely that the superior segment of the right lower lobe remains aerated, but this is not entirely certain since it is possible for the upper lobe to have expanded into this region as well.

If the long, relatively sharp edge in the posterior right eighth interspace on the PA view represents the depressed minor interlobar fissure against the consolidated and atelectatic right middle lobe, why couldn't all the changes be due to atelectasis of the middle lobe? Why is it necessary to invoke atelectasis of the right lower lobe as well?

When the right middle lobe is atelectic, it does not cause enough hyperexpansion of the right upper and lower lobes to account for the observed difference in gray tone between the aerated portions of the right and the left lungs as seen here. Furthermore, atelectasis of the middle lobe alone would not explain the loss of the entire right hemidiaphragm in the lateral view. A combination of middle lobe atelectasis and pleural effusion would explain that, but there is no evidence to suggest significant effusion on the PA view. The shift of the superior mediastinum is far in excess of that which is seen with right middle lobe atelectasis. This shift is commonly seen with right lower lobe atelectasis or, as in this case, with combined right middle and lower lobe atelectasis.

(C–E) Consolidation and Atelectasis of the Right Middle and Lower Lobes Due to or Associated With Pneumonia

This young man had a distal pancreatectomy and pancreaticojejunostomy, duodenostomy, and spincterotomy before these films were taken. Twenty-four hours after surgery he developed a temperature of 38 degrees C and a productive cough. There were decreased breath sounds on the right with rales and rhonchi heard over the lower chest.

(C) PA view shows loss of the right hemidiaphragm and increased tissue density at the right base. The upper margin of the opacity has a long, relatively sharp edge, raising the likelihood of a pleural surface boundary. This edge is the interface between the atelectatic middle lobe and the expanded upper lobe at the minor fissure.

(D) Lateral view shows loss of the sharp right hemidiaphragm-lung interface along its entire anteroposterior extent. This supports the deduction that both the middle and the lower lobe are involved. However, the wavy appearance at the margins of the aerated lung with the opaque zone suggests the presence of pleural fluid. How do we know that some of the lost diaphragm image is not due to associated pleural effusion?

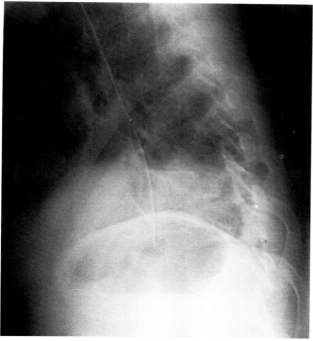

(D)

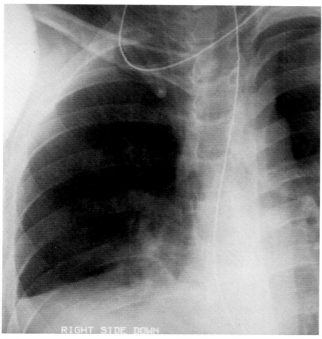

(E)

(E) The right lateral decubitus view, (shown here as though the patient were erect) demonstrates that there is no change in the appearance of the abnormalities at the right base (compare with Fig. C). This indicates that there is no free-flowing pleural fluid.

Sputum cultures grew a coagulase-positive *Staphylococcus* and *Streptococcus pneumoniae.* The patient was started on antibiotics and the fever abated in 12 hours. The atelectatic components took several days to clear radiographically.

From the radiographic appearance alone you cannot tell whether areas of reduction in volume and consolidation are mechanical or pathophysiologic alone, or whether they are accompanied by pneumonia.

Other points to be noted in this patient include:

1. The PA view shows a shift of the upper mediastinal structures to the right (look at the position of the right central line where it traverses the superior vena cava).
2. The lateral view shows the distal end of a nasogastric tube superimposed on a large volume of air in the stomach. You might be tempted to say that the tube tip is in the stomach. However, the PA and right decubitus views show that the tube end is *not* in the stomach but in the region of the distal esophagus. You cannot identify the position of a tube or appliance accurately from only one view.

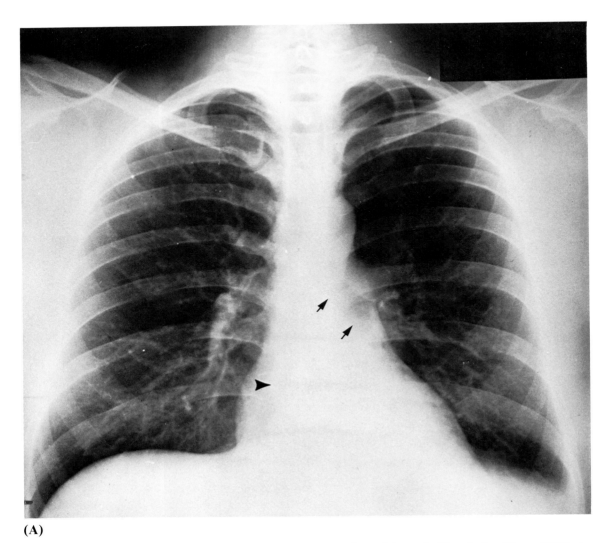

(A)

Fig. 4-21.   Chronic Left Lower Lobe Atelectasis Due to Bronchiectasis Simulating Pleural Effusion

This 24-year-old medical student was sent for examination because something abnormal had been seen on a survey chest film.

(A) PA view. No vessels are seen in the left retrocardiac region in spite of the fact that intervertebral disc spaces (retouched) can faintly be seen through the heart shadow (arrowhead). The left hemidiaphragm is much less sharply defined than the right. Although the ill-defined appearance of the presumed left hemidiaphragm could be caused by pleural effusion, the steep inclination of the left main bronchus (arrows) and the evidence of hyperexpansion of the left upper lobe (increased blackness and fewer visible vessels than on the right) indicate that left lower lobe atelectasis must be a major component of this abnormality. *(Figure continues.)*

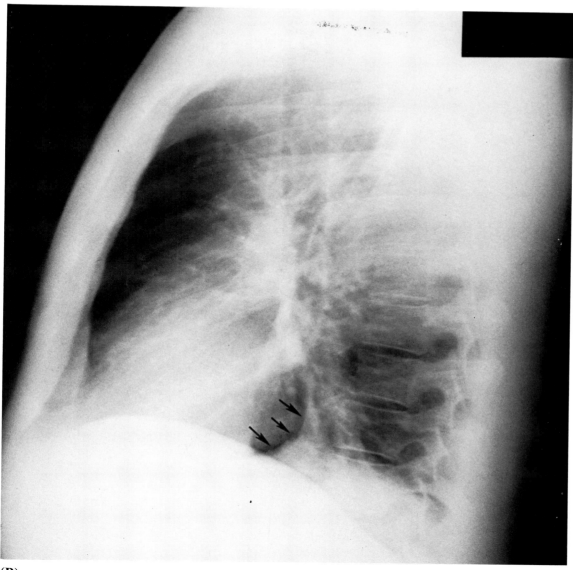

(B)

Fig. 4-21. *(Continued).* **(B)** Lateral view shows an edge shadow (arrows) opposite the image of the posterior heart border, and there is a wedge of increased tissue density extending from the hilum to the diaphragm. The sharp, curved edge is the posteriorly displaced major fissure. The posterior half of the left hemidiaphragm is obscured by the lung consolidation, and the anterior half of the diaphragm is effaced by the adjacent heart. Hence, only the right hemidiaphragm is seen.

These are findings of consolidation and reduction in volume of at least the basilar segments of the left lower lobe. In this example of lower lobe atelectasis the sharp interface of atelectatic lung against the major fissure is seen on the lateral rather than the PA view as in Fig. 4-13A. This difference relates to the orientation of the displaced fissure to the beam in each case.

Upon closer questioning this student recalled that for several years he would often awaken at night and get up to "clear his throat," but otherwise he had no symptoms whatsoever. Eventually a bronchogram was done. *(Figure continues.)*

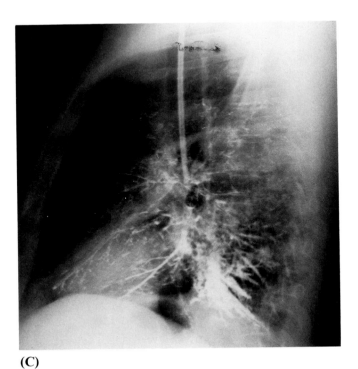

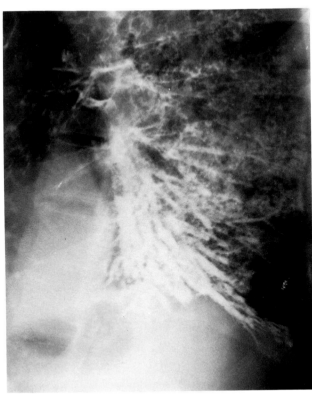

(C)   **(D)**

Fig. 4-21. *(Continued).* **(C)** Lateral view of the bronchographic study shows how the approximated, deformed, and moderately dilated bronchi of the collapsed basilar segments correspond with the abnormalities seen on the lateral chest film.

(D) Coned oblique view shows how these basilar segmental bronchi are approximated and that their walls have beaded marginal contours, they do not taper normally as they approach the periphery, and they appear "pruned" in that the smaller airway branches arising from them do not fill with contrast.

This left lower lobe atelectasis is due to intrinsic alteration of lung structure, the result of chronic inflammation and bronchiectasis. Patients with so-called "dry bronchiectasis" may have few symptoms until an episode of hemoptysis causes them to seek medical aid.

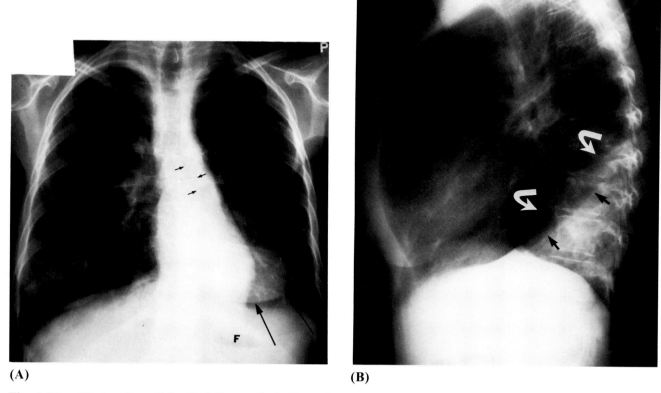

(A) (B)

Fig. 4-22. Obstruction of the Left Lower Lobe Bronchus With Atelectasis And Perilobar Pleural Effusion

This young woman with recurrent Hodgkin's disease has narrowing and partial obstruction of the left main and lower lobe bronchi.

(A) PA view. The left lower lobe bronchus was barely seen between the small arrows on the original film. There is an intensely opaque area behind the left heart with complete loss of vessel images in the lower lobe. There is also a loss of the contour of the left hemidiaphragm and an increased distance between the air in the gastric fundus (F) and the apparent left diaphragm. Do not confuse the left breast image (long arrows) with abnormal lung.

(B) Lateral view. There is a more or less triangular zone of opacity with its apex posteriorly (behind and slightly above the upper white arrow) and its base on the left diaphragm. The image of the diaphragm itself is totally effaced because of the adjacent opacified lung. Only the right diaphragm is seen posteriorly.

There is a sharp anterior edge (black arrows) to this zone of opacity. It represents the lateral edge of the posteriorly displaced and rotated major fissure. (Notice that in this case the major interlobar fissure is also seen sharply on the lateral view, but not on the PA view.) Just anterior to this sharp interface there is another faint edge (white arrows) that follows a similar course except that it curves toward the hilum. This is part of the medial aspect of the major fissure draping toward the so-called mediastinal wedge. *(Figure continues.)*

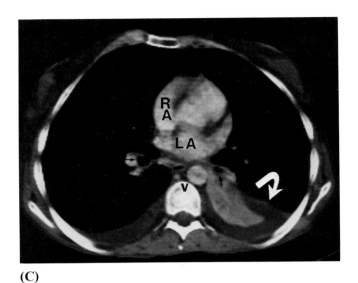

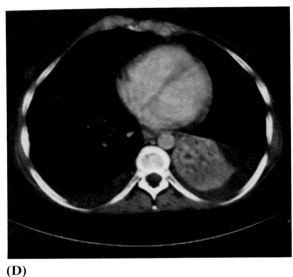

(C)   **(D)**

Fig. 4-22. *(Continued).* (C) CT scan at a level below the tracheal carina. An opacified tongue of atelectatic left lower lobe is surrounded by pleural fluid, which allows the lung to retract completely from the chest wall. In this position the fluid extends into the posteriorly retracted major interlobar fissure (white arrow) and produces a sharp interface with adjacent lung. This scan was photographed at window and level settings such that aerated lungs appear black. (LA, left atrium; RA, right atrium; V, vertebra. The left limb of the V points to the azygos vein just anterior to the vertebral body. The right limb points to the descending aorta.

Just anterior to the azygos vein there is air in the esophagus. Notice the narrow caliber of the left lower lobe bronchus compared to the right (small arrows).

(D) CT scan at a lower level than Fig. C. The opacified, atelectatic left lower lobe has become wider as it extends toward the diaphragm. It is still surrounded by pleural fluid, (F) which extends into the major interlobar fissure. You can understand why the major fissure is seen well on the lateral view of the chest, but is seen more or less en face on the PA view. There is also a right pleural effusion, (F) which appears as a crescent of water density cradled against the right posterior chest wall in both Figs. C and D. The right effusion is not evident on the PA view of the chest, but on the original lateral film the posterior portions of the right hemidiaphragm appeared to curve upward just anterior to the posterior right ribs in the manner of a small subpulmonic effusion. Unfortunately this cannot be seen on Fig. B because it is in a very dark area of the film.

The presence of left pleural effusion in this case is difficult to detect on the chest films because it is perilobar. The large distance between the air in the stomach and the presumed diaphragm on the PA view is a clue.

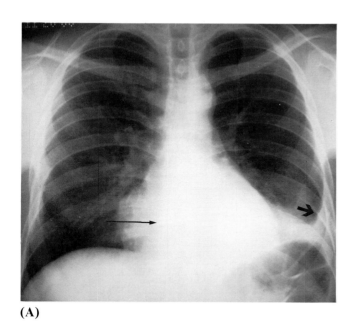

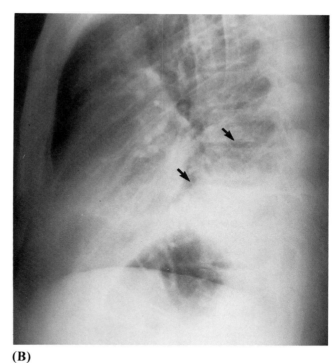

(A)   (B)

Fig. 4-23.   Consolidation of Basilar Segments of the Left Lower Lobe With Pleural Effusion

(A) PA view. An interspace between vertebrae in the retrocardiac region was seen faintly on the original film (long arrow). Under these circumstances one should be able to see vessels in the retrocardiac portions of the left lower lobe, yet in this patient that region is entirely opaque. There is evidence of pleural effusion with fluid extending up along the lower left chest wall (short arrow). Although the hemidiaphragm is not seen, the high position of the gas-filled colon indicates the diaphragm is slightly high.

Although pleural effusion alone could account for these findings, the slight depression of the left hilum, the slightly darker gray of the lung in the left parahilar region compared to the right, and the slightly lesser concentration of small vessels in this zone indicate that there is some hyperexpansion of the left upper lobe. When combined with an elevated left hemidiaphragm this suggests a significant element of atelectasis of the lower lobe in addition to the pleural effusion.

(B) Lateral view shows the image of only one diaphragm: the right. Gas in the splenic flexure of the colon helps to predict the position of the left hemidiaphragm, but the image of the hemidiaphragm itself is effaced.

There are no truly sharp edges to indicate the position of the major interlobar fissure, because the interface between the consolidated, atelectatic lobe and the aerated lobe projects an insufficient tangent to the beam. Sometimes the edge of a rib (arrows) will simulate a displaced major interlobar fissure, but careful analysis will help to avoid that pitfall. For example, in this case there is actually a series of these rib edges ascending towards the thoracic inlet rather than just the one outlined by the arrows. *(Figure continues.)*

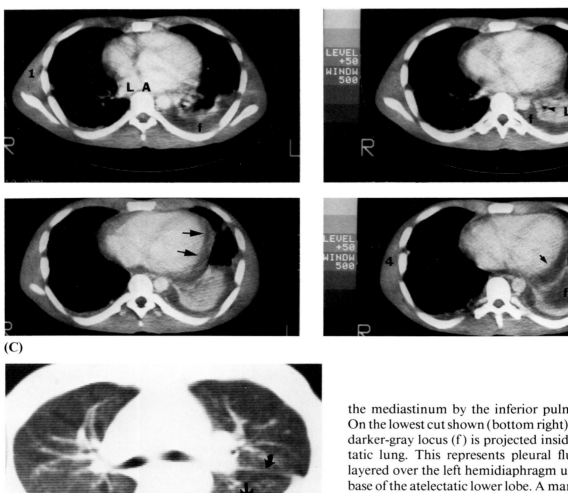

(C)

(D)

Fig. 4-23. *(Continued).* **(C)** Series of CT scans of the same patient. Radiopaque contrast material has been administered intravenously, and the atelectatic left lower lobe has become opacified.

The highest scan (top left) is made at a level well below the tracheal carina. The contrast-filled left atrium (LA) is seen anterior to the spine and the rounded contour of the descending aorta to the left of the spine. A mantle of pleural effusion (f) is cradled along the posterior wall of the left hemithorax. At a slightly lower level (top right) you can see the opacified, atelectatic basilar segments of the left lower lobe surrounded by pleural effusion (f). A small black circle within the medial portions of the basilar segments represents a narrowed left lower lobe bronchus (arrowhead). At a still more caudal level (bottom left), the collapsed basilar segments are seen tethered to the mediastinum by the inferior pulmonary ligament. On the lowest cut shown (bottom right) an irregular oval, darker-gray locus (f) is projected inside a rim of atelectatic lung. This represents pleural fluid that remains layered over the left hemidiaphragm under the concave base of the atelectatic lower lobe. A mantle of pericardial fluid is present at the two most caudal levels (arrows).

In addition to the abnormalities on the left side, there is a thin rind of thickened pleura along the posterior and lateral aspects of the right chest, with a small tag of thickened pleura seen laterally.

(D) CT scan of the chest made at a level just below the bifurcation of the trachea. The right and left main bronchi are seen as oval black images in the center. Window and level settings were chosen to demonstrate lung structure. The curve of the lung-chest wall interface posteriorly on the right side is normal. On the left side an absorber (straight arrow) is interposed between the posterior chest wall and the aerated lung. This proved to be a layer of fluid when displayed at different window and level settings (not shown). This mantle of fluid extends up to the level of the major interlobar fissure (curved arrow), which can be seen as a line extending from the left lateral chest wall to the hilum. This portion of the major fissure is probably seen well because of a thin layer of fluid extending into it and because it has the expanded upper lobe anteriorly and air remaining in the superior segment of the lower lobe behind to serve as contrast.

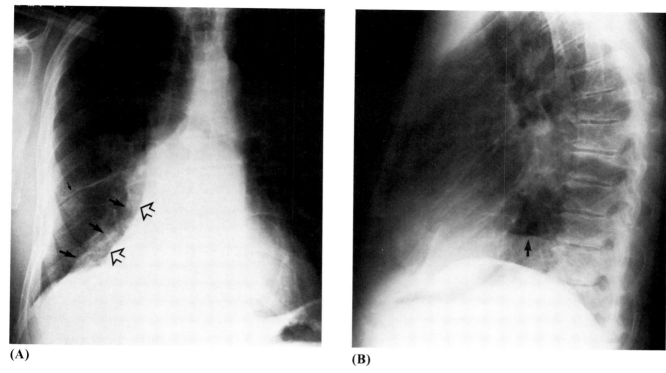

(A)   (B)

Fig. 4-24.   Atelectasis of the Right Lower Lobe Around A Hilar Mass

(A) PA view. The upper lung zones appear black and devoid of vessels largely because of the technique used to make both the original film and this reproduction. However, in part, this appearance is due to the hyperexpansion of the right upper lobe secondary to the marked loss of volume of the right lower lobe.

There is a shift of the trachea and the superior mediastinum to the right. Open arrows point to a very sharp interface that mimics a displaced major interlobar fissure such as is seen in Fig. 4-13. In fact, however, it is the mediastinal pleural reflections over the right side of the heart and an adjacent prominent right cardiac fat pad, as a CT study will show.

Three black arrows point to a slightly undulating interface between a water-density absorber and the adjacent lung. This interface is not as sharply defined as that of the right side of the mediastinum. Above the most cephalad arrow the course of this interface changes so that instead of being gently concave toward aerated lung it is now gently convex. This raises the suspicion of a mass in the lower pole of the right hilum. The right main bronchus is well seen, but the bronchus intermedius and the lower lobe bronchus are not.

A thickened minor interlobar fissure (small arrows) appears slightly caudally displaced. The fact that it is seen as a line shadow indicates that there must be air on both sides of it, in the upper lobe superiorly and in the middle lobe inferiorly.

(B) Lateral view. No sharp edges are seen to help identify the atelectatic, consolidated right lower lobe. However, the posterior third of the right hemidiaphragm is totally effaced. The retrocardiac portion of the diaphragm (arrow) can be seen, but its interface with lung is lost posteriorly. There is a change in the gray tone over the lower half of the posterior portions of the chest such as may be seen with a soft tissue filter in the beam; this is the location of the atelectatic, consolidated right lower lobe. Other than this change in gray tone and the loss of outline of the posterior third of the right hemi-diaphragm, the signal produced by the atelectatic right lower lobe on this view is at best cryptic. Once again, the mediastinal wedge, (i.e., the portion of atelectatic lung that reaches to the hilum) is not at all discernible.

The hilum is lacking in detail, and the individual vessels emanating from it are poorly defined. This is in keeping with the presence of a lower hilar mass that displaces lung and obscures the ordinarily visible vessel-lung interfaces. However, no discrete edges of a mass are seen. *(Figure continues.)*

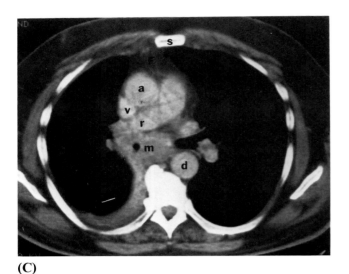

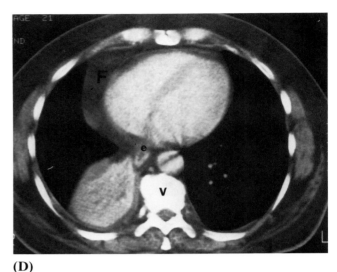

(C)   **(D)**

Fig. 4-24. *(Continued).*   **(C)** CT scan of the high subcarinal region of the chest of the same patient. A rounded mass (m) extends into the right hilum and surrounds and narrows the lumen of the bronchus intermedius (small black hole to the left of m).

The great vessels are partially opacified by intravenous contrast material. There is also partial opacification of a tongue of atelectatic lower lobe that cradles against the right posterior chest wall. This scan was photographed at window and level settings such that aerated lungs appear totally black.

The fat (F) in the anterior portions of the mediastinum has shifted to the right of the sternum (s) as a result of the reduced volume of the right hemithorax (a, ascending aorta; v, superior vena cava; r, right pulmonary artery; d, descending thoracic aorta).

(D) CT scan at a lower level in the same patient. The atelectatic right lower lobe is located posteriorly and paravertebrally, as one would have expected from its plain film appearance. Adjacent to the right side of the heart there is a large fat pad that has a sharp interface with adjacent lung. This tangent, parallel to the beam, accounts for the very sharp interface between the right side of the mediastinum and the lung in the PA projection. The atelectatic lung margin, however, does not present as long a tangent to the beam, and therefore it would account for the faint interface seen and outlined by the black arrows in Fig. A.

The aerated portions of the lungs appear black. A few small vessels are seen end-on in the left lung. The atelectatic right lower lobe is opaque because it is airless and has become opacified with contrast material. Faint streaks of gray are produced by bronchi that still contain air.

A slightly curved, fairly thick gray band separates the opacified blood in the right ventricle from that in the left ventricle; it represents the interventricular septum. A small amount of air is seen within the esophagus (e). A small rounded opacity immediately anterior to the vertebrae (v) represents a cross section of the azygos vein. The very prominent thick, black stripe running across the opacified descending thoracic aorta is an artifact but mimics the flap of an aortic dissection. The vertebra itself is misshapen, and here and in Fig. C there are prominent osteophytes along its right anterior margin. The window and level settings at which these scans were photographed do not adequately display bone detail.

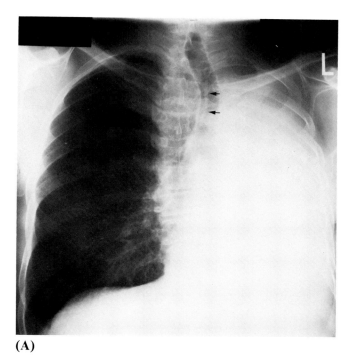

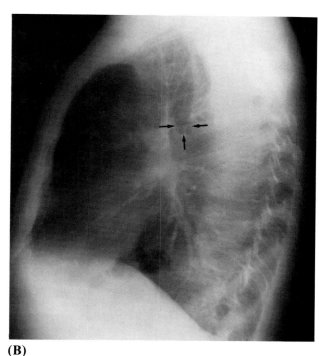

(A)   **(B)**

Fig. 4-25.   Opaque Hemithorax Due to Atelectasis

(A) PA view. There is opacification of the left hemithorax, with a shift of the mediastinal structures to the left. A thin band superimposed on the trachea represents a displaced posterior junction line (arrows). This indicates that the abnormalities on the left side are due not to the patient's having had a pneumonectomy, but rather to massive atelectasis of the left lung. There is just enough aerated left lung remaining in the prevertebral position to allow the posterior junction line to be seen as the interface between the right and left lungs. The right lung looks black because of the filming technique used.

(B) Lateral view of the same chest. The vascular shadows seen anterior to the airways, at the region of the hilum, must all be produced by vessels of the right lung. The ordinarily prominent image of the left pulmonary artery arching over the left upper lobe bronchus is totally effaced by the surrounding opaque left lung. A short segment of the left main bronchus, also visible on the PA view, is seen here to terminate abruptly (arrows).

Only one hemidiaphragm is visible (the right). The posterior two-thirds of the chest has a rather uniform gray tone as through a filter had been placed in the beam. The film is blacker anteriorly, where there has been herniation of the hyperexpanded right lung across the mediastinum to the left. This anterior herniation of lung, in cases of contralateral pneumonectomy or contralateral total-lung atelectasis, is common and indeed can be identified on the original PA view. *(Figure continues.)*

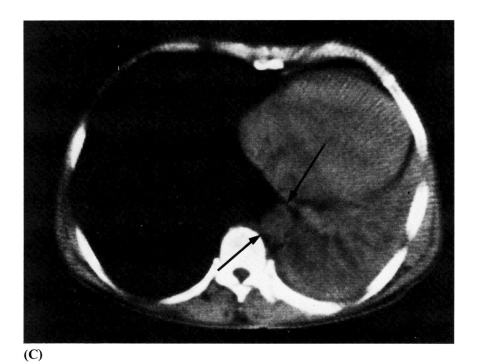

(C)

Fig. 4-25. *(Continued).* **(C)** CT scan of the same patient's chest below the level of the hila and above that of the diaphragm. There is marked shift of the heart (H) into the left hemithorax. The greater density discrimination of the CT scanning technique clearly shows that there is lung in the posterior portions of the left hemithorax, and there are air-filled bronchi (branching, dark gray streaks) visible within this markedly collapsed portion of the lung. The presence of air in peripheral bronchi *cannot* be used as a sign to rule out central bronchial obstruction, especially when seen on CT scan.

The collapsed left lung has the density of soft tissue, whereas the aerated right lung appears black at these CT settings.

The descending thoracic aorta (arrows) can be clearly identified on the CT scan even without use of intravenous contrast injection, but is not detectable on the PA or the lateral view of the chest.

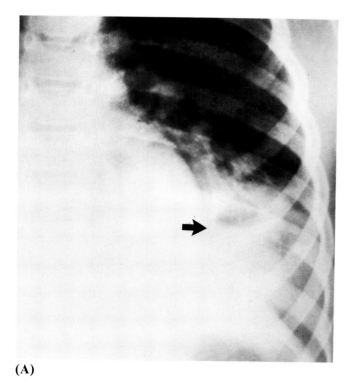

(A)

Fig. 4-26.   Intralobar Pulmonary Sequestration

(A) Coned view of the left lung base in a child with an intralobar bronchopulmonary sequestration. There is extensive opacification of the left lower lung. Even though you can see the intervertebral spaces faintly, no vessel shadows whatsoever are seen in the left retrocardiac area. The arrow points to a fluid level in an air pocket within the zone of consolidation. In a majority of patients the sequestration involves the posterior basilar segments of the left or the right lung; other lobes are much less commonly involved.

(B,C) Later PA and lateral views, respectively, of the same region. There has been considerable reduction in the amount of consolidated lung in comparison to Fig. A, and there is a much larger air-fluid level in the residual parenchymal abnormality in Fig. B (arrows). On the lateral view the abnormality occupies a posterior location, as is usually the case. *(Figure continues.)*

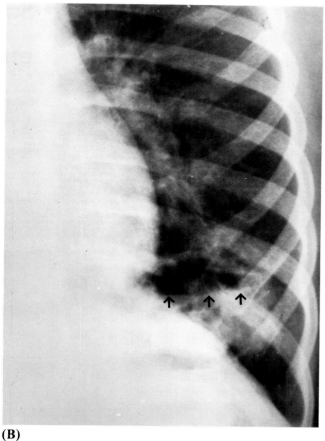

(B)

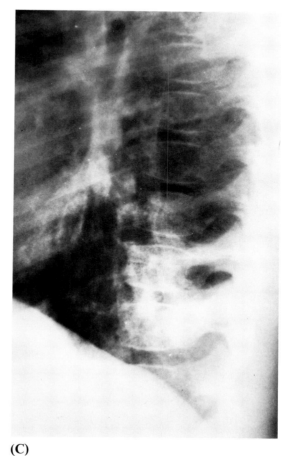

(C)

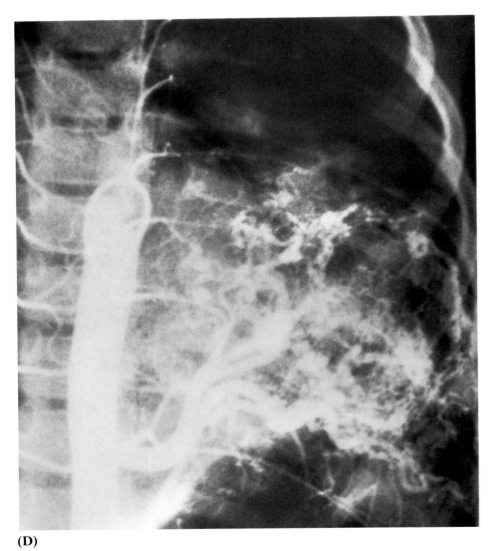

(D)

Fig. 4-26. *(Continued).* **(D)** Arteriogram of the same patient. A very large anomalous vessel originates from the aorta just above the crus of the left hemidiaphragm. There is filling of a large conglomerate of abnormal vessels in this sequestrated portion of the lung. The venous drainage was via the pulmonary veins, as is usual for intralobar sequestration. In some cases venous drainage is via the inferior vena cava or the azygos and hemiazygos system.

Intralobar pulmonary sequestrations are often cystic, but when they have no communication with the bronchial tree — which is the usual case if they are not infected — they contain no air and appear as uniformally dense soft tissue. When infection supervenes, a communication with the bronchial tree may be established, and the patient will often have signs and symptoms of pneumonia accompanied by a productive cough.

Extralobar sequestrations also occur and represent ectopic pulmonary tissue that is enclosed within its own pleura and completely separated from normal adjacent lung. It is most commonly found at the left lung base. As in intralobar sequestration, the arterial supply is from an anomalous vessel originating from the lower thoracic or upper abdominal aorta, and the venous drainage is usually via the systemic veins.

Either intralobar or extralobar sequestrations may communicate with the gastrointestinal tract, although this is uncommon.

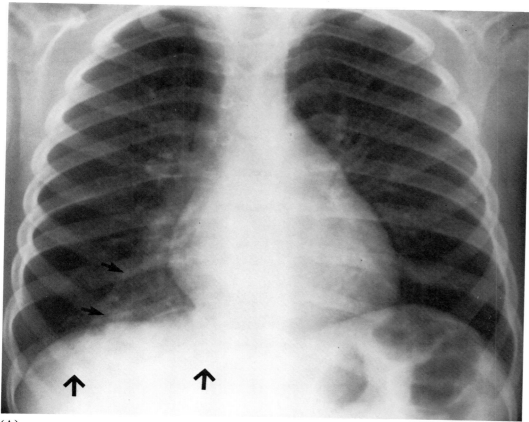

(A)

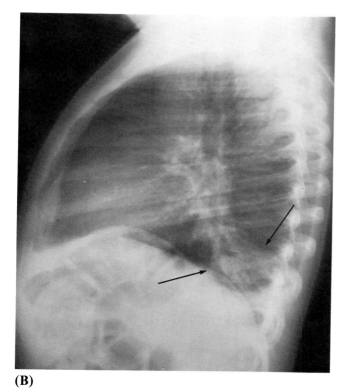

(B)

Fig. 4-27. Atelectasis of Right Lower Lobe Basilar Segments Simulating Posterior Segment Consolidation

(A,B) There is a pie-shaped zone of inhomogeneous consolidation medially (arrows) on the PA view (Fig. A) and posteriorly (arrows) on the lateral view (Fig. B). It resembles the distribution of the consolidation seen in Fig. 4-4D, which was predominantly in the posterior basal segment. Is this the same? Superficially yes, but the width of the consolidation at its base would indicate an unusually large posterior basal segment. In fact, however, this consolidation involves *all* of the basal segments (as was shown on a bronchogram). The basal segments were reduced in volume as a result of bronchiectasis and chronic inflammation, which changed their intrinsic structure. The well-aerated lung seen laterally at the base on the PA view is the overexpanded right middle lobe. The well-aerated lung seen anterior to the consolidation on the lateral view is also the right middle lobe, whereas that seen posterosuperiorly is the hyperexpanded superior segment of the lower lobe.

When the basal segments of either lower lobe lose considerable volume, they can simulate disease in a large posterior basal segment. There is only a minimal mediastinal shift to alert you to the true extent of the abnormality.

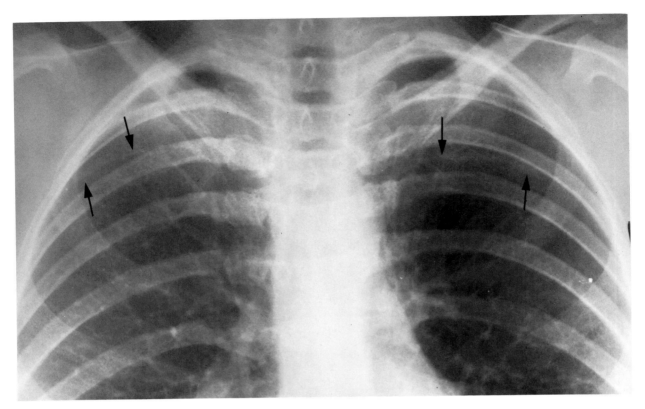

Fig. 4-28. Postirradiation Changes

Coned view of the upper portions of the lungs of a young woman who had received mantle irradiation therapy for nodular sclerosing Hodgkin's disease approximately 10 years before this chest film was taken. Subtle but definite arclike edge images (arrows) are projections of the edges of elevated major interlobar fissures. They are seen either because of pleural thickening extending into the major fissures or because of extrapleural fat along their edges. Although the position of the major interlobar fissures depends on the relative size of the upper and lower lobes, and can be quite variable, it would be unusual for both major fissures to be this high on the basis of anatomic variation alone.

In addition, there is distortion of the upper portions of both hila, which have retracted medially as a result of contraction in volume of the paramediastinal portions of both upper lobes. Such contraction is very common following mantle irradiation therapy and is much more striking in some patients than in others unrelated to treatment dose. Even the degree of apical cap thickening is quite variable from patient to patient. The upper lobe abnormalities can be so striking that they simulate the changes of chronic infection.

Although the reduction in volume of the paramediastinal portions of both lungs is significant, it may be difficult to recognize radiographically. Often it represents reduction in volume without associated consolidation.

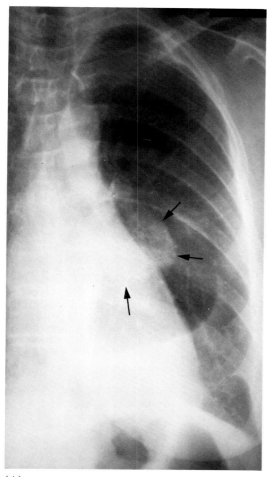

(A)

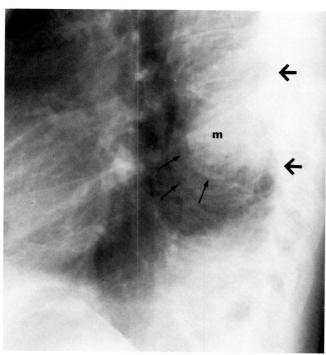

(B)

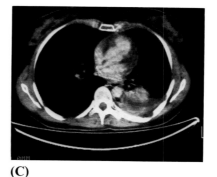

(C)

Fig. 4-29. Round Atelectasis (Trapped Lung)

(A) Coned PA view of the left side of the chest of a woman who had mantle irradiation therapy for Hodgkin's disease approximately 18 years before this film was taken. Approximately 7 years before the film was taken she developed pericarditis and pleuritis, which were probably viral in origin. She was treated conservatively with pericardiocentesis as well as thoracentesis and did well.

A rounded mass is projected in the left hilar region (arrows). There is also a veil-like increase in density over the lower half of the left hemithorax, with a very sharp interface with adjacent aerated lung. This is due to a chronic pleuritis that has been present since her acute episode.

(B) On lateral view the mass (m) is seen far posteriorly. An area of intense pleural thickening (a very white zone) is seen along the inner aspects of the ribs above and below the mass (horizontal arrows). Vessels are seen curving around and then up into the posteroinferior aspects of the mass (thin arrows). This combination of a mass sitting in a field of pleural thickening accompanied by a tether of curving vessels entering its inferior or superior aspect is characteristic of a zone of "trapped lung" or so-called "round atelectasis."

(C) CT scan of the chest at the level of the mass. Intravenous contrast material was administered, and this mass opacified during the systemic arterial phase rather than the pulmonary arterial phase of the passage of the bolus. A layer of thickened pleura is also enhanced. The blood supply to the thickened pleura is probably from branches of the intercostal arteries.

A ball of trapped, atelectatic lung (L) in a field of thickened pleura may follow nonspecific pleuritis or may be seen in patients with asbestos-induced pleuritis. It may simply be an incidental finding on chest films taken for other purposes. Change in size of the mass component has rarely been reported, but in this woman there had been a definite gradual increase in the size of the mass over the preceding few years. This progression was so worrisome that the woman had a thoracotomy to confirm the diagnosis and to rule out the possibility of recurrent Hodgkin's disease in either the pleura or the lung.

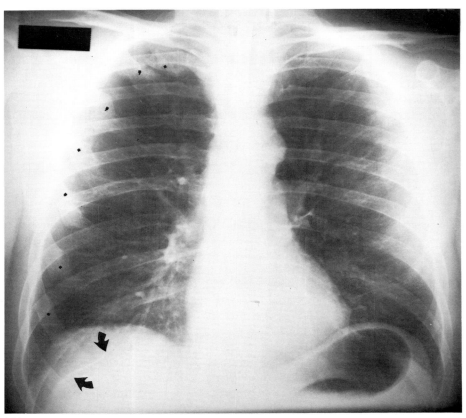

(A)

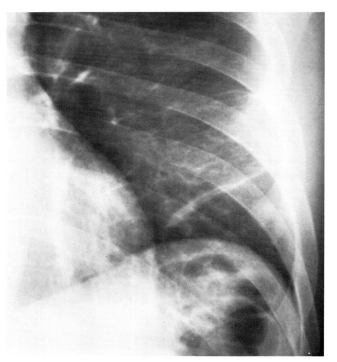

(B)

Fig. 4-30. Peripheral Atelectasis (Plate Atelectasis)

(A) Far caudally, at the right lung base, there is a long line image that neither tapers nor branches (arrows). It is tempting to consider this as scar, but if there are no old films to show stability over time you cannot distinguish it from peripheral atelectasis. Dots mark old rib fracture deformities.

(B) Coned view of the left base made one day after Fig. A. There is a thick band of peripheral (plate) atelectasis laterally. There are also irregular band shadows in a peribronchial and perivascular distribution behind the left heart in Fig. B. The line image at the right base in Fig. A also became much thicker on this follow-up film (not shown).

Bands of peripheral atelectasis are common, nonspecific chest radiographic abnormalities that probably result from hypoventilation of diverse causes.

5

Pulmonary Infection

Pneumonia is a serious cause of morbidity, and for many patients a life-threatening complication of many different types of antecedent disease and treatment regimens. There is frequently a legitimate sense of urgency to establish a precise diagnosis in order to institute specific therapy. This need is most compelling when the patient's signs and symptoms are severe, and especially when the patient is known to be immunocompromised. It is understandable, then, to seek some method of diagnosis that is rapid, disturbs the patient very little, carries no morbidity, and is fairly reproducible. Chest radiography is frequently called upon to serve this function.

The correlation between any given radiographic abnormality and any specific microorganism as a cause of pulmonary infection is not high enough to permit use of the radiographic study alone as a solution. This is a hard fact for both clinician and radiologist to live with. Many articles have described the characteristic roentgenographic appearances of pneumonias produced by a variety of organisms, but "characteristic" and "specific" are not synonymous, and an appearance that is characteristic of infection by one organism may also be part of the radiographic spectrum of appearances of infection with other organisms. *There is no radiographic appearance that is diagnostic for infection with one particular microorganism to the exclusion of others.*

Pulmonary infection is defined in terms of bacteriology; the tissue inflammatory response is defined in terms of histopathology, which is only partially reflected in gross appearance. The chest radiograph can only approximate the gross pathology, and it is unrealistic to expect it to be precise in predicting the bacteriologic cause when there is, of course, not even a hope of seeing a microorganism on a radiograph.

What role can the chest radiograph serve for the patient with suspected pneumonia?[20] Radiographic analysis can:

1. Establish the presence of an abnormality in the lungs consistent with infection
2. Permit estimation of the extent and character of the pulmonary involvement
3. Permit estimation of the rate of change based on serial examination
4. Be correlated with clinical data to elaborate a differential diagnosis and to list the choices in rank-order of likelihood
5. Aid in choosing invasive studies such as bronchoscopy, needle aspiration, or open-lung biopsy
6. Permit recognition of coexisting or complicating factors such as pleural effusion, empyema, bronchopleural fistula, pneumothorax, bronchiectasis, masses causing bronchial obstruction, hilar and mediastinal adenopathy, or involvement of ribs and vertebrae
7. Cast doubt on unlikely diagnoses developed from other data (on rare but important occasions, the conjunction of radiographic and clinical findings are so at odds with the diagnosis derived from laboratory procedures such as sputum cultures that further studies are prompted to explore the likelihood that more than one disease is present or that the first diagnosis is in error)
8. Evaluate resolution and record residual scarring.

In item 1 the words "consistent with" were deliberately chosen rather than "diagnostic of." Infection may well be the most likely explanation of a chest film abnormality, especially when accompanying signs and symptoms are considered. Unfortunately, there are many instances in which pulmonary lesions due to malignant lymphoma, alveolar cell carcinoma, metastatic neoplasm, pulmonary hemorrhage, pulmonary edema, pulmonary infarction, allergic responses to environmental pollutants, reaction to drugs, and noninfectious granulomatous diseases, among others, may be responsible for similar clinical and radiographic abnormalities.

In some patients the chest radiographs may show evidence of pulmonary infection when the clinical signs and symptoms do not—for example, in the elderly, even when the responsible organisms are those associated with acute bacterial pneumonia; occasionally in the patient with altered immunity and infection due to one of the ubiquitous fungi; and notoriously in patients with pulmonary tuberculosis or other infectious granulomatous disease.

On the other hand, there are unusual cases of proven pulmonary infection in patients whose chest films are negative. This has been reported in patients with extreme neutropenia,[52] and perhaps the associated impaired inflammatory response does not permit a radiographically detectable lesion to evolve. Occasionally the initial chest film of a symptomatic patient with pneumonia due to *Pneumocystis carinii* or other microorganisms may appear normal, but surveillance films 24 to 48 hours later show an evolving pneumonitis.

Patients with tracheobronchitis may also have clinical signs and symptoms of pneumonia without any radiographically visible acute parenchymal lesions. Many of these patients suffer from chronic lung disease as well.[28]

ESTABLISHING THE DIAGNOSIS

The best methods for obtaining specimens and establishing the etiology of a given pneumonia are not always simple, nor are they beyond debate.[2,4,5,47] Identification of the responsible organisms in cells of the involved tissue or in the associated inflammatory response, with subsequent retrieval from growth in culture, is the ideal, yet one that often is not satisfied for practical reasons. Retrieval of organisms from accessible secretions, specifically sputum, is a frequent substitute. Both stains of slide preparations and bacteriologic culture of sputum samples may be used.

In many clinical situations the value of sputum cultures is seriously questioned because of false-negative and false-positive results. The disparity of opinion is highlighted by the titles of two articles: "The Diagnostic Value of Sputum Culture in Acute Pneumonia"[44] and "The Non-Value of Sputum Culture in the Diagnosis of Pneumococcal Pneumonia."[3]

Problems arise because some people harbor, in their nose and throat, bacteria that are ordinarily considered pathogenic.[4] *Streptococcus pneumoniae, Staphylococcus aureus, Streptococcus pyogenes,* and *Haemophilus influenzae* are examples of bacteria that may be cultured from nonhospitalized people who have no signs or symptoms of disease. Furthermore, there may be seasonal fluctuations in the carrier rates of these organisms. Hospital personnel may also be colonized but show no signs nor symptoms.

Tillotson and Lerner[45] proposed the following criteria for the diagnosis of pneumonia caused by gram-negative bacilli.

1. Isolation of the same bacteria from two or more consecutive sputa, or
2. Isolation of the same bacteria from cultures of blood and sputum in close proximity, or
3. Isolation of the bacteria from pleural fluid.

To be considered significant, the bacterium had to be present on cultures as the only or the predominant organism, and the clinical course had to be compatible with the diagnosis of parenchymal involvement of the lung. These criteria and minor modifications have been cited by other authors reporting their experience with pulmonary infections.

More global criteria are needed to include pneumonias due to anaerobic organisms, which in the past have been underdiagnosed, and to include infections due to organisms that cannot be cultured or require highly specialized techniques not available in many laboratories.

A discussion of bacteriologic and serologic methods used in the diagnosis of pulmonary infections can be found in references 4 and 5 in the Bibliography for this chapter.

THE COMPROMISED HOST

Any person whose disease or treatment regimen interferes with critical humoral and cellular defenses against infection can be considered a compromised host.[9,14,33,47,48] Common examples are patients who have been treated with steroids or cytotoxic drugs (e.g., transplant recipients) or who suffer from leukemia, malignant lymphomas, hypogammaglobulinemia, or acquired immunodeficiency syndrome (AIDS). However, patients suffering from a large variety of chronic diseases (Table 5-1) are also prone to develop life-threatening pulmonary infections. Although it is tempting to separate disorders of T cell and B cell function and correlate them with specific types of infection, there is so much overlap

TABLE 5-1. Patients Prone to a High Incidence of Pulmonary Infections Because of Altered Defense Mechanisms

General cases
  Patients receiving chemotherapy or long-term, high-dose steroid therapy for lymphoproliferative disorders, malignant neoplasms, connective tissue diseases, or organ transplantation. (The neoplastic diseases and connective tissue diseases may themselves alter host resistance, but pulmonary infections are more common after institution of chemotherapy or steroid therapy.)
  Patients intubated for respirator therapy
  Patients obtunded from any cause (higher incidence of aspiration)

Specific nonneoplastic chronic diseases carrying an increased incidence of pulmonary infection or septicemia
  Cystic fibrosis *(Staphylococcus, Pseudomonas)*
  Sickle cell anemia *(Streptococcus pneumoniae)*
  Absent spleen *(Streptococcus pneumoniae)*
  Diabetes mellitus
  Chronic obstructive pulmonary disease
  Chronic heart disease
  Uremia
  Alcoholism
  Bronchiectasis

Immune deficiency syndromes
  Acquired immunodeficiency syndrome (AIDS)
  Congenital: agammaglobulinemias, hypogammaglobulinemias, dysgammaglobulinemias, and defects in delayed hypersensitivity response (DiGeorge syndrome); disorders of phagocytosis (chronic granulomatous disease of childhood)

of these dysfunctions in patients with altered immunity that there is little practical gain.

LOBAR PNEUMONIA

The majority of bacterial pulmonary infections are due to aspiration or inhalation of microorganisms. Bacteria may multiply in fertile fields because preceding viral infections have altered cellular defense mechanisms or bacterial clearance mechanisms in regions that ordinarily rid themselves of bacteria before infection becomes clinically manifest.[36] However, whether viral upper respiratory infections are a frequent precursor of bacterial pneumonia in adults is unsettled.[18]

The term "lobar pneumonia" is often used to denote a condition in which an inflammatory exudate and edema fluid extend throughout a portion of lung via the pores of Kohn, the canals of Lambert, and other small airway passages while the bronchi themselves suffer little damage.[36] The radiograph is characterized by homogeneous opacification of lung tissue in a lobar or segmental distribution (Fig. 5-1). In fact, however, early in the evolution of the inflammatory process a rather small peripheral focus may be all that is present, and often there is sparing of a portion of the involved lobe or segment even when the consolidation is at its peak.

Air remaining in bronchi that traverse regions of consolidation may be recognized as air bronchograms. Their recognition is important in clearly establishing that the abnormality causing the increased tissue density is in the pulmonary parenchyma, rather than in the pleural space as may sometimes be mistakenly supposed. However, they do not distinguish lobar pneumonia from bronchopneumonia.

Pneumonias caused by almost any microorganism can appear as complete or partial segmental or lobar consolidation at some stage in their radiographic evolution. In community-acquired pneumonias, the bacteria most commonly responsible for lobar pneumonia are *Streptococcus pneumoniae* (pneumococcus) and much less commonly *Klebsiella*, but *Legionella*, other *Streptococcus* sp., *Staphylococcus*, and *Haemophilus*, as well as *Mycoplasma*[41] and viral pneumonias, may produce similar lesions (Fig. 5-2). Even tuberculous pneumonia (Fig. 5-3) or pneumonia associated with infections due to *Histoplasma* or *Coccidioides*[6,7,15] or *Blastomyces*[24] may have an appearance that is indistinguishable from the more common causes of lobar pneumonia.

BRONCHOPNEUMONIA

Some organisms when inhaled or aspirated cause major damage to small airways. Focal patches of peribronchiolar consolidation develop, with several foci evolving simultaneously. Spread into more and more alveolar spaces then occurs until lobules of lung are filled with exudate. When the disease is fulminant, there may also be thrombosis of lobular branches of the pulmonary artery and associated hemorrhagic edema.

The radiographic hallmark of bronchopneumonia is captured in the word "patchy." The consolidations are often patchy and may have peribronchial distributions as well (Fig. 5-4). However, as the lesions progress and become more confluent, the radiographic appearance is indistinguishable from lobar pneumonia, and this can have occurred before the patient seeks medical aid.

Often at the periphery of the consolidation, whether it be lobar or bronchopneumonic in character, there is apparent inhomogeneity, and small foci of increased tissue density, usually under 1 cm in size and with poorly defined margins, may be seen (Fig. 5-5). These represent exudates in small units of lung that are visible because they interface with adjacent interspersed units that are uninvolved. Although sometimes called acinar shadows, their precise anatomic substrate is a matter of controversy.[31] There are instances in which the bulk of the radiographically evident disease appears as clusters of these lesions.

Staphylococcus aureus and *Streptococcus pyogenes* typically produce a bronchopneumonia pattern.

There does not seem to be much benefit in attempting to distinguish lobar pneumonia from bronchopneumonia. The only important function served would be that of predicting the organisms responsible, and unfortunately the same organisms that are associated with classical lobar pneumonia (e.g., *Streptococcus pneumoniae*) may cause lesions similar to those of bronchopneumonia.[21] The sublobular, lobular, and patchy confluent phases of viral, *Mycoplasma*,[43] *Legionella*,[16] and other bacterial pneumonias[52] may also produce indistinguishable radiographic images. Patients with emphysema may have patchy-appearing consolidation due to interspersed foci of emphysematous lung amid consolidated foci. Thus, even lobar pneumonia may have an atypical appearance in these patients.[51]

Patients with pneumonia due to anaerobic organisms[19,23] have zones of consolidation that are indistinguishable from those caused by other bacteria (Fig. 5-6; see also Fig. 5-25), but frequently these patients do not appear as ill as expected and may give a history suggesting an indolent infection. Empyema is a serious complication, and some patients may have empyema without any detectable pulmonary component (see Ch. 3).

BLOODSTREAM DISSEMINATION

Some pneumonias occur as a consequence of bloodstream dissemination from a focus of infection that was primary in the lung or that was extrapulmonary or from an inoculum inadvertently introduced into the bloodstream. These pulmonary infections may then present a diffuse appearance such as occurs in miliary tuberculosis or miliary forms of infection due to pathogenic fungi and, uncommonly, miliary dissemination of other bacteria. Perhaps diffuse viral pneumonias are also consequent to viremia.

Staphylococcal pneumonia may be caused by organisms disseminated from extrapulmonary sites via the bloodstream. Focal lesions may be seen first in one or both lower lobes, or there may be scattered multiple foci in one or both lungs (Fig. 5-7). The lesions may then coalesce. Multiple septic emboli, usually due to staphylococci are often a complication of intravenous drug abuse. Endocarditis may also occur in these patients and become difficult to eradicate.

One form of *Pseudomonas* pneumonia also behaves as though organisms had been disseminated via the bloodstream, resulting in widespread involvement of both lungs.

MASSLIKE ZONES OF CONSOLIDATION

Masslike zones of consolidation may occur with many different bacterial and fungal pneumonias. In cases of rapid onset and rapid progression, as either an increase in size of a single lesion or an increase in the number of areas involved, consider infections with gram-negative organisms, especially *Klebsiella, Escherichia coli,* and *Pseudomonas.*[10] Infrequently, a type III pneumococcus (gram-positive) may produce similar lesions. Hemolytic streptococci may also cause masslike consolidation (see Fig. 5-5). Massive gram-negative organism pneumonia and type III pneumococcal pneumonia may progress rapidly to cavitation. The patients are usually extremely ill, and their clinical course mirrors that of the radiographic progression (Figs. 5-8 and 5-9).

When masslike consolidations occur adjacent to interlobar fissures, the fissures may bulge toward adjacent healthier lung, presenting another radiographic sign that raises the suspicion of necrotizing pneumonia, particularly that caused by gram-negative organisms (see Fig. 5-2).

Patients with *Legionella* pneumonia may also show masslike opacities (Fig. 5-9). Increase in the size of a zone of consolidation or the appearance of new areas of consolidation may occur even after treatment with appropriate antibiotics has begun (Fig. 5-10).[16,22]

Bacteria such as *Pseudomonas* and fungi such as *Aspergillus* and *Mucor* are vascular invaders and cause thromboses that result in areas of necrosis and hemorrhagic infarction. Clinically these events may mimic pulmonary embolic disease and may appear as masslike zones of consolidation or even as nodules.

NODULES (WITH OR WITHOUT CAVITATION)

Noncalcified pulmonary nodules or nodular foci of consolidation may vary from under 1 cm to several centimeters in size. They may be solitary or multiple (miliary lesions are discussed in a later section).

Many organisms may produce focal inflammatory pulmonary lesions that present as solitary or multiple nodules. Tuberculosis, histoplasmosis, coccidioidomycosis, and cryptococcosis are examples of diseases that commonly manifest as nodular foci in the lungs. Any lobe may be involved, but when the lesions are multiple, they are frequently clustered in one or two areas, usually the upper lobes in tuberculosis (Fig. 5-11). Less commonly there may be multinodular involvement of all the lobes.

Nodules or small masses, solitary or multiple are also seen frequently as new lesions due to pulmonary infections in patients with altered immunity. The ubiquitous fungi, such as *Aspergillus, Mucor,* or *Cryptococcus,*[17] or the higher bacterium *Nocardia* are commonly the cause (Figs. 5-12 and 5-13). However, nodules of consolidation may also be due to infection with anaerobes and occasionally other microorganisms.[10,11] Cavitation does not change the differential diagnosis, because lesions due to these organisms can manifest either as solid-appearing nodules or as cavitary nodules.

Uncommonly, pulmonary nodules in patients treated with immunosuppressive drugs may be due to development of a malignant lymphoma (Fig. 5-14). The determination as to whether a new pulmonary nodule (or nodules) is due to the lymphoma or to an infection is usually not feasible without biopsy. Fever and malaise may be a part of the symptom complex of the malignant lymphomas, so that those findings alone cannot be used as clinical indications of infection.

Nodular and cavitary nodular pulmonary lesions may also be seen as roentgenographic manifestations of septic emboli in patients with extrapulmonary infections or who are involved in intravenous drug abuse. Marantic pulmonary artery aneurysms may be due to infections in these people as well. The organisms most commonly associated with these septic emboli or marantic aneurysms are the staphylococci.

Solitary nodules with or without cavitation are most unusual as the initial presentation of infections due to viruses, *Mycoplasma,* gram-negative organisms, or staphylococci. It is tempting to eliminate these from discussion when formulating differential diagnoses for nodules in patients with altered immunity. The facts would be better served if you gave them a low rank-order of probability rather than eliminated them, because uncommon events do occur (Figs. 5-15 to 5-17).

INFECTIONS APPEARING AS DIFFUSE LUNG DISEASE

Small, Irregular Opacities or Reticulonodular Patterns

Small, diffusely distributed, nodular opacities due to peribronchiolar inflammatory foci may be seen during the relatively early stages of pulmonary infection with many organisms. This pattern is especially noteworthy as part of the radiographic spectrum of viral pneumonias (Fig. 5-18A to G). Aside from the influenza viruses, adenoviruses, and other common respiratory viruses in patients with altered immunity, cytomegalovirus, varicella-zoster, and rarely measles virus may cause such lesions. A pattern of small, irregular nodular opacities is also part of the spectrum seen with *Pneumocystis carinii* infections.

Because of their small size and unsharp margins, these nodules can be confused with overlapping vascular shadows and may be difficult to recognize when few in number. Their appearance varies from an often bibasilar granular pattern (Fig. 5-18G) to a more coarsely nodular pattern (Fig. 5-18E) and a larger confluent nodular pattern (Fig. 5-18F). Frequently a reticulonodular pattern is present.

Usually not all portions of both lungs are involved initially as they are in miliary tuberculosis. As the disease progresses, however, the pattern changes (Fig. 5-18C), and radiographic spectra overlap. Viral pneumonias may then resemble each other or even miliary tuberculosis. As confluent, irregular foci evolve, the appearance becomes indistinguishable from that of disseminated pneumonia due to any other organism (Fig. 5-18G).

Occasionally in the case of infection with varicella-zoster, the nodules may not be widespread throughout both lungs but may be clustered in one or two zones. It is likely, however, in these exceptions that the radiographic findings do not actually reflect the true pathologic extent of the disease.

Miliary Lesions

There is a spectrum of radiographic patterns that can be described as "miliary," although at the extremes they do not correspond to millet seeds (think of birdseed) in size. The lesions may vary from a barely detectable granular pattern to nodules 2 to 5 mm in size, with ill-defined borders (Fig. 5-19). All of the organisms included in the infectious granulomatous disease group may produce miliary nodules during the progressive primary or reactivation phase of infection.[6,7,15,40] All portions of both lungs are involved, presumably secondary to bloodstream dissemination. Chest roentgenograms may show a relative sparing of the periphery of the lungs in some cases, but critical analysis will show that these areas are truly involved, although less obviously so. Sometimes, in addition to the miliary pattern, there may be focal abnormalities from antecedent lesions, for example, lesions of chronic tuberculous infection or even cavitation in the apices.

One cannot distinguish miliary tuberculosis from miliary histoplasmosis, miliary coccidioidomycosis, or miliary blastomycosis radiographically. Simply because it is the most common, tuberculosis receives first rank in the list of differential diagnoses when considering this group of infections in most communities.

Although there are many causes of miliary patterns[12]

other than infectious granulomatous disease, seldom are the others so clearly seen to involve all portions of the lungs. Among other infections that may cause a miliary or miliary-like pattern are those caused by *Pneumocystis carinii, Toxoplasma gondii,* various viruses, rarely other bacteria such as *Staphylococcus* or *Salmonella,* or disseminated ubiquitous fungi[30] or *Nocardia.*

Miliary patterns may also be seen in noninfectious disorders and these will be discussed in Ch. 10.

Diffuse Pneumonia in Other Patterns

Diffuse pulmonary infection is often seen on chest films as extensive homogeneous or inhomogeneous consolidation, often with foci of circumscribed radiolucency due to interspersed uninvolved lung or to areas of necrosis and cavitation. These lesions can also be patchy and may be seen to have evolved from more discrete nodular lesions. Almost any organism or, worse, any combination of organisms can result in such patterns, and the responsible pathogen is impossible to predict with any degree of precision in the individual case. *Pseudomonas,* other gram-negative organisms, *Staphylococcus,* tubercle bacillus, anaerobic bacteria, viruses (cytomegalovirus, herpes simplex, varicella, measles), ubiquitous fungi, *Toxoplasma,* and *Pneumocystis* may be found alone or in various combinations (Figs. 5-20 and 5-21). At times, particularly in patients who have been on long-term antibiotics, even open-lung biopsy may not permit recognition of the responsible organisms. You may be left with the diagnosis of nonspecific organizing pneumonia based on histopathology.

Patients who develop the adult respiratory distress syndrome (ARDS) may also show radiographic abnormalities identical to those who have pulmonary infection. In acutely ill patients the diagnosis can be suggested on the basis of a combination of disturbances in physiology and a roentgenographic pattern of diffuse disease that shows little change on sequential films made over a period of several days. Diffuse lung disease due to an untreated acute infection, in contrast, rarely remains stable over several days. Nevertheless, it may be impossible to exclude infection coexistent with ARDS.

Lungs of patients with acute diffuse pneumonia may be massively involved and appear as nearly solidly opaque, except for air bronchograms. The appearance is comparable to that of extreme pulmonary edema. Fortunately, this pattern is uncommon at the time the patient is first seen, and more often is seen to evolve on sequential films of patients with relentless disease progression.

CAVITIES, PSEUDOCAVITIES, AND ABSCESSES

When necrotic lung tissue is expelled into airways, a cavity may be left. When the cavity becomes sufficiently large to be distinguished from surrounding consolidation, it can be seen as a distinct entity. However, uninvolved lobules of lung among others that are filled with exudate, or focal emphysematous changes peripheral to bronchioles that are partially obstructed, may be misconstrued as small cavities. Serial films over a few days may be required to permit a clear distinction. When a cavitary lesion develops in a patient with altered immunity who also has diffuse lung disease, consider the likelihood that more than one cause is responsible (Fig. 5-22).

Abscesses in the lung may not be distinguishable as distinct lesions when they are surrounded by inflammatory change in adjacent lung tissue. If they have not cavitated, abscesses may appear simply as mass lesions and are virtually indistinguishable from mass lesions of any other cause by radiographic criteria alone (Fig. 5-23).

Differential Diagnosis of Single Cavitary Lesions

True cavities occur when necrotic portions of inflammatory or neoplastic masses are expelled through communicating bronchi, and air enters the lesion.

The commonest causes of true cavity formation in the lung can be conveniently grouped under four headings:

1. Infection
   a. Infectious granulomatous diseases
   b. Nongranulomatous infections
2. Neoplasm
3. Noninfectious granulomatous diseases
4. Other.

The last category includes numerous but uncommon causes of pulmonary cavities (Fig. 5-28).

The majority of cavitary lesions you will see fall into one of the first three categories (Figs. 5-22, 5-24 to 5-28). Table 5-2 lists subsets of causes of pulmonary cavitation for each category. Both common and uncommon causes are included, but those that are rare (in the United States) are omitted.

Other causes of "holes" in the lung are not included in the list of differential diagnosis for true pulmonary cavities. These apparent holes are usually, but not always, distinguishable from true cavities by a combination of their radiographic appearance and a knowledge of the circumstances in which they occur.

TABLE 5-2. Causes of Pulmonary Cavities

Infectious diseases

Infectious granulomatous disease: most commonly tuberculosis, but including histoplasmosis, coccidioidomycosis, and blastomycosis, and some forms of cryptococcosis, nocardiosis and actinomycosis

Nongranulomatous infections: Other infections that may cause necrosis of lung tissue
- Gram negative organisms: *Klebsiella, Escherichia coli, Pseudomonas, Proteus,* and less commonly *Legionella* or other gram-negative bacteria
- *Staphylococcus* and uncommonly *Streptococcus pneumoniae* or other gram-positive bacteria
- Ubiquitous fungi: *Aspergillus,* phycomycetes *(Rhizopus, Mucor), Cryptococcus,* and less commonly others
- The higher bacterium *Nocardia*
- Anaerobic organisms

Neoplastic diseases

Most commonly bronchogenic carcinoma (squamous cell type more often than the others, but all types may present as cavities)

Metastasis (especially from a squamous cell primary tumor such as cervical tumor)

Hodgkin's disease and non-Hodgkin's lymphoma

Noninfectious granulomatous disease

Wegener's granulomatosis

Rheumatoid lung nodules

Rarely sarcoid

Conglomerate mass lesions of silicosis and coal miner's pneumoconiosis with or without complicating tuberculosis

Other causes

Cavitating pulmonary infarcts, especially consequent to septic emboli

Parasites
- Ecchinococcosis
- Paragonimiasis
- Amebiasis

Apical cavities in patients with ankylosing spondylitis

Certain pneumonias other than those more commonly known to cause cavitation (see "Nongranulomatous infections," above)
- Viral pneumonias (e.g., cytomegalovirus; infection is not uncommon, but cavitation is rare)
- Bacterial pneumonias that are rare in themselves, but may present as cavitary lesions
  - *Bacillus cereus* (gram-positive rod) pneumonia
  - Rare chronic form of *Pseudomonas aeruginosa* or *Klebsiella* pneumonia (as opposed to the more common acute forms, which may also cavitate)
  - *Pseudomonas pseudomallei* pneumonia
Hamartoma (very rare as a cavity)
Cavitation in an infected pulmonary sequestration

For example, cavitation in granulomatous masses due to sarcoidosis is rare, but cystic spaces develop in the lungs of patients who have distortion of lung architecture from chronic sarcoid lesions, usually in the upper lobes. This also occurs in other chronic lung diseases. However, these lesions and other causes of blebs, bullae, post-traumatic cysts, and cystic bronchiectasis are discussed in Chapters 10 and 11.

Distinctive Radiographic Features of Cavitary Lesions

Attempts have been made to find radiographic characteristics that would permit distinction between benign and malignant cavitary lesions. Lesions having extremely thin walls such that no portion exceeds 1 mm in thickness are almost invariably benign, and lesions in which even segments of the wall exceed 15 mm are almost always malignant.[49] Although these generalizations have statistical validity, they have limited use when applied to an individual patient. Many cavitary lesions have walls that are intermediate in thickness. The walls of neoplastic lesions may be extremely irregular and lobulated, but a significant percentage of inflammatory cavities also have irregular walls. Smooth-walled cavities may be benign or malignant. The presence or absence of fluid in a cavity is of no critical value in distinguishing benign from malignant lesions.

Differential Diagnosis of Multiple Cavitary Lesions

The differential diagnosis of multiple cavitary lesions differs from that of solitary cavitary lesions largely in that multiple, simultaneous primary cavitary bronchogenic carcinomas would be a rare curiosity. The other common causes of pulmonary cavities may produce solitary or multiple lesions.

All of the entities known to cause cavitary lesions present more commonly as noncavitary lesions, and the presence of cavitation within a lesion does not influence the differential diagnosis as much as do other, more important variables. In general, establishing the precise etiology of a cavity encompasses the same combination of diagnostic skills and procedures discussed under the headings of pulmonary infections and pulmonary neoplasms.

Cavity Contents Other Than Fluid

Occasionally ball-like soft tissues may be seen in a cavity and are seen to have shifted position when films in the decubitus positions are compared to those made with the patient either upright or supine. These are commonly intracavitary fungus balls. Usually the mass consists of a collection of mycelia of the fungus *Aspergillus,* and uncommonly other fungi or *Nocardia.* These represent secondary saprophytic invaders of preexisting cavities produced by tuberculosis, old abscesses, or other causes. Usually the lesions are asymptomatic or accompanied by hemoptysis, which prompts the patient to seek medical attention.

In contradistinction, patients with altered immunity may have life-threatening infections caused by invasive *Aspergillus* and other ubiquitous fungi, which result in areas of parenchymal necrosis with subsequent cavitation. The cavitation of the lesion usually corresponds to the return of white blood cells after a period of profound neutropenia. Masslike foci within these cavities may simulate saprophytic fungus balls, but are instead masses of necrotic lung due to invasive fungal disease and require a different treatment (see Fig. 5-12C). These frequently do not shift with changes in the patient's position. Occasionally an intracavitary blood clot may simulate a fungus ball or necrotic lung.

Echinococcus cysts may be solid in appearance until such time as they establish connection with the bronchial tree. Air may then accumulate in the lesion and produce a separation of the endocyst lining so that it floats on the fluid content of the cyst, producing a wavy interface between the air and the fluid contents ("the sign of the camalote," named after a water lily found in the Amazon River).

PLEURAL EFFUSION AND EMPYEMA

Pleural effusion, unilateral or bilateral, small to moderately large in amount, may be seen with any type of pulmonary infection, and the fact that it is more commonly seen in some types than in others is of very little help in radiographic diagnosis of an individual patient. It is likely, judging from experience with CT, that the presence of pleural effusion is underestimated in those cases where only PA and lateral chest films (no decubitus views) are obtained. The underestimation is still more likely in those cases where portable chest films are obtained with the patient supine or semiupright.

Whether an effusion is infected (and thus an empyema), or a sterile parapneumonic exudate or transudate cannot be judged from its radiographic appearance; analysis of pleural fluid specimens is required to make that distinction. Effusions may occur early in the course of pneumonia or later during the clearing phase. A worsening of symptoms and a rise in temperature accompanying late-onset effusion, or rapidly increasing effusion, should raise a suspicion of empyema (see Fig. 5-25 and Ch. 3).

LOCATION AND EXTENT OF THE PULMONARY LESION

If one is studying the radiographic spectrum of a specific pulmonary infection, conclusions may be drawn regarding the relative incidence of involvement (for example, upper lobes compared to lower lobes) or the relative extent (unilateral versus bilateral, unilobar versus multilobar, focal versus diffuse, etc.). As important as these variables are to defining a spectrum, however, none is specific for a given organism. Furthermore, the preponderant localization in one series of patients does not always agree with that derived from another series.

Even though we cannot use these variables to identify specific causative organisms, we recognize that certain groups of organisms are *more likely* to produce disease in certain segments of the lung than others, and likewise disease found in certain segments of the lung is more likely to be produced by one group of organisms than another. For example, postprimary tuberculosis is seen more commonly in the apical and subapical regions of the lung than elsewhere. The apical and posterior segments are commonly involved, whereas the anterior segments are rarely involved alone. Coincidently, infectious disease involving the apices and subapical regions of the lung are more likely due to mycobacteria. However, the fact that they are more commonly the cause of apical and subapical infectious lesions does not mean that they are exclusively so. Other members of the group of organisms causing infectious granulomatous diseases as well as other bacterial pathogens may produce these lesions. In fact, a serious error to be avoided is that of mistaking a lung carcinoma for a lesion of tuberculosis, or lesions of noninfectious granulomatous disease for lesions of tuberculosis (see Figs. 5-26 to 5-28).

Although the superior segments of the lower lobes are also frequent sites of the lesions of postprimary tuberculosis, many other organisms produce disease at those sites as well. Likewise, aspiration pneumonias with anaerobic bacteria are prone to involve the basilar segments of the lower lobes. Many other types of pneumonia, however, behave in similar fashion, and aspiration may occur into the middle or upper lobes, particularly the posterior segments or the axillary subsegments, depending on the patient's position at the time of aspiration.

RATE OF CHANGE

Some organisms produce pulmonary lesions that are relatively slow to progress. Typically, postprimary tuberculosis, chronic histoplasmosis, and coccidioidomycosis are representative of those infections that may evolve slowly and remain relatively stable for days, months, or even years, even though active untreated disease is present. Comparison of films made at long intervals often permits recognition of fluctuation or progression of abnormalities, whereas comparison only of films made at short intervals—days or weeks or months—may lead to the erroneous conclusion of stability.

On the other hand, the necrotizing pneumonias, most often due to gram-negative organism infections, can progress rapidly (see Fig. 5-8). Within days, and sometimes within hours, they can increase markedly in volume and extent or proceed to cavitate. *Legionella pneumophila,* a weakly staining gram-negative organism, may also cause pneumonia that appears masslike when first seen and may progress even while being treated (see Fig. 5-10).

Pneumonia due to anaerobic organisms can also increase in volume but usually does so more indolently (see Fig. 5-25). However, pneumonias due to mixed anaerobes and aerobes, including gram-negative organisms, may also occur.

Pulmonary infections with the ubiquitous fungi or the higher bacterium *Nocardia* have a rate of progression that is variable, but usually of an intermediate time course; they ordinarily do not show striking increases in lesion size or number over 6 to 12 hours. Even at 24-hour intervals there may be only minimal evidence of progression. Some of these lesions may appear to stabilize (Fig. 5-29), but others can show slow, relentless progression day by day, even when treated with appropriate drugs. It is unfortunate that in this group of patients the lesions produced by *Nocardia* have the same appearance as those of the ubiquitous fungi, because treatment is different for the two groups, and often invasive techniques such as needle aspiration, bronchoscopic biopsy, or thoracotomy and biopsy are required to establish the diagnosis and make the distinction. Even when they follow an indolent course in the lungs, these lesions may be life threatening because of their potential to embolize to the brain or other extrapulmonary sites.

SPECIAL SITUATIONS

There are many pulmonary infections and infestations that can be thought of as "special situations." That is, you would ordinarily not give them serious consideration unless some element of the history—particularly one related to geography, living conditions, work, travel, or hobbies—prompted you to do so. Although these are unusual diseases in most communities of the United States and Europe, there are geographic enclaves and occupational groups in which they are endemic. In addition, they may be found as sporadic cases in patients who have traveled from or through endemic regions. Most are treatable if diagnosed in time, but many are fatal if not treated promptly.

A list of such infections and infestations would include

plague pneumonia, pneumonia due to *Rickettsia,* chlamydia (ornithosis), *Echinococcus* disease, amoebic lung or pleural lesions, anthrax, *Strongyloides stercoralis,* schistosomiasis, paragonimiasis, and filariasis, among others. Familiarity with the locales or the type of travel, work, or hobbies that are known to be related to acquiring these infections may serve you well in diagnosing isolated cases. Their roentgenographic appearances in general are not distinctive enough to evoke a presumptive diagnosis in the absence of an appropriate history. Many of them (anthrax, brucellosis, plague, tularemia, etc.) have a high incidence of associated hilar or mediastinal lymphadenopathy.[8]

HILAR OR MEDIASTINAL ADENOPATHY IN ASSOCIATION WITH PNEUMONIA

The presence of even subtle hilar or mediastinal adenopathy in association with a pneumonia should prompt consideration of tuberculosis or other organisms of the infectious granulomatous disease group as the etiology. Atypical mycobacteria (nontuberculous mycobacteria, NTMB) may also cause hilar or mediastinal adenopathy. Such adenopathy need not be present, however.

Adenopathy is seldom manifest in adults with the usual acute bacterial or viral pneumonias or in those with pneumonia due to the ubiquitous fungi. Adenopathy does accompany some cases of *Mycoplasma* pneumonia and frequently the special situation pneumonias, including those produced by *Yersinia pestis* (plague) and *Francisella tularensis* (tularemia). Adenopathy may also be seen in association with chronic or recurrent pneumonia such as may occur in patients with bronchiectasis or cystic fibrosis or in patients with lung abscesses.

Adenopathy may also be present in patients who have neoplasms that obstruct bronchi and cause an obstructive pneumonitis. The adenopathy in these cases may consist predominantly of benign reactive lymph node changes associated with the chronic inflammation. Radiographically, however, there is no way to distinguish reactive adenopathy from metastatic lymphadenopathy, which may or may not also be present (see also Ch. 7.)

INFECTIOUS GRANULOMATOUS DISEASE

The infectious granulomatous diseases are important enough to warrant additional discussion even at the risk of repetition. Tuberculosis is still one of the commonest

causes of morbidity in the world, even though its prevalence in western societies has been on the wane for a few
decades. As the incidence of disease caused by *Mycobacterium tuberculosis* declines in the western world, so it
seems the incidence of infections due to varieties of
NTMB—particularly *Mycobacterium kansasii* and
Mycobacterium avium-intracellulare, but other rapidly
growing mycobacteria as well—is on the rise. Seldom
can reliable distinctions be made on the basis of radiographic findings alone as to which of these organisms is
responsible in any given case. Ultimately the diagnosis
depends on characteristics of the organisms isolated by
culture.

Many of the patients who present with infection and
disease due to atypical mycobacteria have some other
disorder that impairs host tissue defenses, but this is not
invariable. Patients with AIDS are especially susceptible
to diseases caused by NTMB, particularly *Mycobacterium avium-intracellulare* and *Mycobacterium kansasii,*
but they also are prone to *Mycobacterium tuberculosis*
infection.[1,25,27,50] The retrieval of NTMB from patients
with AIDS is usually an indication of disseminated disease regardless of the chest film findings. In immunocompetent people, however, NTMB may colonize without producing overt clinical disease.[25]

Since disease caused by *Mycobacterium tuberculosis* is
communicable and can cause serious morbidity and
death if unrecognized and untreated, and since effective
treatment is available, its diagnosis is important.

In general, the radiographic spectrum of pulmonary
tuberculosis or the pathogenic fungi that comprise the
infectious granulomatous disease group is a reflection of
the various stages of the disease, in accordance with
theories of pathogenesis.[32,37–39] The following is a brief
review.

Negative Chest Film

Theory holds that a positive tuberculin test in a person
who has received neither bacillus Calmette-Guérin
(BCG) prophylaxis nor antituberculous chemotherapy
indicates the presence of viable tubercle bacilli. Nevertheless, the majority of such patients, including those
who are known recent skin test converters, will have
chest radiographs that appear normal. The size of the
primary disease focus in this group is below the recording
system threshold. Rarely, a patient with proven tuberculosis had endobronchial disease demonstrated by bronchoscopy and biopsy, but no detectable parenchymal
component on chest films. Such a patient may go undiagnosed until some physician undertakes the study of

the persistent, disturbing, unexplained cough for which
the patient seeks help. Extrathoracic tuberculous lesions
are also not uncommon in patients who have no detectable pulmonary lesion.

A positive skin test for tuberculin may be used as a
measure of the prevalence of tuberculosis in populations
that have not received BCG. The high percentage of
positive reactors to histoplasmin and coccidioidin, in
areas where histoplasmosis and coccidiodomycosis are
endemic, indicates that there must also be a large number of patients who have been infected with those organisms. Yet many have no current clinical or radiographic evidence of disease. Calcified granulomas in the
spleen may be the only indication of prior infectious
granulomatous disease (usually histoplasmosis or tuberculosis) in some of these patients.

Because skin tests for blastomycosis and cryptococcosis are so unreliable, it is not possible to assess the
prevalence of these organisms in asymptomatic hosts.[5]

Common Residuals of the Primary Complex

The Primary Focus (Ghon's Tubercle) and Other Calcified Lesions

The commonest residual radiographic manifestation
of tuberculous infection is the partially or completely
calcified primary focus. Although more commonly
found in the lower half of a lower lobe, these nodules
may be located in any pulmonary lobe or segment and
may vary from pinhead size to more than 1.0 cm in
diameter (Fig. 5-30).

There are other causes of calcification within solitary
pulmonary nodules besides the infectious granulomatous diseases, but the only other one that occurs with
sufficient frequency to merit frequent consideration is
the hamartoma.

Multiple calcified or partially calcified nodules, frequently clustered, may also be due to tuberculosis and
may still contain viable organisms (Fig. 5-31). Histoplasmosis and to a lesser extent coccidioidomycosis may
also be responsible for calcified pulmonary lesions, and
in certain geographic locations, particularly the Missis-
sippi Valley, Ohio, and St. Lawrence River Valleys, histoplasmosis accounts for many of these lesions. Fairly
large nodules, about 1 to 3 cm in diameter, may occur
and show only a central calcified nidus, the remainder of
the lesion being composed of fibrous tissue and chronic
inflammatory cells. Some nodules may show concentric
rings of calcification. Multiple scattered, calcified pulmonary nodules, in conjunction with multiple calcified

foci visible in the spleen, suggest that dissemination at the time of primary infection is common even in patients with no recall of having had histoplasmosis.

A profusion of *small, completely calcified nodules* disseminated throughout both lungs is nearly diagnostic of old histoplasmosis (Fig. 5-32). In parts of the world where histoplasmosis in unknown, similar calcified nodules have been seen in patients with a history of prior chickenpox pneumonia. There are also rare reports of disseminated, calcified small nodules consequent to coccidioidomycosis, but no cases, to my knowledge, have been documented as representing residuals of miliary tuberculosis.

Infectious granulomatous lesions in many organs, i.e., spleen, liver, kidney, adrenal glands, brain, etc., may leave calcified foci as roentgenographic clues of prior infection.

Pulmonary metastases, especially from bone sarcomas, and rarely other primary sites, may appear calcified because of foci of calcification or ossification. Rarely, amyloid nodules in the lung may appear calcified.[46] Multiple calcified nodules may also be seen in silicosis. Patients with long-standing mitral valve disease may have multiple calcified or ossified nodules of hemosiderosis. Certain parasitic infections, e.g., schistosomiasis, *Armillifer armillatus,* and paragonimiasis may also cause calcified pulmonary nodules.

The Primary Complex

The primary complex is a combination of a pulmonary focus associated with hilar or mediastinal lymph node involvement. Lymph nodes of the pulmonary hila and mediastinum are infected with the tubercle bacillus or other organisms of the infectious granulomatous disease group via lymphatic channels draining the original parenchymal focus. A granulomatous reaction in the nodes ensues, and months later when the nodes are often no longer enlarged, caseous foci within them may undergo organization and calcification and become visible on chest films (see Fig. 5-30).

Hilar and mediastinal calcified lymph nodes may be solitary or multiple and may be seen in the absence of a visible parenchymal focus. Calcified lymph nodes may also occur in silicosis, amyloidosis,[46] treated Hodgkin's disease (postirradiation), and uncommonly in sarcoidosis, but by far the majority are due to chronic infectious granulomatous disease, especially tuberculosis or histoplasmosis.

Noncalcified Nodules

Unfortunately, the spectrum of radiographic appearances of the infectious granulomatous diseases includes noncalcified nodules, often single but occasionally multiple (see Fig. 5-11). The differential diagnosis of solitary or multiple noncalcified pulmonary nodules is discussed further in Chapter 6.

Pneumonia

During the early phase of tuberculous disease there is a parenchymal component of pneumonia. This also occurs with infection by the pathogenic fungi that are members of the infectious granulomatous disease group, and the appearances are indistinguishable. Chest films may show areas of consolidation that are subsegmental, segmental, lobar, or multilobar in distribution and are indistinguishable from pneumonic consolidation due to any other organism (Fig. 5-33; see also Fig. 5-3). The upper, lower, or middle lobes may be involved. The pneumonia may slowly resolve without leaving any clues as to its presence, but there may be signs of scarring, such as peribronchial thickening, linear or bandlike shadows due to fibrosis, or residual nodular foci (Fig. 5-34A and B). A pneumonic presentation of infectious granulomatous disease is frequently, but not always, accompanied by subtle or obvious hilar or mediastinal lymphadenopathy, which serves as a clue to an otherwise difficult diagnosis. This occurs in both children and adults with primary disease. Other pneumonias that may be associated with adenopathy have already been discussed.

A noncalcified parenchymal focus with noncalcified hilar or mediastinal lymphadenopathy due to infectious granulomatous disease is a radiographic combination indistinguishable from that due to bronchogenic carcinoma with nodal metastases.

Pneumonia is often a manifestation of primary infection in the infectious granulomatous diseases, but occasionally it may be seen as a reinfection or postprimary disease in patients with tuberculosis.

Apical and Subapical Foci

In theory, during primary tuberculous infection, there is a phase of "early aborted generalization," from which the vast majority of patients recovered even in the prechemotherapeutic era. In this phase, organisms are disseminated to many organs in the body via the bloodstream. They eventually perish or at least remain idle at these sites. Seeding of the apical regions of the lung occurs in this phase; the organisms may remain dormant or produce foci of disease locally, and then arrest, leaving small linear and nodular scars, which may be visible on chest films. Viable organisms remain quiescent in these lesions until some event, probably associated with a reduction of host resistance, causes proliferation of lesions and signs of advancing disease (Figs. 5-34 and 5-35).

Thus, the apical and subapical regions of the lungs and to a much lesser extent the superior segments of the lower lobes are common sites of disease in cases of postprimary tuberculosis. The majority are believed to be reactivations of latent foci, whereas true instances of reinfection with other strains of mycobacteria are less common.[37,38] Residual apical scars may have nonspecific histopathologic appearances that show no characteristics of tuberculous lesions, yet extracts of these tissues in a substantial proportion of those tested in the past produced tuberculous lesions when injected into guinea pigs.[29] Whether or not that would be true today is not known. When the apical lesions are recognizably fibrocaseous, a still higher proportion will produce tuberculous lesions in guinea pigs. Postprimary pulmonary tuberculosis may also be seen as an amorphous or nodular focus in the subapical regions of the lung, which projects on films as an abnormality in a subclavicular location independent of any visible primary focus and even independent of apical lesions.

Cicatrizing Disease

Many chronic pulmonary infections, and some acute ones as well, leave behind signs of their presence by scarring of the lung. The infectious granulomatous diseases, and particularly tuberculosis, do so notoriously. There is contraction in volume of the involved lung segments, most often those of the upper lobes. The process may be unilateral or bilateral and at times may be severe and produce marked distortion of lung architecture. Bronchiectasis, particularly in the upper lobes, may occur because of alteration of lung structure by chronic disease (Figs. 5-36 and 5-37).

Estimation of Activity in Foci of Chronic Disease

One cannot reliably state on the basis of chest film findings alone whether chronic lesions are inactive. Serial films made over time can be compared to evaluate stability. The correlation between stability and inactivity may be good, but it is imperfect. In fact, before the era of antituberculous drugs, radiographic stability over several years could be seen in patients who continued to have viable tubercle bacilli isolated from sputum. So long as activity is defined in terms of the presence of

viable organisms in tissues or secretions, radiographic data can never suffice in themselves to rule out activity. Sometimes, however, active disease can be predicted with a high likelihood when pulmonary abnormalities, suspect for tuberculosis, are seen as new findings not present on previous films, or when the lesions have an appearance of consolidation more characteristic of an acute type of pulmonary reaction.

Postirradiation Changes in Lung Simulating Chronic Infection

Pleural and parenchymal apical and subapical lesions, combined with hilar distortion and other signs of reduction in volume of the paramediastinal portions of the upper lobes, occur frequently after radiation therapy to these regions and are indistinguishable from similar lesions of tuberculosis and other chronic infections. It is important, therefore, to know whether or not the patient has received irradiation to these zones in the past (Fig. 5-38).

Noncalcified Hilar and Mediastinal Adenopathy

Enlarged nodes in the hilar regions or the mediastinum, or both, may be seen as radiographic signs of infectious granulomatous disease. The hilar involvement may be unilateral or bilateral. A parenchymal component may or may not be detected on the films. Manifest intrathoracic adenopathy is predominantly a sign of primary infection when it occurs in the infectious granulomatous diseases (Fig. 5-39).

In patients with coccidioidomycosis and perhaps blastomycosis, the development of mediastinal lymphadenopathy may be taken as a sign of dissemination and has a serious prognosis. Adenopathy due to infection cannot be differentiated from any other cause of adenopathy in the absence of calcification.

Although mediastinal and hilar lymphadenopathy is not a feature of NTMB infection in immunocompetent hosts, it is an important component in immunocompromised patients, especially those with AIDS. Mediastinal and hilar node involvement by NTMB (most commonly *Mycobacterium avium-intracellulare*) may cause radiographically manifest adenopathy with or without detectable parenchymal components of disease in patients with AIDS. In patients with Kaposi's sarcoma, hilar and mediastinal adenopathy also occurs as a result of involvement with that neoplasm. In some AIDS patients the lymph nodes may be involved with both Kaposi's sarcoma and NTMB.[25,50]

Miliary Disease

Miliary tuberculosis may be a clinically elusive disease. Indeed, some have classified a portion of its clinical spectrum as cryptic. The patient may have a history of several weeks of unexplained fevers, nonspecific malaise, and perhaps a cough. Extensive workup directed toward diagnosis of fever of undetermined etiology may indeed confirm that the patient is subacutely ill, but often does not produce a specific diagnosis. Chest radiographs initially may be normal. Then, after several days or weeks, a clear miliary pattern may appear on follow-up films (see Fig. 5-19). By this time there is multiorgan involvement, the patient is usually more severely ill, and diagnosis and treatment must proceed quickly, preferably within hours, if it is to be successful. Some patients have a severe leukemoid reaction that can be mistaken for acute leukemia.

"Diffuse Indolent Tuberculosis"

Although it is not uncommon for patients with moderately extensive pulmonary tuberculosis to have surprisingly few symptoms, that is very unusual for patients with miliary tuberculosis. However, rare cases of miliary tuberculous lung lesions have been reported in patients with few or no symptoms, in whom the disease is discovered because of lesions seen on chest films obtained for unrelated reasons (Fig. 5-40). Buechner and Anderson[12,13] have proposed the designation of "diffuse indolent tuberculosis" for this entity. Tubercle bacilli are usually extremely difficult to isolate from the sputa of these patients, and large numbers of sputum samples (20 or more) may be necessary. The tuberculin skin test is only weakly positive. Buechner and Anderson reported that many of their cases were given a presumptive diagnosis of sarcoid after an unrewarding search for tubercle bacilli.

The radiographic spectrum of this form of tuberculosis encompasses that which may be seen with the more usual and less cryptic forms of pulmonary tuberculosis in addition to the miliary pattern.

Diffuse Disease That Is Not Miliary

Tuberculosis may be spread by aspiration of infected material from one segment of lung to another via the bronchi or by the discharge of caseous lymph node or cavity contents into an adjacent bronchus after erosion through the bronchial wall (see Fig. 5-24A). Patchy foci of various size may develop in one or both lungs, and large areas of coalescence and consolidation may cause pulmonary function to be severely impaired. Diffuse patchy or reticulonodular patterns of disease may also be seen with other organisms of the infectious granulomatous disease group.

Cavitary Disease

Pulmonary cavities have already been discussed. Cavities due to *Mycobacterium tuberculosis* usually are surrounded by radiographically abnormal lung. Cavities due to atypical mycobacteria, however, may be found in the presence of relatively normal surrounding lung (see Fig. 5-24B and C), and cavities in the small mass lesions of cryptococcosis may also appear in the midst of relatively normal appearing lung. Cavities of coccidioidomycosis may appear in the midst of chronically abnormal lung indistinguishable from tuberculosis (see Fig. 5-36), or they may appear as solitary, thin-walled lesions in a subclavicular location, surrounded by relatively normal lung (Fig. 5-41).

The presence of a tuberculous cavity is presumptive evidence of active disease. However, in the prechemotherapeutic era some tuberculous cavities (about 15 percent) remained open, even though no tubercle bacilli were isolated from them when they were resected.[42] When cavities heal, they may leave no more than stellate or linear scars behind, or they may decrease in size, become inspissated, and remain visible as nodules.

PLEURAL EFFUSION AS A RADIOGRAPHIC SIGN OF TUBERCULOSIS

Pleural effusion may occur as part of the primary disease process in tuberculosis with or without a detectable parenchymal focus. Theory and supportive evidence hold that a caseous focus in the lung periphery extrudes into the pleural space, and effusion is the response to pleural infection with tubercle bacillus. The effusion may be small or large, and rarely bilateral. Organisms may not be present on a smear of even concentrated sediment and may not grow on culture either. Pleural biopsy may be necessary for diagnosis. Pleural effusions, unilateral or bilateral, may also be found as chest film abnormalities in patients with postprimary pulmonary tuberculosis.

Except for coccidioidomycosis, pleural effusion consequent to pleuritis caused by other members of the infectious granulomatous disease group is relatively uncommon.

INVOLVEMENT OF THE CHEST WALL

Involvement of the chest wall (other than the pleura) is uncommon with any type of pneumonia. Organisms of the infectious granulomatous group, especially tuberculosis, actinomycosis, and blastomycosis, may involve the chest wall in continuity with pulmonary lesions in a very small percentage of cases. Actinomycosis also may involve the chest wall in continuity with pleural foci of infection. Often rib destruction is the first radiographic indication of chest wall extension. Draining sinuses may be apparent clinically.

Many organisms may involve bones as a result of septic emboli from pulmonary or extrapulmonary sites of infection, but that is a different mechanism with different radiographic findings.

PULMONARY LESIONS OF DIVERSE ETIOLOGIES RESEMBLING TUBERCULOSIS

Practically all components of the radiographic spectrum of tuberculosis can be duplicated by pathogenic fungi of the infectious granulomatous disease group or by neoplasm. Uncommonly, cases of chronic cavitary disease due to *Klebsiella* or *Pseudomonas* pneumonia (Fig. 5-42) or the chronic form of *Pseudomonas pseudomallei* (melioidosis) may be indistinguishable. Parenchymal disease with or without cavitation may occur as chronic infection due to *Nocardia asteroides.* This form of nocardiosis could be included as a member of the infectious granulomatous disease group. However, as a rule pulmonary lesions due to *Nocardia* are now far more commonly seen as acute or subacute infections in patients with altered immunity. Finally, just as there are patients who have both carcinoma of the lung and tuberculosis, so are there patients who have tuberculosis and simultaneously histoplasmosis or other infectious granulomatous disease. The presence of these organisms in combination ordinarily cannot be deduced from radiographic appearances.

The pulmonary apical lesions seen in patients with ankylosing spondylitis can also mimic tuberculosis. The ability of postirradiation changes to mimic those of tuberculosis has been discussed under the heading of "Cicatrizing Disease."

WHAT ELSE COULD IT BE?

The question, "What else could it be besides infection?" becomes of special importance when considering the clinical and radiographic abnormalities of the immunocompromised patient.

Interstitial edema from fluid overload, early congestive heart failure, or renal failure can mimic diffuse infection from viruses, *Pneumocystis carinii,* or multiorganism pneumonia. Pulmonary hemorrhage in the severely thrombocytopenic patient (e.g., with acute leukemia), leukemic infiltration of the lungs in the patient with very high peripheral white cell counts, or the pulmonary lesions of ARDS can do the same. Acute pulmonary reaction to blood transfusions or a hypersensitivity response to drugs can also produce diffuse lung lesions.

Patients with malignant lymphoma or mycosis fungoides[34] can have extremely rapid infiltration of the lung by neoplasm that precisely mimics pneumonia. Patients with AIDS may have pulmonary lesions of Kaposi's sarcoma that mimic *Pneumocystis carinii* or cytomegalovirus pneumonia.

Patients with bronchoalveolar cell carcinoma may have zones of consolidation similar to those of lobar pneumonia. Pneumonic foci peripheral to endobronchial obstructing neoplasms may resemble pneumonia unassociated with neoplasm (see Ch. 6).

Transplant recipients, particularly bone marrow and heart-lung recipients, may have bronchiolitis obliterans and organizing pneumonia as a graft-versus-host response in the former and probably a rejection phenomenon in the latter. Radiographically these lesions also simulate those of diffuse pulmonary infection.

All of the above conditions may be accompanied by signs and symptoms similar to those occurring in pneumonia. Nevertheless, a detailed knowledge of the history and recent treatment allows you to consider all of these possibilities in a differential diagnosis (see Ch. 10).

SUMMARY

1. The radiographic appearances of pulmonary infections can be classified under three general categories:
   a. Lobar or segmental consolidations or focal nonsegmental consolidation. In general these are caused by bacteria but may also be due to viruses, mycoplasma, or fungi. The precise organism responsible cannot be predicted from radiographic appearances.
      (1) Community-acquired pneumonias* will most commonly be due to *Streptococcus*

---

* This refers to the usual community-acquired infections in patients who are not considered immunocompromised. Immunocompromised patients may develop a larger assortment of pulmonary infections either in the community or while in the hospital (nosocomial infections).

pneumoniae, Mycoplasma, or (probably) *Legionella,* and seasonally to viral infections.

(2) *Mycobacterium tuberculosis* and other organisms of the infectious granulomatous disease group may also cause focal segmental or lobar consolidation. They do not respond to the usual antibiotics, however, and patients may not appear as ill as you might predict from the radiographic extent of their disease.

(3) Patients who have disorders associated with aspiration may have pneumonia due to anaerobic or mixed anaerobic and aerobic organisms.

(4) Patients with emphysema or bronchitis may have, in addition to the pneumonia caused by common organisms of the community, pneumonia or purulent tracheobronchitis due to infection with *Haemophilus influenzae.*

(5) Patients who acquire pneumonia in the hospital or who are immunocompromised have a higher incidence of gram-negative organism pneumonia (*Klebsiella, Pseudomonas, Escherichia coli,* Serratia, *Enterobacter,* Citrobacter, Proteus, etc.), including the weakly gram-negative Legionella. The disease may present as rapidly progressive, masslike zones of consolidation with or without cavitation. Similar mass lesions may be due to streptococci or type III pneumococci.

b. Nodules or small masses, single or multiple (countable and usually greater than 0.5 cm in diameter).

(1) Community-acquired lesions of this type may appear in asymptomatic individuals, and most often the critical determination is whether the lesion is benign or malignant (see discussion in Ch. 6).

(a) Community-acquired infections that present in this manner are predominantly due to organisms of the infectious granulomatous disease group, with tuberculosis being the most common outside of geographic enclaves where histoplasmosis or coccidioidomycosis predominates.

(b) Septic emboli (usually infected with staphylococci) may be seen as nodules with or without cavities in the lungs of intravenous drug abusers, or may be consequent to emboli from bacterial endocarditis or infection elsewhere in the body.

(c) Other community-acquired infections

or infestations that present as nodules or small masses are rare in the United States and have no special features that would predict their etiology (e.g., *Dirofilaria immitis*). Some may fall in the category of "special situations," in which some personal factor or clinical finding alerts you to the possibility of an uncommon infection (e.g., cryptococcosis, echinococcosis, or amebiasis).

(2) Patients with altered immunity may have a nodule or nodules or small mass lesions due to infection with the ubiquitous fungi *(Aspergillus, Rhizopus, Mucor, Cryptococcus, Candida and others)* or the higher bacterium *Nocardia.*

(a) In heart transplant recipients the nodules are frequently due to either *Aspergillus* or *Nocardia.* A smaller percentage will be due to infection with anaerobic bacteria or other fungi.

(b) In patients with acute myelogenous leukemia (AML) these nodular lesions are usually due to *Aspergillus. Nocardia* is actually an uncommon cause of infection in patients with AML. Candidiasis is common in patients with leukemia but is rarely present as pulmonary lesions in the absence of other signs of *Candida* infection.

(c) Bacteria such as *Pseudomonas, Proteus, Legionella, Staphylococcus,* and even *Streptococcus pneumoniae* present infrequently as a solitary nodule or small mass in the lungs of patients with altered immunity.

(d) The presence of a cavity within the lesion does not per se separate one cause from another. However, the presence of a cavity *and* an intracavitary mass in a patient with AML correlates very well with *Aspergillus* infection, especially during the phase of recovery from severe neutropenia. Unfortunately, this is a late sign.

(e) A nodule or nodules may be due to lymphoma developing in immunocompromised patients.

c. Diffuse lung disease due to infection

(1) Community-acquired infections

(a) Viral pneumonias

(b) Disseminated infection due to either miliary or bronchogenic dissemination of organisms of the infectious granulomatous disease group, most commonly tuberculosis

(c) Uncommonly, advanced untreated bacterial pneumonias of the usual community-acquired pneumonia type

(d) *Haemophilus influenzae* pneumonia in patients with chronic obstructive pulmonary disease

(2) Patients with altered immunity; nosocomial infections, or community-acquired infections

(a) *Pneumocystis carinii* pneumonia

(b) Viral pneumonia, especially

(i) Cytomegalovirus

(ii) Varicella-zoster (almost always preceded by disseminated skin lesions)

(iii) Measles (rare, but unaccompanied by any other stigmata of measles; usually a history of exposure to an active case)

(c) Nontuberculous mycobacteria, especially in patients with AIDS

(d) Miliary dissemination of tuberculosis, histoplasmosis, coccidioidomycosis, cryptococcosis, and others of the infectious granulomatous disease group; (uncommonly ubiquitous fungi or *Nocardia*)

(e) Disseminated *pseudomonas, staphylococcus,* or other usual bacterial pneumonia

(f) Disseminated infestation (e.g., with *Strongyloides stercoralis*)

(g) Multiorganism pneumonia.

2. Determining the precise organism or organisms responsible for a given infection is only part of the problem.

a. Some patients, especially those with malignant lymphoma, mycosis fungoides, or Kaposi's sarcoma involving the lungs may have radiographic and clinical signs and symptoms that precisely mimic those of pneumonia. The distinction usually requires some type of lung biopsy to avoid days lost pursuing ineffective treatment.

b. Pulmonary edema or hemorrhage, hypersensitivity pneumonitis, pulmonary embolus and infarction, alveolar proteinosis, and a variety of infiltrating neoplasms or chronic interstitial lung diseases may mimic radiographic patterns of infection.

3. Some pneumonias are caused by more than one organism acting concurrently.

a. Many times there is no radiographic indication that multiple organisms are involved.

b. In some patients there are two or more patterns of lung disease present simultaneously, raising the suspicion of multiple causes.

4. If a patient responds to treatment for one infection but subsequently develops another, we do not assume that the second infection is a recurrence of the first, even if the radiographic appearance is similar. The second (or third, etc.) infection is frequently due to another organism.

5. Pulmonary tuberculosis has a radiographic spectrum:

a. Negative chest film

b. Nodules (solitary or multiple, with or without calcification)

c. Pneumonia

d. Minimal apical or subclavicular opacities

e. Cicatricial lesions with marked lung distortion, usually of one or both upper lobes

f. Cavitary lesions

g. Mediastinal or hilar adenopathy (may calcify late and may be present without a visible parenchymal component)

h. Miliary lesions

i. Diffuse, nonmiliary lesions

j. Pleural effusion with or without visible parenchymal disease.

6. All of the organisms of the infectious granulomatous disease group produce lesions that share in the radiographic spectrum of tuberculosis.

7. Cavitation occurs in pulmonary lesions caused by many different microorganisms (see Table 5-2 for an elaboration of the differential diagnosis).

8. Establishing the precise etiology for a given pneumonia may be difficult.

A variety of special techniques may be required to obtain appropriate specimens for culture and cytologic and histologic study.

Patients who are immunocompromised may be colonized with a variety of organisms that can be identified on culture of the sputa but that are not the cause of the pneumonia.

Correlation of radiographic studies and the clinical condition of the patient allows for a rational choice of invasive studies when they are required.

At times, diagnosis and initial treatment will have to be based on the most likely diagnosis derived from correlating radiographic findings, clinical signs and symptoms, history, and available laboratory data including serologic tests.

BIBLIOGRAPHY

1. Albelda SM, Kern JA, Marinelli DL, et al: Expanding spectrum of pulmonary disease caused by nontuberculous mycobacteria. Radiology 157:289, 1985

2. Bandt PD, Blank N, Castellino RA: Needle diagnosis of pneumonia—value in high risk patients. JAMA 220:1578, 1972

3. Barrett-Connor E: The non-value of sputum culture in the diagnosis of pneumococcal pneumonia. Am Rev Respir Dis 103:845, 1971

4. Bartlett JG: Bacteriological diagnosis of pulmonary infection. p. 707. In Sackner MA (ed): Diagnostic Techniques in Pulmonary Disease: Part II. Marcel Dekker, New York, 1981

5. Bates JH: Evaluation by serological techniques. p. 747. In Sackner MA (ed): Diagnostic Techniques in Pulmonary Disease: Part II. Marcel Dekker, New York, 1981

6. Bayer AS: Fungal pneumonias: Pulmonary coccidioidal syndromes: part I. Chest 79:575, 1981

7. Bayer AS: Fungal pneumonias: Pulmonary coccidioidal syndromes: part II. Chest 79:686, 1981

8. Berkmen YM: Uncommon acute bacterial pneumonias. Semin Roentgenol 15:17, 1980

9. Bisno AL, Freeman JC: The syndrome of asplenia, pneumococcal sepsis and disseminated intravascular coagulation. Ann Intern Med 72:389, 1970

10. Blank N, Castellino RA, Shah V: The roentgenographic manifestations of pulmonary infection in patients with altered immunity. Radiol Clin North Am 11:175, 1973

11. Blank N, Castellino RA: The diagnosis of pulmonary infection in patients with altered immunity. Semin Roentgenol 10:63, 1975

12. Buechner HA: The differential diagnosis of miliary diseases of the lungs. Med Clin North Am 89:112, 1959

13. Buechner HA, Anderson AE: Diffuse indolent tuberculosis. Am Rev Tuberc 71:503, 1955

14. Caldicott WJH, Baehner RL: Chronic granulomatous disease of childhood. Am J Roentgenol 103:133, 1968

15. Castellino RA, Blank N: Pulmonary coccidoidomycosis. The wide spectrum of roentgenographic manifestations. Calif Med 109:41, 1968

16. Dietrich PA, Johnson RD, Fairbank JT, et al: The chest radiograph in Legionnaire's disease. Radiology 127:577, 1978

17. Feigin DS: Pulmonary cryptococcosis: radiologic-pathologic correlates of its three forms. AJR 141:1263, 1983

18. Fiala M: A study of the combined role of viruses, mycoplasmas, and bacteria in adult pneumonia. Am J Med Sci 257:44, 1969

19. Finegold S, Bartlett JG: Anaerobic pleuropulmonary infections. Cleve Clin Q 42:101, 1975

20. Genereux GP, Stilwell GA: The acute bacterial pneumonias. Semin Roentgenol 15:9, 1980

21. Kantor HG: The many radiologic phases of pneumococcal pneumonia. AJR 137:1213, 1981

22. Kroboth FJ, Yu VL, Reddy SC, Yu AC: Clinical radiographic correlation with the extent of Legionnaire's disease. AJR 141:263, 1983

23. Landay MJ, Christensen EE, Bynum LJ: Anaerobic pleural and pulmonary infections. AJR 134:233, 1980

24. Laskey W, Sarosi GA: The radiological appearance of pulmonary blastomycosis. Radiology 126:351, 1978

25. Marinelli DL, Albelda SM, Williams TM, et al: Nontuberculous mycobacterial infection in AIDS: clinical, pathologic, and radiographic features. Radiology 160:77, 1986

26. Miller AC: Early clinical differences between Legionnaire's disease and other sporadic pneumonias. Ann Intern Med 90:562, 1979

27. Murray JF, Felton CG, Garay SM, et al: Pulmonary complications of the acquired immunodeficiency syndrome. N Engl J Med 310:1682, 1984

28. Musher DM, Kubitschek KR, Crennan J, et al: Pneumonia and acute febrile tracheobronchitis due to *Haemophilus influenzae*. Ann Intern Med 99:444, 1983

29. Opie EL, Aronson JD: Tubercle bacilli in latent tuberculous lesions and in lung tissue without tuberculous lesions. Arch Pathol Lab Med 4:1, 1927

30. Pagani JJ, Libshitz HI: Opportunistic fungal pneumonias in cancer patients. AJR 137:1033, 1981

31. Recavarren S, Benton C, Gall EA: The pathology of acute alveolar diseases of the lung. Semin Roentgenol 2:22, 1967

32. Rich AR: Pathogenesis of tuberculosis. 2nd Ed. Charles C Thomas, Springfield, IL, 1951

33. Rosenow EC, Wilson WR, Cockerill FR: Pulmonary disease in the immunocompromised host. Mayo Clin Proc 60:473, 1985

34. Rubin DL, Blank N: Rapid pulmonary dissemination in mycosis fungoides simulating pneumonia. Cancer 56:649, 1985

35. Sider L, Davis T: Pulmonary aspergillosis: unusual radiographic appearances. Radiology 162:657, 1987

36. Spencer H: Pathology of the Lung. 4th Ed. p. 168. Pergamon Press, Oxford, 1985

37. Stead WW: Pathogenesis of a first episode of chronic pulmonary tuberculosis in man: recrudescence of residual of the primary infection or exogenous reinfection. Am Rev Respir Dis 95:729, 1967

38. Stead WW, Bates JH: Epidemiology and prevention of tuberculosis. In Fishman AP (ed): Pulmonary Diseases and Disorders. New York, McGraw-Hill, 1980

39. Stead WW, Kerby GR, Schleute DP, Jordahl CW:

The clinical spectrum of primary tuberculosis in adults. Ann Intern Med 68:731, 1968

40. Stelling CB, Woodring JH, Rehm SR, et al: Miliary pulmonary blastomycosis. Radiology 150:7, 1984
41. Stenstrom R, Jansson E, Von Essen R: Mycoplasma pneumonia. Acta Radiol [Diagn] (Stockh) 12:833, 1972
42. Sutinen S: Evaluation of activity in tuberculous cavities of the lung. Scand J Respir Dis, suppl., 67:1, 1968
43. Tew J, Lalenoff L, Berlin B: Bacterial or non-bacterial pneumonia. Accuracy of radiographic diagnosis. Radiology 123:607, 1977
44. Thorsteinsson SB, Musher DM, Fagan T: The diagnostic value of sputum culture in acute pneumonia. JAMA 233, 894, 1975
45. Tillotson JR, Lerner AM: Pneumonias caused by gram negative bacilli. Medicine 45:65, 1966
46. Wilson SR, Sanders DE, Delarne W: Intrathoracic manifestations of amyloid disease. Radiology 120:283, 1976
47. Wilson WR, Cockerill FR III, Rosenow EG: Pulmonary disease in the immunocompromised host II. Mayo Clin Proc 60:610, 1985
48. Wood RE, Boat TF, Doerskuk CF: Cystic fibrosis. Am Rev Respir Dis 113:833, 1976
49. Woodring JH, Fried AM, Chuang VP: Solitary cavities of the lung: diagnostic implications of cavity wall thickness. AJR 135:1269, 1980
50. Woolfenden MJ, Carrasquillo JA, Larson SM, et al: Acquired immune deficiency syndrome: Ga-67 citrate imaging. Radiology 162:383, 1987
51. Ziskind MM, Schwarz MI, George RB, et al: Incomplete consolidation in pneumococcal lobar pneumonia complicating pulmonary emphysema. Ann Intern Med 72:835, 1970
52. Zornoza J, Goldman AM, Wallace S, et al: Radiologic features of gram-negative pneumonias in the neutropenic patient. Am J Roentgenol 127:989, 1976

Atlas

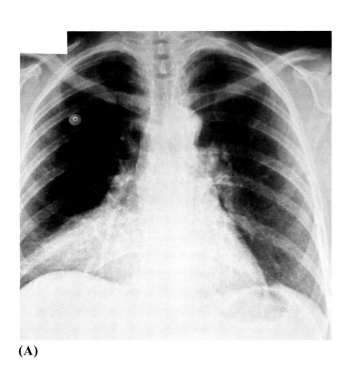

(A)

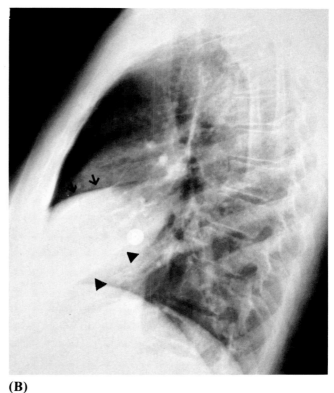

(B)

Fig. 5-1. Right Middle Lobe Pneumonia

Two days before admission this woman noted the onset of fever and cough with thick, whitish sputum. On the day of admission she twice had shaking chills. At admission she had fever of up to 38.6°C, a significant leukocytosis with a shift to the left, and a respiratory rate of 25 per minute. Sputum Gram stain showed many polymorphonuclear leukocytes with intracellular gram-positive cocci in pairs and chains. The presumptive diagnosis was pneumococcal pneumonia. The patient was treated with intravenous ampicillin and the fever abated rapidly.

(A,B) PA and lateral views, respectively. There is reduction in volume of the middle lobe as well as consolidation. The minor interlobar fissure is displaced caudally (arrows in Fig. B). The position of the major fissure is within normal limits (arrowheads in Fig. B). The sharply marginated, target-like opacities are probably caused by EKG leads in place on the skin surface.

The radiographic appearance is characteristic of pneumonia due to *Streptococcus pneumoniae*. However, lobar and segmental consolidations may be caused by a wide variety of microorganisms, and at the same time not all of the pneumonias produced by *Streptococcus pneumoniae* will present as characteristic segmental or lobar zones of consolidation. Pneumococcal pneumonia has a broader spectrum of radiographic appearances, including not only segmental and lobar consolidation but patchy zones of consolidation and even areas of inhomogeneous streaked and mottled opacities.[21] Combinations of these radiographic appearances may be found in the same patient in different areas of the lung.

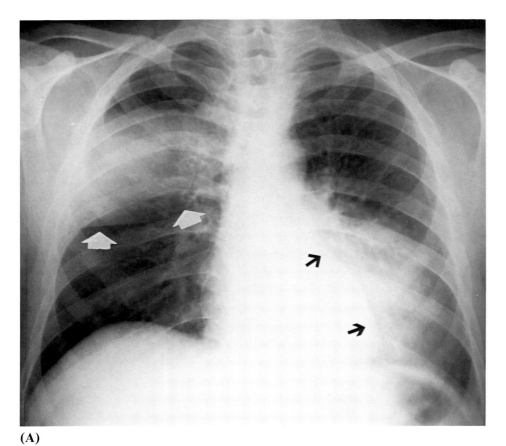

(A)

Fig. 5-2. **(A) Gram-Negative Organism and Type III Pneumococcal Pneumonia of the Right Upper and Left Lower Lobes**

PA chest film of a 30-year-old man who experienced the sudden onset of a shaking chill followed by dyspnea and cough productive of thick, yellow sputum, which later became bloody. The sputum culture was positive for a group B, type III pneumococcus, and a blood culture was positive for Friedländer's bacillus type A *(Klebsiella)*.

There is an intense zone of consolidation in the right upper lobe with slight downward bowing of the minor fissure (white arrows). There is also consolidation of the left lower lobe, against which the left heart border (between black arrows) can still be seen.

The rapid appearance of massive zones of consolidation is characteristic of either of the organisms cultured. Even though the organism retrieved from the blood culture is the more likely offender, there is no reason why both organisms cannot be responsible. This patient died within 3 days of onset of his illness in the preantibiotic era. (Courtesy of Dr. Richard Greenspan, New Haven, Connecticut.)

(Figure continues.)

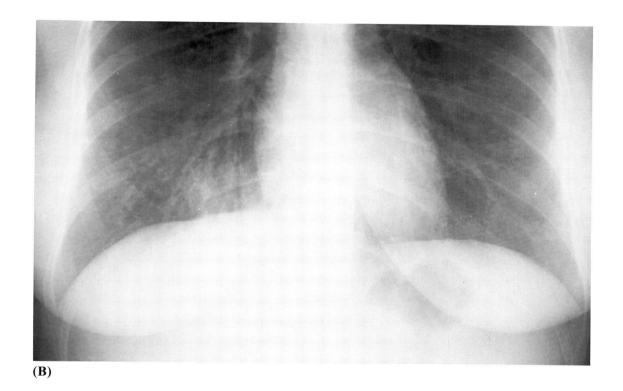

(B)

Fig. 5-2. *(Continued).* **(B,C) Right Lower Lobe** *Mycoplasma* **Pneumonia**

This 42-year-old woman had fever, chills, malaise, and severe dry cough for several days. A chest film showed a right lower lobe pneumonia. She was treated with ampicillin with little improvement. Her chest films 3 days later showed little change.

(B) PA view coned to the lung bases, where a zone of inhomogeneous consolidation with air bronchograms is seen medially on the right.

(C) Lateral view shows consolidation in the posterior basilar segment and some in the medial basal segment (behind the heart) as well.

The patient continued to do poorly, and eventually a *Mycoplasma* titer (1:512) was done. The antibiotics were changed and the patient experienced a slow return to normal. It is of interest that the patient's young daughter had a similar infection 2 months before, and a son developed the same syndrome after the patient's illness.

This patient fits the clinical and serologic pattern of *Mycoplasma* infection. Radiographically, there is no way to distinguish this type of pneumonia from *Streptococcus pneumoniae* pneumonia. It is common for *Mycoplasma* pneumonia to have a reticular and irregular nodular pattern radiographically, but a pattern of segmental or multisegmental opacification alone or along with the reticulonodular pattern is not infrequent (approximately 20 percent of cases).[41]

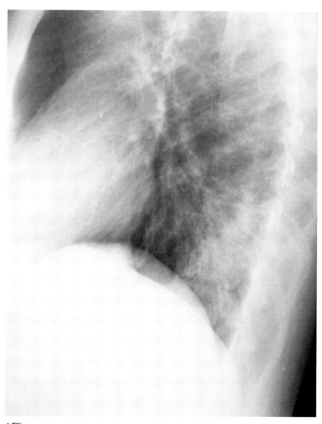

(C)

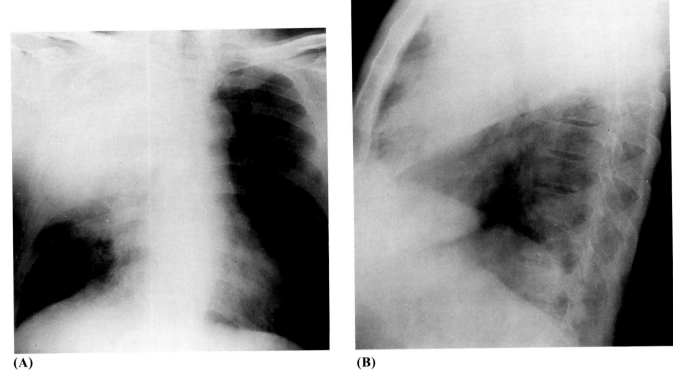

(A)   **(B)**

Fig. 5-3. Lobar Consolidation Due to Tuberculous Pneumonia

(A,B) PA and lateral views, respectively, of a 60-year-old male laborer who had been having chest pain and fever for 6 days, starting with a chill. He did not appear acutely ill in spite of a temperature of 39.5°C. His white blood cell count was 23,000 with 88 percent polymorphonuclear leukocytes. Bronchial breathing over the right upper lobe was noted on physical examination. Sputum cultures grew *Streptococcus viridans.* However, the patient did not respond to treatment, and bronchoscopy showed persistent purulent right upper lobe discharge. Finally, three successive smears were positive for acid-fast bacilli.

There is massive consolidation of the right upper and right middle lobes. (The small white specks scattered over the PA view are artifacts.)

A large variety of pulmonary pathogens can produce this pattern of consolidation. There is nothing specific about its appearance that would lead you to include tuberculous pneumonia in the differential diagnosis other than the knowledge that such consolidation is part of the radiographic spectrum of pulmonary tuberculosis. Most patients presenting with such massive consolidation due to gram-negative organisms, streptococci, or type III pneumococci would appear more severely ill.

Tuberculous pneumonia can result from extensive parenchymal reaction to the mycobacteria or to obstructive pneumonitis caused by tuberculous involvement of a bronchus or compression of bronchi by enlarged tuberculous lymph nodes. In fact, at times the lymph nodes may spill their caseous contents into the bronchi and produce a tuberculous pneumonia in that fashion. The role of *Streptococcus viridans* in this particular pneumonia is indeterminate.

Subsequent chest films showed gradual clearing of the consolidation, with scarring and reduction in volume of the involved lung. This type of resolution supports the contention that the tuberculous infection played a major role in the pulmonary abnormality.

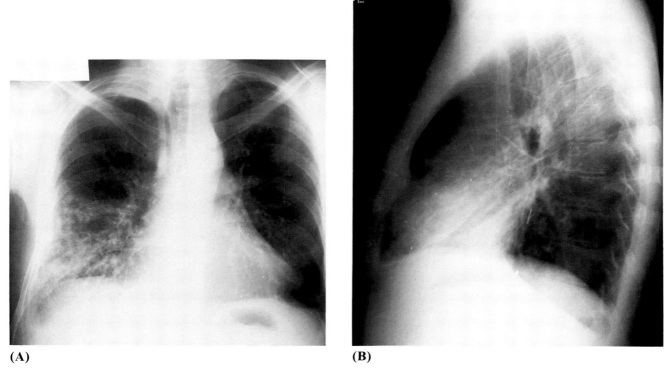

(A)   (B)

Fig. 5-4.   Mixed-Organism Pneumonia in an Immunocompromised Host

This patient is a young male heart transplant recipient who developed a slowly progressive right middle and right lower lobe patchy consolidation.

(A) PA view. Multiple circumscribed, rounded lucencies are seen in the area of consolidation. These simulate cavities but are due to areas of relatively uninvolved lung interspersed among the patchy foci of consolidation rather than true cavitary lesions. This appearance is not at all uncommon in patients with bronchopneumonia. That distinction, however, is not as important as determining the responsible organisms and their susceptibility to antibiotics.

A heavy growth of *Enterobacter aerogenes* was cultured from sputum and transtracheal aspirates. A moderate growth of *Staphylococcus,* coagulase positive, was also grown from sputum and transtracheal aspirates. A few *Candida* organisms were grown from sputum and transtracheal aspirates, and a small number of *Haemophilus influenzae* organisms were grown from the sputum only. The patient was treated with appropriate antibiotics, and the pneumonia cleared. However, none of the antibiotics used would be expected to have controlled an infection with *Candida.* It is likely that this organism was colonizing but not causing tissue-invasive disease. Otherwise, any or all of the other three pathogens could have caused this pneumonia.

Patients who have been hospitalized for even a short time may have their noses and throats colonized by a variety of gram-negative pathogens such as *Klebsiella* and other enterobacteria, or they may harbor *Staphylococcus aureus, Staphylococcus pyogenes,* and other gram-positive bacteria or a variety of the ubiquitous fungi such as *Candida* or *Aspergillus.* Patients who have endotracheal tubes or tracheostomies may also have their tracheas colonized. Thus, microorganisms retrieved from sputa may not be the ones responsible for the pulmonary infection.

There is distortion of the mediastinum due to the previous surgery, and there is fat deposition due to treatment with steroids. There is also extensive pleural thickening over the apices, greater on the right than on the left.

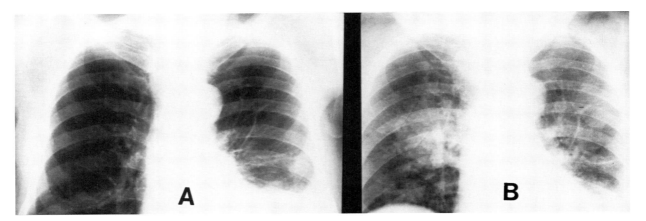

Fig. 5-5. Masslike Consolidation Due to Hemolytic Streptococcal Pneumonia

(A,B) There is a rounded, massive consolidation in the right perihilar zone of this man with malignant lymphoma (Fig. B). A film taken 1 day earlier (Fig. A) showed this region to be clear.

The small foci of consolidation around the periphery of the larger zone have been called "acinar" shadows, although the acini are not likely to be their precise anatomic substrate.

This type of fulminant, masslike consolidation is characteristic of necrotizing pneumonia, due most often to gram-negative organisms but possibly also to streptococci and type III pneumococci.

(From Blank et al.[10] and Blank and Castellino,[11] with permission.)

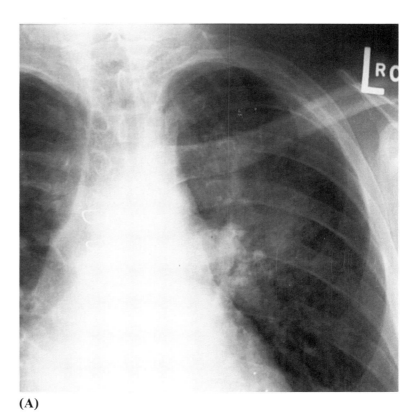

(A)

**Fig. 5-6. Anaerobic Organism
Pneumonia**

(A) PA view of a heart transplant recipient
who developed a large zone of consolidation in the posterior portions of the left
upper lobe.

(B) On lateral view the consolidation
has a long axis against the posterior chest
wall.

An anaerobic bacterium *(Propionibac-
terium acnes)* was recovered by percutaneous needle aspiration under fluoroscopic
control. The diagnosis of anaerobic organism pneumonia cannot be made from
sputum cultures, because anaerobes are
part of normal oropharyngeal flora.

Patients with anaerobic organism pneumonia may produce a putrid, foul-smelling sputum that should prompt consideration of the correct diagnosis. Often a
mixture of anaerobes is responsible for the
infection, or there may be a mixture of
anaerobic and aerobic organisms.

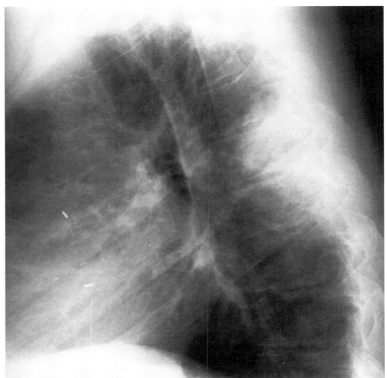

(B)

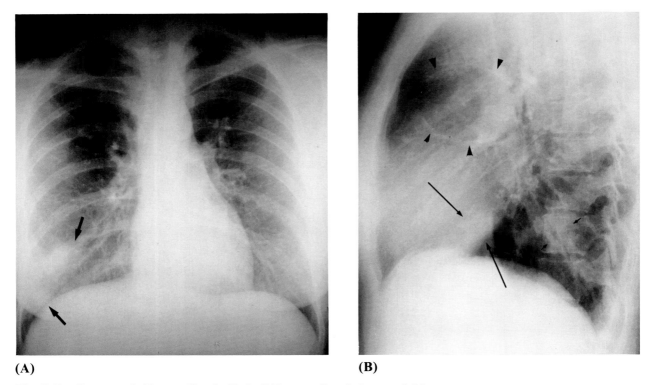

(A)　　　　　　　　　　　　　　　　　　　　**(B)**

Fig. 5-7.　Pneumonia Due to Septic Emboli From a Staphylococcal Abscess

This 28-year-old woman developed an abscess in her left axilla. Five days before having these films taken, she drained this abscess herself. Gross pus returned. A day later she noticed fever of up to 102°F with shaking chills, myalgias, and arthralgia. The episodes of fever and chills lasted 2 hours and occurred every 6 to 8 hours. She denied any skin rash or history of drug abuse.

(A,B) PA and lateral views of the chest, respectively, on admission to the hospital. **(A)** An ill-defined zone of patchy opacification is seen in the right lower lobe (arrows). **(B)** On the lateral view one poorly marginated focus is seen superimposed on the spine (short arrows), and another is superimposed on the posteroinferior aspects of the heart just anterior to the inferior vena cava (long arrows).

Multiple blood cultures were positive for *Staphylococcus aureus.* In spite of prompt institution of antibiotic treatment, the patient maintained hectic fevers over the next several days. *(Figure continues.)*

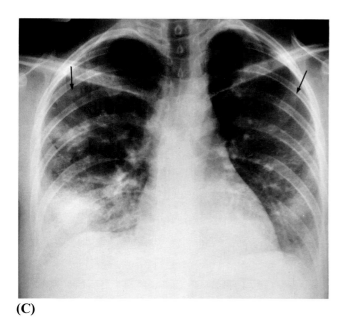

(C)

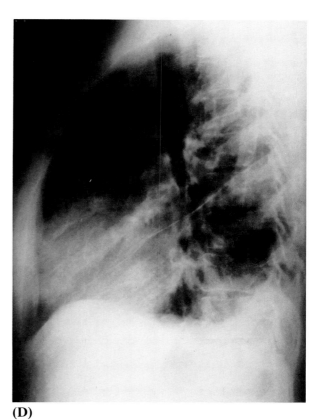

(D)

Fig. 5-7. *(Continued).* **(C,D)** PA and lateral views, respectively, made 3 days after Figs. A and B. There has been a marked change in the number of lesions present as well as an increase in the size of the original foci at the right base.

(C) On the PA view there are numerous small, ill-defined, nodular opacities scattered throughout both lungs. A few of the smaller ones are denoted by arrows. **(D)** On the lateral view, the right posterior gutter is effaced by a moderate pleural effusion. Thoracentesis produced a serosanguineous fluid specimen that had the qualities of an exudate, although cultures were sterile.

This sequence of events is representative of the pulmonary abnormalities that may occur with septic emboli and hematogenous dissemination of staphylococci. Fortunately, the patient responded to antibiotics and tube drainage of the right pleural space over a prolonged course of therapy.

Note. Arrowheads mark two curving pulmonary vessels in Fig. B. If you mentally completed the ring these vessels seem to outline, you could make a spurious observation of a large, thin-walled cavity. Vessels can be projected on planar images in a manner that may be confused with cavity formation.

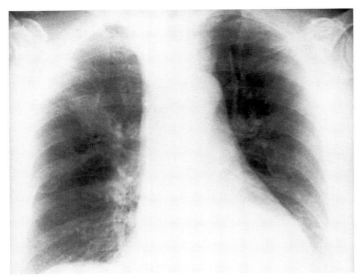

(A)

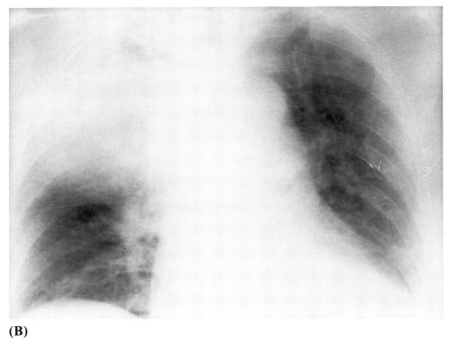

(B)

Fig. 5-8. (A,B) Rapidly Progressive Pneumonia Due to Pseudomonas

(A) An oval zone of consolidation has developed in the right upper lobe of this woman with acute leukemia, whose chest film 3 days earlier was negative.

(B) Within 48 hours the consolidation has become massive and spares only the lowest portions of the lobe. At autopsy the same day a massive hemorrhagic pneumonia due to infection with *Pseudomonas* was found to be the cause.

This alarming rate of progression is most suggestive of pneumonia due to gram-negative organisms with hemorrhagic necrosis. This sequence may be seen with pneumonias due to *Klebsiella, Escherichia coli,* and *Pseudomonas* as well as other gram-negative organisms. Less commonly, a type III pneumococcus *(Streptococcus pneumoniae)* or *Staphylococcus pyogenes* or *Legionella* may cause such explosive, massive pneumonia.

The appearance of the original lesion is nonspecific; a distinction between bacterial pneumonia and pneumonia due to ubiquitous fungi could not be made. The rate of change, however, would be unusual for infection due to the ubiquitous fungi. *(Figure continues.)*

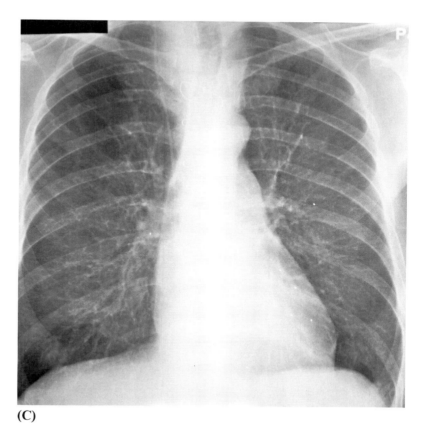

(C)

Fig. 5-8. *(Continued).* **(C–F)** **Rapid Progression of Left Lower Lobe Pneumonia Due to E. Coli**

This man is a heart transplant recipient. Numerous sputum cultures over 3 days grew *Escherichia coli,* which was also grown on cultures of transtracheal aspirates and of blood. He was colonized with *Aspergillus,* which was not thought to be responsible for his pneumonia, nor was it cultured from transtracheal aspirates. He also had oral cytomegalovirus infection.

(C,D) PA views of the chest taken 1 day apart. On Fig. D there is an increase in left retrocardiac opacity with effacement of vessel images behind and lateral to the heart. This represents a striking change from Fig. C in only 1 day. *(Figure continues.)*

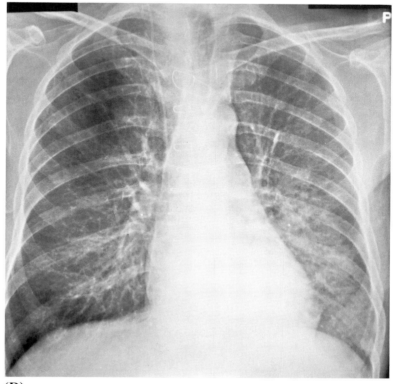

(D)

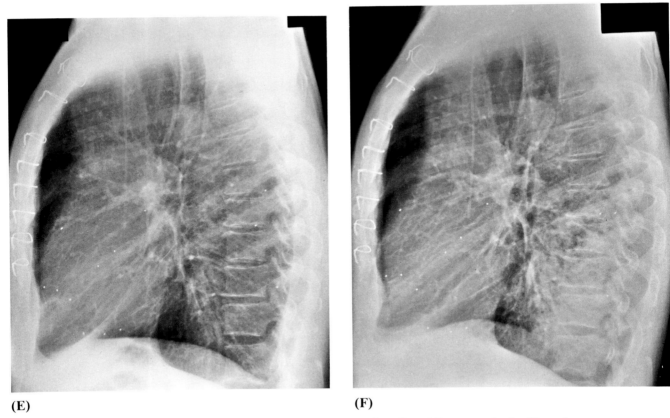

(E)   **(F)**

Fig. 5-8. *(Continued).* **(E,F)** Lateral views corresponding to Figs. C and D, respectively. There has been rapid consolidation of the left lower lobe. Notice the complete effacement of the posterior third of the left hemidiaphragm, the loss of vessel images, and the opacification of the lung superimposed on the lower thoracic vertebrae on Fig. F, taken 1 day after Fig. E.

These patients are usually critically ill. This combination of clinical and radiologic evidence makes the diagnosis of gram-negative organism pneumonia strongly suspect even before bacteriologic confirmation.

The small metallic densities seen in the heart on the lateral view are tantalum screws placed at the time of surgery to compute wall motion, from fluoroscopic recordings, after transplantation.

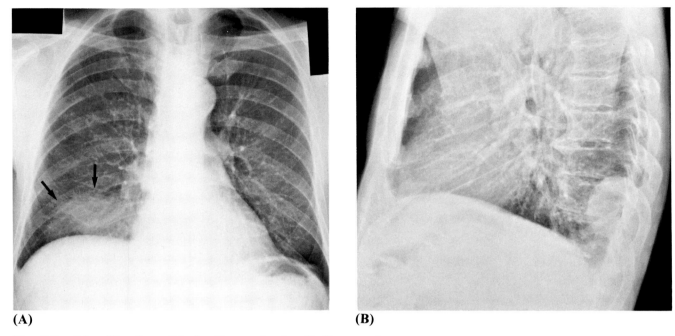

(A)   **(B)**

Fig. 5-9.   Masslike Consolidation Due to *Legionella* Pneumonia

(A) PA view. There is a large area of increased opacity with poorly defined edges at the right base (arrows).

(B) Lateral view. The edges of this right lower lobe lesion are sharply defined except where there is intimate contact with the right posterior chest wall. Open-lung biopsy specimens showed this consolidation to be due to infection with *Legionella,* a fastidious gram-negative bacterium. This patient had chronic lymphocytic leukemia.

Although the lesion simulates an extrapleural mass, it is not. On the lateral view the pleura does not drape over its upper edge in the fashion characteristic of extrapleural mass lesions.

Pneumonia caused by *Legionella pneumophila* may first appear as a patchy peripheral focus of consolidation, which in many cases progresses to involve larger zones of one or more lobes over a few days' time. Multilobar involvement may also be seen initially. At times the foci of consolidation may appear rounded and masslike, as with other gram-negative organism pneumonias. Cavitation may occur, particularly in patients with serious underlying disease. Diffuse, patchy patterns or a pattern of small, irregular shadows may also be seen. Resolution is usually prolonged over several weeks and sometimes months, and residual scarring may occur. Abdominal or gastrointestinal symptoms and mental confusion are commonly associated.[26]

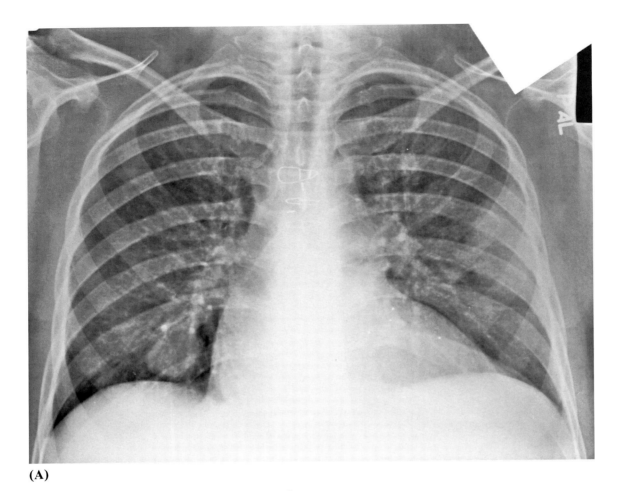

(A)

Fig. 5-10. Progressive *Legionella* Pneumonia

This cardiac transplant recipient had a diagnosis of *Legionella* pneumonia based on identification of organisms from a fluoroscopically guided percutaneous needle aspiration of one focus of consolidation.

(A) PA view. There is a rounded, masslike consolidation in the right lower lung and a larger area of consolidation with a long axis adjacent to the chest wall in the left lung. *(Figure continues.)*

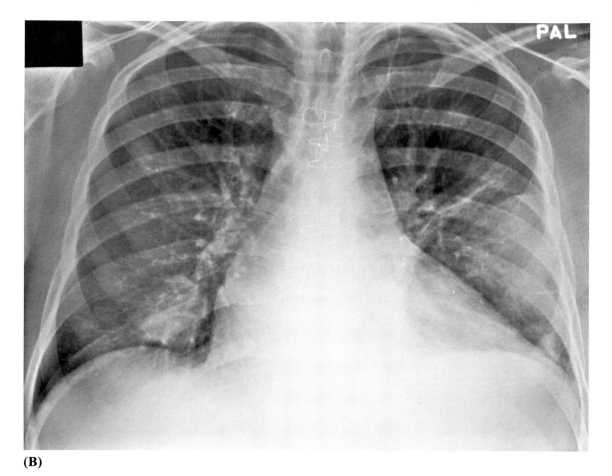

(B)

Fig. 5-10. *(Continued).* **(B)** PA view 3 days later shows both regions of consolidation to be slightly larger. Nevertheless, the rate of change is not rapid. There is also a nonspecific band of peripheral atelectasis more medially on the left.

The radiographic appearance and the rate of change of these lesions are consistent with pneumonitis due to *Legionella* infection. It is radiographically indistinguishable from infection due to anaerobes, the ubiquitous fungi, or the higher bacterium *Nocardia*. Since the treatment is different for these groups of organisms, it is important to establish the etiology as precisely as possible. Other gram-negative organism pneumonias may also appear as masslike zones of consolidation, but if untreated would usually progress more rapidly. If treated, however, their rate of progression is modified.

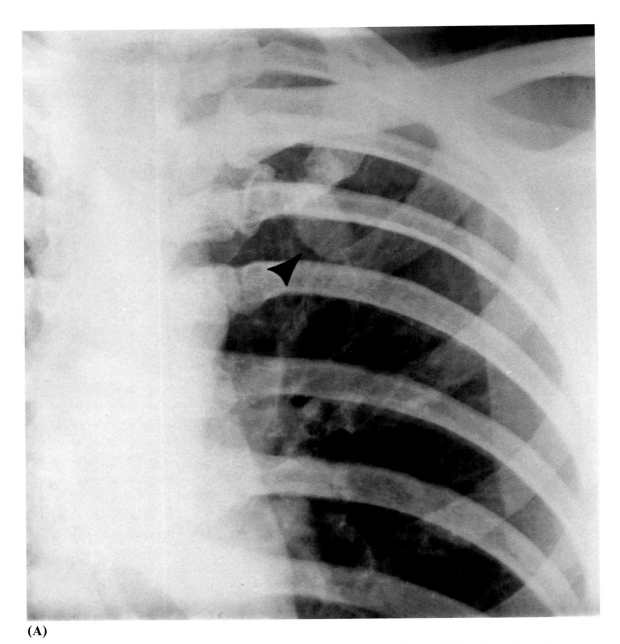

(A)

Fig. 5-11. (A). Solitary Noncalcified Pulmonary Nodule as a Sign of Infectious Granulomatous Disease

A well-defined, well-circumscribed nodule is projected between the anterior ends of the first and second ribs (arrowhead). This is a nummular or nodular form of pulmonary tuberculosis. It is a common location for such lesions. However, as long as nodules due to infectious granulomatous diseases are noncalcified, there is no way to distinguish them with any degree of reliability from nodules due to primary or secondary malignant neoplasms or from hamartomas. Further studies and procedures are necessary to make that distinction. Whenever possible, older chest films should be obtained for comparison. If, in retrospect, the lesion can be judged to have been present and unchanged for a minimum of 2 years, it is likely to be benign. Further workup and follow-up can be planned on that presumption. The fact that a nodular focus of tuberculosis (or of any of the infectious granulomatous diseases) remains stable does *not* mean viable organisms are not present. *(Figure continues.)*

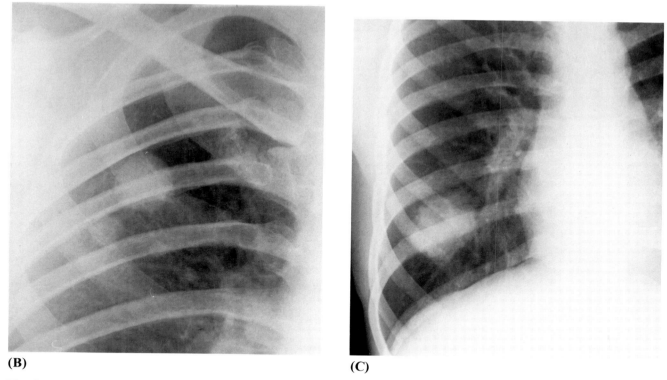

(B)

(C)

Fig. 5-11. *(Continued).* **(B) Clustered Nodules—Part of the Radiographic Spectrum of Tuberculosis**

There are clustered nodules (you can count at least three) in the right upper lung. They vary in size and none of them show calcification. This appearance of clustered nodules is another part of the radiographic spectrum of pulmonary tuberculosis. However, there is nothing specific about these abnormalities, and further studies or procedures are necessary to eliminate other possibilities such as metastases.

How could you determine that any one of these nodules is not a neoplasm? From this examination alone, you cannot make that determination.

Note the calcifications of the costal cartilage of the right first rib. It is important that this not be mistaken for a pulmonary lesion.

(C) Small Mass Due to Cryptococcal Infection

This young man was a pigeon raiser. There is a rounded mass with lobulated margins in the right lower lobe. The lesion was removed and was shown to be due to infection with *Cryptococcus.* Later the patient developed disseminated disease involving other portions of the lung as well as numerous lesions of bone.

Pulmonary lesions due to *Cryptococcus neoformans* may appear as nodules or small masses, solitary or multiple, or as segmental consolidations. Cavitation may occur, as may hilar lymphadenopathy. In addition, diffuse, small, poorly defined nodules and interstitial patterns have been described in a few cases. *Cryptococcus* infection may also contribute to the diffuse lung lesions seen in patients dying of multiorganism pneumonia.

Cryptococcal meningitis may occur and bones may also become involved. Many but not all patients with pulmonary cryptococcosis have other diseases or conditions associated with altered immunity.

Some patients with positive sputum cultures for *Cryptococcus* have reportedly had no radiographic pulmonary lesions and presumably had only airway colonization.

Although the history of exposure to pigeons in this instance is a real factor, such a history is by no means necessary for diagnosis. *Cryptococcus* is a ubiquitous organism.

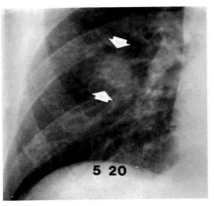 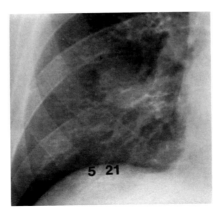 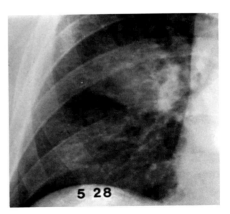

(A)

Fig. 5-12.   (A). Nodular Consolidation Due to *Nocardia*

Series of coned views of the right lung base of an immunocompromised man. A nodule with poorly defined margins is seen on the May 20 film. A needle aspiration specimen revealed *Nocardia*. On May 21 the nodule is slightly larger; on May 28 it has more than doubled in size while the patient was on appropriate treatment. This rate of change, although rapid, is not as explosive as that which can occur with untreated gram-negative organism pneumonia.

In patients with altered immunity, *Nocardia* infection is commonly due to *Nocardia asteroides*. The lesions may vary from a discrete solitary pulmonary nodule or mass, with or without cavitation, to multiple pulmonary nodules or masses, with or without cavitation, or solitary or multiple patchy foci of consolidation. The lesions progress at a variable rate, but usually with an intermediate time course similar to that of pulmonary infection due to ubiquitous fungi. Rarely, miliary lesions occur in the lungs. Dissemination of the organisms to many body sites may occur just as with infections due to ubiquitous fungi.

Patients may have little in the way of signs and symptoms, or they may have the entire spectrum of clinical signs and symptoms common to pulmonary infections in general.

Heart transplant recipients, renal recipients, patients with malignant lymphoma or chronic renal failure, and those who have been treated with steroids and immunosuppressive drugs are among those most commonly affected. Patients with pulmonary alveolar proteinosis who have been treated with steroids are also reported to have a propensity for pulmonary infection due to *Nocardia*.

In our hospital, however, patients with acute myelogenous leukemia rarely have pulmonary infections with *Nocardia*, although they commonly have infections with *Aspergillus*, which has an almost identical radiographic spectrum of appearances.

Nocardia pulmonary infection occurs uncommonly in patients who are not known to be immunocompromised; in these patients it may appear quite similar to tuberculosis.

(From Blank and Castellino,[11] with permission.) *(Figure continues.)*

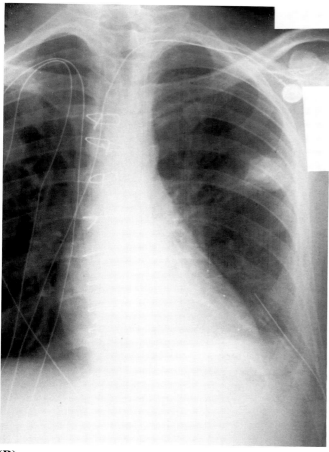

(B)

Fig. 5-12. *(Continued)* **(B) Nodular Consolidation Due to *Aspergillus* in an Immunocompromised Host**

This cardiac transplant recipient developed a nodular zone of consolidation in the left lung. He was afebrile. A diagnosis of *Aspergillus* infection was based on organisms retrieved from a fluoroscopically guided percutaneous needle aspiration specimen.

Aspergillus, usually *Aspergillus fumigatus,* may involve the lungs as:

1. Invasive aspergillosis, rarely occurring in patients without altered immunity but common in those with impaired immune mechanisms. Radiographically the infection may appear as one or more zones of consolidation, often due to infarction consequent to vascular invasion by the fungus, but indistinguishable from pneumonia, or as one or more nodules or masses, with or without cavitation. When subacute the lesions may resemble those of chronic infectious granulomatous disease.

2. Allergic aspergillosis, causing a characteristic form of bronchiectasis, with focal dilatation of proximal segments of the bronchi while the peripheral segments are spared. Afflicted individuals usually, but not always, have a history of asthma or atopy. Mucoid impaction may coincide with these lesions.
3. Saprophytic invaders of previously existing cavities presenting as "fungus balls."
4. Uncommonly, a nodular or focal consolidation due to indolent infection with *Aspergillus* in an immunocompetent, asymptomatic host.[35]

Occasionally the presence of *Aspergillus* infection may be suggested by the appearance of focal pleural thickening that is disproportionate to adjacent parenchymal disease, particularly when seen in the apices of patients with impaired immunity. In patients who are clearly immunocompromised, there is a justifiable reluctance to base the diagnosis of pulmonary aspergillosis on retrieval of the fungus from sputum alone, since colonization can occur in the absence of invasive disease. *(Figure continues.)*

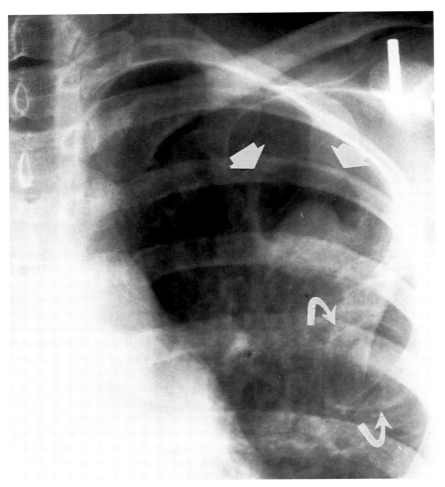

(C)

Fig. 5-12. *(Continued).*   **(C) Cavitary Lesions Due to Invasive Aspergillosis**

Coned view of the left upper lung of a woman being treated for acute myelogenous leukemia (AML). There is a cavity present in the axillary region of the left upper lung, and in the bottom of the cavity there is a small mass. The top of the cavity (short arrows) happens to superimpose on the superior cortex of the posterior fourth rib and may be difficult to see.

In patients with invasive aspergillosis these intracavitary masses represent necrotic lung tissue mixed with organisms. This lesion is to be distinguished from a true fungus ball consisting of the mycelia of *Aspergillus,* which behave as saprophytic invaders of preexisting chronic cavitary lesions.

Invasive aspergillosis often becomes manifest at a time of profound neutropenia in patients with AML. The lesions appear as solid nodules or masses or as solid zones of consolidation, which often undergo necrosis and cavitation. The cavitation usually occurs at a time when the bone marrow is recovering and neutrophils reappear in the blood. The lesions may expel much of their necrotic contents and end up as thin-walled cavities. These lesions may cause hemoptysis.

Notice that in this figure another very thin-walled cavity is seen laterally in the left midlung zone (curved arrows).

Cavitary lesions with ball-like contents occurring in patients with AML are almost diagnostic of *Aspergillus* infection, but the diagnosis should be considered and treatment begun before the characteristic air crescents become obvious.

Cavities within nodules or small masses in patients with altered immunity may also be caused by *Mucor, Nocardia,* anaerobic bacteria, and less often other microorganisms.

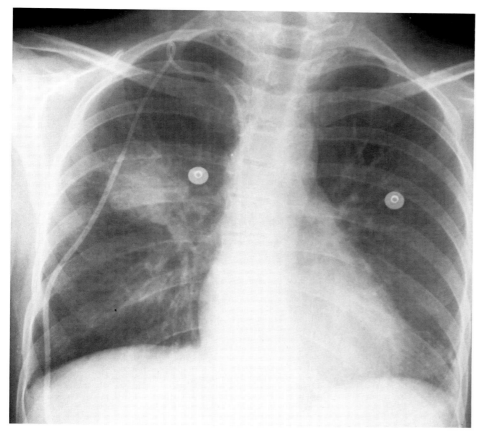

Fig. 5-13. Unusual Fungus Resembling *Aspergillus*

There is a rounded zone of consolidation in the right perihilar region. You could call it a "masslike" zone of consolidation, or you could call it a large nodule. There are no agreed-upon criteria that distinguish a "mass" from a "nodule" on the basis of size. This type of lesion may appear like a rounded mass in one projection and like a segmental or wedge-shaped opacity in another. A nodule, however, should look like a nodule in all views. The description often has to be based on the appearance of the lesion on a frontal view, since an AP view is usually all that is obtained when patients are very ill and portable x-ray equipment is used.

This lesion was caused by an infection with a fungus, *Pseudoallescheria boydii,* which morphologically resembles *Aspergillus* but is culturally distinct and requires different treatment. The patient was a young girl suffering a relapse of acute leukemia.

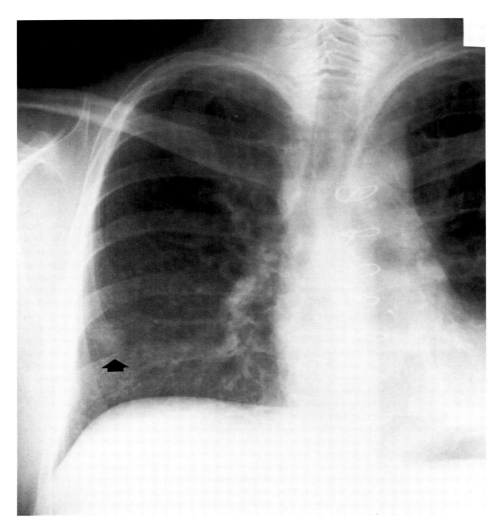

Fig. 5-14. Pulmonary Nodule Due to Malignant Lymphoma in an Immunocompromised Host

This cardiac transplant recipient developed an immunoblastic lymphoma approximately 3 months after transplantation. He received combined-modality treatment. Approximately 7 months later he developed a nodule in his right lower lobe (arrow) and became febrile. Cytologic study of a percutaneous needle aspiration specimen of this lesion indicated that it was due to his immunoblastic lymphoma. No microorganisms were present, nor were any cultured from the specimen.

Pulmonary nodules are part of the radiographic spectrum of lesions due to malignant lymphoma. They cannot be distinguished from nodular lesions due to ubiquitous fungi such as *Aspergillus* or to *Nocardia* or anaerobic bacteria, which are all more common in this patient group.

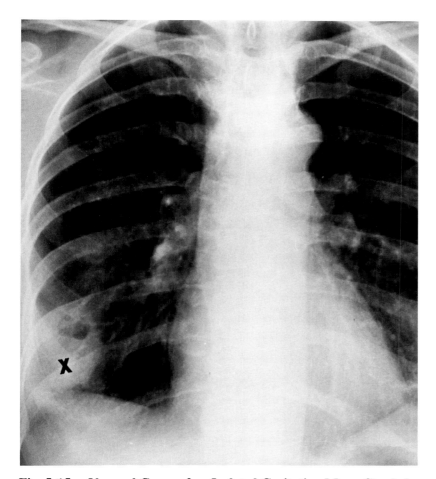

Fig. 5-15.   Unusual Cause of an Isolated Cavitating Mass: Staphylococcal Infection

This 35-year-old woman was an immunocompromised renal transplant recipient. There is a fairly well circumscribed, small, masslike zone of consolidation (X) laterally at the right base. A lucency in its upper third is due to cavitation. *Staphylococcus aureus* was recovered from this lesion by needle aspiration. It is unusual for *Staphylococcus* infection to present in such a well-defined, localized fashion in patients who are immunosuppressed. In this cohort of immunocompromised patients, lesions such as this are more commonly due to ubiquitous fungi or *Nocardia.*

Focal staphylococcal abscesses in the lung are more likely to occur as a result of hematogenous dissemination from an extrapulmonary site or as a result of bloodstream contamination such as occurs in intravenous drug abusers.

(From Blank et al.,[10] and Blank and Castellino[11] with permission.)

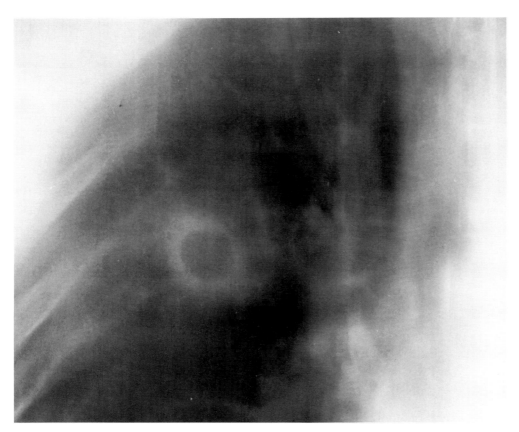

Fig. 5-16. Unusual Cause of an Isolated Cavitary Nodule in a Patient With Altered Immunity

Coned view of a tomographic scan from a heart transplant recipient almost a year after surgery. He was relatively asymptomatic at the time the lesion was first seen on a routine surveillance chest film.

There is a cavity in the right lung greater than 2.0 cm in diameter. Usual causes of a small pulmonary cavity in a cardiac transplant recipient include infection with one of the ubiquitous fungi or *Nocardia*. A percutaneous needle aspiration specimen from this lesion grew three varieties of *Pseudomonas* and produced a small growth of *Streptococcus pneumoniae*. These are unexpected organisms for this type of asymptomatic lesion but serve to remind us that uncommon things do occur and should be ranked accordingly in formulating a differential diagnosis rather than simply ignored as possibilities.

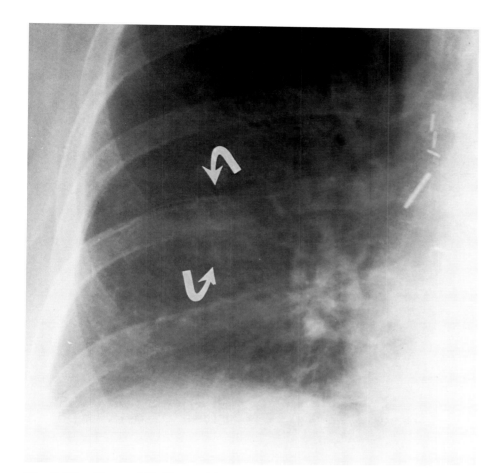

Fig. 5-17. Unusual Radiographic Presentation of Cytomegalovirus Pneumonitis as a Focal Lesion

This woman is a heart and lung transplant recipient who developed a fever. On the chest film a circumscribed, low-density focus of consolidation is seen in the right midlung (arrows). Percutaneous needle aspiration of this lesion was performed under fluoroscopic control. Cytomegalovirus (CMV) was cultured from this specimen.

It is very unusual for CMV pneumonia to present as a solitary, circumscribed focus. It is likely that other lesions were present in both lungs but were unrecognizable on the chest film. Nevertheless, at the time of diagnosis this was considered the only significant lesion.

Several days later a follow-up chest film (not shown) showed multiple, poorly defined, low-density nodules randomly distributed in both lungs. This was a more usual appearance for CMV pneumonitis. One of the nodules was removed and again was shown by culture and histopathology to be due to CMV. The patient was treated with DHPG, an analog of guanine, and showed remarkable clinical and radiographic improvement.

The problem of CMV infection in patients with altered immunity is challenging because it is difficult to distinguish between colonization (or infection without tissue disease) and infection with tissue disease. Even when CMV is recovered from the urine, that does not mean that a concomitant pulmonary infection is due to the same organism.

Proven CMV pneumonia usually appears as a disseminated granular pattern or as small (approximately 5 mm) nodules throughout both lungs, often with bibasilar predominance (see Fig. 5-18). Seldom is CMV pneumonia diagnosed when in a localized form. CMV pulmonary infection may coexist with *Pneumocystis carinii* pneumonia and other, often fatal, multiorganism pneumonias.

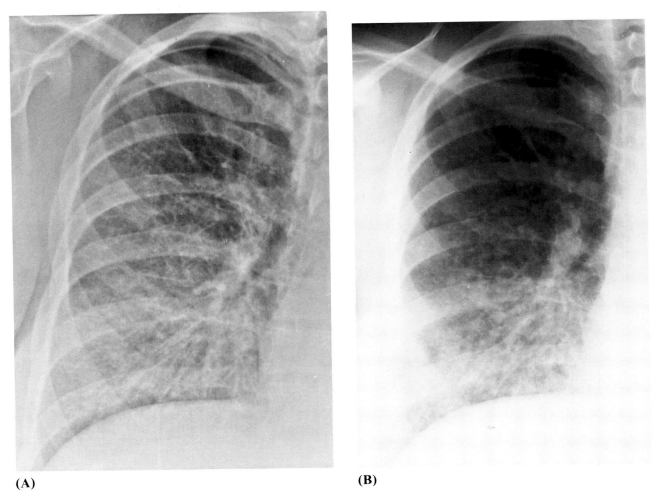

(A)   **(B)**

Fig. 5-18. (A – C) Cytomegalovirus Pneumonitis

This 17-year-old girl had recently been operated upon for an embryonal cell carcinoma of the ovary. She had a blood transfusion at that time but did not have multiple transfusions. She later had one course of chemotherapy.

(A) Coned view of the right lung (the left appeared similar) shows a loss of definition of the fine vascular shadows throughout, as well as numerous septal lines visible as linear opacities that neither branch nor taper. These lines correspond to Kerley-A lines. This is an appearance of interstitial edema. Small, vague, poorly defined nodules are also present. A film taken 4 days earlier was normal.

The patient was febrile and suffering from moderately severe respiratory distress.

(B) Coned view from a film 1 day later shows a pattern of small, coarse, ill-defined nodules in the middle and upper lung zones with greater profusion and coalescence at the bases. In addition, there is a background of fine reticular shadows that may not be visible on this reproduction. A lung biopsy showed Cowdry type A viral inclusion bodies but no cytoplasmic inclusion bodies diagnostic of cytomegalovirus (CMV). However, CMV virus was cultured from the lung, and CMV immunoglobulin M titers were positive. The patient was treated with DHPG and eventually recovered. *(Figure continues.)*

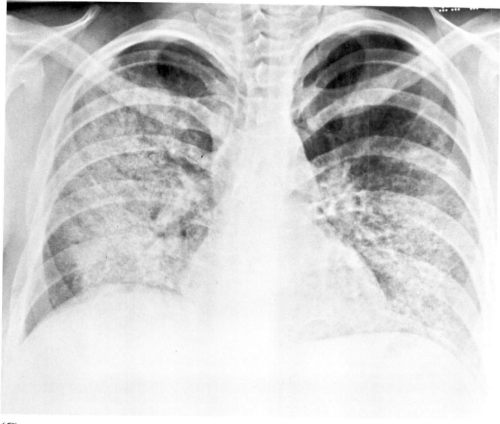

(C)

Fig. 5-18. *(Continued).* **(C)** Before clearing of the pulmonary lesions began, they progressed to the point where there was extensive consolidation of the lungs with only relative sparing of the periphery.

The appearance of interstitial pulmonary edema at onset **(A)** is not surprising in view of the pathogenesis of viral and *Pneumocystis carinii* pneumonias. Clinically it can be a problem because pulmonary edema due to intravenous fluid overload is not uncommon in these patients while undergoing intensive chemotherapy. Early on these two causes, fluid overload and infection, are easily confused.

This series shows how a pneumonitis may change its appearance with time and how one should anticipate a spectrum of radiographic possibilities for any given infection dependent in part on the extent of pulmonary involvement when the patient is first seen. (*Figure continues.*)

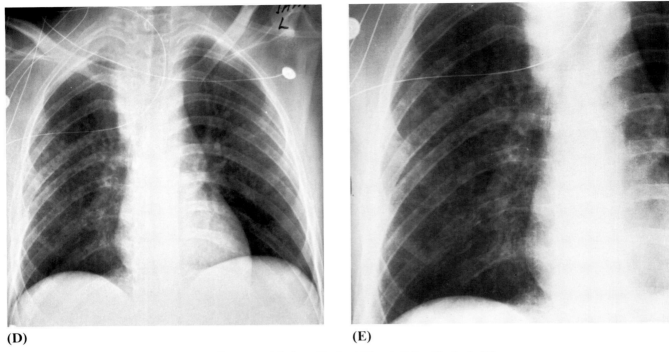

(D)   **(E)**

Fig. 5-18. (D,E) Varicella-Zoster Pneumonitis in a Patient Treated for Crohn's Disease

This young man was being treated with steroids for Crohn's disease of the bowel when he developed fever and intense back pain. He was immediately referred with a tentative diagnosis of retroperitoneal abscess. However, he began to develop a diffuse skin rash characteristic of chickenpox, and it soon became apparent that varicella-zoster viral infection was responsible for his clinical signs and symptoms. His chest film shows a diffuse, small, coarse nodular pattern in both lungs, which is best seen in the right middle zone.

(E) Coned view shows innumerable low-density, small nodules (approximately 5 mm or less). These are the radiographic counterparts of the foci of hemorrhagic necrosis that occur in the lung in cases of varicella-zoster pneumonia.

Notice in Fig. D that a mantle of soft tissue separates the lung from the extreme apex of the hemithorax. In addition, the right superior mediastinum is wide, and the trachea is shifted to the left. These distortions are caused by blood in the mediastinal and extrapleural spaces due to bleeding from an unsuccessful attempt to pass a central line. There was spontaneous resolution of this complication. *(Figure continues.)*

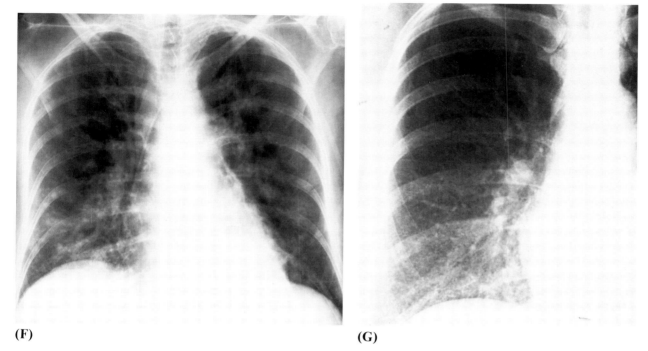

(F)   **(G)**

Fig. 5-18. *(Continued).*   **(F) Confluent Nodular Lesions of Varicella-Zoster Pneumonia**

This woman had a 2-year history of diffuse histiocytic lymphoma stage IVb. She had been treated with chemotherapy and prednisone. Approximately 3 weeks before this radiograph was taken she noted cutaneous vesicles over the anterior chest wall. In that 3-week period the lesions disseminated to multiple dermatomes. Approximately 4 days before this radiograph was taken she noted the onset of fever.

There are multiple coarse nodular densities of varying size distributed throughout both lungs. The nodules have poorly defined margins. In some areas there is a thickening of the peribronchial tissues. A diagnosis of varicella-zoster pneumonia was confirmed on lung biopsy.

Initially the nodules of varicella-zoster pneumonia usually are smaller (see Fig. E) than those shown here. When they progress and become confluent, this radiographic pattern may result. The pulmonary manifestations of varicella-zoster infection are very rare in the absence of disseminated skin lesions.

Measles pneumonia may cause diffuse, small nodular opacities in the lungs even in the absence of skin lesions or other stigmata of measles in patients with impaired immunity. Fortunately, it is a rare complication. Exposure to an active case of measles is apparently catastrophic to patients with severely impaired host defenses.

(G) Coexistent Cytomegalovirus and *Pneumocystis carinii* Pneumonia

Coned view of the right lung of a woman with acute lymphocytic leukemia. Innumerable small nodules permeate the lower lung zone (similar lesions were present on the left), and there is also effacement of the images of small and medium-sized vessels. This reproduction was filmed to emphasize the lesions of the lung base, and the upper lung is therefore lacking in detail. On the original films the upper zones appeared within normal limits, but it is likely that the radiograph understates the true extent of the disease.

Both cytomegalovirus and *Pneumocystis carinii* were found on lung biopsy. Either of these organisms alone can produce a similar pattern.

Although leukemic infiltrates do occur in the lungs of patients with leukemia, they present radiographic abnormalities far less often than does infection in these patients. When leukemic infiltrates cause radiographic changes, there is usually a very high count of blast forms and leukemic cells in blood.

Patients with chronic lymphatic leukemia, however, may have pulmonary lesions, in the absence of high numbers of leukemic cells in the blood, similar to those seen in patients with diffuse, well-differentiated lymphoma.

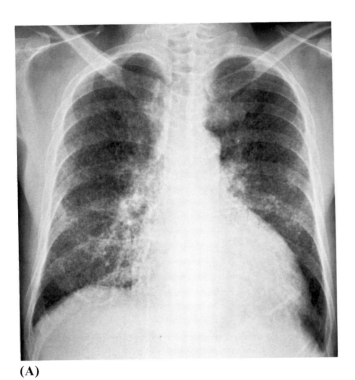

(A)

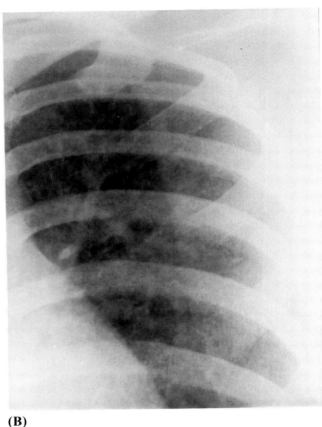

(B)

Fig. 5-19.   (A – E) Miliary Tuberculosis

(A) PA chest film of a patient with miliary tuberculosis. There are fine, fairly discrete, nodular opacities distributed throughout all portions of both lungs.

   (B – E) Series of coned views of the lungs of four different patients showing a spectrum of "miliary" nodules. The appearance depends on the size of the lesions, their profusion, their degree of coalescence, and the film technique used. The areas shown are representative of disseminated lesions present throughout both lungs.

   (B) There is a fine nodular pattern that is difficult to see on this reproduction. None of the small vessel images are seen distinctly because of the diffuse lung disease. The black area medially appears relatively spared, but if you viewed the original film with a bright light you would see that sparing to be more apparent than real. *(Figure continues.)*

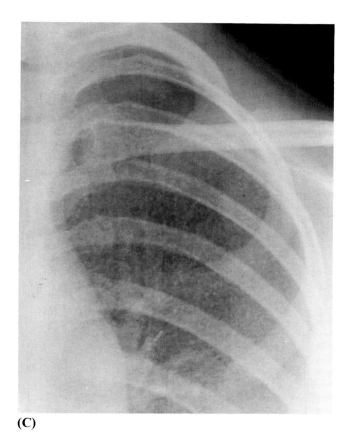

(C)

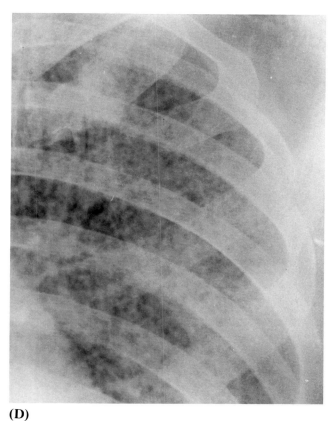

(D)

Fig. 5-19. *(Continued).* **(C)** Myriad tiny nodules permeate the lung. They are quite discrete considering their size.

(D) In this case the nodules are larger and in some places do not appear discrete because of summation and coalescence.

(E) Here the nodules are even larger and again show foci of coalescence.

Often, affected adults have other underlying diseases or conditions that alter their immune mechanisms. Tubercles may be widespread in the bone marrow, abdominal viscera, peritoneum, eyes, and meninges. *(Figure continues.)*

(E)

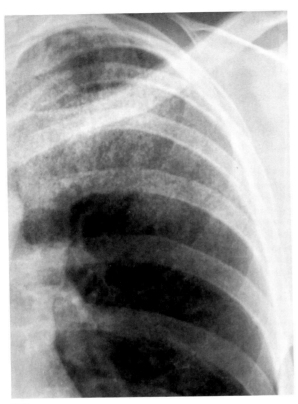

(F)

Fig. 5-19. *(Continued).* **(F) Miliary Histoplasmosis**

Coned view of the left upper and midlung zones of a 29-year-old man who was critically ill at the time this film was made. He had a known occupational exposure to pigeon and chicken dung during the process of fertilizer manufacture.

The radiograph shows a very finely stippled nodular pattern, which is most marked in the left apical and subclavicular region. However, all portions of both lungs were involved with a similar but less heavily concentrated granular pattern. There is no way to distinguish the miliary lesions of any of the infectious granulomatous diseases from one another radiographically.

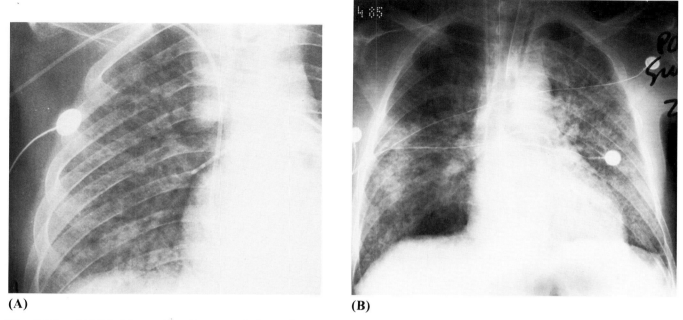

(A)   **(B)**

Fig. 5-20. (A) Multiorganism Pneumonia in an Immunocompromised Host

Coned view of the right lung (the left lung looked the same) of a young man with end-stage cardiomyopathy. He had been treated with steroids and other immunosuppressive drugs.

The lungs are diffusely abnormal, but it is difficult to choose adequate words to describe the pattern. No portion of the lung appears spared. This appearance correlates with the biopsy, which showed all alveoli in the specimen filled with large quantities of eosinophilic foamy material as well as occasional histiocytes and lesser numbers of polymorphonuclear leukocytes. There were also histopathologic changes characteristic of cytomegalovirus infection, large numbers of *Pneumocystis carinii*, and budding yeasts whose morphologic appearance was most consistent with *Cryptococcus.* Any one of these three organisms alone could have produced a similar appearance of advanced-stage infection, but it is not rare for them to occur together in the lungs of desperately ill, immunocompromised patients.

(From Blank and Castellino,[11] with permission.)

(B) *Pneumocystis carinii* **Pneumonia in a Patient With Hemophilia**

This 64-year-old man with well-controlled hemophilia developed a febrile illness and progressive respiratory failure.

On admission his chest film showed extensive bilateral abnormalities indistinguishable from pulmonary edema with alveolar flooding. His heart is not enlarged, a cardiac catheterization study showed no evidence of left heart failure, there was no evidence of renal failure, and there had been no excessive parenteral fluid administration. *Pneumocystis carinii* was retrieved from a tracheal aspirate.

It is not surprising that florid *Pneumocystis carinii* pneumonia resembles pulmonary edema, since alveolar flooding is a common histopathologic abnormality among the spectra of changes that can be seen in each of these conditions.

Severe intrapulmonary hemorrhage could also cause this appearance but should cause a drop in hematocrit when this marked. When due to thrombocytopenia, pulmonary hemorrhage is often accompanied by signs of bleeding elsewhere (e.g., petechiae, guaiac-positive stools) even though hemoptysis may be absent.

The diagnosis of *Pneumocystis carinii* pneumonia in a patient with hemophilia should alert one to the likelihood that the patient has AIDS resulting from virus-contaminated blood transfusions. *(Figure continues.)*

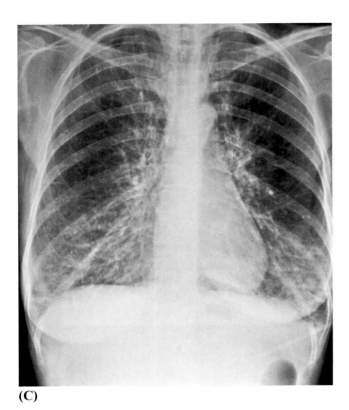

(C)

Fig. 5-20. *(Continued).* **(C)** *Pneumocystis carinii* **Pneumonia After Chemotherapy**

This 57-year-old nurse had an oat cell carcinoma of the lung, for which she had been treated with five courses of chemotherapy, radiotherapy, and whole-brain irradiation. For 3 weeks before admission she had symptoms of sore throat, cough, and "sinus drainage" along with increasing shortness of breath. Her temperature was 37.5°C, 37°C, and 37.5°C on three successive occasions, respirations were 35 per minute but were not labored, PO_2 was 47 mmHg, and PCO_2 was 33 mmHg.

This chest film was made the day after admission. It shows bilateral disease manifested by reticulonodular opacities, coarser conglomerate nodular foci at both bases, and loss of definition of small and medium-sized vessels, most marked at the bases but extending cephalad to include marked loss of sharpness of the hilar vessels. Not only have the vessels in the lower zones lost their sharp outlines, but in addition there are thick, irregular opacities that ramify in peribronchial distributions.

An open-lung biopsy showed interstitial pneumonitis, and silver stains demonstrated *Pneumocystis carinii* both in clusters and as individual microorganisms. No other organisms were recovered from cultures of the lung biopsy specimen.

Pneumocystis carinii pneumonia has a broad radiographic spectrum of appearances and a considerable range of clinical signs and symptoms. Classically the pneumonia is seen as a bilateral, relatively symmetrical opacification of both lungs, often with striking air bronchograms visible, and a distribution like that of intense alveolar edema. Profound tachypnea, hypoxemia, fever, and malaise are often associated with this pattern. Some patients may have cough, sore throat, or abdominal distress.

In some patients the first radiographic manifestations may be so subtle that they escape recognition, unless there is a prior film for comparison to show that there is a loss of definition of small, fine pulmonary vessels and a granular appearance of the lung bases that barely exceeds the background noise of the film. Patients may have a profound tachypnea and hypoxemia in spite of the paucity of radiographic findings.

Other patients may show a focal zone of patchy consolidation in a lower or upper lobe as the first chest film finding. This commonly progresses over 24 to 48 hours to a bilateral, diffuse, relatively symmetrical pattern. Some of these patients may not appear very ill and may have much less respiratory distress than expected for the degree of measured hypoxemia. Not all patients are severely hypoxemic.

At times there may be sparing of peripheral or central lung zones. Septal lines can be striking (both Kerley-A and -B types) and indistinguishable from those of interstitial edema without infection. *(Figure continues.)*

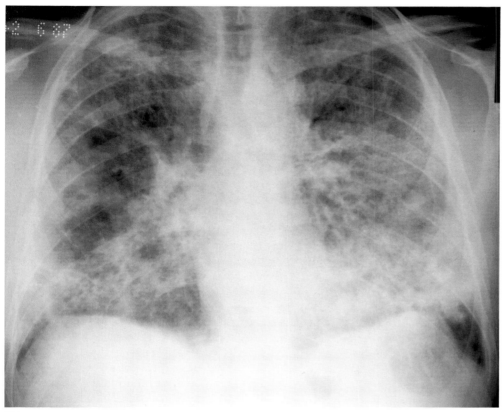

(D)

Fig. 5-20. *(Continued).* **(D,E)** *Pneumocystis carinii* **Pneumonia and Pulmonary Lesions of Kaposi's Sarcoma in a Patient With AIDS**

This homosexual man has both *Pneumocystis carinii* pneumonia and Kaposi's sarcoma. This is not an uncommon combination of pulmonary abnormalities in patients with AIDS.

(D) PA chest film shows a widespread, bilateral, inhomogeneous opacification of both lungs with areas of relative sparing in the lateral portions of the right midlung zone. The minor interlobar fissure is slightly elevated.

(E) Coned view of the left upper lung at the same magnification as the original chest film. There is a finely granular pattern of lesions. In addition, however, there are irregular linear and bandlike opacities. On the full view of the chest you can see that there is thickening of peribronchial structures emanating from the left hilum, producing an appearance of thick-walled bronchi. At the bases some irregular, clustered nodular foci are present, and at the right base there are foci of honeycombing as well.

Kaposi's sarcoma produces both nodular lesions and extensive interstitial lesions in the lungs. It is virtually impossible to separate the contribution of the *Pneumocystis carinii* pneumonia from that of the Kaposi's sarcoma to this radiographic appearance.

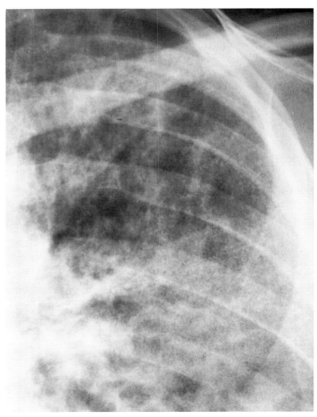

(E)

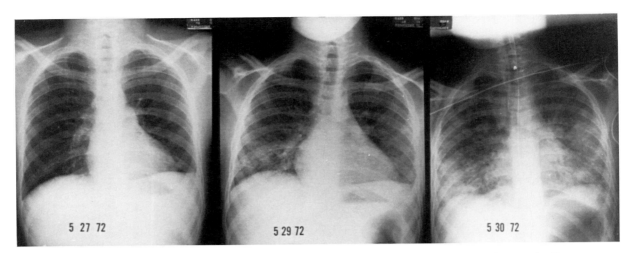

Fig. 5-21. Progressive Staphylococcal Pneumonia in a Patient Treated for Systemic Lupus Erythematosus

Chest films of a 21-year-old man with systemic lupus erythematosus who had been treated with steroids. On the day of the first film (May 27), he had developed fever and cough and produced brownish sputum. There is obliteration of the left costophrenic angle by a fixed chronic pleuritis, but there is no pulmonary consolidation. In approximately 48 hours the film in the middle was obtained; now there is a sizeable zone of inhomogeneous patchy and nodular consolidation. *Staphylococcus* was cultured from sputa and transtracheal aspirates. The film taken 1 day later shows rapidly progressive patchy, rounded, and amorphous zones of consolidation, which predominate in the lower lungs but extend into the middle and upper lung regions bilaterally. Although the patient was profoundly ill during this pneumonia, he eventually recovered after appropriate antibiotic treatment.

Staphylococcal pneumonia may be segmental, lobar, or multilobar in distribution. In adults it is frequently bilateral and may cause abscess formation with subsequent cavitation. Pneumatoceles, commonly seen in children with staphylococcal pneumonia, are seldom seen in adults. Empyema is a common complication of staphylococcal pneumonia in adults.

(From Blank and Castellino,[11] with permission.)

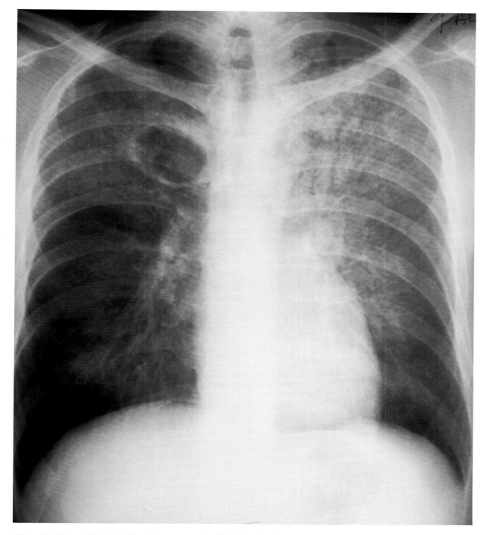

Fig. 5-22. *Klebsiella* **Pneumonia With Cavity in a Bisexual Male With** *Pneumocystis carinii* **Pneumonia**

The patient is a 49-year-old bisexual man who had been having daily fevers (up to 105°F) and night sweats for the past 9 months. For the past 3 weeks he had also noted increasing shortness of breath and nonproductive cough along with his continuing fevers. He then went to see his private physician, and three morning sputa all showed *Pneumocystis carinii* organisms on GMS stain.

This PA view of the chest shows inhomogeneous consolidation extending from the subapical regions of the left upper lobe caudally down to the left heart border, but there is sparing of the basilar segments of the left lower lobe. Air bronchograms can be seen in the upper portions of the left-sided consolidation.

On the right, inhomogeneous consolidation extends from the subapical regions approximately down to the level of the hilum. There is a parahilar component, but there is sparing of the right lower lung zones.

A large cavity with moderately thick walls is seen in the right subclavicular region. On the lateral view (not shown), this was seen to be in the anterior segment of the right upper lobe. A cavity this size would be rare or nonexistent in *Pneumocystis carinii* pneumonia. A heavy growth of *Klebsiella* was cultured from sputum. This organism in all likelihood accounts for the cavity. Cavitation is common in gram-negative organism pneumonias.

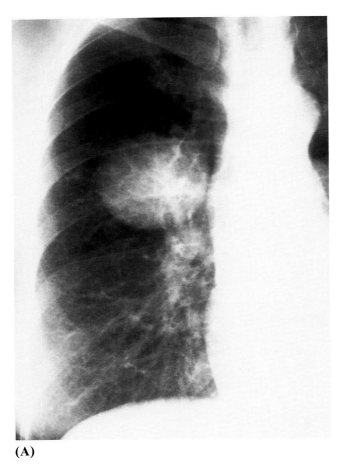

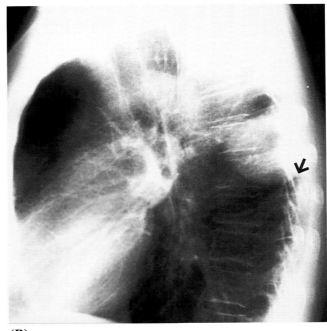

(A)   (B)

Fig. 5-23. Indolent Lung Abscess Due to Anaerobic Bacteria

(A) PA view. This 55-year-old woman was referred because of a persistent mass seen on chest films. About 10 days before she had noted pleuritic right-sided chest pain. She had an elevated white blood cell count and a shift to the left. She was treated for pneumonia with broad-spectrum antibiotics at an outside hospital, but the lesion persisted.

Needle aspiration of the lesion was inconclusive. Bronchoscopy was negative. At thoracotomy a necrotic mass was found in the superior segment of the right lower lobe. A single culture grew anaerobic bacteria. Histopathologically this was a lung abscess containing necrotic débris, neutrophils, and occasional pairs of plump gram-positive cocci. There was a wall of fibrous tissue and interstitial fibrosis in the surrounding parenchyma, with numerous intra-alveolar macrophages.

(B) On lateral view the mass is seen to be in apposition to the posterior chest wall and could be mistaken for an extrapleural mass. However, the inferior angle between the mass and the chest wall (arrow) is sharper than expected for an extrapleural mass. The appearance fits best with a peripheral lung mass.

It is surprising how abscesses due to anaerobic organisms can produce indolent lesions in patients who frequently do not appear critically ill.

Fig. 5-24. (A) Cavity Due to *Mycobacterium tuberculosis*

Chest film of a 49-year-old Latin American man with an 8-day history of fever and hemoptysis. Sputa were positive for acid-fast bacilli.

There is a thick-walled oval cavity in the left upper lobe, and there is mottled inhomogeneous consolidation extending into the lingula. The distribution was confirmed on a lateral view (not shown). The pericavitary and lingular consolidation cleared within a few days, but the cavity persisted. This mottled consolidation of the left upper lobe was probably due to aspiration of blood from the bleeding cavity.

Blood can be cleared rapidly from the lung and leave little trace. This serves as an example of how tuberculosis can be spread by expulsion of cavity contents into bronchi followed by transbronchial spread to other pulmonary segments.

In addition to the disease on the left side, there are small, irregular opacities in the right apical and subclavicular region consistent with residuals of old tuberculous infection; however, "old" does not equal "inactive."

The low position and flattened appearance of both hemidiaphragms indicates some element of chronic obstructive pulmonary disease in this patient. (*Figure continues.*)

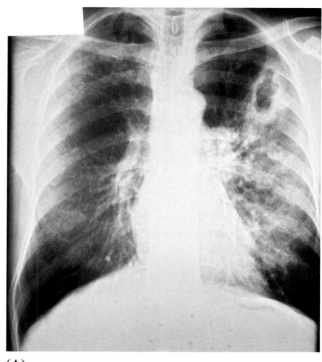

(A)

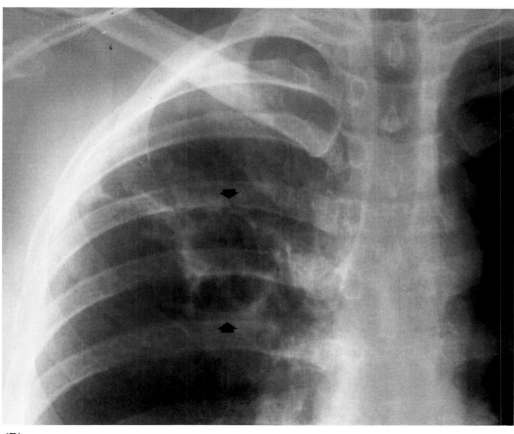

(B)

(See legend p. 272)

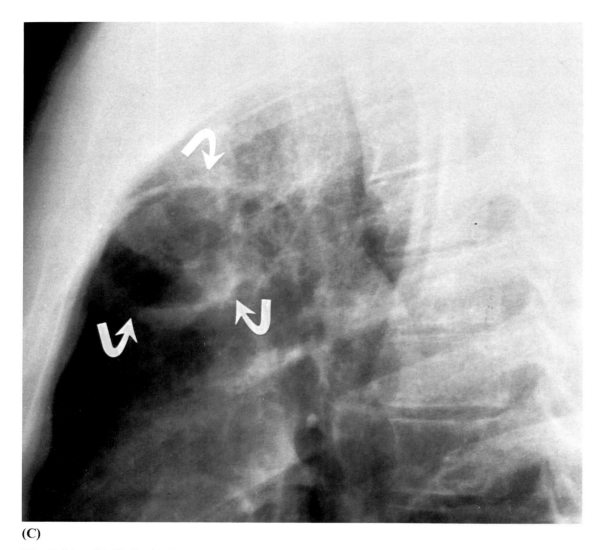

(C)

Fig. 5-24.   (B,C) Cavity Due to *Mycobacterium intracellulare*

There is a cavity in the anterior segment of the right upper lobe (arrows in Fig. C) caused by infection with *Mycobacterium intracellulare.* The posterior segment showed no involvement. Notice that the surrounding lung shows only a small amount of inhomogeneous consolidation, with a focal extension to the pleura seen on the PA view (Fig. B). The patient was a young man who felt well but sought care because of recurrent hemoptysis. The lesion did not respond to a long trial on multiple drug therapy and eventually was resected. Cavitation is common in pulmonary lesions caused by atypical mycobacteria but indistinguishable from those caused by *Mycobacterium tuberculosis.*

Cavitation in the anterior segments of the upper lobes, with no detectable disease in the posterior or apical segments, can occur in cases of atypical mycobacteria infection and also with progressive primary infection due to *Mycobacterium tuberculosis.*

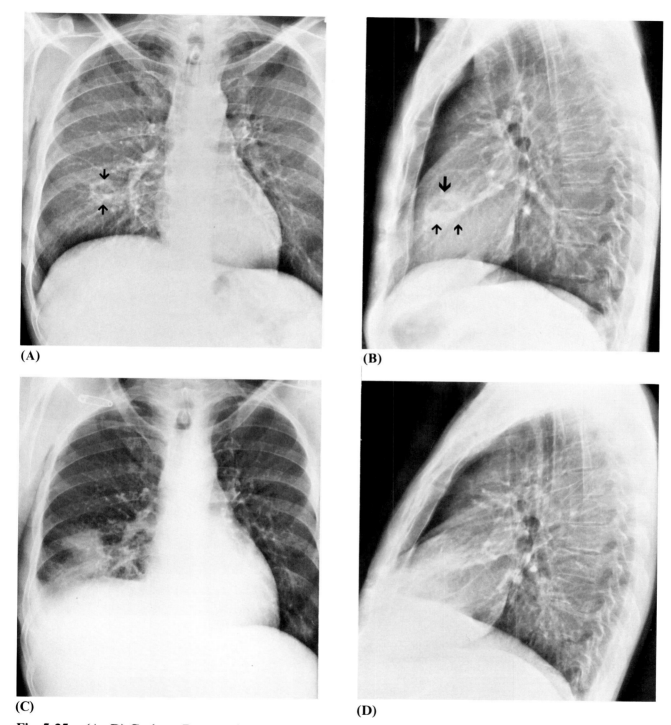

(A)

(B)

(C)

(D)

Fig. 5-25.   (A – D) Cavitary Pneumonias Due to Anaerobic Organism Pneumonia

(A,B) This patient had received radiation therapy for a carcinoma of the larynx and later developed perichondritis and an abscess of the larynx. While on prednisone and penicillin, he developed a cavitary pneumonia of the right middle lobe (arrows) with, surprisingly, no symptoms referable to the chest. The pneumonia became subacute in spite of antibiotic treatment.

(C,D) The cavity is not seen, but the pneumonia has progressed and there is now a large zone of consolidation with irregular margins occupying a portion of the right middle lobe. The right costophrenic angle is filled in, and the lateral margin of the right diaphragm is obscured by a moderate pleural effusion.

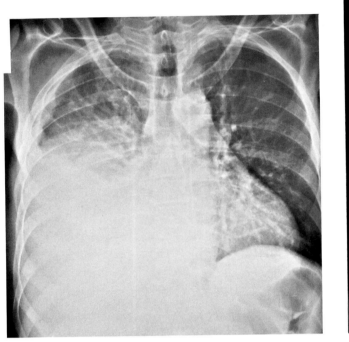

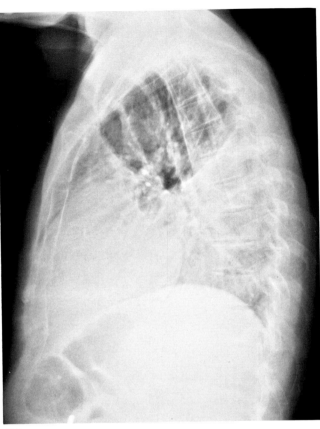

(E)

(F)

Fig. 5-25. **(E,F) Empyema and Anaerobic Organism Pneumonia**

PA and lateral views of the chest taken 1 day after those in Figs. C and D. There has been a marked increase in pleural fluid, which totally obscures the right lower and middle lobes. This very rapid increase in pleural fluid associated with a pneumonia is strong evidence of empyema. Cultures of the pleural fluid grew mixed anaerobes. These had also been cultured from the laryngeal abscess, along with gram-negative bacilli (three varieties of *Serratia*). However, only the mixed anaerobes were recovered from the pleural fluid. The patient responded to long-term antibiotic treatment, but eventually a decortication of the right lung was required.

Anaerobic organism pneumonia can be quite indolent, but development of empyema is still a serious complication. The diagnosis of pneumonia caused by anaerobes cannot be made from sputum studies, because these bacteria are part of the normal oropharyngeal flora.[19,23] Specimens for culture should be obtained from lower in the airway or directly from the lungs or pleura. Blood cultures are seldom positive in patients with anaerobic organism pneumonia.[4]

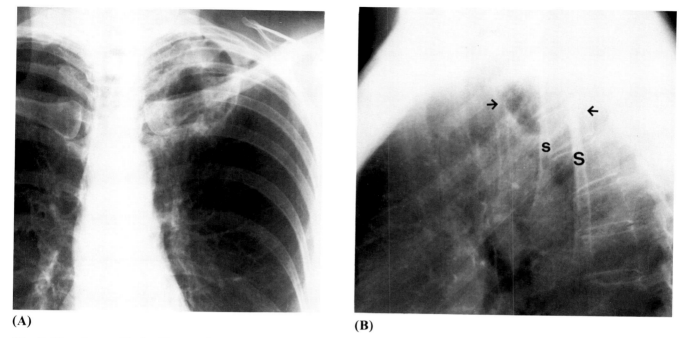

(A)   **(B)**

Fig. 5-26.   Large Cavity Due to Adenocarcinoma

(A) PA view. There is a large cavity in the apicoposterior segment of the left upper lobe. Its upper margins blend with adjacent foci of parenchymal consolidation, which extend to the pleural surface and the chest wall superiorly.

(B) On lateral view the cavity (arrows) is seen in the apicoposterior segment of the left upper lobe. Two scapulae are superimposed over the spine and the prespinal region, respectively. One scapula (s) is superimposed over the center of the cavity, and the other (s) on its posterior margin. *(Figure continues.)*

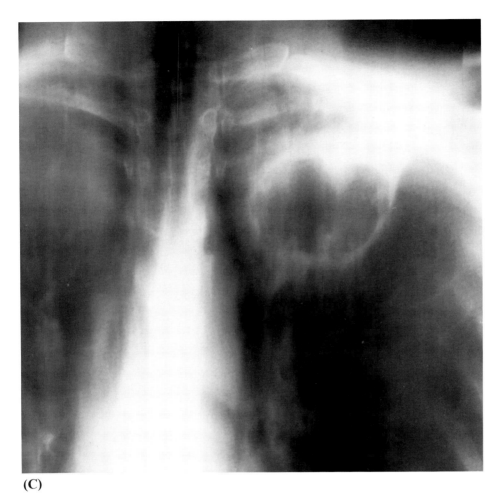

(C)

Fig. 5-26. *(Continued).* **(C)** Tomographic cut shows the margins of the cavity more clearly because of selective blurring of images above and below the plane of the cut, but offers no data that change the differential diagnosis.

The appearance of this lesion is indistinguishable from that of tuberculosis. Many years ago a patient with this radiographic lesion, a positive tuberculin skin test, and cough, hemoptysis, and fever might have been placed in a sanitorium and treated for a presumptive diagnosis of tuberculosis without bacteriologic or histopathologic proof. Modern techniques of diagnosis make such presumption unnecessary, and the correct diagnosis can be arrived at before thoracotomy through a variety of procedures with low associated morbidity.

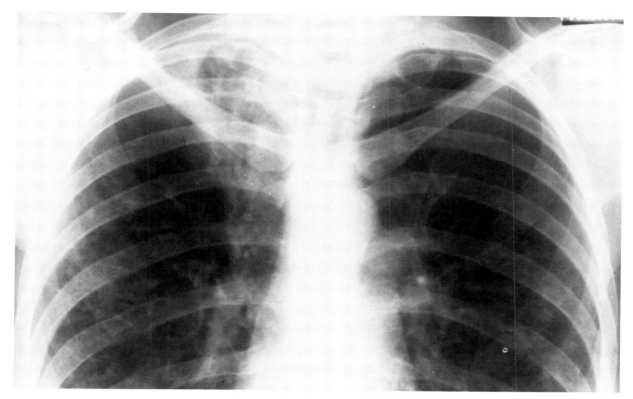

Fig. 5-27. Cavitation Due to Wegener's Granulomatosis

PA view of the upper zones of the chest of a 23-year-old woman who had noted insidious weight loss, spotty alopecia, and fatigue over the past year, with aching and drainage from the left ear for 6 months. This was followed by similar difficulties in the right ear and swelling of the bridge of the nose along with a discharge of blood and tissue. Urinalysis showed microscopic hematuria, red blood cell casts, and 2 + protein. Sinus films showed evidence of pansinusitis. A diagnosis of Wegener's granulomatosis was based on histopathology of nasal biopsy specimens.

The film shows bilateral apical lesions and small nodular opacities along the peripheral portions of both lungs, with sparing of the perihilar zones. The nodules in the periphery of the lungs are difficult to see on the reproduction, but the abnormalities in the right apex are readily identified.

In the left apex a cavity with a well-defined inferior rim is projected against adjacent lung. The wall is on the order of 2 to 3 mm in diameter. The superior margin of the cavity is not visible because it has an interface with the soft tissues of the apex of the chest. There was also a thick-walled cavity in the right lower lobe, which is not shown.

After chemotherapy there was marked improvement in the pulmonary lesions. The consolidation in the right upper lobe regressed to the point where there were only linear and bandlike residuals.

The cavity in the left apex became so thin walled that it was indistinguishable from a bulla. The nodules in the peripheral lung zones resolved.

The radiographic spectrum of the pulmonary lesions that may be seen in cases of Wegener's granulomatosis includes focal zones of consolidation with or without visible air bronchograms, multiple nodular densities or small masses in both lungs, and, less commonly, a solitary pulmonary nodule. The nodules or masses may be solid or may show cavities. Miliary and interstitial nodular patterns have also been described. (See also Ch. 10.)

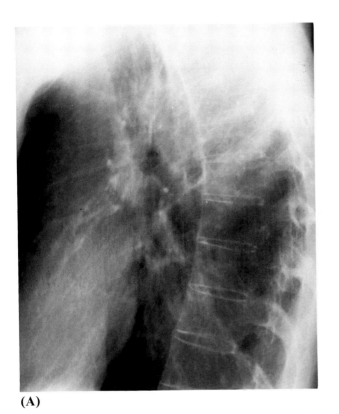

(A)

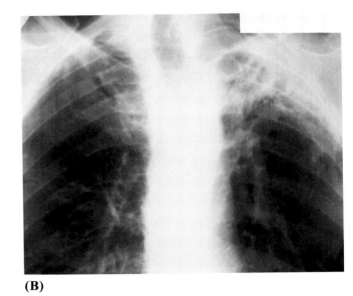

(B)

Fig. 5-28.   Apical Pulmonary Cavitation in a Patient With Ankylosing Spondylitis

(A) Lateral view of the chest shows the marked abnormalities of the thoracic spine characteristic of involvement with ankylosing spondylitis. Notice that there is ligamentous bridging of the anterior aspects of the intervertebral spaces, but an absence of osteophytes. There is also osteopenia, so that the superior and inferior plates of the vertebrae appear light gray in comparison to the less dense (dark gray) vertebral bodies.

(B) Coned PA view of the upper portions of the chest of this man shows that there is contraction in volume of the upper lobes. The abnormalities are more marked on the left, where there is considerable upward retraction of the hilum. In addition, there is biapical pleural thickening, and there are multiple circumscribed lucencies, consistent with cavities, within the contracted portions of the left upper lobe.

A small percentage of patients with ankylosing spondylitis develop a profound pulmonary fibrosis that frequently is more marked in the upper lung zones and is accompanied by emphysematous and bullous changes in the lung as well as areas of cavitation. These patients are thoroughly studied for the presence of infectious granulomatous disease because the radiographic appearances are so similar to those of chronic tuberculosis. It appears, however, that this type of pulmonary abnormality may be a consequence of the primary connective tissue disorder itself. As with other bullous or cavitary lesions, these can become secondarily invaded by saprophytes such as *Aspergillus* or even by atypical mycobacteria.

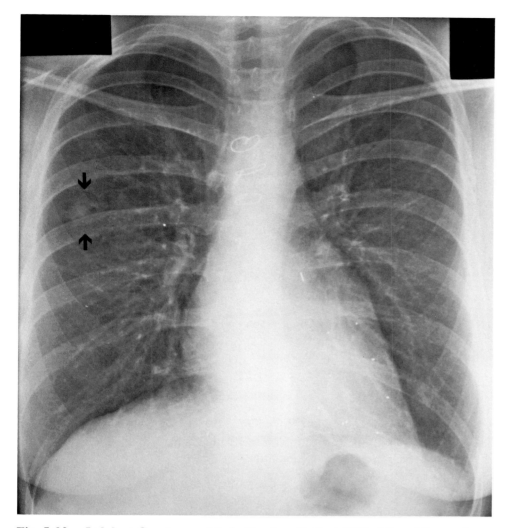

Fig. 5-29. Indolent Cryptococcal Infection in a Patient With Altered Immunity

This young woman was a heart transplant recipient who developed a small nodule in the right upper lobe. She was attending college at the time and was reluctant to take time away from her studies to have this lesion investigated. She had no signs or symptoms to indicate pulmonary infection. Finally, after several months she consented to have a needle aspiration of the lesion (arrows), which fortunately had grown very little. This was done under fluoroscopic control, and a diagnosis of *Cryptococcus* infection was made from the material aspirated.

Although nodules are a common sign of pulmonary infection with the ubiquitous fungi in patients with altered immunity, it is unusual to have the clinical and radiographic course quite this indolent. Pulmonary nodules, solitary or multiple, may also be caused by malignant lymphoma in immunosuppressed transplant recipients. The incidence of malignant lymphoma in these patients, however, is very much less than that of infection.

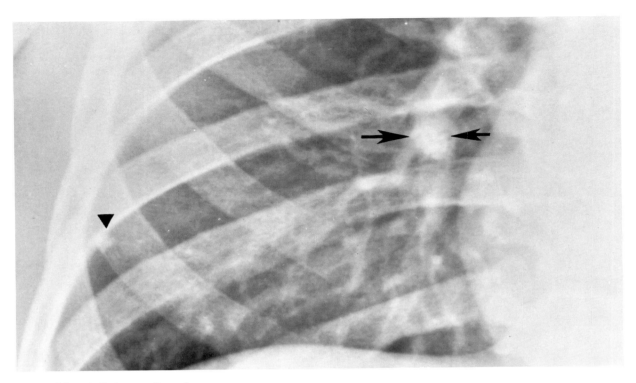

Fig. 5-30. A Primary Complex

Coned view of the lower portions of the right lung and right hilum of a young asymptomatic man. There is a 5-mm nodular opacity with somewhat angular margins laterally in the lower lung (arrowhead). It is very dense for its size. This appearance is typical of a small, calcified granuloma. The granulomas may be single or multiple.

Hilar nodes are commonly involved in cases of primary infection with organisms of the infectious granulomatous disease group, and calcification of dystrophic changes within the nodes may occur. Calcifications in hilar or mediastinal nodes are radiographic signs of prior disease, most commonly tuberculosis or histoplasmosis.

The hilar node calcifications (arrows), may be difficult to recognize on high-kilovoltage films, but careful attention to hilar and mediastinal detail usually permits their recognition.

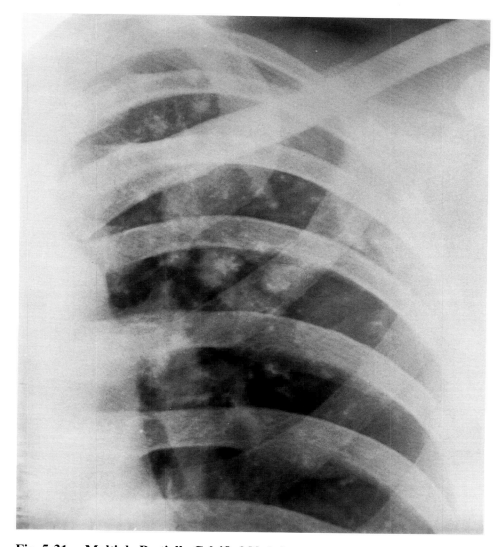

Fig. 5-31. Multiple Partially Calcified Nodules

There are many nodules of varying size in the left upper lobe. Relatively small, dense foci are present within many of the nodules, the result of patchy calcification. This is part of the radiographic spectrum of infectious granulomatous disease, especially of tuberculosis and histoplasmosis. You cannot predict whether or not tuberculosis is inactive by looking at the radiograph. Tubercle bacilli can be cultured from partially calcified nodules. The untreated patient may live in an apparently arrested disease state until some alteration of immune status permits a recrudescence.

Calcific foci are more difficult to recognize on films exposed at high kilovoltage (e.g., 120 to 150 kV) than on films exposed at low kilovoltage (approximately 60 kV). Low-kilovoltage techniques provide for more contrast between calcified and noncalcified foci and can serve that function for selected cases, but in general, high-kilovoltage techniques are preferred for routine chest radiography.

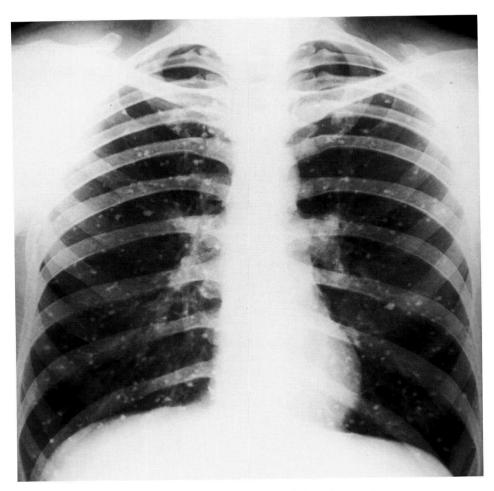

Fig. 5-32. Classical Calcified Nodules Due to Histoplasmosis

There are numerous small, irregular, very dense nodules scattered throughout both lungs. The density of the nodules in relation to their size is indicative of calcification. In addition, the entire nodule is calcified rather than only a portion. This is a very characteristic appearance of old, healed histoplasmosis and probably represents the healed phase of multiple granulomatous lesions consequent to inhalation of a large inoculum of the organisms.

In regions of the world where histoplasmosis is unknown, similar opacities have been reported in the lungs of patients who had a prior history of chickenpox pneumonia. There are several other causes of multiple calcified nodules in the lung, but rarely would they precisely mimic this radiographic appearance and distribution.

Although this radiographic appearance is characteristic of old, healed histoplasmosis, there are other multinodular forms of histoplasmosis in which the nodules are larger and either noncalcified or only partially calcified.

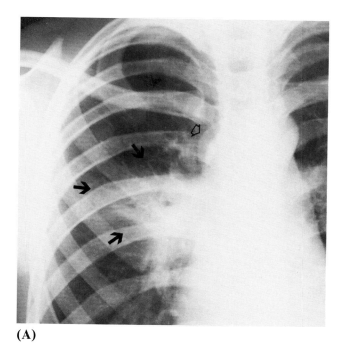

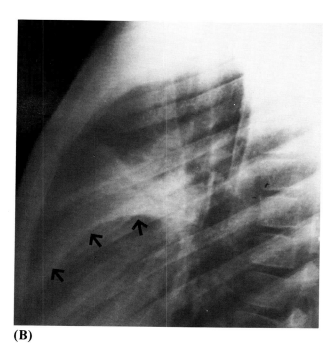

(A)

(B)

Fig. 5-33.   Tuberculous Pneumonia

Coned views of the lungs of a teenage girl with a presumptive diagnosis of tuberculosis. (A) PA view. A dense zone of consolidation is seen in a perihilar distribution (arrows). (B) The consolidation is shown to be in the anterior segment of the right upper lobe on this lateral view, which shows a sharp inferior delineation by the minor interlobar fissure (arrows), which is bowed sharply upward due to some contraction in volume of the anterior segment of the right upper lobe. An air bronchogram is visible in a portion of the consolidation on the lateral view.

The rounded edge of the developing manubrium is seen projected in the right paratracheal region of the PA view (open arrow) and should not be confused with lymphadenopathy. The image of the azygos vein seen superimposed on this portion of the manubrium is within normal limits. At the time this diagnosis was made there was no chemotherapy or antibiotic therapy available for pulmonary tuberculosis. (Courtesy of Dr. Richard Greenspan, New Haven, Connecticut.)

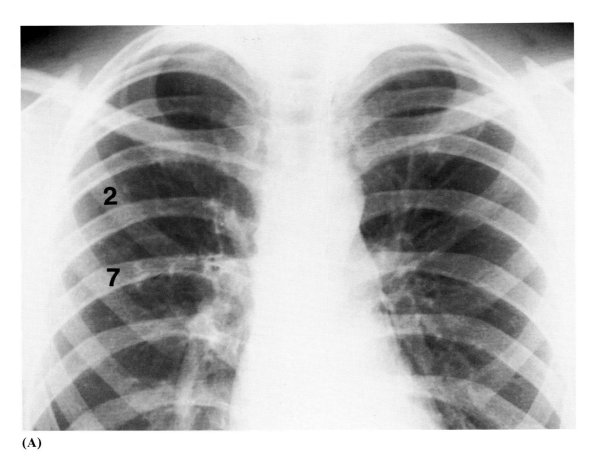

(A)

(B)

Fig. 5-34. Residual Scarring and Recurrent Apical Disease Due to Tuberculous Pneumonia

(A,B) PA and lateral views, respectively, of the chest of the young woman in Fig. 5-33, 3 years later. She had been treated in a local sanitorium and was asymptomatic at this time. The anterior segment pneumonia has resolved but scarring remains.

(A) The residual scarring is seen on this PA view as small, irregular opacities superimposed on the posterior seventh rib (7) lateral to the hilum, and a small nodule is projected above the anterior second rib (2). There is also some thickening of bronchi seen end-on in the upper right hilum.

(B) In the lateral view the residuals are more pronounced. Irregular bands of varying thickness and length are present in a peribronchial distribution extending from the hilum to the anterior chest wall.

These are rather characteristic findings for residuals of chronic pulmonary infection. They can be seen in patients who have no knowledge of ever having had tuberculosis or any of the other infectious granulomatous diseases. Nevertheless, positive skin tests indicate that they did indeed have such infections, which went unrecognized in the primary phase. You cannot predict the presence or absence of viable organisms within these areas on the basis of their radiographic appearance. *(Figure continues.)*

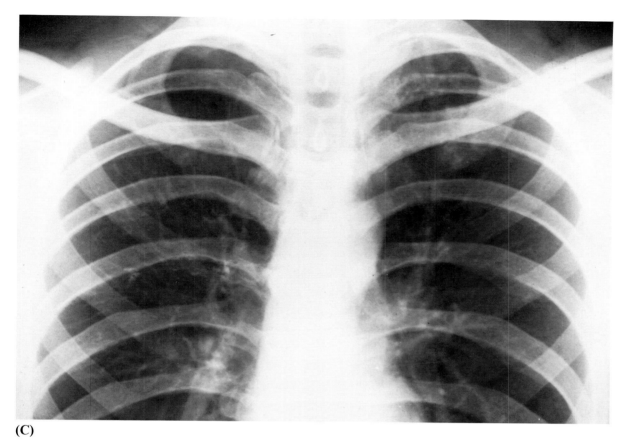

(C)

Fig. 5-34. *(Continued).* **(C)** A more heavily exposed PA view of the same woman's chest taken 5 years after that in Fig. A. The small, irregular opacities in the lung lateral to the right hilum have changed little in the interim. However, now compare the apices with their appearance on the earlier film. There is a striking change in the appearance of the left apex. There are now new, small, clustered nodules present, many of which are superimposed on the posterior third rib.

The apices are a common site of radiographic evidence of reactivation of pulmonary tuberculosis. However, the patients may have little in the way of symptoms, and the organisms may be difficult to recover from the sputum. In this case, the patient had noticed some swelling in her neck. Material was aspirated from enlarged lymph nodes and injected into guinea pigs. The diagnosis of reactivation of tuberculosis was confirmed by this test. (Courtesy of Dr. Richard Greenspan, New Haven, Connecticut.)

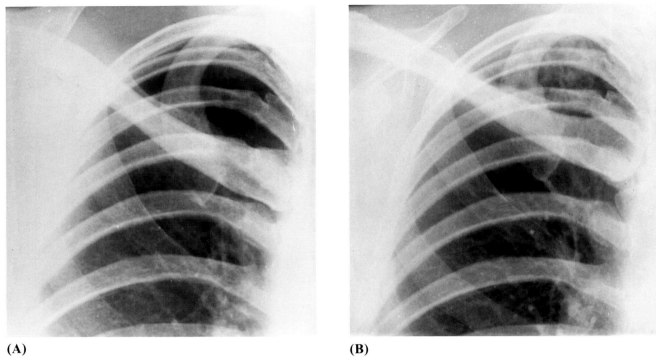

(A)   **(B)**

Fig. 5-35.   Tuberculosis With Minimal Apical Involvement

(A) This 26-year-old nurse had a routine surveillance chest film. This is a coned view of the right apex, which is normal.

(B) Sixteen months later there is considerable right apical parenchymal disease, which is composed of short, irregular, clustered opacities. This sequence commonly represents reactivation of tuberculosis. Today the retrieval of tissue or secretions from which to recover the organisms would be pursued vigorously and appropriate treatment begun. In the past, however, such patients were often treated presumptively on the basis of the radiographic findings in conjunction with a positive skin test. Since young patients with a positive PPD (purified protein derivative) now usually receive chemotherapy for tuberculosis even when the chest film is negative, this type of reactivation should become uncommon.

You will still see asymptomatic patients who have smaller and fewer irregular nodules and short, linear opacities in one or both apices that are residuals of infection with tuberculosis. When there are no earlier films for comparison you cannot assess the age, stability, or activity of these lesions or their current clinical significance from the radiographic findings alone.

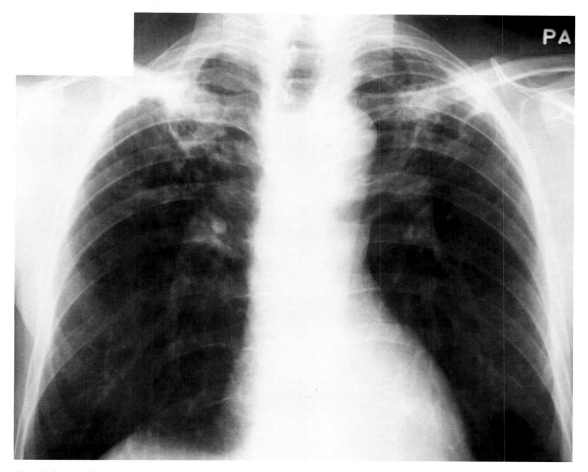

Fig. 5-36.   Chronic Coccidioidomycosis

PA film of the chest of a 58-year-old man who had had five episodes of massive hemoptysis over the past 4 years. He was known to have had pulmonary coccidioidomycosis.

There is severe contraction in volume of both upper lobes with elevation of the hila, splaying of the middle and lower zone vessels due to compensatory expansion of these portions of the lung, and gross distortion of lung architecture. Multiple ill-defined cavities and bronchiectatic changes along with nodules and linear opacities are present within the contracted upper lung zones. These findings are characteristic of changes due to chronic granulomatous infection, most commonly tuberculosis, but in this case due to chronic coccidioidomycosis. The radiographic appearances, as in this case, are indistinguishable, and bacteriologic or histopathologic proof is required to make the distinction. Uncommonly, other infectious granulomatous diseases, e.g., blastomyeosis, histoplasmosis, and others may cause similar lesions.

Severe hemorrhage may occur in patients with cavitary lesions from almost any cause as a result of erosion of bronchial arteries. Resection of the involved segments or lobes may be necessary to prevent exsanguination.

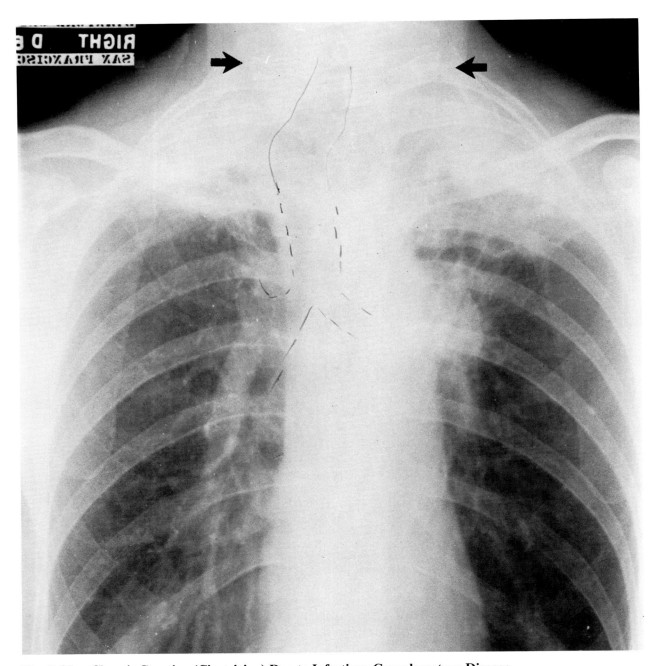

Fig. 5-37. Chronic Scarring (Cicatrizing) Due to Infectious Granulomatous Disease

This is an example of the marked scarring that can occur in the lungs as a result of chronic granulomatous infection (commonly tuberculosis). Ordinarily, lung extends to the extreme apices (arrows). Instead, opaque zones occupy the apices and subclavicular regions because of a combination of pleural thickening and extensive, destructive, inflammatory pulmonary parenchymal changes. There is marked reduction in volume of the upper lobes, and often there is bronchiectasis as well.

The hilar vessels and major bronchi are retracted upward, and the trachea (outlined) buckles to the right because of traction from adjacent scarred lung. The superior mediastinal contours are distorted and partially effaced by the adjacent lung disease. Vessels in the lower lobes appear very prominent because they are elongated and separated from one another by the compensatory lower lobe hyperexpansion.

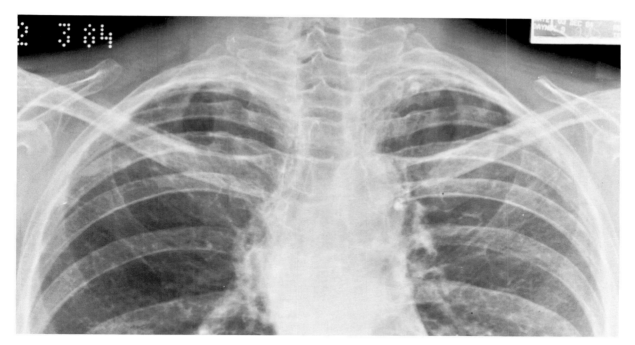

Fig. 5-38.   Postirradiation Reaction

This woman had had radiation therapy for Hodgkin's disease. The lung apices, the mediastinum and the hilar, and the paramediastinal portions of both lungs were included in the treatment portals.

There is thickening of the apical pleura bilaterally, but it is not very marked. Irregular linear and nodular opacities are present in both apices and subclavicular regions. There is upward and marked medial retraction of the vessels and bronchi of both hila, with loss of sharp lung-mediastinum interfaces as well.

Post-treatment scarring from radiation is quite variable from patient to patient even when the same dose has been delivered. It begins early after treatment with signs that at first are very subtle. Progressive changes can occur for several months, but usually after a year the lesions appear stable.

Radiographically these postirradiation changes are indistinguishable from those caused by tuberculosis or other chronic infectious granulomatous disease. This is particularly so when the scarring is asymmetrical. A history of irradiation, correlation with treatment portals, comparison with prior chest films, and clinical assessment usually suffice to make the distinction. At times, however, a more elaborate investigation may be required.

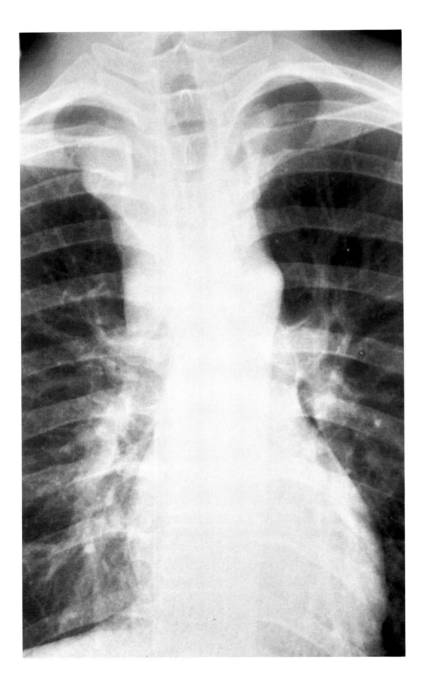

Fig. 5-39. Mediastinal Lymphadenopathy Due to Tuberculosis

Coned view of the mediastinum and perimediastinal portions of both lungs of a 22-year-old man who sought medical help because of a subacute febrile illness. The altered contours of a widened mediastinum begin just above the upper margins of the right upper lobe bronchus and extend up to the level of the clavicle. The mediastinum on both sides of the trachea is abnormal. These findings are indicative of lymphadenopathy. A lymph node biopsy from the right paratracheal chain showed necrotizing granulomas and acid-fast bacilli. *Mycobacterium tuberculosis* was cultured from the specimen.

Mediastinal and/or hilar lymphadenopathy with or without a detectable parenchymal component is part of the spectrum of radiographic appearances of the infectious granulomatous diseases. This may be the sole radiographic sign of disease during the phase of primary infection. Sometimes patients present clinically with a flulike syndrome.

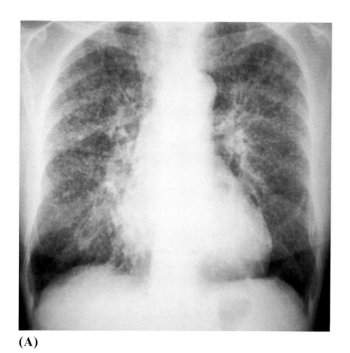

(A)

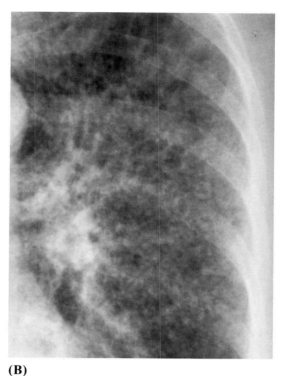

(B)

Fig. 5-40.　Chronic Indolent Tuberculosis

The patient is a 64-year-old woman who denied having any symptoms of pulmonary or systemic disease. She had a routine chest film taken as part of a physical examination. Because of the abnormality seen on the chest film she was referred to the chest clinic. Her PPD and physical examination were entirely negative, as were her pulmonary function studies. She had a slightly elevated serum calcium and a slightly elevated serum phosphorus with an elevated blood urea nitrogen and creatinine.

(A) Her chest film shows disseminated, small (2 to 4 mm) nodular opacities distributed throughout both lungs with relative sparing of the extreme lateral bases.

(B) Coned view of the left lung at approximately the same magnification as the original chest film. It shows that the nodular opacities are fairly discrete, but there are also some incomplete, ringlike structures suggesting dilated distal air spaces. No definite hilar or mediastinal adenopathy was recognized. The hila are lacking in detail because of the extensive lesions in the surrounding lung.

On the full view of the chest, the heart appears moderately enlarged, and there is a larger (about 1 cm), dense nodule superimposed on the right posterior seventh rib that may represent a calcified granuloma. There is also a deformity of the left ninth rib in the posterior axillary line, most likely due to an old, healed fracture. There were no old films for comparison, but the patient recalled having had a normal chest film 7 years ago.

These extensive abnormalities seen in a virtually asymptomatic patient suggest sarcoidosis or eosinophilic granuloma of the lung as the most likely etiology. From the radiographic standpoint alone one could not distinguish this from miliary tuberculosis or miliary infections with the pathogenic fungi, or even from miliary metastases from an unknown primary.

The patient had a gallium-67 scan, which was 4+ positive for lung activity; in addition, there was associated activity in the parotid and lacrimal glands, which was felt to be compatible with but not specific for sarcoid.

Because of the activity shown on the gallium scan, the patient had a transbronchial lung biopsy. The histopathologic diagnosis was noncaseating granulomas consistent with sarcoidosis. However, cultures of the bronchial washings and the biopsy specimen grew *Mycobacterium tuberculosis*. The question now is whether this is a case of a woman with sarcoidosis who incidentally has pulmonary tuberculosis, or a case of diffuse indolent tuberculosis as described by Buechner and Anderson?[13]

Regardless of the answer, this case dramatically emphasizes the importance of obtaining cultures of bronchial washings and tissue specimens from patients with histopathologic findings compatible with those of the noninfectious granulomatous diseases, because the infectious granulomatous diseases can produce similar histopathologic changes. It is not possible to rule out these infections in the absence of the results of specimen cultures. (Courtesy of Drs. James McCort and Gordon Yenokida, San Jose, California.)

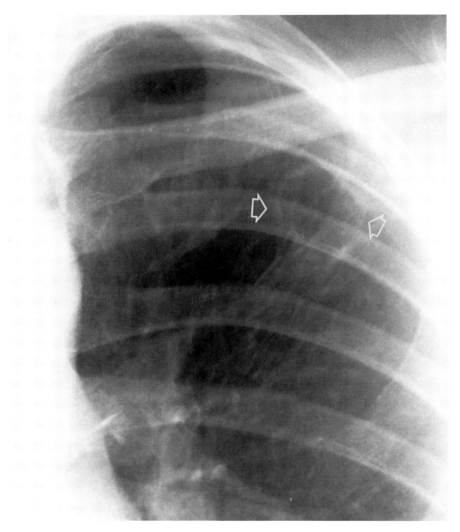

Fig. 5-41. Cavity Due to *Coccidioides immitis*

There is a relatively thin-walled cavity (arrows) in the left upper lobe of this 33-year-old agricultural consultant who lived and worked in California. He had been having hemoptysis of about 2 table-spoons of red blood approximately twice a week for 5 months. He had no fever, night sweats, or malaise. Physical examination and laboratory studies were normal except for a positive serologic test for *Coccidioides* infection.

The lesion was removed, and examination showed a cavity wall approximately 0.2 cm thick. The organisms of *Coccidioides immitis* were recovered by culture as well as by histopathologic examination of the specimen. Caseating and noncaseating granulomas were also found in lung tissue a short distance from the cavity.

Epidemiologic evidence indicates that the majority of cases of primary coccidioidomycosis have no radiologic residuals of the disease. A small percentage of patients, however, may be left with a coccidioidal lung nodule or a peripheral coccidioidal cavity. The majority of these cavities are found when the patient has a chest film taken for some unrelated purpose. However, some patients have hemoptysis or low-grade fevers. Characteristically these cavities are found in the upper lung zones. The majority resolve spontaneously, but some may be colonized by *Aspergillus* or bacteria, and some may rupture into the pleural space and produce pyopneumothorax. Whether or not asymptomatic residual coccidioidal cavities need to be removed surgically is a matter of controversy.[6,7]

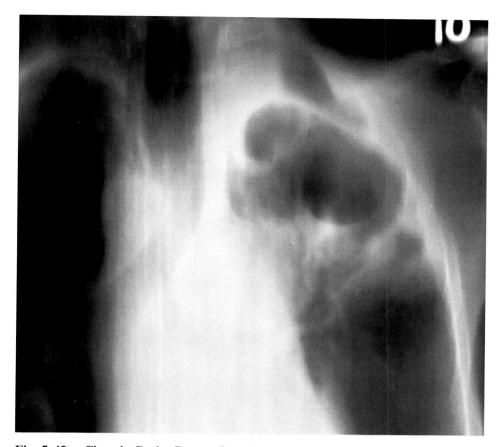

Fig. 5-42. Chronic Cavity Due to *Pseudomonas* Pneumonia

This 48-year-old woman had a history of weight loss, fever, and productive cough for over a month. Sputum cultures and all skin tests were negative. She underwent bronchoscopy, and *Pseudomonas* and mixed alpha streptococci were recovered from the bronchial washings. She was placed on broad-spectrum antibiotics but did not improve.

Because of persistent symptoms and the lack of response to antibiotic treatment, the patient underwent an upper lobectomy. The resected lung contained a large, thin-walled, necrotic cavity. *Pseudomonas* was cultured from the cavity and the adjacent lung.

This tomographic cut shows a large, somewhat lobulated cavity in the left upper lobe with thickening of adjacent pleura and mottled irregular zones of consolidation in subadjacent parenchyma. There is also marked distortion of the hilum and the left side of the mediastinum.

Notice that there is a rounded soft tissue "mass," which impinges upon the right side of the trachea just above the level of the takeoff of the right upper lobe bronchus. This is the classic appearance of a right aortic arch, which was an incidental congenital anomaly in this woman. She had been operated upon in childhood to correct a tetralogy of Fallot anomaly.

Chronic cavitary lesions from gram-negative organism infections such as *Pseudomonas* and *Klebsiella* are known but uncommon entities.

6

Nodules and Neoplasms

Pulmonary neoplasms have a diversity that reflects all of the different types of tissue that occur in the lung. If you think about all the types of tissue that are found in the lung — including blood vessels, lymphatics, nerves, bronchial walls, alveolar walls, and interstitium — sooner or later you are bound to discover reports of benign or malignant neoplasms originating from those tissue components or their primitive precursors. Hence, there is no need to remember long lists of different pulmonary neoplasms; you can deduce them by becoming familiar with the histology of the lung.

Concentrating on what does occur rather than what could occur, however, narrows the range. The majority of primary pulmonary neoplasms will be bronchogenic carcinomas of various histopathologies, bronchoalveolar carcinomas, bronchial gland carcinomas (bronchial adenomas), and, less commonly, malignant lymphomas. All of the other possible primary neoplasms such as sarcomas, hemangiopericytomas, pulmonary blastomas, and a variety of benign mesenchymomas are uncommon or rare.

Primary malignant neoplasms anywhere in the body may metastasize to the lungs, of course, and at times metastases to the bronchi or the lungs may be mistaken for primary neoplasms.

Malignant neoplasms that commonly are multifocal at the time of initial diagnosis, such as multiple myeloma, lymphomas, and leukemias, can share the same radiographic spectrum as metastases. They can also mimic certain primary pulmonary neoplasms and a variety of infections.

THE SOLITARY, NONCALCIFIED PULMONARY NODULE OR MASS

Extrapulmonary Structures Simulating Pulmonary Nodules

In considering the diagnosis of a solitary (and to a much lesser extent multiple) noncalcified pulmonary nodule (SNPN), first be certain that the lesion is in the lung and not on the skin or in the chest wall (Fig. 6-1). This can be accomplished by inspection and palpation. If you find a skin surface mole or other protuberance, especially the nipple, that might be in a position to account for the suspect shadow, you can identify it with an opaque marker. You can then fluoroscope the patient and determine precisely the relationship of the marked surface structure to the suspected lesion. As an alternative, you could obtain stereoscopic films to determine whether the marked structure retains a precise spatial relationship to the suspect shadow. Using these methods you can always satisfy yourself that the superficial protuberance does indeed account for the radiographic finding or that it does not.

Other images can be mistaken for pulmonary nodules, and the following list includes those that are often confusing:

1.* Exuberant calcification or ossification of the costal cartilage and the costochondral junctions of the first ribs (easily mistaken for pulmonary lesions when the appearance on one side of the chest is

295

conspicuously different from that on the other side)

2.* Compact islands of sclerosis ("bone islands") in the ribs, the clavicle, or the thoracic spine (Fig. 6-2C and D), infrequent in occurrence but easily misidentified when present

3. Callus about nondisplaced rib fractures

4. Large hypertrophic spurs about intervertebral discs, especially when seen end-on in a lateral view of the chest

5. Transverse processes of thoracic vertebrae, especially those projecting behind the heart

6. Large vessels seen end-on

7. The venous confluences adjacent to the left atrium

8. A variety of artifacts associated with EKG leads, tubing for central lines or respirators, and opaque material in dressings

9. Long hair or braids hanging over the apices

10. Plastic buttons or clasps on clothing

Many of these pseudolesions are seen in the illustrations throughout this text. Usually all of the pitfalls can be recognized by remaining aware of the problem and employing careful analysis of the radiographic image. When doubt remains, fluoroscopy, stereoscopic views, or comparison with prior films can be used to resolve the issue. Occasionally tomograms, CT scans, or MRI studies may be required.

With good-quality stereoscopic PA chest films and high-quality lateral views, fewer than 10 percent of significant solitary nodules should remain invisible. However, that is not the same as saying they will be seen. The error rate in the detection of peripheral nodules by competent observers is high.[25]

Differential Diagnosis of SNPNs

I know of no commonly agreed-upon distinction between a nodule and a mass. Some observers use 4.0 cm as a size threshold; others use a higher limit. Perhaps it suffices to measure the lesion, at least in its greatest dimension if not in all three. Thus, a reported 4.0-cm "nodule" and a 4.0-cm "mass" would describe the same image.

A variety of benign conditions and all types of malignant neoplasms may present as solitary, noncalcified pulmonary nodules (SNPN). Frequently there are no clinical signs, symptoms, elements of personal history,

or laboratory data to aid in distinguishing benign from malignant nodules. The patient may or may not have symptoms referable to the chest.

In day-to-day practice, the differential diagnosis of an SNPN involves three probable causes and a much larger number of less likely possibilities. The probable causes are:

1. Neoplasm (the vast majority of nodular pulmonary neoplasms are malignant and more commonly primary than metastatic; a small percentage are benign)

2. Infectious granulomas (most commonly tuberculosis, histoplasmosis, or coccidioidomycosis, depending on geographic history; Figs. 6-1A and B, 6-2 A to D)

3. Hamartoma.

Approximately 90 to 95 percent of all noncalcified nodules will fall into one of these three groups. Hamartoma is by far the least common of the three, but is more common than any one of the possibilities constituting the remaining 5 to 10 percent. These "other" SNPNs have a large number of etiologies; the precise number depends on whether you are a lumper or a splitter. A list of some of these is included in the "uncommon causes" category of Table 6-1, but in general these diagnoses are not arrived at until special studies or histopathologic analyses of the lesion have been performed.

Arteriovenous malformations can present as pulmonary nodules and sometimes have characteristic features that will be discussed later.

Foci of consolidated, atelectatic lung trapped in zones of pleural thickening may project as rounded masses (round atelectasis) simulating neoplasm. Frequently these round atelectases can be recognized by:

1. Their location in the periphery of the lung

2. Their location adjacent to conspicuous pleural thickening

3. The appearance of a curved vessel or bundle of vessels entering the lower margins usually, or the upper margin occasionally (see Ch. 4).

The rank-order of the probabilities for neoplasm and infectious granuloma changes depending in part on the age and sex of the population studied. If you were to survey an entire community, the incidence of noncalcified nodules would be expected to vary in accordance with the prevalence of certain infections such as histoplasmosis, coccidioidomycosis, and tuberculosis. The greater the prevalence of such infections in the community, the more likely it is that any nodules detected would be benign. However, if you surveyed only that portion of

---

* The loss of contrast between calcified and noncalcified structures is part of the price to be paid for the otherwise beneficial aspects of high-kilovoltage techniques in modern chest radiography. This loss of contrast makes it difficult to recognize thin calcified or ossified structures as calcium-containing radiodensities.

TABLE 6-1. Causes of Solitary, Noncalcified Pulmonary Nodules or Masses

Common Causes

Neoplasm
    Bronchogenic carcinoma (any cell type)
    Bronchioloalveolar cell carcinoma
    Metastasis from any primary

Granulomas due to tuberculosis, histoplasmosis, coccidioidomycosis, and indeterminate causes

Hamartoma (sometimes referred to as chondroma)

Uncommon Causes

Primary neoplasms other than bronchogenic carcinoma
    Lymphoma limited to the lung
    Carcinoid tumor and bronchial gland carcinoma
    Any tissue occurring in lung may have a neoplastic counterpart (e.g., lipoma, leiomyoma, fibroma, hemangiopericytoma, hemangioma, papilloma, chemodectoma, neurogenic tumor); many have both benign and malignant variants.
    Pedunculated mesothelioma mimicking a pulmonary nodule
    Plasmacytoma

Vascular lesions
    Arteriovenous malformation
    Pulmonary vein varix
    Aneurysm of a pulmonary artery branch

Inflammatory disorders (other than tuberculosis, histoplasmosis, or coccicioidomycosis)
    Ubiquitous fungi
        Aspergillus
        Rhizopus, Mucor
        Cryptococcus
        Candida
        Others
    Nocardia
    Parasites
        Ascaris
        Amoeba
        Echinococcus
        Dirofilaria immitis (dog heartworm)
        Filaria
        Schistosoma
    Pyogenic abscess
    Organizing pneumonia ("cholesterol" pneumonia)
    Lipoid aspiration pneumonia
    Plasma cell granuloma

Benign intrapulmonary lymph node

Amyloid nodule or mass[38]

Bronchogenic, duplication, or neurenteric cyst

Hematoma

Fibrin ball

Trapped lung adjacent to an area of pleural thickening (round atelectasis)

Conglomerate mass due to pneumoconiosis

Scarred residual of a pulmonary infarct

Noninfectious granulomatous disease (uncommon as a *solitary* nodule)
    Sarcoid
    Rheumatoid nodule
    Wegener's granulomatosis

Mucus-filled obstructed bronchus

a population that was male and over 45 years old, a large portion (but still less than 50 percent) of the SNPNs found would be malignant.[18] Moreover, if you surveyed only those patients above the age of 50 years who had chest radiographs upon admission to tertiary care hospitals (regardless of whether or not there were symptoms or signs related to the chest), the possibilities of a nodule being benign or malignant would be roughly equal.[16] Others have also shown an increase in the prevalence of malignant nodules with age.[35] A host of recognized and unrecognized selection factors separate these populations.

Distinguishing Benign from Malignant SNPNs

Reliable determination of the benign or malignant nature of an SNPN from its radiographic appearance alone would be of tremendous importance to the patient's psychological, physical, and financial well-being. Many attempts to find critical radiographic variables have been made, but no unassailable criteria have survived. Thus, there are no criteria of size, shape, marginal contour, sharpness of outline, or position in the lung that permit distinction of a benign from a malignant SNPN with enough reliability to permit the planning of definitive therapy based on radiographic appearance alone. There are, to be sure, criteria that are felt to favor one choice over the other. They are useful in analyzing series of cases, but require much reservation when applied to an individual. A brief discussion of some of the concepts that have been investigated follows.

Size

The larger the lesion, the more likely it is to be malignant.[32,37] This is a useful concept, but is not without many exceptions. In certain granulomatous diseases both infectious and noninfectious, certain infections with ubiquitous fungi, and some benign tumors, nodular lesions reach sizes in excess of 3 cm with just enough frequency to impair the usefulness of the concept.[28]

The corollary—*the smaller the lesion, the more likely it is to be benign*—will help you to select the benign lesions from among a series of a hundred cases, but even if you use cutoff size of 1.0 cm you will not exclude all malignant nodules (Fig. 6-3). In any case, you will not have many nodules under 1 cm in diameter in your series. It is theoretically possible to detect an SNPN as small as 3 mm in diameter. However, the resection of lesions this small, solely because of an appreciation of their malignant potential, is rare indeed. It is infrequent for resection of nodules under 1½ cm in diameter to be reported even in the largest surgical series. This seems to indicate that the majority of physicians have extreme difficulty in detecting the miniscule nodule, or, having done so, encounter difficulty in convincing themselves and their colleagues of its potential. It is my general impression, unsubstantiated by tested data but not contradicted by experience, that the tiny nodule of about 3 to 5 mm diameter, when very dense, sharp, and obvious on the films, is a calcified granuloma (Fig. 6-4).

Nodules of such small size that are not radiodense, sharp, and obvious severely test the interpreter's ability, for they fall in a portion of the spectrum where one's ability to distinguish true lesions from anatomic noise from vessels is sorely tested. In a retrospective study, one may easily be convinced that where there is currently an obvious sizeable nodule or mass, there was on an older roentgenogram a 3-mm nodule. This only enhances one's intuitive judgment that retrospection is more accurate than prediction. Size alone is an unreliable criterion for differentiating a benign from a malignant lesion.[35]

Marginal Contours

Do smooth, sharp margins indicate a benign lesion? Benign nodules frequently have smooth, sharp margins, but there are far too many exceptions to this rule. Some malignant nodules may be sharply defined, and some benign nodules may not. Thus, this concept is not safe to apply to an individual patient.[4,5]

Do spiculated margins or linear extensions along the margins indicate a malignant lesion? Spiculated margins or linear extensions (Fig. 6-5) are a useful sign of malignancy[32]—not perfect, but very good. However, similar appearances have been associated with lesions that proved to be granulomas or even conglomerate silicotic mass lesions.[15]

Does a nodule with a line or bands superimposed or appearing to pass through the nodule or appearing as a "tail" indicate a malignant lesion? Linear shadows due to infolding of visceral pleura or focal septal edema, fibrosis, or tumor infiltration in association with an adjacent nodule have been identified and characterized as a sign of malignancy (Fig. 6-5). Unfortunately, such linear shadows have also been reported with scarring associated with benign lesions, so again the finding is not diagnostic.[37]

Is there notching or umbilication of a margin? Such features are probably a reflection of the lobulated contour of the lesion. Enough such resected lesions prove to be benign to prevent acceptability of the sign as diagnostic of a malignant nodule.

Satellite Nodules

The presence of small nodules (satellite nodules) in the immediate vicinity of a larger nodule has been proposed as a sign of benignity but has also proven to be unreliable in the individual case.

Calcification in a Nodule

Concentric rings of calcification within a nodule can be accepted as a sign of an infectious granuloma. Scattered foci of calcification occupying most of a nodule seen on a radiograph may also be accepted as a sign of a benign lesion due to either infectious granuloma or hamartoma (so-called popcorn calcification; Fig. 6-6). In fact, the vast majority of solitary nodules that have any clear-cut foci of calcification demonstrated on plain chest films, fluoroscopic spot films, low-kilovoltage tomograms, or CT scans will be benign provided one is precise about what one is willing to call calcified as opposed to simply relatively dense, and provided the relative sizes of the calcified focus and the whole nodule are not disproportionate (see Fig. 6-4).

Serious errors can occur, however, when a small focus (or foci) of calcification is seen radiographically in the periphery, or rarely even in the center, of a nodule or mass or consolidation that is several times larger than the focus of calcium. A malignant tumor can grow about and engulf a benign calcified focus. Therefore, it seems best to pursue these rare situations as though the lesion were not calcified.

There is a rare ossifying bronchial carcinoid that can be mistaken for a calcified nodule.[36] I do not know how to avoid that error in an asymptomatic patient. In a patient who has signs or symptoms of bronchial obstruction, a calcified nodule or mass impinging upon or distorting a major bronchus would prompt consideration of this entity as part of the differential diagnosis. Fortunately this lesion is rare.

Pathologists may find scattered foci of dystrophic calcification on microscopic studies of malignant pulmonary neoplasms, but these microscopic foci ordinarily are not recognizable on radiographs.

Metastases from some neoplasms, especially those of bone, may show calcified foci radiographically, but the fact that the patient has a known extrapulmonary primary tumor is almost always apparent from history or clinical findings.

CT scans are more sensitive than plain films in demonstrating calcified foci. In addition, a cohort of computer-generated numbers (Hounsfield units derived from x-ray linear attenuation coefficients) can be plotted for the nodule. If meticulous care is used in performing the study, it is possible to separate pulmonary nodules into two subsets. One subset includes those nodules with high linear attenuation coefficients, probably due to diffuse calcification in the nodule, which identify the nodule as benign with rare exceptions. The other subset includes those for which linear attenuation coefficients do not reach a certain minimum level. This subset includes nodules that may be either benign or malignant. Unfortunately, not all CT scanners are programmed so as to permit universal application of a single testing method.[40,41] However, as methods are explored and software is modified, a more universally applicable test should evolve. Eventually that subset of patients with nodules that can be shown to test as benign lesions will be spared unnecessary thoracotomy, provided errors remain rare after large-scale testing. Since there are reports of rare primary lung cancers showing calcification on CT study, periodic follow-up examinations could be planned to monitor the stability of unresected calcified lesions; or needle aspiration biopsy could be performed on those nodules that do not show calcification patterns typical of benign lesions. Low-kilovoltage (approximately 65 kV) tomographic cuts can also be used to assess the presence or absence of calcification within a pulmonary nodule, but not as sensitively as CT.

CT scans have also been used to diagnose the presence of low-density foci of fat in a pulmonary nodule to make a presumptive diagnosis of hamartoma. The usefulness of this finding may be limited to the study of nodules under 2.5 cm in diameter in order to avoid error occasioned by low-density foci of necrosis that may be seen in larger malignant nodules.[33]

Use of Conventional and Computed Tomography

CT scans are more sensitive in demonstrating small lesions about the periphery of the lungs than are chest films or tomographic cuts. Metastases have a propensity for the periphery. Some of the peripheral lesions seen on CT scans, however, are only incidental scars.[9] Nevertheless, the net gain in useful information from CT studies compared to chest films and tomograms can be important in treatment planning. There are times when the increased visibility of lesions on CT scans over chest films is astonishing (Fig. 6-5B to E). CT is still not perfect in demonstrating all small lung nodules; when surgical resections of metastases have been undertaken, more lesions have been removed in some cases than were seen on the imaging studies. On the other hand, some nodules seen on CT scan will not be found by the surgeon and yet will be shown to be true lesions on follow-up studies.

CT scans are also useful to make certain that a nodule being studied is indeed solitary. This is important because the discovery of more than one nodule would change the rank-order of the differential diagnosis and would alter treatment planning.

Once a solitary pulmonary nodule has been found on routine films of patients who are being followed because they have had or have a known primary malignancy anywhere in the body, full-lung tomography has an estimated 20 percent chance of showing other nodules not seen on the chest films,[26] and CT is even more sensitive in serving that function.

Time as a Predictive Variable

Time is another variable that can be used effectively to predict the benign or at least nonneoplastic nature of a pulmonary nodule or mass. If a newly discovered nodule was not present on yesterday's or last week's comparison chest films, and if the nodule is of a size and location such that detection would not have been the problem, then the lesion is not malignant. Malignant neoplasms do not appear de novo in days, but inflammatory nodules do. Of course, it is extremely rare to have such recent prior chest films available for the usual patient. It is only the postoperative patient, or the symptomatic patient who is being followed closely because of unexplained symptoms or signs, or the patient who is being treated with drugs that are known to be associated with pulmonary complications, or the patient with altered immunity who is at risk for infection that is followed so closely. Nevertheless, for that select group this variable is useful.

For others, one of the most useful and least expensive services you can perform is to attempt to retrieve any earlier chest films of the patient that may be available for comparison. If a lesion can be shown to have been present and absolutely stable for a minimum of 2 years, the likelihood of its being malignant is low enough that you could rationally choose a noninvasive periodic surveillance program as a means of further evaluation, provided there are no clinical findings to dictate otherwise.

Of course, the key word in the preceding sentence is "absolutely." Comparing size is obvious, but not sufficient. Marginal contours, radiodensity, internal inhomogeneities, apparent migration toward the hilum, and changes in adjacent lung and pleura must all be assessed. This complex judgment based on comparison of radiographs is subjective and open to observer error. It must be done with care. Many reports of malignant pulmonary lesions changing very slowly over 2, 3, or more years are available. Bronchoalveolar carcinoma has been shown to be present for up to 15 years, but so far I have not seen any such cases that met the criteria of absolute stability (Fig. 6-5B to E). Do not substitute reports of earlier radiographs for comparison of the films themselves. The lesion of current concern may have been present but unreported. A lesion in an anatomically noisy area of the film such as the apices, the extreme bases, or the perihilar, retrocardiac, and paraspinal regions could have been overlooked.

Lesions that are subsequently proven to be malignant on rare occasion may appear temporarily to be improving on comparison follow-up films taken at short intervals (Fig. 6-7).

Uncommonly, benign nodules may slowly increase in size, but when uncalcified they are not distinguishable from malignant nodules until they are biopsied (see Fig. 6-2). Any increase in size of a nodule of unknown etiology is a compelling reason to pursue some invasive procedure calculated to provide a definite diagnosis even in an asymptomatic patient.

Solitary Pulmonary Nodules in Patients With Known Extrathoracic or Thoracic Primary Carcinoma

Whenever a solitary pulmonary nodule is found in the lung of a patient known to have had a primary malignant tumor elsewhere in the body or even in the chest, it is logical to consider metastasis as the likely explanation. However, data indicate that in the adult the likelihood that the new nodule is a second primary (see Fig. 6-3) is high and close to or exceeding the likelihood that it is a metastasis.[1,7] This is particularly true if the original neoplasm was a squamous cell cancer of the head and neck region. If the patient is a child or young adult with a primary sarcoma, the assumption of metastasis is more likely to be correct, but even then it is not absolute.

A small but important percentage of nodules in the lungs of patients known to have had previous extrathoracic primary neoplasms will turn out to be benign lesions[7] such as a hamartoma (Fig. 6-8) or even a granuloma, in spite of the fact that the lesion may not have been present on films made one or two years before. Hamartomas often appear de novo in the adult and are seldom found in children. Therefore, it is important to investigate thoroughly the nature of an SNPN in a patient with a known primary malignancy, particularly if the nodule represents the only clinical or laboratory evidence that the primary may have metastasized. The impact on prognosis and treatment is formidable, and one cannot *assume* that the solitary pulmonary nodule is due to metastasis.

In the event that a solitary pulmonary nodule is found in the chest simultaneously with the discovery of a primary malignancy elsewhere in the body, it is important to investigate the pulmonary nodule in accordance with the dictates of the clinical situation. In the event that establishing the nature of the pulmonary lesion — that is, whether it is truly a metastasis or an incidental benign lesion or a synchronous second primary — would alter

treatment radically, then the pursuit of the definitive nature of the pulmonary lesion may take precedence over the corrective surgery planned for the known primary malignancy. On the other hand, if the primary malignancy would require surgical correction regardless of the nature of the incidental pulmonary lesion, then often attention is directed first to the known primary.

Since CT scans are more sensitive in showing pulmonary metastases than are chest films or full-lung tomograms, it is worthwhile to consider chest CT for any patient who is to have mutilating radical surgery in an attempt to cure a malignant neoplasm. The discovery of an otherwise occult pulmonary nodule would lead to different planning and different priorities.[9,26]

Patients With Altered Immunity

In the case of patients with altered immunity from disease or from treatment with steroids or other immunosuppressive drugs, the rank-order of differential diagnoses of solitary pulmonary nodules is changed. The likelihood of infection with the ubiquitous fungi (especially *Aspergillus*) or *Nocardia* is moved into the common consideration category. In fact, in those patients with altered immunity where it can be shown that the lesion is new (i.e., by comparing recent previous chest films), infection with these organisms becomes the most likely diagnosis. Many of these patients will have signs or symptoms of infection, but not all (see Ch. 5). Much less commonly, a pulmonary nodule may be the first sign of lymphoma in an immunosuppressed patient.

MULTIPLE PULMONARY NODULES

In considering the differential diagnosis of multiple pulmonary nodules it is helpful to distinguish two different classes, even though the distinction is not always sharp. One class can be defined as "countable" (Fig. 6-9A). In such cases the nodules are of sufficient size and are sufficiently separable from one another that you *could* count them if you so desired. The other class is defined as "uncountable" and consists of lesions the majority of which are so small and so inseparable that you *would not* rationally decide to count them (Fig. 6-10).

Almost all of the diseases or conditions that cause "countable" nodules may also present as "uncountable" nodules as part of their radiographic spectrum. Thus, the latter group has a larger, more complex differential diagnosis, which is discussed in detail in the chapters on diffuse lung disease (Ch. 10) and pulmonary infections (Ch. 5). The following discussion does not cover the "uncountable" nodules spectrum.

Chapter 5 also contains a brief discussion of multiple calcified nodules.

Differential Diagnosis of Multiple Noncalcified Pulmonary Nodules

The differential diagnosis of multiple noncalcified pulmonary nodules is quite similar to that of the solitary noncalcified pulmonary nodule. The major difference is in the order of likelihood. For example, primary bronchogenic carcinoma is among the three most common causes of an SNPN, but is a rare cause of multiple pulmonary nodules. The radiographic spectrum for bronchoalveolar cell tumor, however, includes multiple nodules as one pattern that may be seen even at the time of initial diagnosis. Otherwise, multiple synchronous pulmonary nodular squamous cell carcinomas or adenocarcinomas are curiosities, and are multiple only in the sense that two, or at the outside three, lesions may be present simultaneously.

Multiple hamartomas occur, but they are rare (Fig. 6-11A).

Pulmonary metastases, on the other hand, commonly present as multiple pulmonary nodules. Approximately 80 percent of these patients will have known primary malignancies or clinical findings strongly suggesting an extrathoracic primary site. Even multiple pulmonary leiomyomas may be metastases from well-differentiated lesions in the uterus.[24] Rarely, carcinoma of the lung, other than bronchioloalveolar cell carcinoma, can present with multiple pulmonary metastases coincident with the primary lesion (Fig. 6-10B). Therefore, the common causes of multiple pulmonary nodules include metastases from primary neoplasms anywhere outside the brain, infectious granulomatous disease, noninfectious granulomatous disease, and, in immunocompromised patients, infection due to ubiquitous fungi or *Nocardia*.

Patients with Hodgkin's disease or non-Hodgkin's lymphoma also may develop multiple pulmonary nodules or masses; they may occur at the time of initial diagnosis, or more commonly as a manifestation of recurrent disease following treatment. However, radiographic appearances do not permit a distinction between pulmonary nodules due to recurrent lymphoma and nodules due to infection in patients with known malignant lymphoma.

Arteriovenous Malformations

Arteriovenous (AV) malformations may appear as solitary (Fig. 6-11B and C), or multiple nodules (Fig. 6-11D, E).[11] They can be recognized on chest films when they have prominent feeder vessels or draining veins (Fig. 6-11D). Characteristic signs, which are not always present, include clubbing of the fingers, cyanosis of the nail beds, and erythrocythemia. These may alert you to the diagnosis in a patient who also has a nodule in the

TABLE 6-2. Causes of Multiple Pulmonary Nodules

Neoplasm
    Metastases from any primary, usually extrathoracic
    Malignant lymphomas, especially as recurrent disease in patients being followed for known Hodgkin's disease and non-Hodgkin's lymphoma, less commonly as the initial manifestation of lymphoma, or as lymphoma developing in patients on long-term immunosuppressive therapy
    Uncommonly, bronchoalveolar cell tumor or intravascular bronchoalveolar cell tumor
    Rarely, benign mesenchymal neoplasms (lipomas, fibromas, etc.)

Infection
    Infectious granulomatous disease (tuberculosis, histoplasmosis, coccidioidomycosis, blastomycosis, etc.)
    In the immunologically altered host, ubiquitous fungi, *Nocardia*, anaerobic organisms, staphylococci, gram-negative organisms
    Parasites, under special circumstances related to the patient's occupational or geographic history

Noninfectious granulomatous disease
    Sarcoid
    Wegener's granulomatosis and variants
    Rheumatoid lung nodules
    Pneumoconioses
    Eosinophilic granulomas

Vascular deformities (arteriovenous malformations)

Others (uncommon or rare)
    Multiple hamartomas (see Fig. 6-11A)
    Bronchial papillomas secondary to juvenile laryngeal papillomatosis[29,34]
    Amyloid nodules[38] (correlate with rectal biopsy)
    Lipoid pneumonia
    Septic emboli

chest (Fig. 6-11B). Pulmonary AV malformations may also occur in patients with multiple telangiectases. Rarely a pulmonary vein varix may project as a nodule in lung adjacent to the left atrium.

Dynamic CT scans are very useful for distinguishing vascular malformations from granulomas or neoplasms, and pulmonary arteriography can be used to resolve any doubts. Multiple lesions that are not seen on the chest films may become apparent on vascular studies.

Table 6-2 is a more comprehensive list of the causes of multiple pulmonary nodules.

Integrating Radiographic, Clinical, and Laboratory Studies

Ultimately the precise diagnosis of the cause of multiple pulmonary nodules in an individual patient depends on microscopic and bacteriologic studies of the involved tissues or secretions, or on imaging studies identifying the vascular nature of lesions such as AV malformations.

Integrating radiographic data, clinical signs and symptoms, laboratory data, known underlying or antecedent diseases, and a complete environmental history including all drugs used or abused permits a critical rank-ordering of diagnostic possibilities. This integration serves as a guide to the selection and orderly sequencing of diagnostic procedures.

Clinical urgency — for example, in a case of presumptive infection in a patient with altered immunity — may dictate commencement of treatment before definitive diagnosis, and the treatment plan must be based on integration of all the available data. The radiographic abnormalities and their interpretation are often critical elements of this data base.

BRONCHOGENIC CARCINOMA AND BRONCHOALVEOLAR (BRONCHIOLOALVEOLAR) CARCINOMA

Bronchogenic carcinoma may occur in any part of the lung, although it is most common in the upper lobes. The radiographic appearance of primary carcinoma of the lung depends on four key variables:

1. Visualization of the tumor itself (Figs. 6-12 and 6-13)
2. Secondary effects of tumor on the pulmonary parenchyma (Figs. 6-14, 6-15D–F, 6-16 to 6-19)
3. Secondary effects of tumor on hilar and mediastinal nodes, pleura, or bone (Figs. 6-15A to C, 6-20, and 6-24A to C)
4. A negative chest film when the lesion is entirely intrabronchial or hidden by anatomic structures.

Each of these variables plays a role in the classification and staging of the disease.

Visualization of the Tumor Itself

When the tumor itself can be visualized (Fig. 6-12), it commonly manifests as a parenchymal nodule or mass with or without cavitation. It may vary in size from barely visible to obvious. Other parenchymal manifestations include nonspecific focal areas of homogeneous or inhomogeneous consolidation, which may, especially in the case of alveolar cell carcinoma, assume a segmental, multisegmental, lobar, or multilobar distribution indistinguishable from pneumonia (see Fig. 6-26). Air bronchograms may be seen in these areas of consolidation.

At times a bronchial wall or lumen deformity produced by a neoplasm may be detected by careful inspection of roentgenograms, but it is far more common to see these changes on tomograms, CT scans, or bronchograms (see Figs. 6-16C, 6-17, 6-19D, and 6-32B).

A bronchogenic carcinoma may also present as a unilateral hilar mass due to a large exophytic component accompanying an endobronchial lesion or due to involvement of neighboring lymph nodes.

Although a pulmonary mass will invoke consideration of bronchogenic carcinoma, there are other relatively common causes of pulmonary masses. These include nonbronchogenic neoplasms (Fig. 6-13), lung abscesses, cysts, conglomerate mass lesions due to pneumoconioses such as silicosis, and all the other conditions listed as considerations for the noncalcified pulmonary nodule.

Secondary Effects on the Pulmonary Parenchyma

A neoplasm may cause partial or complete obstruction of a major bronchus, with areas of atelectasis or homogeneous or inhomogeneous consolidation of lung due to interference with bronchial drainage. The neoplasm itself may not be visible when largely intrabronchial (Fig. 6-14).

Thus, the atelectasis consequent to neoplastic bronchial obstruction may be indistinguishable from atelectasis from any other cause. At times when there is an extrabronchial mass component, there are clear signs that the atelectasis is occurring around the mass. The compliant lung collapses in the expected fashion, but the noncompliant tumor mass bulges out from a portion of the collapsed lobe and is a telltale sign of the presence of tumor (see Ch. 4).

Areas of pneumonia peripheral to obstructing or partially obstructing bronchial neoplasms are common. Not all instances of obstructive "pneumonia" are associated with bacterial or viral organisms. Many show only chronic nonspecific inflammatory changes (Figs. 6-7 and 6-14). However, in some patients pathogenic organisms are isolated, and there are associated clinical signs and symptoms of pneumonia. In fact, after a course of appropriate antibiotics the patient may feel quite well, and patient and doctor may both suffer the illusion of having dealt with a pneumonia pure and simple. Radiographs may show substantial, but seldom complete clearing. In those cases where the true situation is not recognized, the pneumonia will usually recur in a short period, or atelectasis may supervene without infection or with chronic low-grade inflammation or "cholesterol (golden) pneumonia." Although neoplasms are not the only cause of repeated episodes of pneumonia or atelectasis in the same segments of lung, they are of sufficient incidence to warrant further investigation in such patients (Figs. 6-16 and 6-17).

The lung peripheral to a bronchial obstruction may be so filled with secretions that it does not lose volume, but rather maintains volume due to consolidation even without concomitant infection. This phenomenon has been described as the "drowned lung" effect.

When there is focal chronic infection beyond the site of bronchial obstruction, it may not be possible to tell from radiographic studies how much of the lesion is neoplasm and how much is inflammation (Fig. 6-14).

Occasionally the bronchi peripheral to the obstructing tumor may become distended with mucus and have the same radiographic appearance as mucoid impaction or allergic aspergillosis (Fig. 6-18).

Evidence of air trapping and hypoxic vasoconstriction, the so-called "obstructive emphysema," is an earlier manifestation of bronchial obstruction that may be detected by careful inspection of routine films and confirmed on films made during the expiratory phase of respiration. It is, unfortunately, one of those signs more easily recognized retrospectively (Fig. 6-19).

Bronchial obstruction may also result from metastases, benign tumors, and nonneoplastic conditions. Chronic infection, particularly tuberculosis and the other chronic infectious granulomatous diseases, as well as sarcoidosis and even silicosis may cause inflammatory bronchostenosis or obstructive tumefaction.

Fibroma, lipoma, chondroma, and granular cell myoblastoma are examples of benign tumors that may present as intrabronchial masses. They are rare but may simulate findings of bronchogenic carcinoma. The imaging features of these lesions cannot generally be distinguished from those of carcinoma. Inhaled foreign bodies may lodge in and obstruct bronchi, but this is largely a problem in young children, the mentally disturbed, the inebriated, or rarely a consequence of lost pieces of fillings or crowns during dental procedures.

Secondary Effects on Hilar and Mediastinal Nodes, Pleura, or Bone

Metastases to hilar or mediastinal nodes may cause masses that become apparent on plain films or tomograms or both (see also Ch. 7 for a discussion of mediastinal adenopathy). CT scans may show enlarged mediastinal nodes before they are large enough to be seen on plain films. On occasion, extensive mediastinal and hilar adenopathy may be seen on an initial radiographic study while the site of the primary is obscure. This is not an uncommon manner in which oat cell carcinoma may present, but squamous cell and other undifferentiated carcinomas may also present in this way (Figs. 6-15, 6-20, 6-21A and B, and 6-24). Sometimes the mediastinal adenopathy is subtle yet more apparent than the primary site, which may be hidden in an anatomically noisy area or within a central bronchus.

Metastases to pleura may produce pleural effusion that is indistinguishable radiographically from pleural effusion from other causes. Occasionally, pleural metastases produce nodular excrescences on the pleural surfaces that may be seen with or without associated effusion (Fig. 6-21C).

Destruction of portions of the bony thorax may occur in direct continuity with the primary neoplastic mass or may be discovered at a distance from the primary tumor as a result of hematogenous metastasis. In the Pancoast type of carcinoma the diagnosis is often not established before visible destruction of adjacent ribs or vertebrae has occurred (Fig. 6-22).

Not all tumors that occur in the apices are Pancoast tumors. Neurolemmomas (Fig. 6-23), neurofibromas, and meningoceles can present characteristic soft tissue apical masses. However, bone destruction (as opposed to erosion) is not associated with these benign tumors.

Rarely, tumoral forms of actinomycosis or blastomycosis may produce apical or subapical lesions, including bone destruction, that simulate Pancoast tumors. A draining fistula from these lesions may provide material for culture. However, biopsy may be necessary to distinguish these lesions from cancer.

RADIOGRAPHIC CHARACTERISTICS OF DIFFERENT HISTOPATHOLOGIC TYPES OF LUNG CANCERS

Lung carcinoma is most commonly one of five histopathologic types. The relative frequency varies across reported series, depending to some extent on whether only surgical cases are included or whether autopsy data are cited as well. The common histopathologic types are:

1. Epidermoid or squamous cell carcinoma
2. Adenocarcinoma
3. Anaplastic small cell carcinoma (oat cell carcinoma)
4. Anaplastic large cell carcinoma
5. Bronchiolar (bronchioloalveolar, or alveolar cell) carcinoma

Some pathologists recognize an additional category of mixed cell type when there is not sufficient predominance of histopathologic characteristics to warrant clear choice of one of the above groups. Some also identify categories such as carcinosarcoma and other uncommon subtypes. In addition, there does not seem to be a clear dividing line separating certain squamous cell types from the anaplastic carcinomas. It is likely that pathologists vary in their interpretation of these tumors, which may explain some of the observed discrepancies in the clinical behavior of squamous cell carcinomas, in particular.

The Bronchogenic Carcinomas

Expectations have evolved concerning the radiographic characteristics of the predominant mode of presentation of bronchogenic carcinomas. It is tempting to attempt to distinguish one histopathologic type from the other on the basis of chest film appearances. For example, small cell (oat cell) carcinomas most commonly manifest are by abnormalities in and about the hila due to early metastases to lymph nodes (Fig. 6-24). Adenocarcinomas are most commonly seen as a parenchymal nodule or mass away from the hila (see Fig. 6-12). Large cell carcinoma also commonly presents as a parenchymal mass, often a large one (over 4 cm in diameter) when first detected (Fig. 6-25). Squamous cell cancer may also be large and may be either peripheral or central. However, the data clearly show that there is much overlap between the radiographic appearances of the different histopathologic classifications of bronchogenic carcinoma.[4,5,6,22] The predominant mode of presentation of one variety may be the uncommon mode for another type, but all types share the same spectrum. It is true that you could appear clever by predicting that a new, peripheral nodule in a 50-year-old, nonsmoking female will be an adenocarcinoma, since this is the histologic type that is most common in the female and correlates least with smoking. Even here, however, you could be wrong; the lesion could also be a bronchiolar cell carcinoma, a histologic type that occurs less frequently than adenocarcinoma, but that occurs about equally in males and females. Therefore, your prediction would have little practical use.

All histopathologic types of carcinoma may present as a peripheral nodule or mass; cavitation has been observed in each variety, although it is most common in the squamous cell carcinoma and rare in the bronchiolar cell carcinoma; hilar masses alone or in conjunction with a parenchymal lesion have been observed in each; pleural effusion, usually associated with other radiographic manifestations, can be present in any; and Pancoast-type carcinoma may be due to any of these cell types.

Bronchoalveolar Cell Tumor (BAT)

The radiographic spectrum of bronchoalveolar cell tumors is fairly broad[2,17] and includes (a) a solitary nodule or mass (see Fig. 6-6); (b) multiple nodules or masses; (c) foci of inhomogeneous consolidation (Fig. 6-26A and B) that may be present on radiographs for many months; and (d) intense consolidation of segments or lobes (Fig.

6-26C and D). If the lesions are multiple, one of the lesions may be larger than the remainder and predominates. The theory is that the other nodules represent metastases from the larger primary tumor. On the other hand, a multifocal origin of this neoplasm would also serve to explain the presence of multiple lesions in both lungs at the time of original diagnosis.

There are a number of cases in which focal lesions have been shown to be present for many years (Fig. 6-5B and C). If you carefully compare the radiographs made at variable intervals during the period of observation, you will see that the lesions do not remain absolutely stable but rather fluctuate; for example, there are times when the radiographic lesions actually look as though there has been a partial clearing in comparison with an antecedent film. In other instances there is a relentless but indolent progression, which may not be easily appreciated when the films being compared have been made within a short interval of one another. You can be misled into believing that the lesion is benign because of its rather indolent course. Solitary bronchoalveolar cell tumors may be present for years, remain resectable, and have a reasonably good prognosis.

When there is segmental or lobar consolidation with visible air bronchograms, the distinction from pneumonia cannot be made. However, the extensive radiographic lesions, disproportionately greater than the clinical signs and symptoms would warrant, prompt one to consider bronchoalveolar cell neoplasm in the differential diagnosis (Fig. 6-26C and D).

Diffuse calcification rarely may be seen on CT in the consolidated form of BAT due to the presence of calcified psammoma bodies, and there is at least one report of a case in which similar calcification on CT was present in metastases to mediastinal lymph nodes.[23]

Intravascular bronchoalveolar cell tumor characteristically presents as multiple pulmonary nodules 0.5 cm to 1.0 cm in size—a radiologic appearance identical to that of pulmonary metastases. The patients are often young and asymptomatic, may be male or female, who have chest films done as part of preemployment or routine physical examinations. Some have common but nonspecific symptoms of pulmonary disease. Although the name implies a variant of alveolar cell carcinoma, it is more likely that this is a tumor of pulmonary vessel origin (Fig. 6-27).[10]

Scar Carcinoma

There are instances in which proven lung carcinoma exists in an area that histopathologically also shows scarring from chronic inflammatory disease. Retrospective analysis of preceding serial chest films may show irregular linear shadows or a cluster of small, irregular, abnormal opacities that are not readily classified as to shape, or some combination of focal reticular or reticulonodular shadows. It is not possible to know in each case whether these lesions are truly early evidence of the neoplasm itself or whether the neoplasm represents a so-called "scar carcinoma." A scar carcinoma theoretically is one that has arisen and grown in a portion of lung that suffered from previous postinflammatory or chronic inflammatory foci or scarring (see Fig. 6-6).

Carcinoid Tumors and Bronchial Gland Carcinomas

Carcinoid tumors and bronchial gland carcinomas have been referred to as "bronchial adenomas."[3] That terminology, however, does not adequately reflect their behavior. There are four principle histopathologic types: carcinoid (both typical and atypical), adenoid cystic (cylindromatous), mucoepidermoid, and rare true mucous gland adenoma. Only the last of these behaves as a benign tumor.[21] The other types exhibit invasive growth characteristics, may recur locally, and may metastasize to regional lymph nodes. These neoplasms are reported to constitute from 2 to 5 percent of all primary lung tumors, although the incidence may be as high as 10 percent in series that include only resected lesions. Ninety percent are of the carcinoid type. The majority occur in major airways. The atypical forms of carcinoid tumor are those most likely to metastasize to lymph nodes and extrathoracic sites; for example, carcinoid tumor may rarely be a cause of osteoblastic metastases to bone.

Even while behaving as malignant lesions, this group of neoplasms differs markedly from bronchogenic carcinomas. They occur with roughly equal frequency in males and females. They may occur in children and teenagers in whom bronchogenic carcinoma would hardly be considered as a diagnosis. Clinical and radiographic evidence indicates that these neoplasms may be present for several years and even decades without metastasizing. The prognosis for long-term survival in patients with proven nodal metastases or pleural involvement by direct extension is still reasonably good. Late recurrences 10 or more years after primary resection are known to occur. These recurrent lesions may be successfully resected. Repeated endoscopic resections of lesions affecting major airways have been performed with substantial palliation and symptom-free intervals spanning periods of years. In spite of long-term survival, however, death from late recurrences may occur.

Mistaken histopathologic diagnoses of oat cell carcinoma have been made from biopsy specimens in cases shown to be carcinoid tumors on resection. This can be a grievous error because the treatment and prognosis are remarkably different.

Radiographically, carcinoid tumors and bronchial gland carcinomas may manifest as central masses of varying size, with or without associated evidence of bronchial obstruction. Often part of the tumor is endobronchial, while a larger component protrudes outside of the bronchial lumen. The majority of these neoplasms are detectable on bronchoscopy and are found in the main bronchi, less commonly in the trachea, and still less commonly in segmental bronchi. Bronchial obstruction may be responsible for repeated episodes of pneumonia in the same segment or lobe of the lung (Figs. 6-16 and 6-17). Long-standing bronchial obstruction can cause bronchiectatic changes peripheral to the tumor mass. Rarely, these bronchi may become deformed and enlarged by the endobronchial tumor component, and there may be inspissated secretions in the more peripheral branch bronchi. This combination may produce the radiographic appearance of a cluster or string of connected, masslike opacities extending peripherally from the hilum, similar in appearance to mucoid impaction of the bronchus or allergic aspergillosis. A small percentage may present as a peripheral mass or a nodular lesion in the lung.

Cylindromas may occur in the trachea and can easily be missed unless you develop a routine of careful inspection of the trachea on chest films, particularly in the lateral view. Because they are so uncommon they are seldom considered clinically in the evaluation of the patient who presents with asthma-like symptoms or symptoms of chronic obstructive pulmonary disease.

Carcinoid syndrome may rarely occur in a patient with a carcinoid tumor.

Bronchogenic carcinoma in the first and second decades of life is so rare as to be a curiosity. However, carcinomas do occur in young people and are known to occur even in childhood, with the youngest reported case being that of a 5½-year-old. Carcinoid tumors and bronchial gland carcinomas comprise most of the rare primary bronchial tumors of childhood.[20] Bronchoalveolar carcinoma is also known to occur in young adults.

Plasma cell granuloma, although an uncommon pulmonary lesion, is one of the more common mass lesions of the lung seen in children. Plasma cell granuloma can rarely present as a primary endobronchial mass.

CAVITATION IN NEOPLASMS

Cavitation may occur in any of the histopathologic types of bronchogenic carcinoma but is most common in the squamous cell variety, involving approximately 10 percent of these lesions. The cavity occurs within the

TABLE 6-3. Classification of Lung Cancer

Primary tumor (T)

TX   Tumor proven by the presence of malignant cells in bronchopulmonary secretions but not visualized roentgenographically or by bronchoscopy, or any tumor that cannot be assessed (as in a retreatment staging)

TO   No evidence of primary tumor

TIS   Carcinoma in situ

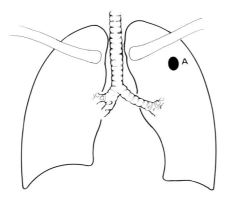

T1

Single tumors 3.0 cm or less in greatest dimension that are surrounded by lung or visceral pleura, and that show no evidence of invasion proximal to a lobar bronchus at bronchoscopy (A). (The uncommon case of a superficial tumor of any size whose invasive component is limited to the bronchial wall is also classified as T1, even if the invasion extends proximal to the main bronchus.)

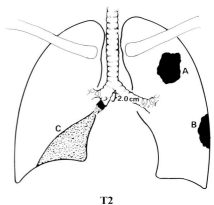

T2

Single tumors more than 3.0 cm in greatest dimension (A), or single tumors of any size that invade the visceral pleura (B) or that have associated atelectasis or obstructive pneumonitis extending to the hilar region. At bronchoscopy, the proximal extent of demonstrable tumor must be within a lobar bronchus or at least 2.0 cm distal to the carina. Any associated atelectasis or obstructive pneumonitis must involve less than an entire lung (C).

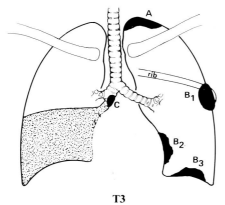

T3

Single tumors of any size with direct extension into the chest wall (A) (including superior sulcus tumors), the diaphragm, or the mediastinal pleura or pericardium (B$_{1-3}$) without involving the heart, great vessels, trachea, esophagus, or vertebral body; or single tumors in the main bronchus within 2.0 cm of the carina but not involving the carina (C).

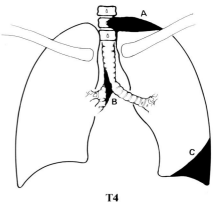

T4

Single tumors of any size that invade the mediastinum, or involve the heart, great vessels, trachea, esophagus (not shown), vertebral body (A), or carina (B), or the presence of malignant pleural effusion (C).

Nodal involvement (N)

N0   No demonstrable metastasis to regional lymph nodes

N1   Metastasis to lymph nodes in the peribronchial or the ipsilateral hilar region, or both, including direct extension

N2   Metastasis to ipsilateral mediastinal lymph nodes and subcarinal lymph nodes

N3   Metastasis to contralateral mediastinal lymph nodes, contralateral hilar lymph nodes, ipsilateral or contralateral scalene or supraclavicular lymph nodes

Distant metastasis (M)

M0   No (known) distant metastasis

M1   Distant metastasis present—specify site(s)

Pleural effusions. Most pleural effusions associated with lung cancer are due to tumor. There are, however, some few patients in whom cytopathologic examination of pleural fluid (on more than one specimen) is negative for tumor, and the fluid is nonbloody and is not an exudate. In such cases, where these elements and clinical judgment dictate that the effusion is not related to the tumor, the patients should be staged T1, T2, or T3 excluding effusion as a staging element.

Invasion of contiguous structures. The determination of invasion of pleura, chest wall, pericardium, heart, or diaphragm is most reliably made at surgical exploration. Imaging studies may show an intimate juxtaposition of a neoplasm with neighboring anatomic structures. The distinction between contiguity and actual invasion based on assessment of the presence of an intervening tumor-free plane is unreliable under those conditions.

Modified from: Mountain CF: A New International Staging System for Lung Cancer. Chest 89:225S–233S, 1986

neoplasm itself or rarely as part of an abscess in parenchyma beyond an obstructed bronchus. Characteristically, cavities within pulmonary neoplasms are described as having thick walls, eccentric lumina, or protruding portions of outer wall and irregular or nodular excrescences of inner wall. These are useful signs, but they are not specific when applied to an individual. In addition, you will rarely encounter a very thin walled cavity, regular in outline and inner contour, that nevertheless contains malignant cells in the wall and represents true bronchogenic carcinoma. Fluid levels may also be seen in malignant cavitary lesions (Fig. 6-28).

STAGING OF CARCINOMA OF THE LUNG

It is very difficult to gather unbiased data concerning the prognosis of patients with carcinomas of the lung. A more widespread use of classification factors pertaining to the size and location of the primary lesion (T), the presence or absence of adenopathy (N), and the presence or absence of metastases (M) may serve to make different series more amenable to comparison. The TNM classification can be used in clinical and surgical staging of an entire population of patients. Perhaps staging can lead to a better understanding of those factors that radically alter prognosis and permit critical comparison of different populations of patients (Tables 6-3 and 6-4; Fig. 1).

WHAT USES DOES THE CHEST RADIOGRAPH SERVE WELL?

First of all, chest radiography is currently the only practical way of detecting a pulmonary neoplasm in the asymptomatic individual. Cytologic study of sputa also has merit as an atraumatic screening method, but logistics apparently prevents its widespread use for this purpose so far.

Second, the chest radiograph may provide the first objective evidence that a pulmonary neoplasm is the likely explanation for the signs and symptoms of an individual patient. The symptoms of bronchogenic carcinoma, when present, are nonspecific. They encompass any or all those symptoms common to pulmonary disease in general: cough, sputum production, fever, night sweats, chest pain, dyspnea, and weight loss. Patients may also present with a variety of paraneoplastic syndromes[14] such as dermatomyositis, Cushing's syndrome, hyponatremia, and psychological and neurologic disorders. Although the carcinoid syndrome is rare, even when a bronchial carcinoid is present, the syndrome may also occur in patients with oat cell carcinoma.[31]

Bone and joint pain associated with pulmonary osteo-

TABLE 6-4. Stage Grouping of TNM Subsets

Stage	Primary Tumor	Nodal Involvement	Metastasis
Occult carcinoma	TX	N0	M0
Stage 0	TIS	Carcinoma in situ	
Stage I	T1	N0	M0
	T2	N0	M0
Stage II	T1	N1	M0
	T2	N1	M0
Stage IIIa	T3	N0	M0
	T3	N1	M0
	T1-3	N2	M0
Stage IIIb	Any T	N3	M0
	T4	Any N	M0
Stage IV	Any T	Any N	M1

(From Mountain CF: A new international staging system for lung cancer. Chest 89:225S–233S, 1986, with permission.)

arthropathy may be a presenting clinical complaint in a patient with a pulmonary neoplasm. Sometimes bone pain or central nervous system disturbances consequent to metastatic lesions may be the presenting complaint. Elaboration of the cause of the profound disturbance in

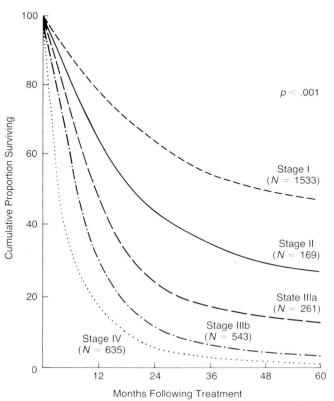

Fig. 1. Cumulative proportion of patients surviving 5 years by clinical stage of disease. (From Mountain CF: A new international staging system for lung cancer. Chest 89:232S–233S, 1986, with permission.)

these patients often depends on the objective evidence first provided by chest imaging studies.

Third, the constellation of abnormalities seen on chest film and subsequent CT scans, or MRI scans can aid in planning and sequencing of further studies likely to establish the precise nature and extent of the lesion. Bronchoscopy, needle aspiration, scalene node biopsy, mediastinoscopy, parasternal approach to mediastinal node biopsy, adrenal needle biopsy, thoracentesis, pleural biopsy, or other studies are planned according to the results of imaging studies.

CT AND MRI IN PRIMARY LUNG CANCER

CT scans of patients with suspect or proven carcinoma are valuable to detect mediastinal adenopathy that may be occult on plain films.[27] CT scans can also be used to demonstrate possible chest wall invasion or unsuspected pulmonary metastases.

Identification of ipsilateral hilar adenopathy can be important in deciding whether a lobectomy or a pneumonectomy will be required to eradicate the disease. Detection of extensive ipsilateral mediastinal adenopathy or definite contralateral mediastinal adenopathy may contraindicate attempts at curative surgery without prior biopsy of the enlarged nodes. Since the CT criteria for evaluating mediastinal lymph nodes are largely limited to determining their size and number, biopsy is important to prove involvement by metastases. This topic is discussed in Chapter 7.

Unsuspected adrenal masses demonstrated on CT may indicate the need for needle biopsy to rule out metastases as opposed to incidental benign adrenal adenoma. CT scans are also useful in assessing the extent of disease before radiation treatment planning for those patients who are not considered able to benefit from surgery.

MRI studies serve similar purposes to CT in the evaluation of the mediastinum and are discussed further in Chapter 7. In general they have no proven advantage over CT for these purposes. They do not require exposure to ionizing radiation, however, and the distinction between hilar or mediastinal vessels and nodal masses can usually be made without the use of intravenous contrast agents.

BRONCHOGRAPHY IN THE DIAGNOSIS OF CARCINOMA OF THE LUNG

In the past, bronchography was commonly used in the investigation of patients with suspected bronchogenic

neoplasm. Several bronchographic abnormalities had high correlations with the presence of malignant neoplasm. Nevertheless, the diagnosis was still inferential. Fiberoptic bronchoscopy, augmented by bronchial brushings, bronchial biopsy, or needle aspiration of accessible lesions, are techniques used to obtain specimens for histologic and cytologic study to arrive at more definitive diagnoses. They eliminate the need for bronchography in the diagnosis of carcinoma of the lung.

HODGKIN'S DISEASE AND NON-HODGKIN'S LYMPHOMA IN THE LUNG

Hodgkin's disease and non-Hodgkin's lymphomas may present as pulmonary lesions indistinguishable from those of other pulmonary neoplasms. The lymphomas may present as endobronchial lesions and cause atelectasis or consolidation peripherally. They may present as discrete nodules (either single or multiple), as masses or cavities (Fig. 6-29), or as areas of pulmonary consolidation with or without air bronchograms. Involvement of lung alone, at the time of initial presentation, is rare in Hodgkin's disease, but occurs with enough frequency in non-Hodgkin's lymphoma to at least warrant consideration in differential diagnoses of pulmonary nodules or masses (Fig. 6-30) or unexplained zones of consolidation.[13] In Hodgkin's disease there is at least concomitant hilar or mediastinal lymphadenopathy. However, pulmonary involvement, as the first or only sign of *recurrent* Hodgkin's disease or non-Hodgkin's malignant lymphoma, is not uncommon.[8]

Mycosis fungoides is a T cell lymphoma with primary skin involvement. The chest can become involved, however, and the lesions can appear as nodules, a mass, patchy zones of consolidation, reticulonodular diffuse bilateral lesions, or pleural effusion. Hilar adenopathy may occur with these other lesions. The radiographic spectrum is shared by other neoplasms, metastases, lymphoma, and pulmonary infections.[30]

KAPOSI'S SARCOMA

Until the outbreak of acquired immune deficiency syndrome (AIDS), Kaposi's sarcoma was a relatively uncommon neoplasm primarily involving the skin. Since the onset of the AIDS epidemic, Kaposi's sarcoma has become a frequent cause of diffuse pulmonary disease in addition to the skin lesions.[12] Radiographically, there may be a diffuse pattern of small, irregular nodules throughout both lungs (Fig. 6-31A and B) or a predominant interstitial pattern with septal lines or a combined reticulonodular pattern.

Unfortunately, AIDS patients frequently suffer from *Pneumocystis carinii* pneumonia as well as pulmonary disease from *Mycobacterium avium-intracellulare* and other microorganisms. These infections share their radiographic spectra with Kaposi's sarcoma and indeed often occur simultaneously. The presence of hilar or mediastinal adenopathy does not separate Kaposi's sarcoma from infection. *Mycobacterium avium-intracellulare, Mycobacterium tuberculosis,* and *Cryptococcus* infection can also cause such adenopathy separately or concurrently.

Gallium-67 citrate scans have a high sensitivity for detection of *Pneumocystis carinii* pneumonia but are also positive with other pulmonary infections. However, there has not been any significant uptake of this isotope in the lesions of Kaposi's sarcoma. Therefore, a *negative* isotope scan would be of help in distinguishing these possibilities when invasive studies are contraindicated or undesired.[39]

PULMONARY METASTASES

The majority of pulmonary metastases are due to primary malignancies of the breast, the gastrointestinal system, the osseous system, or the genitourinary system, but any primary malignant tumor can metastasize to the lungs. Often these patients do not appear seriously ill in spite of the alarming appearance of their chest films. As more and more lung becomes involved, however, dyspnea occurs. Metastases adjacent to pleura may account for chest pain or even pneumothorax. Occasionally a patient with bronchogenic carcinoma may present with symptoms from widespread pulmonary metastases while the primary lesion remains occult in a bronchus.

Approximately 80 percent of patients with pulmonary metastases will have a known underlying malignancy or signs and symptoms indicating the likelihood of an extrathoracic primary tumor. A small percentage of patients who have pulmonary metastases — probably fewer than 20 percent — will present with the metastases as one of the first signs of illness. The true nature of the pulmonary lesions in these patients may not be appreciated at first examination.

Nodular Lesions

Metastases to the lung may present as multiple pulmonary nodules of either the countable or the noncountable type, or less commonly as a solitary pulmonary nodule. These have been previously discussed.

Nodular metastases may be discrete and sharply marginated (see Fig. 6-9), or they may be small, poorly defined, and irregular of contour, and at times have barely discernible margins (Fig. 6-31C). Metastases, particularly from squamous cell primaries (e.g., from the uterus), may also present as cavities.

Complete mapping of lesions is important for those patients who are to have thoracotomy and attempted resection of all metastases. The use of full-lung tomography and CT scans for this purpose has been discussed. These special studies are expected to show more lesions than the chest films in 20 to 35 percent of patients with pulmonary metastases.

Miliary patterns or micronodular patterns of distribution may also be produced by pulmonary metastases (see Fig. 6-10A).

Lymphangitic Metastases

Lymphangitic patterns of metastasis are seen as lines of varying thickness produced by deposition of tumor cells in septal lymphatics and perilymphatic spaces. They may be seen as typical Kerley-B, -A, or -C lines. In addition, small nodular components or reticulonodular shadows may be seen. Hilar or mediastinal lymphadenopathy may or may not be present or recognized.[19] Patients with lymphangitic metastases may have dyspnea because of decreased lung compliance. In the absence of lymphadenopathy, the plain-film findings of lymphangitic metastases can be mistaken for pulmonary edema or chronic interstitial pneumonia. (See also Ch. 10)

Metastasis to a Bronchus

Metastasis to a bronchus from an extrathoracic primary neoplasm may cause secondary changes — bronchial obstruction or a hilar mass — indistinguishable from those caused by primary pulmonary neoplasms (Fig. 6-32). Metastases to the trachea, although uncommon, can cause severe dyspnea (see Ch. 7).

In this chapter I have tried to give an overview of pulmonary neoplasms. In the next chapter additional examples will be presented, but the emphasis will be on the hilar and mediastinal extensions of neoplasms and the nodal components due to metastases.

SUMMARY

1. The majority of primary pulmonary neoplasms consist of bronchogenic carcinomas, bronchoalveo-

lar carcinomas, carcinoid tumors, bronchial gland carcinomas, and a smaller number of malignant lymphomas. All other primary neoplasms that may arise from any of the tissues of the lung or their embryologic precursors are uncommon or rare.

2. The differential diagnosis of a solitary noncalcified pulmonary nodule (SNPN) involves a long list of possibilities. However, at least 90 percent of all of the SNPNs that you are likely to see in day-to-day practice are either neoplasms, granulomas, or hamartomas. Of these three, hamartoma is by far the least common, yet it is more common than any of the other lesions comprising the remaining long list of differential diagnoses.

3. The least expensive and probably the most effective service that you can perform for a patient with an SNPN is to retrieve all available earlier chest films for comparison.

4. There are no radiographic characteristics of the marginal contours or the size of an SNPN that allow you to predict whether it is benign or malignant in an individual patient. Sometimes the clear recognition of the feeding or draining vessels of an arteriovenous malformation provides an exception to this rule. Recognition of all of the characteristic features of a zone of trapped lung or round atelectasis is another (see Ch. 4).

5. Unequivocal calcification seen within a nodule on imaging studies is a generally accepted criterion that the nodule is benign, provided there is an appropriate spatial relationship between the calcification(s) and the nodule. Exceptions are rare, see test.

6. Carefully performed CT scans can be used to obtain density measurements of SNPNs, and two classes of lesions can thus be distinguished. One class consists of those nodules with high radiodensity, which are considered to be benign and can be merely followed by periodic examination. The other group consists of those nodules whose overall radiodensity is insufficient to classify them as either clearly benign or clearly malignant. Adherence to strict technique and strict criteria is necessary.

7. Absolute stability in the radiographic appearance of an SNPN over at least 2 years' time is a generally accepted criterion for benignity. When the criterion of absolute stability cannot be satisfied, then it is best to consider the lesion as indeterminate. Ambiguity remaining after careful evaluation of all available data is still preferable to a false-positive or false-negative diagnosis.

8. An SNPN discovered in a patient with a known extrathoracic malignancy cannot simply be assumed to represent a metastasis. Under certain circumstances, the possibility that the nodule is a separate primary (or less likely a benign lesion) is at least as great as the chance of its being a metastasis.

9. The rank-order of the differential diagnosis of a newly discovered SNPN is different in an immunocompromised patient, in that infection is given first rank. Such nodules are often due to infection with ubiquitous fungi or with *Nocardia,* and less commonly with other microorganisms. Much less commonly, non-Hodgkin's lymphoma may present as a nodule or mass in the lung of a patient who has been chronically treated with immunosuppressive drugs.

10. The differential diagnosis of multiple, noncalcified pulmonary nodules is quite similar to that of SNPNs, but the rank-order of possibilities is changed. Simultaneous primary bronchogenic carcinomas are rare, whereas metastases from extrathoracic neoplasms are common. Nodular forms of the infectious granulomatous diseases may present as either solitary or multiple lesions. However, solitary nodules as initial manifestations of the noninfectious granulomatous diseases, such as sarcoidosis, Wegener's granulomatosis, or pneumoconioses, are rare, whereas multiple nodules are more common manifestations of these entities. Hamartomas are the third most common cause of solitary pulmonary nodules, but they are rare as a cause of multiple pulmonary nodules.

Multiple nodules in the immunocompromised patient have much the same differential diagnosis as do SNPNs in this group.

11. CT studies are useful in the evaluation of a patient with known multiple pulmonary metastases when surgical removal is contemplated. They frequently show more lesions than are apparent on the chest films. Whereas many of these additional lesions are due to the neoplasm, some are incidental scars or other benign lesions, and they may be indistinguishable. However, CT provides a "map" to guide the surgeon in the exploration.

12. The majority of bronchogenic carcinomas are classified as either epidermoid carcinomas, adenocarcinomas, anaplastic small cell carcinomas, or anaplastic large cell carcinomas. These entities share a common radiographic spectrum, although some are more commonly seen as peripheral nodules or masses, whereas others predominate as central lesions.

13. The radiographic spectrum of malignant primary pulmonary neoplasms includes:
   a. A pulmonary parenchymal nodule or mass
   b. A unilateral hilar mass
   c. Atelectasis or pneumonia, or an appearance of "stuffed bronchi" peripheral to an endobronchial mass

d. Evidence of air trapping and decreased perfusion of lung peripheral to an endobronchial neoplasm

e. Patchy, segmental, or lobar consolidation due to parenchymal permeation by neoplasm in patients with bronchoalveolar cell carcinoma or malignant lymphoma

f. Hilar and mediastinal adenopathy, or pleural effusion, usually (but not invariably) due to metastases when present in patients with bronchogenic carcinoma

g. Bone destruction in continuity with the pulmonary neoplasm in cases of Pancoast tumor or chest wall invasion.

14. Bronchoalveolar cell carcinoma has a broad spectrum of radiographic appearances. This cell type is usually separated from the bronchogenic carcinoma group, but some consider it a class of adenocarcinoma.

15. Cavitation within a nodule or mass changes the differential diagnosis surprisingly little. All types of neoplasms involving the lung, including Hodgkin's disease, may show cavities, and many infections may present as cavitating nodules or masses.

16. Carcinoid tumor and bronchial gland carcinoma are best considered malignant lesions that have a good prognosis. Long-term survival is common even after recurrence. Late recurrences (many years after the original lesion has been removed) may occur and cause death.

17. Pulmonary metastases may appear as discrete pulmonary nodules or masses, or as small, poorly defined, and often barely perceptible irregular nodules, or as miliary lesions, or as reticulonodular lesions with septal lines, common to many forms of diffuse lung disease.

BIBLIOGRAPHY

1. Adkins PC, Wesselhoeft CW, Newman W, et al: Thoracotomy on the patient with previous malignancy: metastasis or new primary? J Thorac Cardiovasc Surg 56:351, 1968

2. Berkman YM: Many faces of bronchiolo-alveolar carcinoma. Semin Roentgenol 12:207, 1977

3. Burcharth F, Axelsson C: Bronchial adenomas. Thorax 27:442, 1972

4. Byrd RB, Miller WE, Carr DT, et al: The roentgenographic appearance of squamous cell carcinoma of the bronchus. Mayo Clin Proc 43:327, 1968

5. Byrd RB, Miller WE, Carr DT, et al: The roentgenographic appearance of large cell carcinoma of the bronchus. Mayo Clin Proc 43:333, 1968

6. Byrd RB, Miller WE, Carr DT, et al: The roentgenographic appearance of small cell carcinoma of the bronchus. Mayo Clin Proc 43:337, 1968

7. Cahan WG, Shah JP, Castro ELB: Benign solitary lung lesions in patients with cancer. Ann Surg 187:241, 1978

8. Castellino RA, Blank N, Cassady JR, Kaplan HS: Roentgenologic aspects of Hodgkin's disease II. Role of routine radiographs in detecting relapse. Cancer 31:316, 1973

9. Chang AE, Schaner EG, Conkle DM, et al: Evaluation of computer tomography in the detection of pulmonary metastases. A prospective study. Cancer 43:913, 1979

10. Dail DH, Liebow AA, Gmelich JT, et al: Intravascular, bronchiolar, and alveolar tumor of the lung (IV BAT). Cancer 51:452, 1983

11. Dines DE, Arms RA, Bernatz PE, et al: Pulmonary arteriovenous fistulas. Mayo Clin Proc 49:460, 1974

12. Fauci AS, Macher AM, Lougo DL, et al: NIH Conference. Acquired immunodeficiency syndrome: epidemiologic, clinical, immunologic, and therapeutic considerations. Ann Intern Med 100:92, 1984

13. Filly R, Blank N, Castellino RA: Radiographic distribution of intrathoracic disease in previously untreated patients with Hodgkin's disease and non-Hodgkin's lymphoma. Radiology 120:277, 1976

14. Gomez-Uria A, Pazianos AG: Syndromes resulting from ectopic hormone-producing tumors. Med Clin North Am 59:431, 1975

15. Heitzman ER, Markarian B, Raasch BN, et al: Pathways of tumor spread through the lung: radiologic correlations with anatomy and pathology. Radiology 144:3, 1982

16. Higgins GA, Shields TW, Keehn RJ: The solitary pulmonary nodule. Ten year follow-up of Veterans' Administration — Armed Forces cooperative study. Arch Surg 110:570, 1975

17. Hill CA: Bronchioloalveolar carcinoma: a review. Radiology 150:15, 1984

18. Holin SM, Dwork RE, Glaser S, et al: Solitary pulmonary nodules in a community-wide chest roentgenographic survey. Am Rev Tuberc 79:427, 1959

19. Janower ML, Blennerhassett JB: Lymphangitic spread of metastatic cancer to the lung. Radiology 101:267, 1971

20. Lack EE, Harris GBC, Eraklis AJ, et al: Primary bronchial tumors in childhood. Cancer 51:492, 1983

21. Lawson RM, Ramathan L, Hurley G, et al: Bronchial adenoma: review of an 18-year experience at the Brompton Hospital. Thorax 31:245, 1976

22. Lehar TJ, Carr DT, Miller WE, et al: Roentgenographic appearance of bronchogenic adenocarcinoma. Am Rev Respir Dis 96:245, 1967

23. Mallens WMC, Nijhuis-Heddes JMA, Bakker M: Calcified lymph node metastases in bronchioloalveolar carcinoma. Radiology 161:103, 1986

24. Martin E: Leiomyomatous lung lesions: a proposed classification. AJR 141:269, 1983

25. Muhm JR, Miller WE, Fontana RS, et al: Lung cancer detected during a screening program using four-month chest radiographs. Radiology 148:609, 1983

26. Neifield JP, Michaelis LL, Doppman JL: Suspected pulmonary metastases. Correlation of chest X-ray, whole lung tomograms, and operative findings. Cancer 39:383, 1977

27. Osborne DR, Korobkin M, Ravin CE, et al: Comparison of plain radiography, conventional tomography, and computed tomography in detecting intrathoracic lymph node metastases from lung carcinoma. Radiology 142:157, 1982

28. Ray JF III, Lawton BR, Magnin GE, et al: The coin lesion story: update 1976. Chest 70:332, 1976

29. Rosenbaum HD, Alavi SM, Bryant LR: Pulmonary parenchymal spread of juvenile laryngeal papillomatosis. Radiology 90:654, 1968

30. Rubin DL, Blank N: Rapid pulmonary dissemination in mycosis fungoides simulating pneumonia. Cancer 56:649, 1985

31. Said S: Endocrine role of the lung in disease. Am J Med 57:453, 1974

32. Siegelman SS, Khouri NF, Leo FP, et al: Solitary pulmonary nodules: CT assessment. Radiology 160:307, 1986

33. Siegelman SS, Khouri NF, Scott WW, et al: Pulmonary hamartoma: CT findings. Radiology 160:313, 1986

34. Singer DB, Greenberg SD, Harrison GM: Papillomatosis of the lung. Am Rev Respir Dis 94:777, 1966

35. Toomes H, Delphendahl A, Manke H-G, et al: The coin lesion of the lung—a review of 955 resected coin lesions. Cancer 51:534, 1983

36. Troupin RH: Ossifying bronchial carcinoid—A case report. AJR 104:808, 1968

37. Webb WR: The pleural tail sign. Radiology 127:309, 1978

38. Wilson SR, Sanders DE, Delarne NC: Intrathoracic manifestations of amyloid disease. Radiology 120:283, 1976

39. Woolfenden JM, Carrasquillo JA, Larson SM, et al: Acquired immune deficiency syndrome: Ga-67 citrate imaging. Radiology 162:383, 1987

40. Zerhouni EA, Boukadoum M, Siddiky MA, et al: A standard phantom for quantitative CT analysis of pulmonary nodules. Radiology 149:767, 1983

41. Zerhouni EA, Spivey JF, Morgan RH, et al: Factors influencing quantitative CT measurements of solitary pulmonary nodules. J Comput Assist Tomogr 6:1075, 1982

Atlas

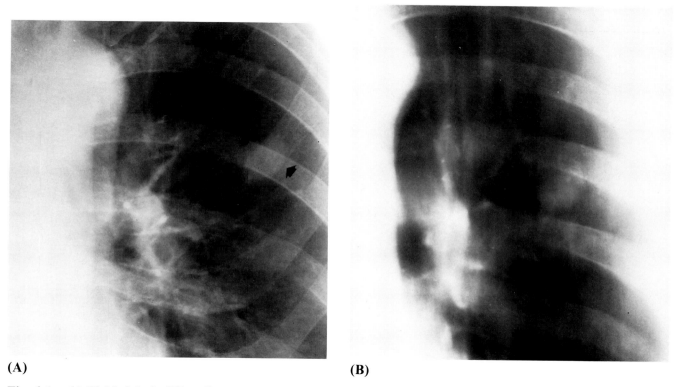

(A)   (B)

Fig. 6-1. (A,B) Nodule in Rib or Lung

(A) Coned PA view. An oval or flame-shaped nodule is superimposed on the anterior left third rib. Is it in the rib or in the lung? The possibility that it was a pulmonary nodule was considered, and further studies were undertaken. No earlier films were available for comparison.

(B) Tomogram of the same lesion. Here the lesion is projected between two posterior ribs, which are still slightly in focus, indicating that it is a nodule located in the posterior portions of the lung. In fact, one can still see the out-of-focus medial edge of the scapula in the lateral portion of this coned view.

The nodule was removed and found to be a partly caseating nodule. Periodic acid-Schiff and acid-fast stains were negative for fungi and acid-fast bacilli. Tubercle bacilli, however, were cultured from the specimen.

Stereoscopic views of the chest can also be used to distinguish lesions in ribs from lesions in the lung. The movement of the x-ray tube between the two exposures will not permit the lesion to maintain precisely the same relationship to anatomic structures on each film unless they are in the same plane. The solution could also be achieved by fluoroscopy. *(Figure continues.)*

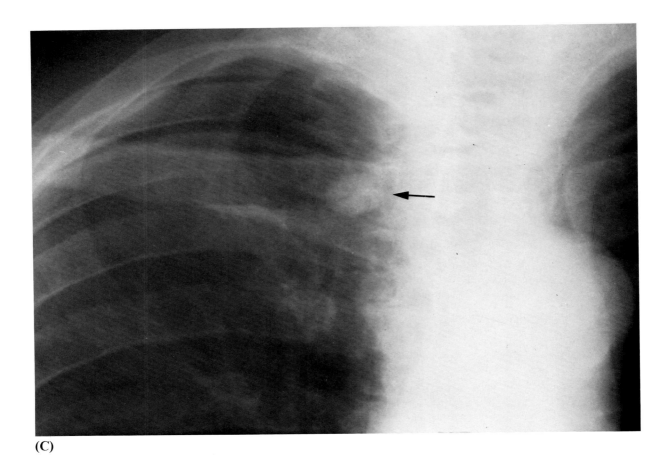

(C)

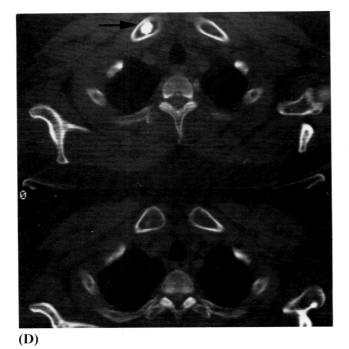

(D)

Fig. 6-1. *(Continued).* **(C,D) Differentiation Between a Bone Island and a Lung Nodule**

(C) Coned view of a PA film of the chest shows a nodule greater than 1 cm in diameter in the medial portion of the subapical region of the right upper lobe. It was not clearly identified on a lateral view. The patient had no symptoms referable to the chest. There were no old chest films for comparison.

(D) Limited CT scan of this region done to localize the nodule and determine whether it was calcified. The nodule is actually a focus of sclerosis in the medial end of the clavicle — a benign bone island. It is seen very well on the top scan, but a small portion is still seen on the bottom scan made 1.0 cm caudad.

CT scans are not necessary to prove that this nodule is in bone and not in lung, but the outcome is graphic, leaves no doubt, and requires little time or excessive cost if the study is limited to the region in question. Fluoroscopy or stereoscopic views could have accomplished the same objective, however.

These CT scans were photographed at settings that accentuate bone detail. Compare the appearances of the medial ends of the clavicles.

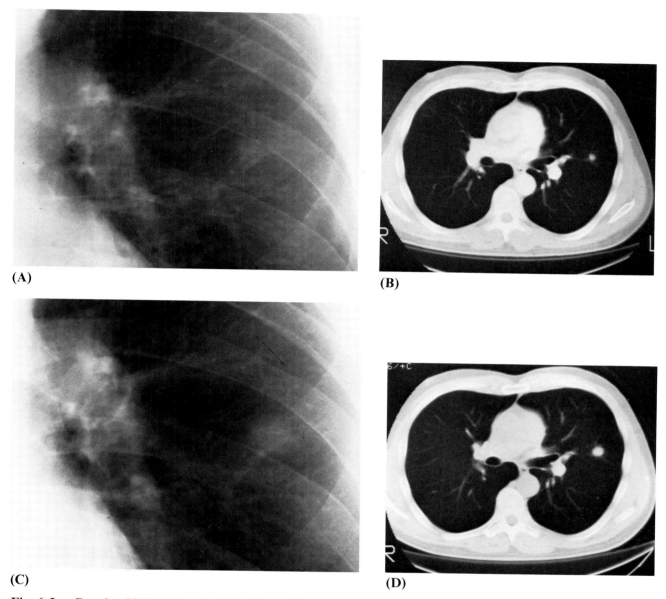

(A)

(B)

(C)

(D)

Fig. 6-2. Growing Nodule Due to Histoplasmosis

(A) Coned view of the midzone of the left lung of a 56-year-old man who was undergoing workup for suspected coronary artery disease. The nodule was an incidental finding. He had no symptoms of lung disease. The nodule has poorly defined margins.

(B) CT scan shows the nodule well. It produces a much stronger signal in relation to the background than the lesion seen on the chest film. The entire chest was scanned and no other nodules were seen.

(C) Coned view of the area in Fig. A 2 months laters. The nodule has grown.

(D) CT scan 2 months after the scan in Fig. B. It confirms that there has been an increase in the size of the nodule, from 0.9 cm to more than 1.5 cm. Again the complete series showed no other nodules. (Assuming the lesion is spherical, what is the change in volume?)

The nodule was removed; it was a necrotizing granuloma with large numbers of *Histoplasma* organisms seen on GMS stain.

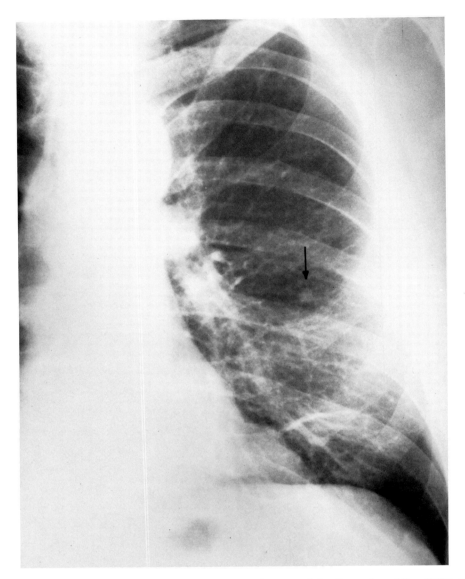

Fig. 6-3. **New Nodule Due to Adenocarcinoma of the Lung in a Man With Prior Seminoma of the Testicle**

This 57-year-old man had had an orchiectomy for seminoma approximately 6 years before this chest film was made. He had been receiving regular follow-up, including chest films, and now a new nodule is seen in the left midlung (arrow). The nodule is less than 1 cm in diameter. Fortunately, it is not hidden by superimposed ribs, and it is clearly distinguished from surrounding vessels. On other films made at the same time, however, the lesion was difficult to see because it was hidden by overlapping rib and vessel shadows.

Overlapping anatomic structures probably account for many peripheral nodular neoplasms being missed or misinterpreted on chest radiographs. Comparison with earlier films is extremely helpful in determining that a small opacity is a new abnormality rather than a normal anatomic structure.

Full-lung tomograms were done to confirm the location of the nodule and to search for other nodules; none were seen. In many imaging centers, CT examinations have replaced tomograms for evaluation of pulmonary nodules. This nodule was removed and was diagnosed as a well-differentiated adenocarcinoma. Ten hilar and mediastinal lymph nodes were removed, and all were negative for tumor.

Incidentally, there is a small fat pad next to the heart. The crossed band shadows in the adjacent lung are peripheral atelectases or scars.

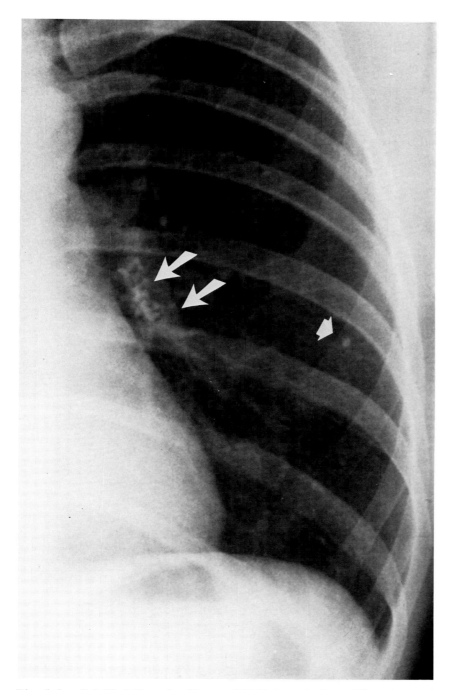

Fig. 6-4. Calcified Complex Due to Old Tuberculosis or Histoplasmosis

Coned view of the left lung of a 51-year-old woman who was being followed after treatment for carcinoma of the breast 4 years before. A nodule about 2 to 3 mm in diameter is superimposed on the anterior left fifth rib (short arrow). It is very dense for its size. It is too big to be a vessel seen end-on this far peripherally in the lung.

This is a common appearance for a small, calcified granuloma due to tuberculosis or histoplasmosis (some people may have nodular residuals of both). Also, there are clustered, stippled foci of high density in the left hilum — a common appearance for calcifications in hilar lymph nodes consequent to tuberculosis or histoplasmosis (paired arrows).

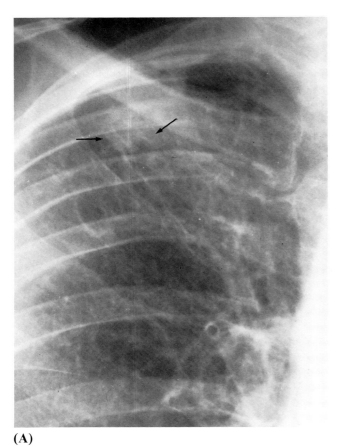

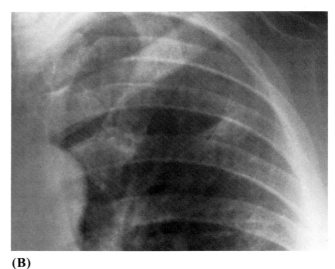

(A)   (B)

Fig. 6-5.   (A) Spiculated Nodule Due to Squamous Cell Carcinoma

This 63-year-old man had been having intermittent interscapular spine pain for many years following a fall from a horse. A recent episode of recurrent, but somewhat different, pain prompted him to seek medical aid, and a chest film was made.

A nodule with irregular margins and peripheral spikes or spiculations is partly hidden by overlying bones in the right subclavicular region (arrows). This was confirmed by CT (not shown), which showed no other nodules and no enlarged hilar or mediastinal nodes. A chest film made 2 years before showed no nodule at this site, but there was some apical cap thickening that appeared stable.

The nodule was removed. Histopathologic study showed it to be a moderately well differentiated squamous cell carcinoma infiltrating into the surrounding pulmonary parenchyma, with a marked desmoplastic response. The remainder of the lobe showed scarring and cystic changes.

(B–E) Nodule With Linear Extensions and Slow Growth (Bronchoalveolar Carcinoma)

(B) Coned view of the left upper zone of patient's chest radiograph. A small, flame-shaped opacity is superimposed partly upon the anterior first interspace and partly on the adjacent anterior second rib. It is a subtle lesion that could easily be missed or, if seen, dismissed as a scar. In fact, since the patient had a positive tuberculin test, it was considered a strong possibility that this lesion represented the residual of a tuberculous infection. The patient was asymptomatic, and there were no earlier films for comparison. He was advised, however, to have further studies, which he did not elect to have at the time. *(Figure continues.)*

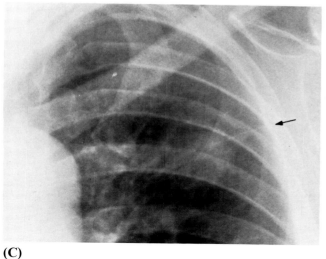

(C)

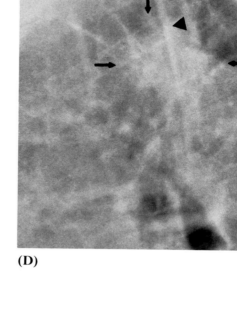

(D)

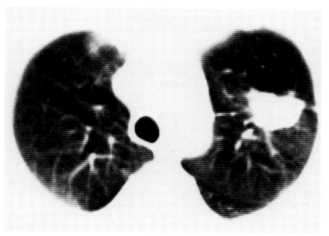

(E)

Fig. 6-5. *(Continued).* **(C)** Coned PA view of the same region of the lung 6 years after Fig. B. The patient had no symptoms referable to the chest. The lesion is larger but still very poorly defined. It appears to be of low density and has margins that blend imperceptibly with adjacent lung. Note, however, that there is a fine linear band that continues laterally from the lesion to the chest wall (arrow).

(D) Lateral view made at the same time as Fig. C. The opacity (arrows) has more visible bulk here than on the PA view. Its margins in this projection are also very poorly defined and appear spiculated. Although this nodule is superimposed on the aortic arch, the trachea, and one of the scapulae, (arrowheads), it can still be easily identified.

(E) CT scan. Notice how obvious the lesion appears on the CT scan compared to the chest films. Because of the increased sensitivity to differences in tissue density inherent in the CT technique, the lesion stands out from the adjacent lung.

The CT scan also shows a short linear band that radiates from the lesion to the lateral chest wall and another from the lesion to the mediastinum.

The rather indolent progress of this neoplasm is part of the spectrum of behavior of bronchoalveolar cell tumors. This neoplasm might be considered as a "scar" neoplasm in that the neoplasm grew in an area of lung scarring. On the other hand, many neoplasms are associated with the production of foci of fibrous reaction and are indistinguishable from so-called scars; therefore, it is very difficult to prove that any given carcinoma of the lung is truly a scar carcinoma.

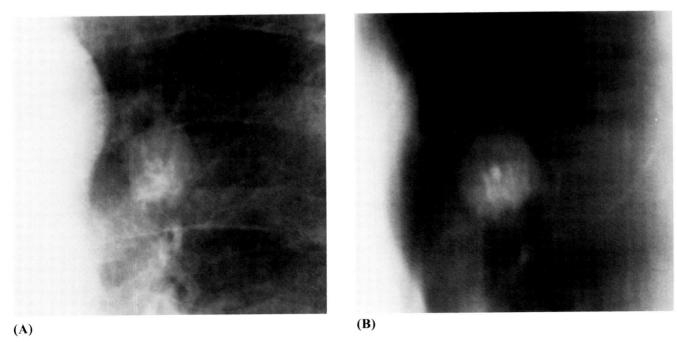

(A)   **(B)**

Fig. 6-6.   Hamartoma With Stippled (Popcorn) Calcification

(A) This nodule lateral to the aortic arch and above the left pulmonary artery was an incidental finding on chest films of a man who had had a spontaneous pneumothorax on the right side.

(B) Tomographic scan shows a central calcified nidus and smaller stippled foci of calcification within the nodule. These findings are quite reliable as signs of a benign lesion. Nevertheless, the patient and his physicians elected to have the nodule removed. It was a hamartoma as was predicted from the radiographic findings.

The tomogram confirms the presence of calcific foci within the nodule and prevents an interpretive error that occurs when vessel images either in front or behind the nodule simulate dense foci within the nodule on chest films. Spot films obtained in multiple projections at fluoroscopy would also serve this purpose.

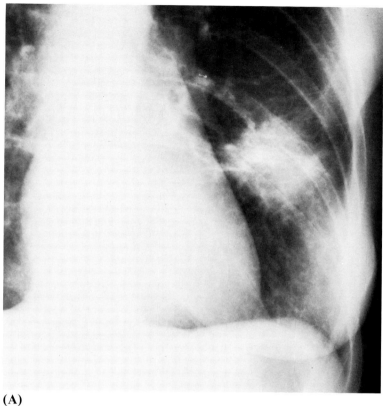

(A)

Fig. 6-7. Partial Clearing of Perifocal Inflammatory Changes Associated With Carcinoma of the Lung

(A,B) Coned views of the left lower lobe of a 70-year-old woman who had fallen and fractured her right hip and right arm. The chest films were made as part of a routine preoperative workup. There is a large, rounded lesion in the left lower lobe that has poorly defined, irregular margins, inhomogeneous internal architecture, and linear extensions to the pleural surfaces both posteriorly and laterally. Because of the urgency of her fractures it was elected to defer the investigation of the pulmonary lesion until she recovered from surgery. *(Figure continues.)*

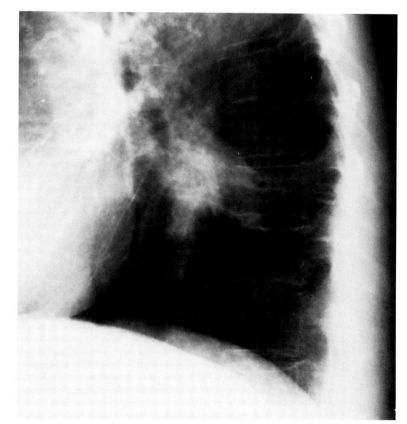

(B)

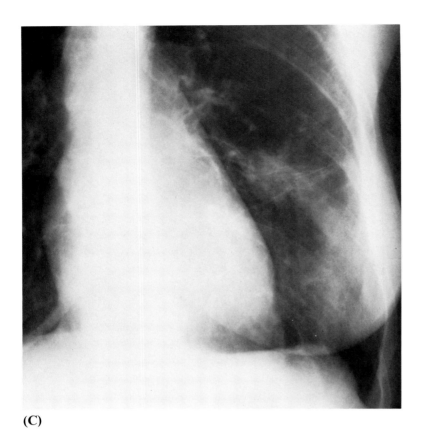

(C)

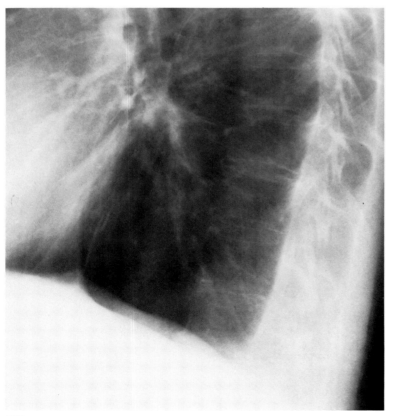

(D)

Fig. 6-7. *(Continued).* **(C,D)** Coned views of the patient's left lower lung 4 months later. There has been a remarkable decrease in size of the consolidation, but a significant residual remains, including the extensions to the pleura. The patient had had an intermittent cough and intermittent hemoptyses over the preceding 6 months. *(Figure continues.)*

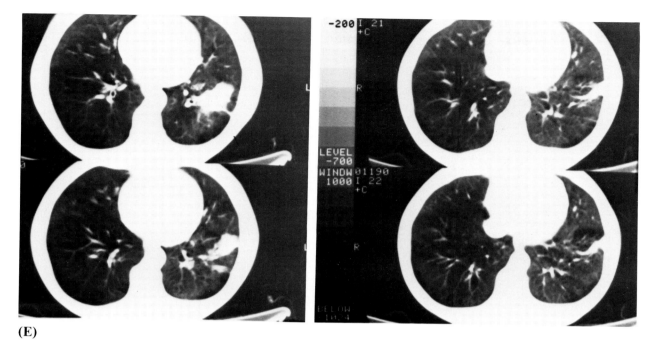

(E)

Fig. 6-7. *(Continued).*   (E) CT scans made a short time before Figs. C and D. The left lower lobe mass is very easy to recognize. The sequential scans confirm that portions of the lesion extend to and are intimately associated with the pleural surfaces along the lateral and posterolateral chest wall.

Under fluoroscopic guidance a biopsy was obtained through a bronchoscope, and the diagnosis of carcinoma was confirmed. A left lower lobectomy was performed. The lesion was a well-differentiated squamous cell carcinoma arising from a small bronchus, extending along multiple bronchi, and producing an obstructive pneumonitis along with focal abscess in the adjacent parenchyma. Pleural fibrosis was found in the specimen, but no actual pleural invasion by neoplasm. All of the removed nodes were negative for tumor.

This case illustrates a few important points: First, even peripheral neoplasms involving the lung may have both neoplastic and inflammatory components due to partial obstruction of small airways by the neoplasm. The abnormality may be seen to undergo partial resolution (reduction in volume) as the inflammatory components decrease. In my experience, this behavior is more common in cases of bronchoalveolar cell tumor, and it is rare in a squamous cell carcinoma such as that shown here.

Second, a lesion that is contiguous with or appears inseparable from another portion of the anatomy such as the pleural surfaces, the mediastinum, or adjacent bones has not necessarily invaded those structures. Clear invasion may be detectable, particularly on CT scans, when a lesion completely transgresses the chest wall or mediastinum and goes through multiple fat planes. That is not the same thing as having the lesion contiguous with and inseparable from those structures, in which case you cannot predict whether a dissection plane free of neoplasm is present or not.

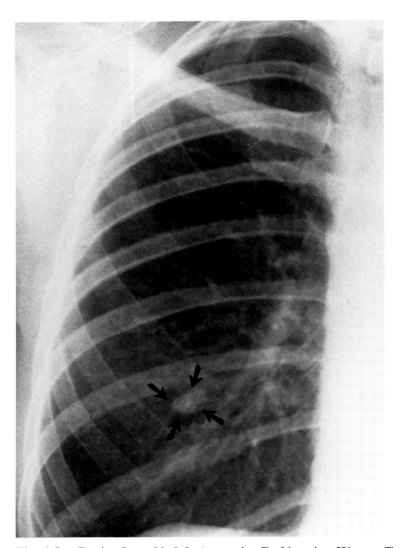

Fig. 6-8.   Benign Lung Nodule Appearing De Novo in a Woman Treated for Carcinoma of the Breast

Coned view of the right lung of a woman who had been treated for carcinoma of the breast 4 years before demonstrates a nodule measuring greater than 1 cm in the right lung (arrows). It was not present on a film made 3 years before. She had no other evidence of recurrent breast carcinoma and no symptoms referable to the chest. The nodule was removed and the histopathologic diagnosis was leiomyoma or possible hamartoma.

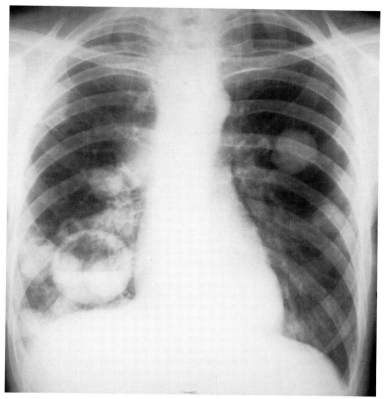

Fig. 6-9. Sharply Circumscribed Nodular Metastases From Undifferentiated Carcinoma of the Thyroid

The nodules seen in the left midlung zone are very sharply defined. On the original films the several nodules in the right lung were also sharply defined. From the PA and lateral views one could actually have counted them had one wished to do so. Besides the solid nodules there are also cavitary lesions. The cavitating mass adjacent to the right heart border has a long fluid level. Cavitary metastases are most commonly due to squamous cell carcinomas, but any type of neoplasm can cavitate.

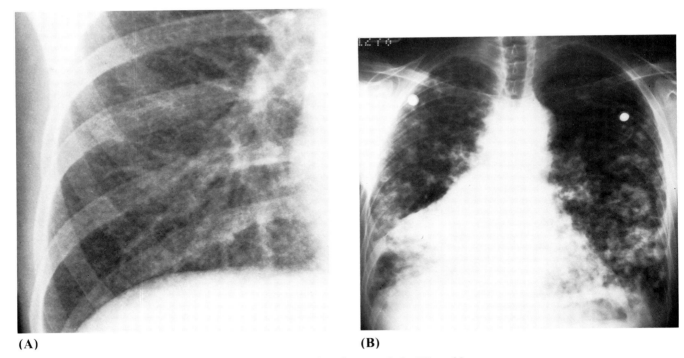

(A)   **(B)**

Fig. 6-10.   **(A) Miliary Nodular Metastases From Carcinoma of the Thyroid**

Coned view of the right lower lobe of a child who is being followed for a known carcinoma of the thyroid with miliary metastases to the lung. There are very small nodular opacities distributed throughout the visualized portions of the lung. They obliterate the details of the smaller vessels and are so numerous that one would not consider counting them.

Miliary metastases to the lungs may occur infrequently from a variety of solid tumors, among which carcinoma of the thyroid is one of the most frequent. However, the more common causes of miliary lesions in the lung are the infectious granulomatous diseases, *Pneumocystis carinii* pneumonia, and viral pneumonia. Uncommonly, fungal pneumonias such as those due to cryptococcosis or to the parasite *Toxoplasma* may produce similar appearances. Rarely, some of the bacterial pneumonias have been reported to present with an indistinguishable radiographic appearance.

If one looks long and hard enough, it seems that there are very few lung abnormalities that may not have a miliary pattern as part of their radiographic spectrum, depending on how one defines "miliary" (see Ch. 5).

(B) Extensive Pulmonary Metastases From Large Cell Undifferentiated Carcinoma of a Bronchus

This 43-year-old man had a 5-month history of hoarseness and a 2-month history of shortness of breath and dyspnea on exertion. He was otherwise well. He had reportedly been seen elsewhere and had a lower lobe opacity that lasted at least 4 months. He now has a right vocal cord paralysis.

Bronchoscopic biopsy of a lesion in the right bronchus intermedius revealed a large cell undifferentiated infiltrating carcinoma. This entity usually presents as a parenchymal mass, and much less commonly as a lesion originating in a central bronchus.

This PA view of the chest shows a large zone of opacification and reduction in volume of the right middle and lower lobes. There are also multiple irregular nodules and small masses distributed throughout both lungs.

This case is an example of a bronchogenic carcinoma that presents with multiple pulmonary metastases at the time of initial diagnosis. It is an unusual presentation that is probably related to the delay in diagnosis in this patient. (The very dense nodular shadows in both subclavicular regions represent surface EKG leads.)

Fig. 6-11.   (A) Multiple Hamartomas

PA view of the right side of the chest of a middle-aged woman. The fairly large nodules seen laterally at the level of the anterior third and fifth interspaces were incidental findings on this preoperative chest film. After a brief negative workup, the patient underwent a thoracotomy. In addition to the two large nodules, a dime-sized, flat lesion was found on the posterior surface of the right lower lobe, and a 5-mm lesion along the posterior visceral pleura at the right apex. All four lesions were hamartomas.

Hamartomas are tumors that probably have their origin in embryologic development and contain the same cellular elements that are present in the organ of origin. The majority of them are seen in adults, and they may be found de novo even in patients who have had previous high-quality radiographs on which a nodule was not visible. Most hamartomas are small nodules, but lesions as large as 8.0 cm have been reported. Calcified hamartomas are seldom removed surgically because the calcified foci within them identify them as benign.

Multiple hamartomas are uncommon, and this patient is quite unusual. Multiple noncalcified hamartomas are radiologically indistinguishable from pulmonary metastases. *(Figure continues.)*

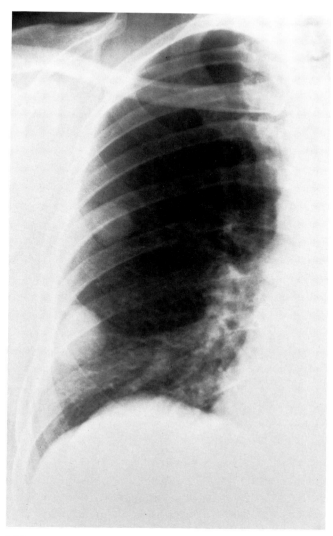

(A)

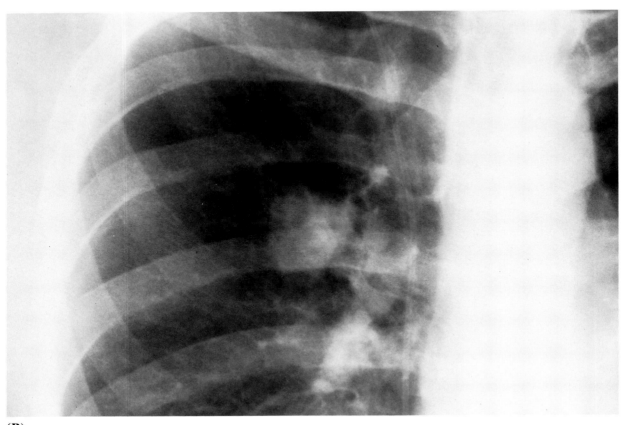

(B)

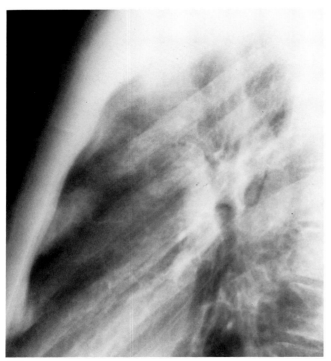

(C)

Fig. 6-11. *(Continued).* **(B,C) Arteriovenous Malformation Associated With Brain Abscess**

(B) Coned view of the right upper lung of a 21-year-old man who developed stiff neck, papilledema, and a fever to 102°F. He became comatose. A head CT scan showed an enhancing lesion in the thalamus. He was also noted to have an erythrocytosis with a hematocrit of 63. His nail beds were cyanotic.

There is an irregular nodule measuring approximately 3 cm in diameter in the medial portions of the right subclavicular region. The margins are not sharply defined and no calcification is seen.

(C) Lateral view. The lesion is very poorly defined, partly because it is superimposed on the anterior ends of the ribs. It appears as a vague area of increased tissue density projected just behind the sternal angle of Louis and the subjacent anterior rib. A pulmonary arteriogram was done (not shown), and the lesion was proven to be an arteriovenous (AV) malformation.

Brain abscesses due to shunts through pulmonary arteriovenous malformations are a recognized complication of this lesion. The persistent hypoxemia (PO_2 of 65 mmHg), the nail bed cyanosis, and the high hematocrit are due to the venous admixture from this AV shunt.

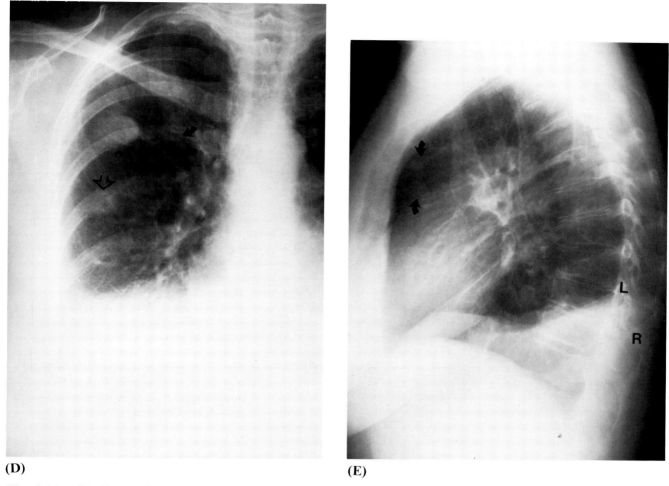

(D)   **(E)**

Fig. 6-11.   (D–I) Arteriovenous Malformations With Pleural Hemorrhage

Approximately 6 days before this examination, this 45-year-old woman with Rendu-Osler-Weber syndrome went to her doctor because she had developed pleuritic chest pain. Chest films and physical examination revealed that the patient had a right pleural effusion, which was determined upon thoracentesis to be a hemothorax.

(D) PA view shows an elongated or oval nodular opacity in the right subclavicular region, and two very large vessels are seen curving from the right hilum toward this nodule (black arrows).

At the level of the posterior right seventh rib there is another faint nodular opacity (open arrow). The diaphragm is effaced and the costophrenic angle obliterated by the residual right pleural effusion (hemothorax).

(E) Lateral view. The right pleural fluid is evident. The nodular opacities are subtle, but two are seen in the retrosternal region. One is projected posterior to the sternal angle of Louis and the other is caudal to it (arrows). *(Figure continues.)*

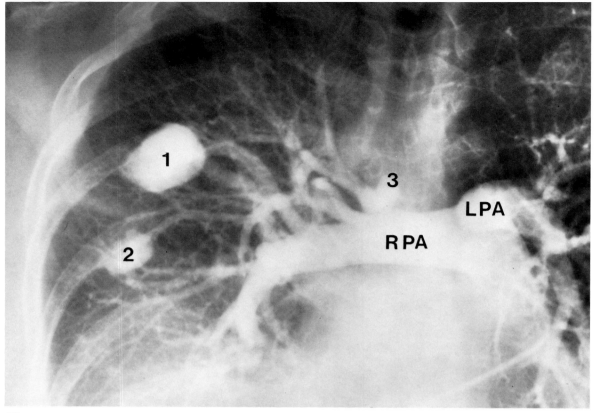

(F)

Fig. 6-11. *(Continued).* **(F)** Coned view of the pulmonary arterial phase of an arteriogram. Three pulmonary AV malformations are seen (1 – 3); 1 and 2 correspond to the lesions seen on the PA chest view, and 3 is a small AV malformation projected over the spine. It is totally obscured on the PA view of the chest.

Ordinarily, one superior branch arises from the undivided portions of the right pulmonary artery (RPA) as it passes through the mediastinum. In this patient, however, there are at least four branches. Two large branches course to the first pulmonary AV. Branch vessels from both the pars interlobaris and one of the anomalous upper lobe branches supply the second AV malformation, and the third is probably supplied by the first branch off the right pulmonary artery.

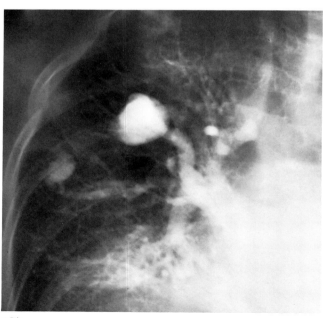

(G)

(G) Pulmonary arteriogram made during the venous filling phase, although there is still some contrast material seen in branches of the pulmonary artery. A large draining vein is seen associated with AV malformation 1, and a vein is also seen passing from the inferior aspect of the second malformation back toward the hilum. If you review the vessels seen in the arterial phase, you can also see these draining veins. They are filled early because of the extremely rapid flow through the low-pressure circuit of the malformations. Malformation 3 is not included on this reproduction. *(Figure continues.)*

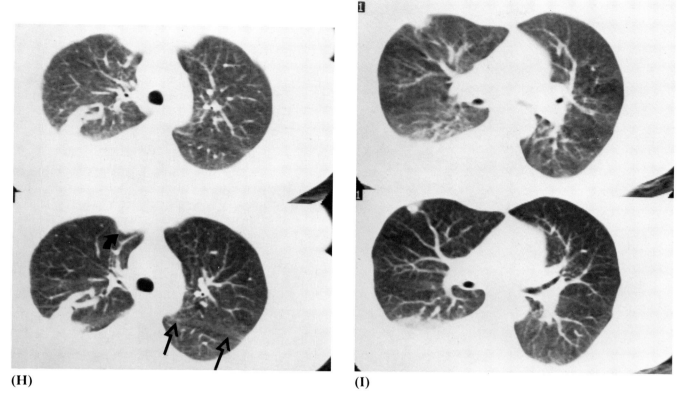

(H)   **(I)**

Fig. 6.11. *(Continued).* **(H,I)** CT scans. **(H)** A large AV malformation located in lung against the posterior chest wall on the right. Two large vessels extend from it toward the right hilum. This is malformation 1 and is probably the lesion responsible for the hemothorax.

In Fig. E one cannot locate this lesion with certainty, even in retrospect. The lesion seen anteriorly on the lateral view is malformation 2. Malformation 3, which is seen medially on the arteriogram, is also far anterior in the lung. In Fig. H its edge is seen projected into the right lung from the anterior chest wall (curved arrow). On films exposed with different window and level settings it was shown to better advantage.

As an anatomic exercise, note the faint bandlike shadow of the left major interlobar fissure (open arrows) and a small portion of its counterpart on the right side (not marked). At this height in the chest, the fissures are oriented so that their lateral ends are posterior to their medial ends.

(I) CT scans made at the level of malformation 2, also located far anteriorly. A large feeding vessel passes from the hilum to the lesion. At this level, the increased opacification of the posterior portions of the right hemithorax compared to the left is due to layering of pleural fluid against the posterior chest wall with the patient in the supine position.

These scans show the anatomic positions of the lesions much better than either the chest films or the pulmonary arteriograms. Malformation 1 is obscure on the lateral view of the chest, and its posterior location is not appreciated on the angiogram because lateral views were not made. In patients with suspected AV malformations, it is important to perform pulmonary arteriography because lesions that are cryptic or not seen at all on the plain-film studies may become apparent on the arteriographic studies. (Pulmonary angiograms courtesy of Dr. Martin Spellman, Fremont, California.)

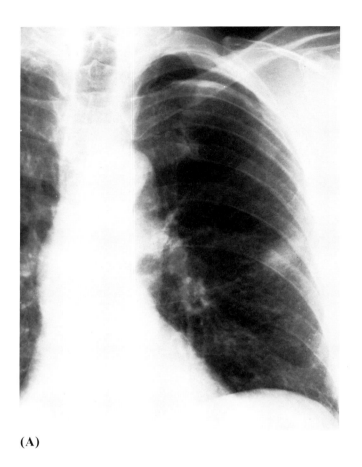

(A)

Fig. 6-12. Adenocarcinoma

(A) Coned view of the chest shows a flame-shaped nodular opacity with very poorly defined margins in the lateral aspect of the left lung. There is no visible hilar or mediastinal lymphadenopathy.

(B) CT scans of the same patient. The parenchymal lesion appears poorly defined and has irregular margins just as it does on the chest film. From its position on the CT scan, the lesion is located in the junctional region between the anterolateral aspects of the superior segment of the left lower lobe and the posterolateral aspects of the superior division of the lingula of the left upper lobe. It may transgress the major fissure to involve both of these segments. The upper right scan shows the takeoff of the superior segmental bronchus from the left lower lobe bronchus (the central portions of the left main bronchus are still visible).

As a peripheral lesion this meets our expectations for an adenocarcinoma of the lung. This diagnosis was confirmed by needle aspiration under fluoroscopic guidance. (In A, see the thickened visceral pleura visible over the left third posterior rib because of an induced pneumothorax.) No mediastinal or hilar lymphadenopathy was detected on the complete CT examination. From the radiographic standpoint, this patient seems to be a good candidate for curative resection. Unfortunately CT of the head demonstrated multiple masses in the brain, presumably metastases.

Of incidental anatomic interest is the very thin anterior junction line on the upper three scans. It becomes slightly thicker on the most caudal scan (bottom right). This appearance is due to deposition of fat in the caudal recesses of the anterior mediastinum.

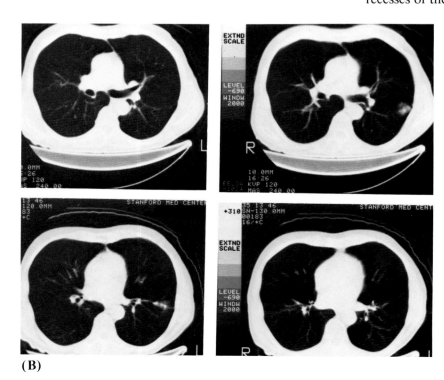

(B)

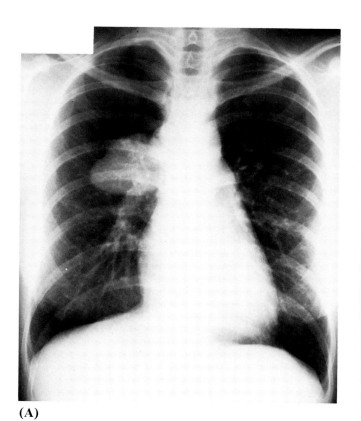

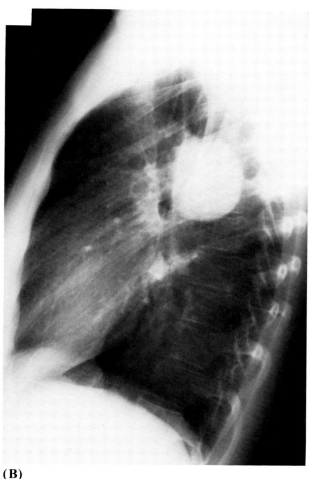

(A)   (B)

Fig. 6-13. Hemangiopericytoma of the Lung

The patient is a 31-year-old woman who had an expiratory wheeze. She coughed up some particulate matter, put it in the freezer, and several weeks later brought it to the clinic. It was sent for pathologic study, and a diagnosis of spindle cell mesenchymal neoplasm was made with the comment that there was not enough tissue to characterize the neoplasm more precisely. The diagnosis was confirmed by bronchoscopy and biopsy of the right upper lobe mass.

(A,B) PA and lateral views, respectively, both show a large, slightly polylobulated mass immediately posterior to the right hilum. The right side of the mediastinum is also abnormal in the region of the azygos node and azygos vein. At operation, an abnormally large azygos vein was found, but there were no metastases to the mediastinal nodes from this hemangiopericytoma.

The larger hemangiopericytomas that are primary in the lungs often prove to be malignant. Although uncommon pulmonary lesions, they characteristically present as solid centrally located masses with sharp margins. However, these characteristics do not really distinguish them from bronchogenic carcinomas.

Hemangiopericytomas may also occur anywhere in the body, and those that are malignant may metastasize to the lungs.

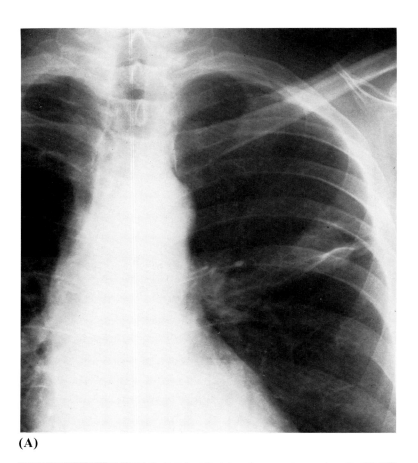

(A)

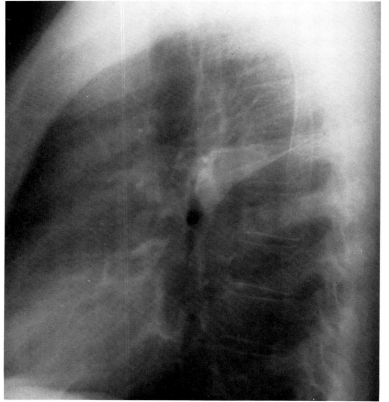

(B)

Fig. 6-14. Small Intrabronchial Squamous Cell Carcinoma With Obstructive Pneumonitis

(A) Coned PA view of the left lung showing a low-density, oval zone of consolidation in the axillary region, with some dense band shadows extending both laterally and medially. The hilum and mediastinum appear normal.

(B) Lateral view shows a pie-shaped zone of consolidation extending posteriorly from the hilum and tapering peripherally. The very sharp posteroinferior margin of this zone conforms to the major interlobar fissure. Judging from its location on both views, this consolidation is in the axillary subsegment of the apicoposterior segment of the left upper lobe. *(Figure continues.)*

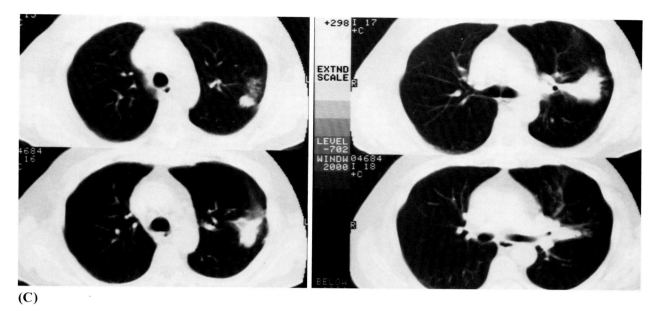

(C)

Fig. 6-14. *(Continued).* **(C)** CT scans showing components of this lesion (read from top left to bottom left, to top right, to bottom right). At the level of the carina (top right), a bronchus is seen end-on in the left hilum (the apical subsegment of the apicoposterior segment of the left upper lobe. Slightly more caudally (bottom right), the left main bronchus is seen extending laterally from the carina with a branch of the upper lobe bronchus (past the takeoff of the apical subsegment) disappearing into the lesion.

The patient underwent bronchoscopy. An endobronchial lesion was biopsied and determined to be a squamous cell carcinoma. The surgical specimen was a $1.2 \times 0.8 \times 0.5$ cm exophytic bronchial tumor causing obstruction, with chronic pneumonia in the lung peripherally. Thus, the bulk of the radiographically visible lesion is the inflammatory process beyond the small neoplasm. Some patients with obstructive pneumonitis have symptoms of acute bacterial pneumonia, whereas others with chronic pneumonitis — without bacterial infection — may have few signs or symptoms.

It is important to consider an endobronchial lesion as a possible cause of a segmental or subsegmental consolidation in order to include bronchoscopy as a diagnostic procedure when clinically warranted. A needle aspiration biopsy of the parenchymal consolidation in this case could have been misleading.

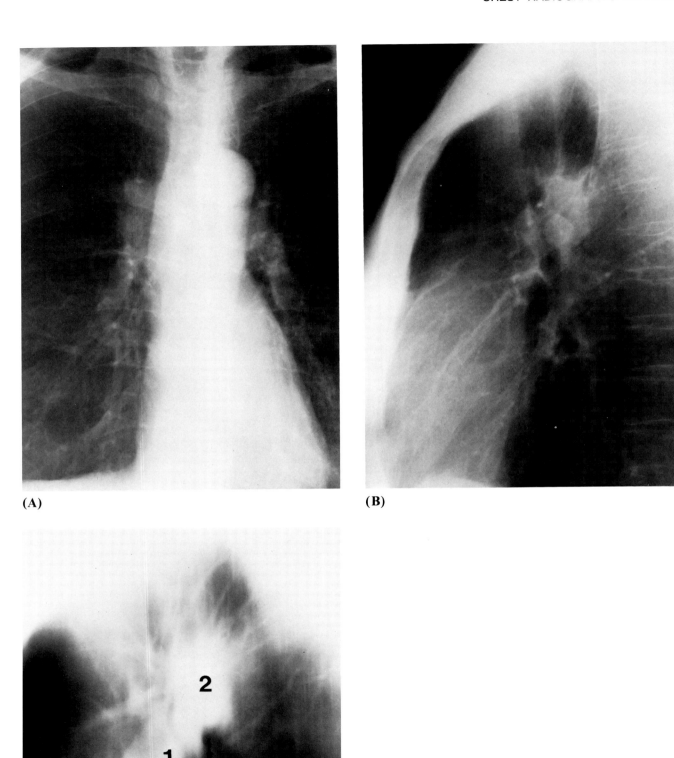

(A)

(B)

(C)

Fig. 6-15. *(Legend on p. 337.)*

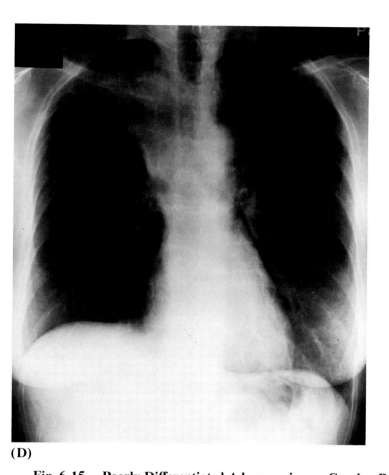

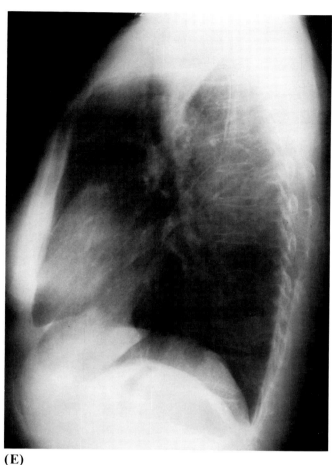

(D)   (E)

Fig. 6-15.   Poorly Differentiated Adenocarcinoma Causing Bronchial Obstruction

(A,B) PA and lateral projections, respectively, show a right hilar and suprahilar mass. On the lateral projection, a portion of the mass is seen to intrude upon the airway.

(C) Lateral tomographic scan confirms the location of the mass. Notice (1) the right pulmonary artery and (2) the tumor mass, which narrows the airway a centimeter or so above the level of the takeoff of the middle lobe bronchus (oblique arrow) and the superior segment of the lower lobe (vertical arrow). Thus, the mass affects both the right main bronchus and the bronchus intermedius. Complex central masses often represent the combined effect of the primary neoplasm and extension to local lymph nodes.

(D,E) One month later there is now atelectasis and consolidation of the right upper lobe due to bronchial obstruction. (D) PA view shows a sharp interface between the lower border of the atelectatic upper lobe and the adjacent overexpanded middle lobe at the minor interlobar fissure. (E) On lateral view there is a very sharp interface between the atelectatic upper lobe and the overexpanded superior segment of the lower lobe at the major interlobar fissure. *(Figure continues.)*

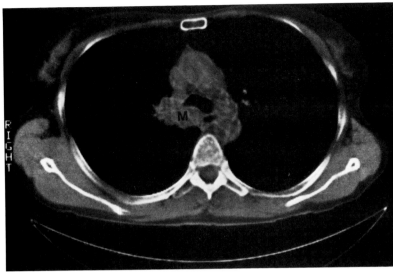

(F)

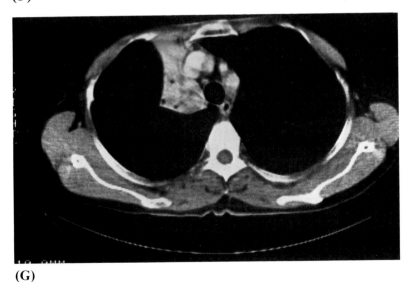

(G)

Fig. 6-15. *(Continued).* **(F)** CT scan at a level just above the transverse aortic arch. The atelectatic right upper lobe is located anteriorly and medially against the mediastinum. At this level the major fissure marks the interface between atelectatic and aerated lung. There is a sharp angle at the posterolateral aspect of the atelectatic lung. Displaced bronchi are seen as air-containing, fairly sharply defined structures within the atelectatic lung.

(G) CT scan at the level of the tracheal bifurcation. It shows marked indentation of the airway at the takeoff of the right upper lobe bronchus, and an irregular mass (M) extends laterally and posteriorly. The oval lucency behind the airway represents air in the esophagus.

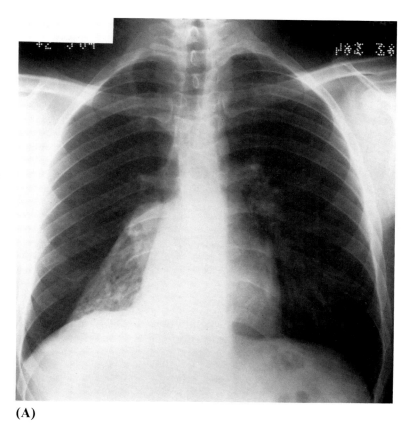

(A)

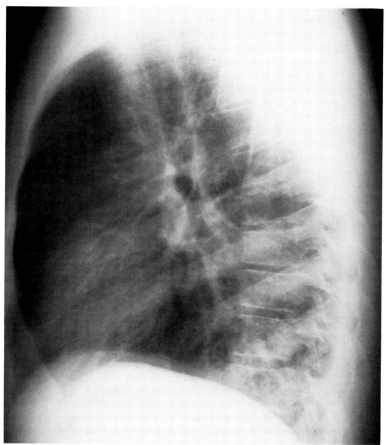

(B)

Fig. 6-16. Carcinoid Tumor of the Bronchus Intermedius

The patient is a 25-year-old man with a history of repeated bouts of pneumonia in the right lower lobe.

(A) PA view demonstrating right lower lobe collapse. The major fissure has moved posteromedially and rotated so that it presents a tangent to the x-ray beam. It accounts for the sharp lateral edge of the collapsed basilar segments. Air bronchograms are still visible within the atelectatic lower lobe.

(B) Lateral view shows the right lower lobe atelectasis as well. The posterior third of the right hemidiapragm image is effaced by the air space consolidation in the contracted lower lobe, and the gray tones over the posterior aspect of the chest are inappropriate. *(Figure continues.)*

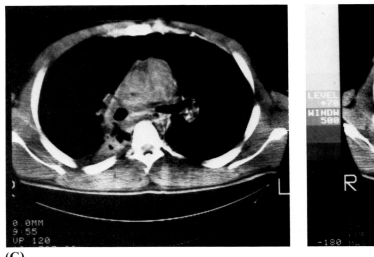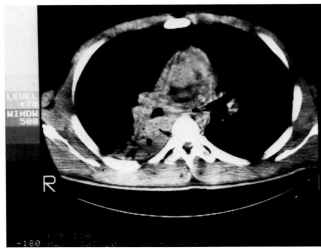

(C)

Fig. 6-16. *(Continued).* **(C)** CT scans of the chest through the level of the bronchus intermedius. The image on the right is 1 cm caudal to that on the left. The consolidation and reduction in volume of the basilar segments of the right lower lobe and the posteromedial shift of the major interlobar fissure are seen well. Multiple black holes within the consolidation are dilated bronchi, which may be seen commonly in patients with acute pneumonitis. However, there is indentation of the posterior wall of the bronchus intermedius shortly past its origin (arrow), and a soft tissue mass extends posterior, medial and lateral to the bronchus intermedius.

At bronchoscopy a carcinoid tumor was found in the bronchus intermedius at the level of the origin of the right lower lobe bronchus. One hilar node and two subcarinal lymph nodes were positive for metastases at the time of a subsequent bilobectomy. However, enlarged lymph nodes may also be due to benign reactive changes from repeated or chronic infection in cases of obstructive pneumonitis peripheral to bronchial neoplasms.

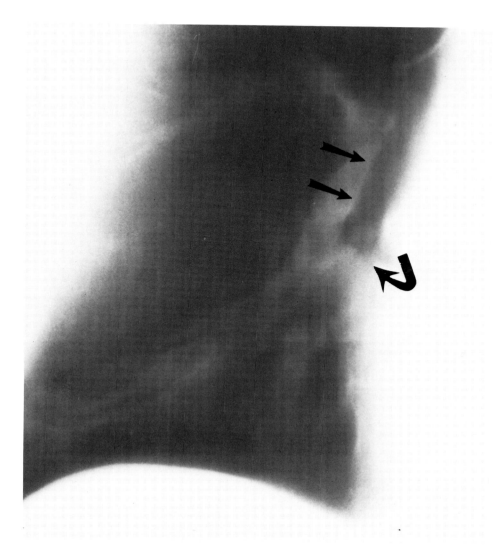

Fig. 6-17. Mucoepidermoid Tumor of the Bronchus Intermedius

Coned view of the distal bronchus intermedius (straight arrows) and the adjacent lung from a tomogram of a 40-year-old physician. Notice that the air column of the bronchus intermedius appears to end abruptly in a soft tissue mound that has an edge that is slightly convex upward (curved arrow). This is a rather characteristic appearance for an endobronchial tumor. It may be of any histopathologic variety, but it is one of the known common ways of presentation of bronchial gland carcinoma.

The study was prompted by one incident of hemoptysis while the patient was recovering from a right lower lobe pneumonia. The patient underwent bronchoscopy and chest surgery after discovery of this lesion, and a mucoepidermoid tumor was removed. The prognosis for this variant of neoplasm is good.

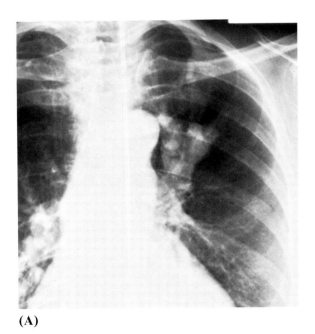

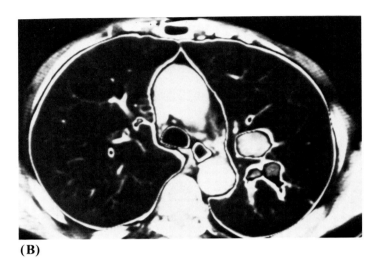

(A) **(B)**

Fig. 6-18. Squamous Cell Carcinoma and Mucoid Impaction of Bronchi

(A) Coned PA view of the left lung of a woman with squamous cell carcinoma. Thick, branching structures radiate into the lung from the superior portions of the left hilum. These are dilated bronchi filled partly with tumor and partly with mucus and inflammatory exudate beyond the obstructing neoplasm.

(B) CT scan of the same woman, displayed with an edge-enhancing technique. On the left side there are enormously dilated bronchi that contain a lumen-filling soft tissue. These represent the CT equivalent of the "stuffed" bronchi seen in the medial portions of the left upper lobe on the PA view.

Normal-caliber bronchi are seen on the right side as small rings with black centers. A normal bronchus is also seen anterior to the large, plugged bronchus on the left.

This appearance of stuffed bronchi may also be seen in patients who have bronchial atresia with impaction of mucus proximal to the site of obstruction, and in patients who have allergic bronchopulmonary aspergillosis or mucoid impaction from other causes. Bronchoscopy is often required to establish the correct diagnosis.

Usually an obstructing broncial lesion causes collapse of the segment or lobe involved. Distended bronchi are lost within the image of the collapse. However, peripheral lung units can remain aerated by collateral ventilation from adjacent unobstructed units through the pores of Kohn and the canals of Lambert. Hence, the distended bronchi remain visible because they are surrounded by aerated lung. (CT scan courtesy of Dr. Warren Becker, Fresno, California.)

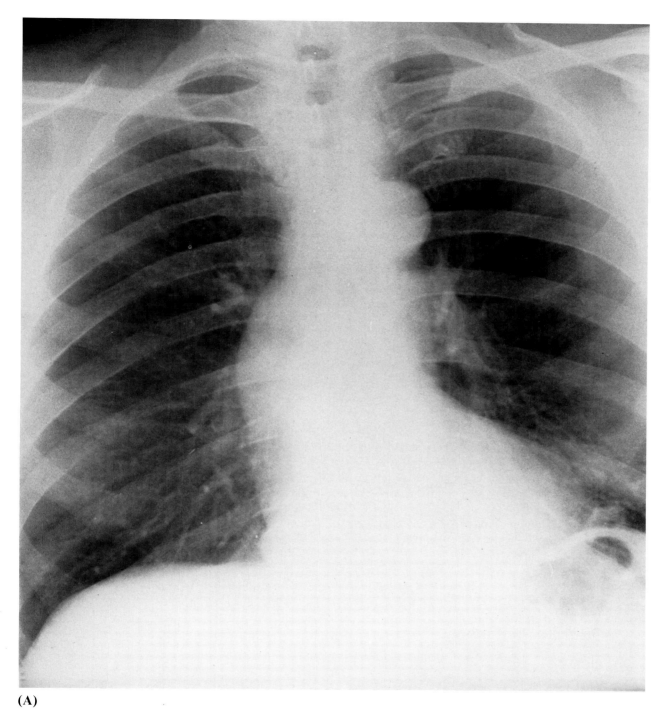

(A)

Fig. 6-19. Air Trapping as a Sign of Endobronchial Neoplasm

(A) PA view of the chest of a man with a carcinosarcoma of the left main bronchus. There is a subtle difference in film density between the right and left upper lung zones. The left side, particularly in the parahilar distribution, appears slightly blacker than the right. There is also a small, inhomogeneous area of consolidation in the lung adjacent to the left heart border, and a slight elevation of the left hemidiaphragm. The convex contour of the right side of the mediastinum is due to dilatation of the ascending aorta, which ordinarily is not border forming on the right side of the chest. *(Figure continues.)*

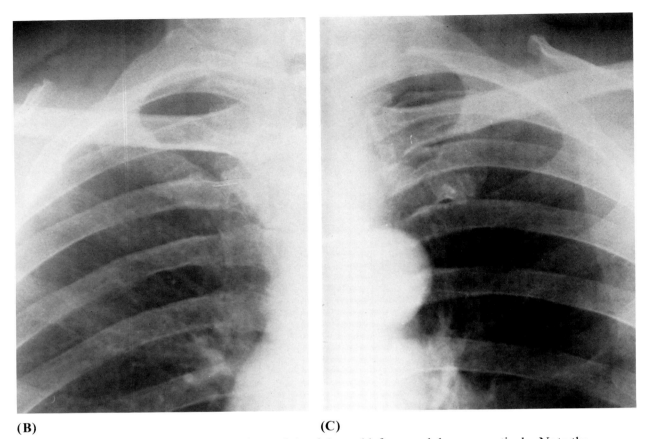

(B)   **(C)**

Fig. 6-19. *(Continued).* **(B,C)** Coned views of the right and left upper lobes, respectively. Note the difference in relative radiodensity. The films also show a relative reduction in the number and caliber of small vessels visible in the parahilar zones on the left side, indicating that the density differences are pathologic rather than technical. (Air trapping in the lung can be accentuated at fluoroscopy or on a chest film exposed after a maximum expiratory effort.) *(Figure continues.)*

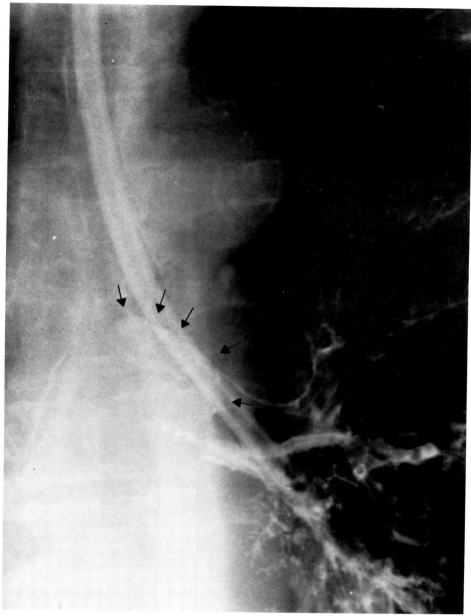

(D)

Fig. 6-19. *(Continued).* **(D)** Bronchogram. Unfortunately, the tube used to instill the contrast material has been passed beyond the rather long, sessile lesion seen along the inferomedial wall of the left main bronchus (arrows). This neoplasm caused the partial obstruction.

Patients with central, partially obstructing, bronchial lesions often give a history of a wheeze that they can hear themselves. Some patients can actually tell you from which side they think the sound is coming. On auscultation, wheezes may be heard in both inspiration and expiration.

Since the advent of fiberoptic bronchoscopy, bronchography is not necessary to diagnose obstructing bronchial neoplasms. A CT scan or tomograms or heavily exposed chest films would also have shown this lesion in the bronchus.

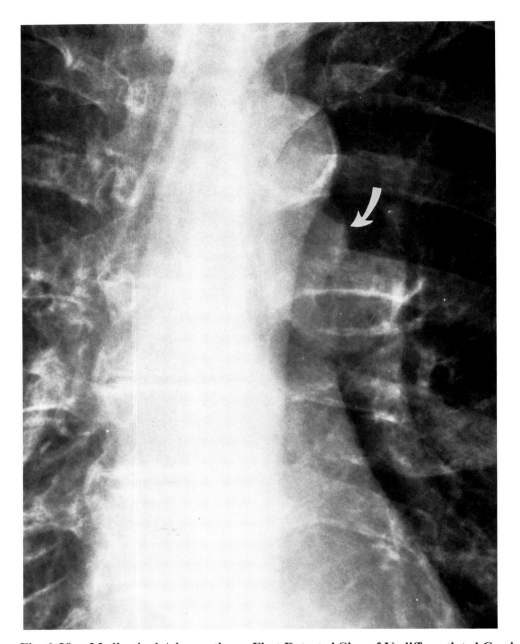

Fig. 6-20. Mediastinal Adenopathy as First Detected Sign of Undifferentiated Carcinoma

Coned view of the mediastinum of a patient with large cell undifferentiated carcinoma of the lung. A small mass (arrow) distorts the mediastinal pleural reflection between the level of the aortic arch and the left pulmonary artery. This is a classic location for the ductus node. It was the discovery of this abnormality on the original radiographs that led to further investigation.

The primary lesion was not located. Clinically silent lung cancer may not be found until metastases have occurred. The patient was being evaluated for severe coronary artery disease, which he had, and the chest film was ordered because of that diagnosis. There were no symptoms of pulmonary disease at all. However, the patient had involuntarily lost 8 pounds over the preceding 4 months.

The diagnosis was made from biopsy of a left suprabronchial node. The ductus node itself is not retrievable ordinarily by the mediastinoscopy approach (see Ch. 7).

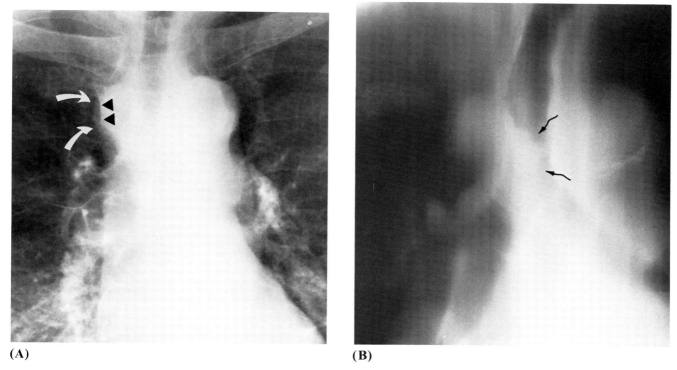

(A)   **(B)**

Fig. 6-21.   (A,B) Carcinoma of the Trachea Presenting as a Mediastinal Mass

(A) Coned view of the central portion of a PA chest film of a patient with carcinoma of the trachea. The technique used does not permit recognition of the intratracheal component of the patient's neoplasm. However, the convex contour of the right superior mediastinum (arrows), which extends lateral to the image of the manubrium (arrowheads) above the level of the azygos vein, is abnormal; it is indicative of a mediastinal mass or adenopathy.

(B) Tomogram at this level shows not only that the mass is inseparable from the right lateral wall of the trachea, but that there is also an intraluminal component (arrows) that partially obstructs the trachea above the level of the carina. The patient received high-dose radiation therapy to this squamous cell carcinoma of the trachea and 4 years later was doing well.

There is no way to tell whether the paratracheal component is due to adenopathy or to direct extension of the primary cancer. *(Figure continues.)*

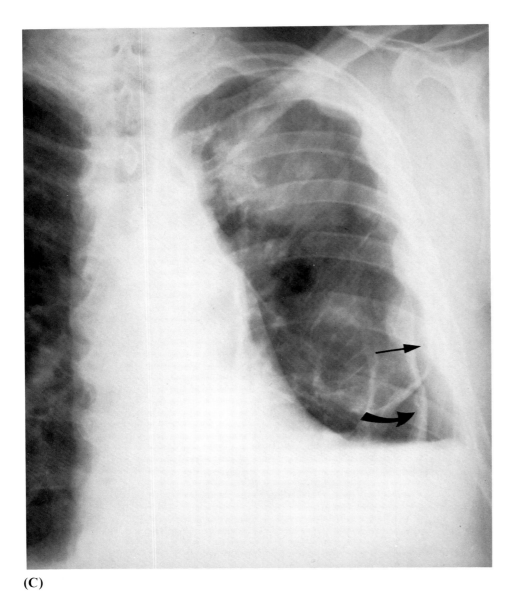

(C)

Fig. 6-21. *(Continued).* **(C) Pleural Metastases From Carcinoma of the Lung With Negative Pleural Fluid Cytology**

This 58-year-old man had a 2-month history of dyspnea. Chest films demonstrated a left upper lobe mass and a left pleural effusion. Thoracentesis on several occasions produced fluid negative for tumor cells on cytologic analysis.

There is a rounded mass in the left upper lobe and a lobulated pleural surface along the periphery of the lung. A residual hydropneumothorax with thickened visceral (curved arrow) and parietal (straight arrow) pleura is visible. Pleural biopsy showed undifferentiated squamous cell carcinoma involving the parietal pleural, with fibrin deposition on the visceral pleura.

A pleural or extrapleural mass or lobulated pleural surface seen in association with carcinoma of the lung is a strong indication of tumor spread. In such cases, pleural biopsy is indicated when pleural fluid samples are negative for malignant cells. A curative resection of lung carcinoma associated with distant pleural metastases is not feasible.

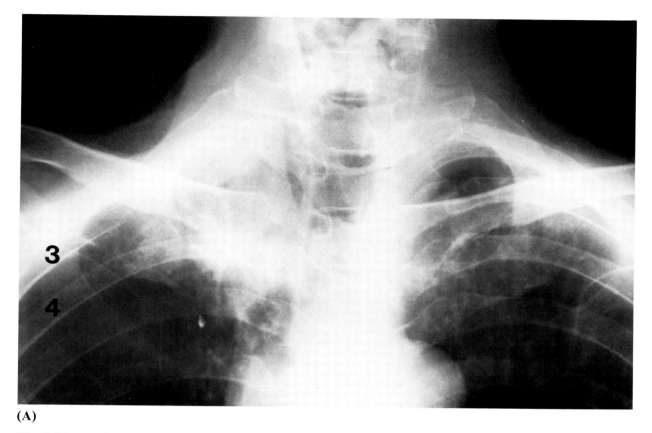

(A)

Fig. 6-22. Apical Mass With Bone Destruction—Pancoast Tumor

(A) Coned view of the upper third of the chest of a 54-year-old man with a history of intractable pain in the right shoulder of 6 months' duration. The tissue density of the right apex is much greater than that of the left, resulting in a lighter gray appearance.

If you scrutinize the bones, you can see that the posteromedial end of the right third rib (3) is no longer present (compare to the opposite side). Just beneath the middle of the right clavicle you see the axillary continuation of the third rib, but its posteromedial extremity is missing. Similarly, a portion of the posterior right second rib is missing, although its transverse process is present.

An apical mass in association with destruction of adjacent bones, usually ribs or vertebrae, is a common set of findings in patients with Pancoast tumor. The name does not imply a specific histopathologic subtype, but rather the location of the lesion. At this site squamous cell carcinoma is the most common, but any of the histologic varieties may occur in this region and warrant the name Pancoast tumor. Horner's syndrome is a common complication of Pancoast tumor, but its occurrence is not limited to such neoplasms. *(Figure continues.)*

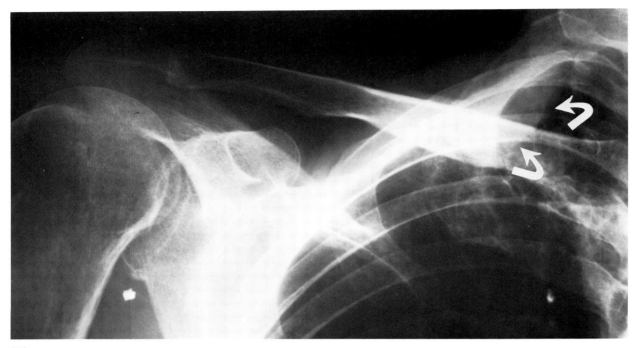

(B)

Fig. 6-22. *(Continued).* **(B)** AP radiograph of the right shoulder taken 9 months before Fig. A. An abnormal soft tissue mound is projected into the right apex. It is partly hidden by the superimposed image of the clavicle. Its visible interface with adjacent lung has an arc that is convex toward the lung (arrows). The overlying ribs are intact at the time of this film.

It is quite easy to underestimate the clinical significance of a lesion located in the apex by assuming it to be due to pleural thickening secondary to prior inflammatory disease, rather than considering the possibility of a mass in the pulmonary parenchyma immediately adjacent to the pleura. In this case the soft tissue component is not located in the extreme apex but is slightly more lateral. One edge is convex toward the lung.

The complaint of ipsilateral shoulder pain associated with even the most subtle apical mass should raise the possibility of Pancoast tumor as the cause.

Rarely, infection of the pulmonary apex with actinomycosis (and probably blastomycosis as well) can cause a radiographic appearance, including rib destruction, similar to that of Pancoast tumor. When there is also a fistulous tract to the skin from which the organisms can be retrieved, the distinction is simplified.

Multiple metallic foreign body densities seen in this patient in the soft tissues about the shoulder and medially in the subclavicular region have the appearance of particles of shrapnel.

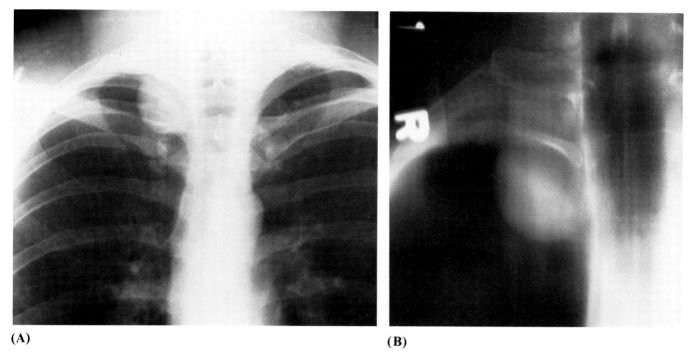

(A)　　　　　　　　　　　　　　　　　　　　　　　(B)

Fig. 6-23.　Neurolemmoma as an Apical Mass

(A) Coned view of the upper right chest. There is a mass in the apex, whose interface with the adjacent lung is very sharp. The interface with the chest wall cannot be defined. On the lateral view (not shown) one could barely make out the inferior aspect of this mass in the high posterior apical region.

(B) Tomogram shows a very sharp margin of the mass against adjacent lung. The margins also taper toward the periphery.

This radiographic appearance is characteristic of an extrapleural neurolemmoma, but there are other tumors that can occur in this region and present indistinguishable images. A meningocele, for example, can present an identical radiographic appearance. An aneurysm or extreme tortuosity of the subclavian artery can also be seen as an extrapleural apical mass.

Tomography has largely been replaced by CT in the examination of the chest, but for illustrative purposes tomograms are useful to display details of plain film images.

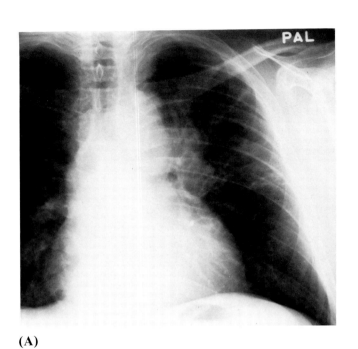

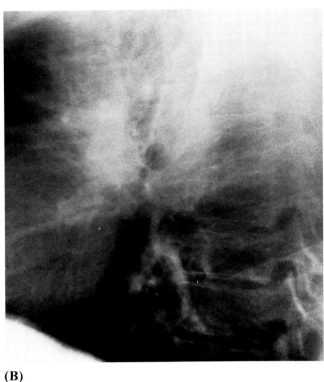

(A)

(B)

Fig. 6-24.   Oat Cell Carcinoma

(A) Coned view of the left lung of a patient with oat cell carcinoma. The enlarged left hilum has polylobulated contours and shows loss of definition of normal hilar vessels. Ill-defined band shadows extend peripherally into the lung. The mediastinal pleural reflection between the aortic arch and the left pulmonary artery is abnormally convex to the left. (See Ch. 7 for a discussion of mediastinal contours.)

(B) Lateral view. The left upper lobe bronchus, seen end-on, is very well defined. Ordinarily this bronchus is outlined superiorly by the left pulmonary artery as it passes from anterior to posterior. Here the bronchus is surrounded by soft tissues that have no particular form and lack the contours of normal vessels. Tumor masses in the hilum distort the interface between lung, bronchus, and left pulmonary artery; the bronchus is surrounded, both above and below, by soft tissue masses and hence stands out as an air column in a "water bath" of soft tissue. *(Figure continues.)*

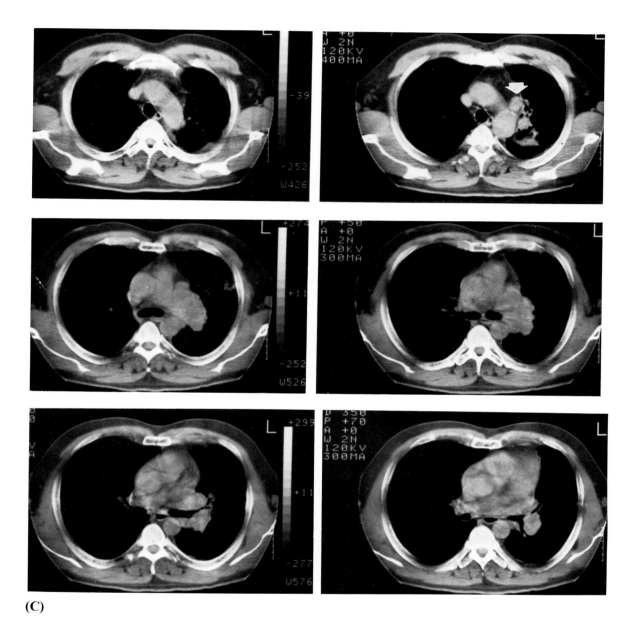

(C)

Fig. 6-24. *(Continued).* (C) CT scans of the same patient. They extend from the region of the aortic arch (top left scan) down to below the tracheal carina (bottom right scan). A well-defined, rounded mass (arrow) is seen in the second scan (top right) within the mediastinal fat at a level that cuts just through the bottom of the aortic arch. This is an enlarged left prevascular lymph node. On subsequent scans you can see that the image of the left pulmonary artery has been replaced by a bulbous mass that preserves none of the contours of a normal left pulmonary artery (see Ch. 7).

The two lowest scans (bottom left and right) show the left upper lobe bronchus surrounded by abnormal masses. The scan at lower left shows the origin of the lingular bronchus, whereas the scan at lower right shows the origin of the superior segment bronchus of the left lower lobe. A large, polylobulated mass is situated between the takeoff of the superior segment of the lower lobe and the lingular bronchus.

This case meets all our expectations for an oat cell carcinoma of the lung in that there are large central masses at the time of the initial diagnosis. Many times the central components — usually a combination of primary tumor and enlarged nodes due to metastases — are even more florid than in this example. (CT scans courtesy of Dr. James Crane, San Jose, California)

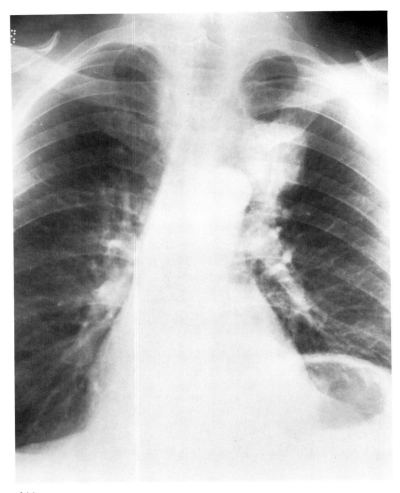

(A)

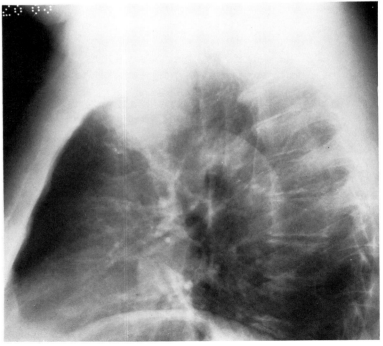

(B)

Fig. 6-25. Large Cell Undifferentiated Carcinoma of the Lung

(A,B) PA and lateral projections, respectively, of a 65-year-old man who had noticed the fairly recent onset of an irritative cough. A large mass with irregular borders is present in the posterior portions of the anterior segment of the left upper lobe. There is also considerable elevation of the left hemidiaphragm.

A needle aspiration of the left upper lobe mass showed that it was malignant. Fluoroscopy of the left hemidiaphragm showed considerable reduction of its excursion. *(Figure continues.)*

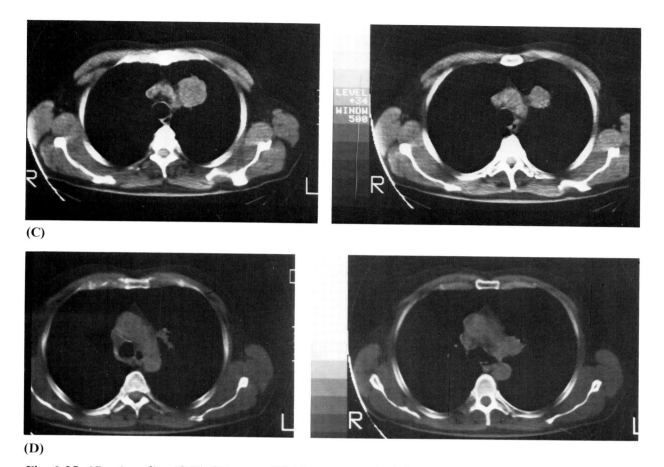

(C)

(D)

Fig. 6-25. *(Continued).* **(C,D)** CT scans. **(C)** The scan on the left, at a level corresponding to the origins of the left subclavian artery, shows the large, lobulated pulmonary mass very well. The mass diminishes in size on sequential caudal cuts.

(D) The scan on the right, just under the aortic arch, however, shows a second mass extending into the left side of the mediastinum (under the aortic arch and on top of the left pulmonary artery) in the region of the ductus nodes.

The left upper lobe was resected, but it was necessary to remove neoplasm from the pulmonary artery by dissection. The lesion was an undifferentiated large cell carcinoma, and mediastinal nodes were involved.

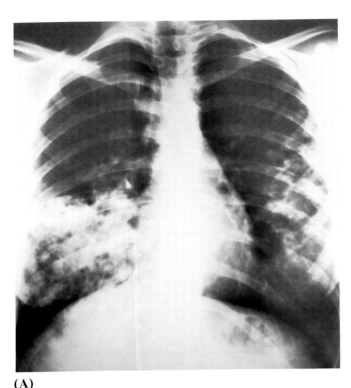

(A)

Fig. 6-26. (A,B). Bronchoalveolar Cell Carcinoma

(A) PA chest film of an asymptomatic 19-year-old woman. The film was taken as part of a preemployment chest survey. There is extensive, inhomogeneous consolidation of portions of both lower lungs.

(B) Tomograms show interspersed, circumscribed, rounded foci of lucency simulating cystic bronchiectatic changes. She had no symptoms or signs of bronchiectasis. A lung biopsy showed these lesions to be due to alveolar cell carcinoma of the lung. (Courtesy of Dr. J. Hentzen, San Leandro, California.) *(Figure continues.)*

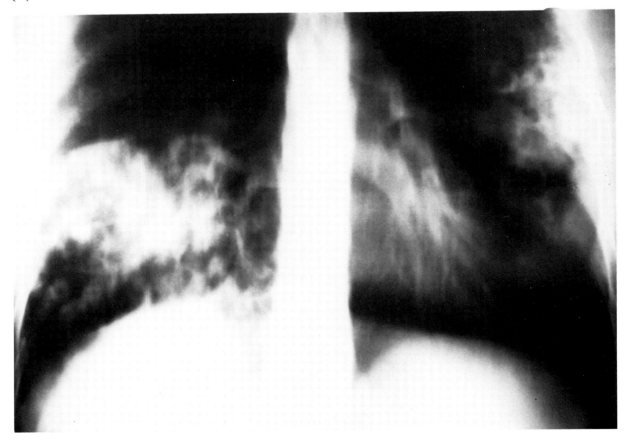

(B)

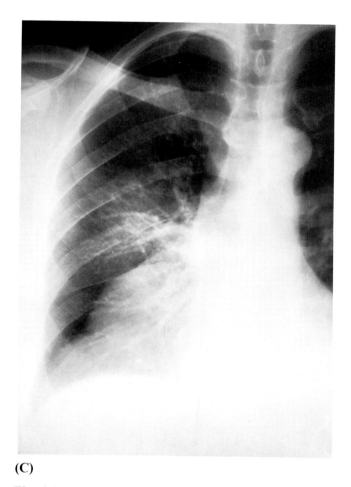

(C)

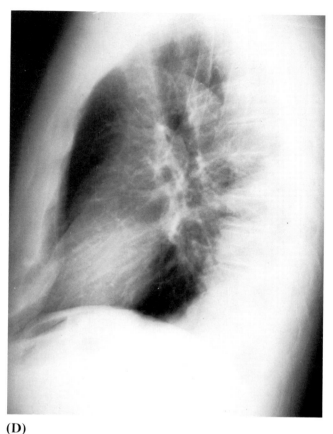

(D)

Fig. 6-26. *(Continued).* **(C,D) Right Lower Lobe Consolidation and Atelectasis Due to Bronchoal-veolar Cell Carcinoma**

This 51-year-old man developed an annoying, nonproductive cough.

(C) PA view. There is intense consolidation of the right lower lobe with reduction in volume. The atelectatic lower lobe has a long, sharp lateral edge due to medial displacement and posterior rotation of the major fissure, which now presents a tangent to the beam. There is moderate shift of the mediastinum and the trachea to the right. There is also an ill-defined perihilar zone of increased tissue density that is not located on the lateral view (Fig. D). That this represented additional disease in the posterior segment of the right upper lobe was confirmed on subsequent studies.

(D) Lateral view. The collapsed, consolidated right lower lobe is seen as a zone of markedly increased opacity superimposed on and effacing detail of the lower thoracic spine.

The patient underwent bronchoscopy, but no transbronchial biopsies of the right lower lobe were taken, and the bronchoscopy was nondiagnostic. The magnitude and character of the radiographic abnormalities and the minimal clinical symptoms (the patient remained afebrile) raised suspicions that malignant neoplasm was the cause.

Bronchoalveolar cell carcinoma and, less frequently, non-Hodgkin's lymphoma can present in just this fashion. Sarcoid lesions can involve the lung extensively in patients with few symptoms, but you would not expect lobar consolidation and atelectasis as the presenting lesion. Infections due to organisms of the infectious granulomatous disease group are rare causes of massive silent lesions.

At operation the patient was found to have a bronchoalveolar cell carcinoma permeating the right lower lobe and extending into the posterior segment of the upper lobe. A pneumonectomy was performed.

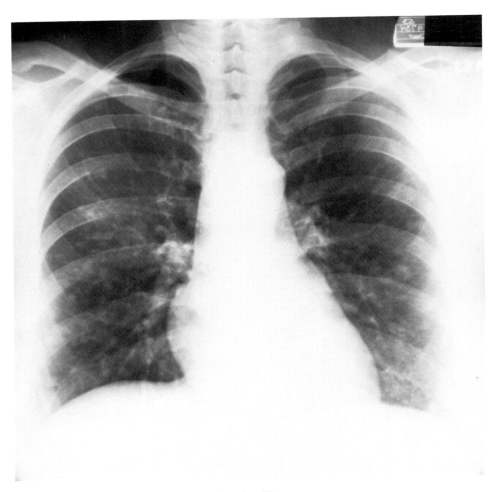

Fig. 6-27. Intravascular Bronchoalveolar Tumor

Preemployment chest radiograph of an asymptomatic 39-year-old woman. Multiple nodules are distributed throughout both lungs; they are most numerous in the middle and lower lung zones and measure approximately 1 cm or less in diameter. This is an example of a very uncommon neoplasm known as intravascular bronchoalveolar tumor. It is likely this is not a bronchoalveolar tumor at all; more likely it is a neoplasm originating in the small vessels of the lungs.

The radiographic appearance is characteristic, but of course since the tumor is so uncommon it is unlikely that the diagnosis is ever made from the radiographic findings alone. Many of the patients with this neoplasm are young and asymptomatic at the time it is first discovered. However, patients who have multiple metastases from an unknown primary tumor, or multiple nodules due to noninfectious granulomatous disease, such as sarcoid or eosinophilic granuloma, may also be asymptomatic.

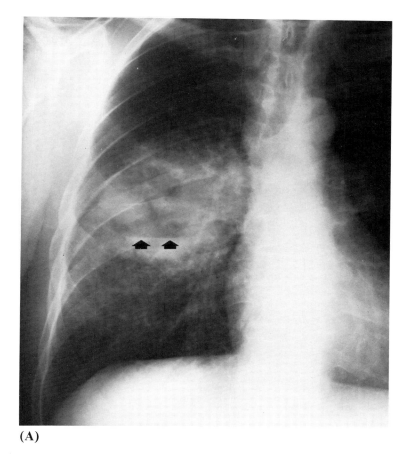

(A)

Fig. 6-28. **Cavitating Adenocarcinoma of the Right Lower Lobe With Metastases to the Right Paratracheal Nodes**

(A,B) PA and lateral views, respectively, show a massive zone of consolidation occupying the superior segment of the right lower lobe, but all around its periphery there is an inhomogeneous infiltration into adjacent lung. A large cavity shows a fluid level on both views (arrows). *(Figure continues.)*

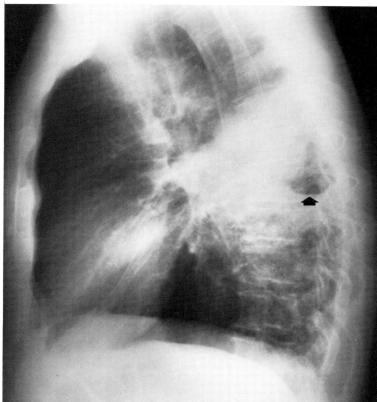

(B)

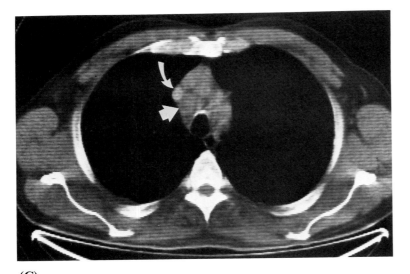

(C)

Fig. 6-28. *(Continued).* **(C)** CT scan just at the top of the aortic arch. There is contrast material in the superior vena cava (curved arrow). A large mass (short arrow) fills the space between the superior vena cava laterally and the wall of the trachea posteriorly and medially. (On the PA film there is a corresponding abnormal convexity of the right side of the mediastinum.) This mass is due to enlarged right paratracheal nodes. These were biopsied at mediastinoscopy and were positive for neoplasm.

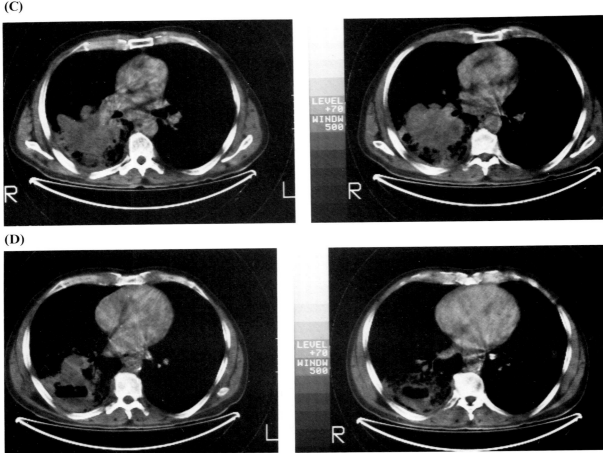

(D)

(E)

(D) CT scans made at more caudal levels show that a solid mass occupies the right lower lobe behind the hilum. This mass surrounds the bronchus intermedius.

(E) On still more caudal scans the large cavity is also easy to see. The inner surface of the cavity wall has a lobulated contour outlined by the air within. Although the irregular outer margins of the tumor extend to the pleura posteriorly and laterally, one cannot infer that the chest wall is invaded, but neither can one say it is not.

Squamous cell carcinoma is the most common form of bronchogenic carcinoma to undergo cavitation. However, this tumor was a poorly differentiated adenocarcinoma. This case emphasizes that all histopathologic types of bronchogenic carcinoma may undergo cavitation.

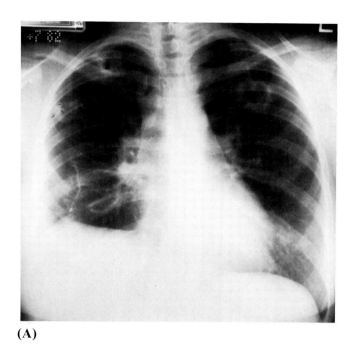

(A)

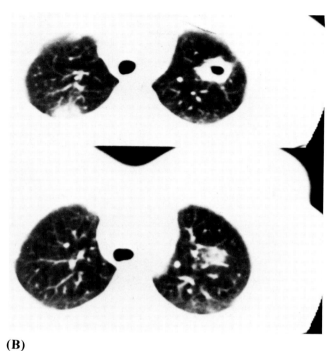

(B)

Fig. 6-29. Cavitating Pulmonary Masses Due to Hodgkin's Disease

(A) PA chest film of a young woman with recently diagnosed Hodgkin's disease. A large cavity in the left upper lobe has walls that vary in thickness. Nodular foci are also present in the right apex and laterally in the right upper lobe. The right hilum is distorted. A long vertical row of surgical staples marks a biopsy site in the right lower lobe. There is pleural thickening at the right base medially and laterally.

Cavitary lung lesions in patients with Hodgkin's disease are not rare. There is always the question as to whether they are due to the disease itself—usually the case when seen at the time of initial diagnosis—or to infection, especially after the patient has been treated. Biopsy is frequently required to make the distinction.

(B) CT scans photographed at settings to show pulmonary details. The left upper lobe cavity is shown well, and a portion of a mass in the posterior segment of the right upper lobe is also seen. CT scans photographed at other settings (not shown) demonstrated that mediastinal lymphadenopathy was also present.

(C) CT scans at and just below the level of the tracheal carina. Another cavity is seen in an axillary subsegment of the right upper lobe, and there is a peripheral nodule along the anterolateral chest wall. The lower scan shows pulmonary consolidation in the juxtamediastinal portions of the right upper lobe (arrows). This accounts for the opaque appearance of the right hilum on the PA chest film, which is due to superimposition. *(Figure continues.)*

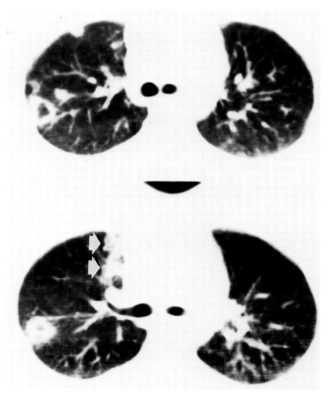

(C)

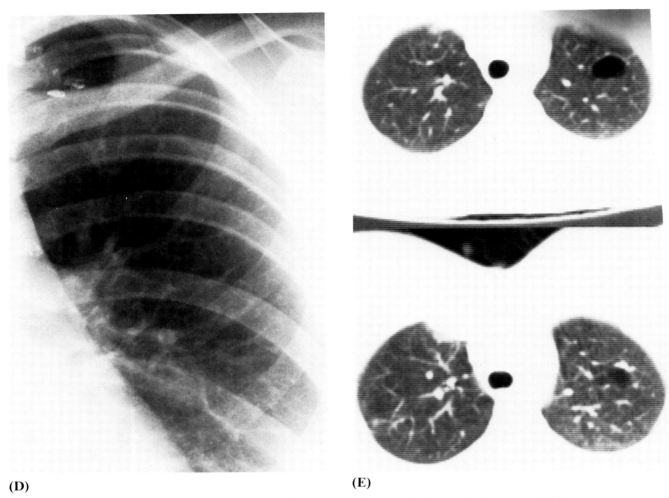

(D)   **(E)**

Fig. 6-29. *(Continued).* **(D)** Coned view of the left upper lung 10 months later, after treatment. There is no recognizable remnant of the upper lobe cavity. The small, white densities above the clavicle medially are lymph nodes, which are opacified from a prior lymphangiogram.

   (E) CT scan showing that there is still a residual cavity with imperceptible (perhaps thin) walls in the left upper lobe at the site of the original cavity. It is not unusual for CT scans to show more lung disease than is anticipated from plain-film analysis, especially when differences in tissue density between the lesion and the adjacent lung are small.

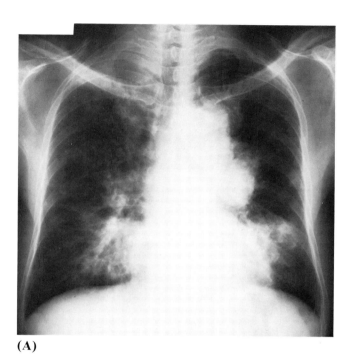

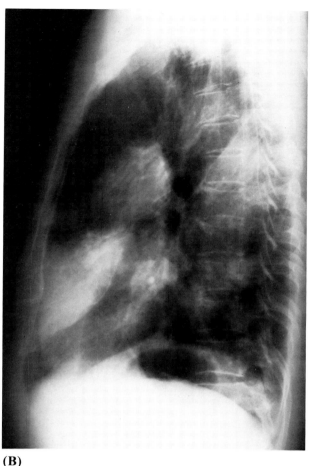

(A) **(B)**

Fig. 6-30. Non-Hodgkin's Lymphoma With Extensive Pulmonary Involvement at the Time of Initial Diagnosis

This 60-year-old man was in good health until 1 year ago, when he noted the onset of a nonproductive cough. Recently he had become easily fatigued and had experienced a 20-pound weight loss over the past 6 months. The physical examination was essentially negative except for a palpable, mobile, 1-cm left supraclavicular lymph node.

(A,B) PA and lateral views of the chest, respectively, made when the patient was first seen. There are bilateral zones of pulmonary consolidation, some of which appear segmental in distribution whereas others appear masslike. The lesions extend into both hilar regions. Biopsy of the right middle lobe revealed small, cleaved cell lymphoma of the B cell type.

Very extensive radiographic pulmonary abnormalities associated with few symptoms generally favor a diagnosis of neoplasm over infection. This presentation would be most unusual for a primary bronchogenic carcinoma, and would be equally unusual for metastases from an extrathoracic primary. Alveolar cell carcinomas and non-Hodgkin's lymphomas, however, may have this presentation. Hodgkin's disease rarely presents initially with pulmonary lesions in the absence of manifest mediastinal and hilar lymphadenopathy.

Pulmonary lesions of sarcoidosis and eosinophilic granuloma may also occur in patients who have few symptoms. Although sarcoid lesions may be disseminated throughout both lungs, they are seldom this conglomerate at the time of initial clinical presentation. They may become so later in the course of the disease, however. Wegener's granulomatosis can present in this fashion, but the pulmonary manifestations are not this marked in a patient with so few symptoms. Regardless of your acumen in elaborating differential diagnoses, the correct diagnosis cannot be established without biopsy.

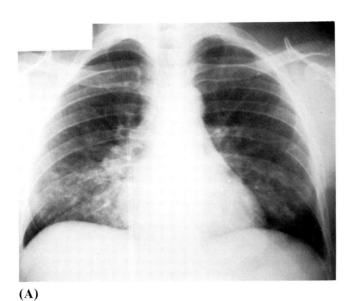

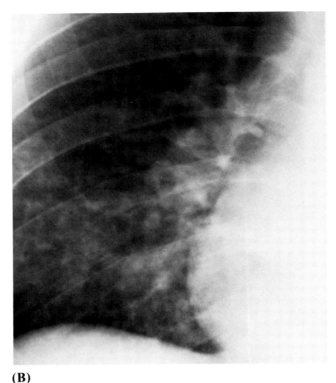

(A)

(B)

Fig. 6-31. (A,B). Kaposi's Sarcoma

(A) PA chest film of a 26-year-old homosexual male who was admitted with a 3-week history of diffuse tender lymphadenopathy associated with fevers, drenching sweats, rigors, nausea, anorexia, and weight loss. He also had a cough that was productive of brownish sputum, associated with bilateral pleuritic chest pain.

Multiple irregular, poorly marginated nodules about 5 mm in diameter are scattered through both lungs. The nodules are most heavily concentrated in the right middle and lower lung zones and to a lesser degree in the left middle and lower lung zones. The right hilum is enlarged, a finding compatible with the presence of lymphadenopathy.

(B) Coned view of the right lower lung shows better the character of the irregular nodules.

Nodules of Kaposi's sarcoma were found on open-lung biopsy. They were located adjacent to bronchi or pulmonary vessels, and some were within lymphatic spaces. Multiple perivascular aggregates of chronic inflammatory cells, predominantly lymphocytes and plasma cells, were also present. Gram stain, acid-fast bacillus stain, and GMS stain for fungus all failed to reveal any microorganisms. This suggested that the foci of inflammatory cells and histiocytes in proximity to the nodules of Kaposi's sarcoma represented a sarcoid-like reaction to the tumor. A cervical lymph node biopsy and biopsy of a skin lesion were also diagnostic of Kaposi's sarcoma.

The pulmonary manifestations of Kaposi's sarcoma may consist of disseminated, small, irregular nodular opacities with or without an accompanying reticular pattern. In some patients the predominant pulmonary manifestation is one of linear interstitial opacities.

Patients with AIDS are subject to a group of pulmonary infections that have elements of a radiographic spectrum similar to that of pulmonary Kaposi's sarcoma. These conditions may coexist in the same patient, making diagnosis difficult. *(Figure continues.)*

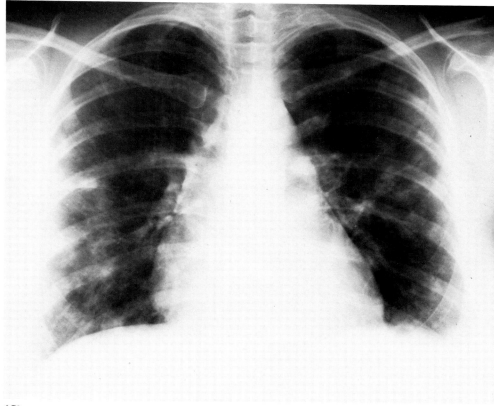

(C)

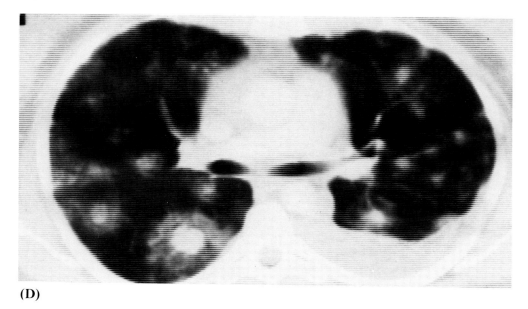

(D)

Fig. 6-31. *(Continued).* **(C – E) Hemorrhagic Margins About Metastatic Nodules**

Chest film of a young woman immediately postpartum. Nodules are present in both lungs. The nodules have poorly defined margins and varying densities; some have a dense central portion and a less dense periphery. The heart appears slightly enlarged even for a young woman postpartum.

(D) CT scan showing the nature of the parenchymal nodules — their radiodense core and less dense peripheral mantle. There is also a left pleural effusion. *(Figure continues.)*

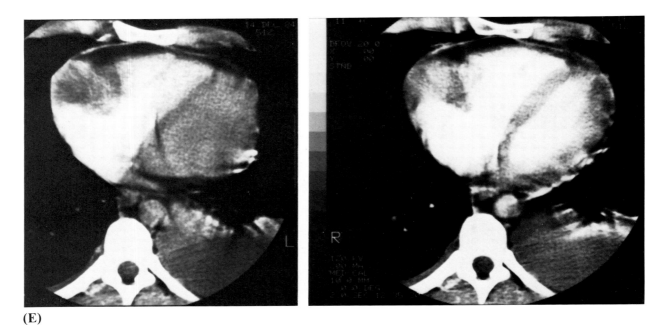

(E)

Fig. 6-31. *(Continued).* **(E)** CT scans taken following intravenous contrast injection. The right atrium and ventricle are opacified, but there is a filling defect in the right atrium. The scan on the right shows that contrast material has progressed to the left ventricle, which is separated from the right by the less opacified interventricular septum. There is still an unopacified zone in the right atrium.

The patient had no known primary neoplasm; a tentative diagnosis of angiosarcoma involving the heart, with metastases to the lung, was made. An alternative possibility of metastases to the lungs and heart from a hitherto undiagnosed choriocarcionoma was also considered.

At thoracotomy a mass was palpated in the right atrium, but the heart was not opened for biopsy. One of the pulmonary lesions was removed, and the diagnosis of angiosarcoma was confirmed histologically.

Nodules in the lungs with dense centers and less dense peripheries are seen with metastases that have zones of peripheral hemorrhage, and these may also occur in patients with metastases to the lungs from choriocarcinoma. Some of the rapid radiographic changes seen in these nodular metastases over a short time are due to a decrease or increase in the amount of peripheral hemorrhage rather than to change in the size of the metastatic deposit itself. Hemorrhage into the lungs may be cleared very rapidly.

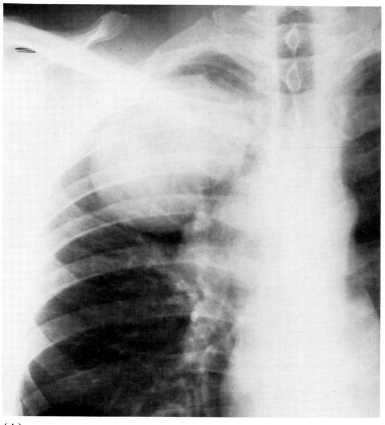

(A)

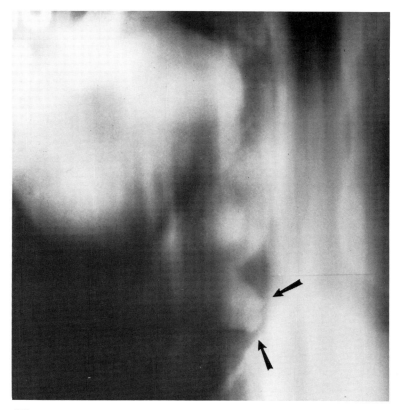

**Fig. 6-32.   Metastasis   to   a   Bronchus
From Carcinoma of the Testis**

(A) Coned view of the upper right lung of a
37-year-old man who had been treated for
a known malignant teratoma of the left
testicle approximately 2 years before this
study. Approximately 4 months before
this chest film, the patient had a bout of
hemoptysis and the onset of mild dyspnea.

A large, slightly lobulated mass occupies
much of the right upper lobe. The mediastinal pleural reflection in the region of the
azygos node is abnormal, and there is enlargement of the upper portions of the
right hilum.

(B) Tomogram shows a fairly large nubbin of tumor (arrows) extending into the
right main bronchus, where it is outlined
by air. A needle biopsy of the large mass
revealed malignant teratoma consistent
with metastasis from the testicle.

(B)

7

The Mediastinum

IMAGING ANATOMY AND DETECTION OF LYMPHADENOPATHY

Anatomic Definition

The mediastinum is an intrathoracic compartment extending from the thoracic inlet to the diaphragm between the right and left lungs. Its lateral boundaries are formed by pleura, which surrounds the mediastinum except for relatively short segments anteriorly and posteriorly.

Anatomists commonly divide the mediastinum into superior and inferior parts through a plane extending from the sternomanubrial junction backward to the lower border of the fourth thoracic vertebra. The inferior part is further subdivided into anterior, middle, and posterior compartments. The anterior compartment extends from the sternum to the pericardium; the middle compartment from the anterior pericardium backward to include the bifurcation of the trachea, the two main bronchi, and the central pulmonary veins; the posterior compartment from the posterior margins of the tracheal bifurcation and the pericardium backwards to the anterior margins of the vertebral column.

You may find it useful to apply these subdivisions to radiographic descriptions, but often mediastinal abnormalities cross these arbitrary dividing lines and do not lend themselves to such tight compartmentalization. Felson[9] proposed dividing the mediastinum into anterior, middle, and posterior portions extending from the diaphragm to the neck. In his configuration, however, on the lateral view the plane demarcating the anterior from the middle mediastinum extends from the diaphragm to the thoracic inlet along the posterior curvature of the heart inferiorly, but continues cephalad anterior to the trachea. The middle mediastinum is separated from the posterior mediastinum by a plane passing from diaphragm to apex approximately 1 cm posterior to the anterior margins of the vertebral column. You can thus see that according to the compartmentalization of the classical anatomists the heart and the trachea would be in the middle mediastinum, whereas according to Felson's compartmentalization the heart would be in the anterior mediastinum while the trachea and main bronchi remain in the middle mediastinum.

Any system that helps you to organize your concepts of the relative position and frequency of mediastinal lesions can be used effectively. I find it most useful to localize mediastinal disease in reference to prominent anatomic landmarks rather than arbitrary compartments, and I use the terms "superior" and "inferior" or "posterior" and "anterior" only as modifiers in the usual general sense. As for the types of lesions that occur at a given location, a knowledge of the structures that "live" in the region of concern or that have passed through the region during embryogenesis provides an understanding of abnormalities that can occur, whereas a study of pathology provides an understanding of lesions that do occur and their relative frequency.

Radiographic Study

Radiographic analysis of the mediastinum and hila is challenging and rewarding. Success requires mastery of much detail. Many medical students will find more detail in this chapter than they care to work to retain. They may prefer to read this chapter only to gain an idea of how the study of the mediastinum can be approached when they are ready to do so. Radiology residents, on the other hand, must become masters of interpretation of the mediastinum and the hila, and it is hoped that this chapter will help them along that path.

This chapter emphasizes the radiographic anatomy of the mediastinum and the detection of mediastinal lymphadenopathy. On chest films and even on tomograms, the mediastinum can be compared to a white box whose important contents, except for the trachea, cannot be seen except where they mold and shape their wrapper—the mediastinal pleura. The air-water interface that occurs at the boundary between the mediastinal pleura and adjacent lung permits the marginal contours of the mediastinum to be seen on chest films. Therefore, in order to use chest films to assess the presence or absence of mediastinal disease, it is critical that you acquire an appreciation of the spectrum of appearances of the mediastinal pleural reflections that may be seen in normal individuals.[4,5,16,17,18,23,27,28,29] This is no small task because the appearance of one's mediastinum seems to be as individual in its nuances as are one's fingerprints. Nevertheless, there are important useful generalizations to be made about mediastinal contours that are applicable to imaging studies.

Basic Landmarks

Figures 7-1 through 7-7 are a series of illustrations of normal mediastinal contours, useful anatomic landmarks, and the locations of important lymph node groups. Many mediastinal recesses are more conspicuous in the living human being than in the cadaver.[12] The boundaries of these recesses can frequently be seen on chest films, and both the boundaries and the contents are demonstrated beautifully on CT and MRI scans. Mediastinal masses and inflammatory processes can cause changes in the contours of mediastinal pleura at its interface with adjacent lung. These include changes from concave contours to straight or convex contours; loss of sharp margins about such anatomic structures as the aortic arch, the origin of the left subclavian artery, and the superior vena cava; and widening of spaces between mediastinal boundaries and mediastinal contents, for example, the relationship between the trachea and the right paratracheal boundary of the mediastinum. These contour changes will be illustrated. However, for the sake of brevity these contour changes will be simply referred to here as "distortions."

Analysis of Radiographic Appearance

An analysis of the mediastinum should answer three basic questions, two of which have subsets of four questions each:

1. Is the mediastinum normal or abnormal?
2. Is the abnormality due to mass or masslike lesions?
   a. Is the lesion vascular or nonvascular?
   b. Is the lesion solid or cystic?
   c. Is the lesion composed of fat?
   d. Is the lesion solitary or multiple?
3. Is the abnormality other than a mass or a masslike lesion?
   a. Are there abnormal air shadows in the mediastinum?
   b. Are there abnormal fluid collections?
   c. Are the major airways intrinsically abnormal?
   d. Is the esophagus intrinsically abnormal?

The importance of the answer to the first question is obvious. Unfortunately, most often the answer must be based on an analysis of images made with the imaging technique that is least sensitive for the task: standard chest roentgenograms. Pragmatic considerations dictate that this be so. Further imaging studies such as fluoroscopy, tomography, CT scans, MRI scans, or radionuclide scans are usually recommended because of lesions initially detected or considered suspect on chest film analysis. Often mediastinal abnormalities on chest films are so compelling that no analyst would knowingly pass them by. On the other hand, some important mediastinal lesions may be so subtle as to defy recognition on chest films by any but the most experienced observers. Furthermore, a significant percentage (perhaps more than 20 percent) of mediastinal lesions that may be seen on CT or MRI scan cannot be recognized, *even in retrospect*, on high-quality chest films made at or near the same time. Therefore, for patients known to have diseases or conditions whose treatment would be modified by determining the presence of mediastinal involvement (e.g., malignant lymphomas or carcinoma of the lung), one might advocate the use of CT scans even when routine films show no evidence of mediastinal extension or nodal disease.

Computed Tomography

CT offers a marvelous opportunity to examine the contents of our "white box." This technique is much more sensitive than chest radiography in demonstrating differences in tissue density and in detecting mediastinal lymphadenopathy.[8,24,27] In most adults the mediastinal contents are outlined by fat. This fat serves as a natural contrast against which blood vessels and other mediastinal soft tissues stand out. (It is regrettable that the differences in density between mediastinal organs and surrounding fat are not sufficient to be of critical use in routine chest radiography.) With CT it is also possible to enhance the radiodensity of blood vessels by the intravenous injection of iodinated contrast material in concentrations that would not produce diagnostic images on a chest film.

Careful timing of CT exposures and bolus injections of contrast material often permits distinction between normal and abnormal mediastinal or hilar blood vessels and neoplasms, and may even permit differentiation among solid tumors, necrotic tumors, and cysts, by showing differences in their x-ray attenuation patterns before and after contrast enhancement. CT also permits the identification of lymphadenopathy within abundant mediastinal fat, and this is a significant contribution (Figs. 7-8 and 7-9).

When chest films are rigorously interpreted, and particularly when old chest films are available for comparison, the diagnosis or at least the strong suspicion of mediastinal lymphadenopathy should be possible in the majority of patients in whom it is subsequently shown to be present on CT scan or MRI. However, enlarged nodes can be seen on CT scan that defy recognition on chest films even on careful retrospection, and CT (or MRI) frequently shows more extensive adenopathy or more nodal groups involved than is anticipated from chest film analysis.

When precise localization is sought to aid in the choice of biopsy technique or surgical approach, or when complete mapping is desired in order to plan the size of radiation therapy portals, CT or MRI scans may be very beneficial even for patients in whom lymphadenopathy is clearly evident on chest films.

Magnetic Resonance Imaging of the Mediastinum

MRI allows mediastinal structures to be examined without the burden of x-irradiation.[3,15,35] The great vessels of the mediastinum and the hila, which contain relatively rapidly flowing blood, can be recognized and distinguished from abnormal masses without the use of intravenous contrast agents (see Fig. 7-3). This is another advantage of MRI studies over CT. However, the spatial resolution of some MRI units in the transverse axial format is not as good as that of CT in the transverse axial

format.[35] The MRI examination usually takes longer and is more expensive, and patients fairly often experience a sense of claustrophobia while in the gantry—more often than with CT scanning. The true contribution of MRI studies to the evaluation of mediastinal abnormalities is still incompletely known. However, if MRI remains equal to CT in evaluating the mediastinum, it may become the preferred method of study, because x-irradiation is avoided, intravenous contrast material is not used, and the acquired data permit image constructions in coronal, sagittal, and oblique planes more easily and with better spatial resolution than is obtained with CT (see Fig. 7-3).

MRI does not permit as critical evaluation of the lungs as does CT.[15] Some patients must be excluded from study because they have cardiac pacemakers or prosthetic devices containing ferrous metals that would be affected adversely by high magnetic fields or would adversely affect the images.

Lymph Nodes of the Mediastinum and the Hila

At present there are no reproducible, clinically practical techniques to opacity the lymph nodes of the mediastinum. Lymphangiography, performed by injecting contrast material into the lymphatics of the dorsum of the feet, is ordinarily used to study the retroperitoneal lymph nodes. Occasionally, however, lymph nodes of the mediastinum fortuitously are opacified by this procedure (see Fig. 7-7).

Our understanding of the lymph node anatomy of the mediastinum and of the parietal intrathoracic lymph nodes has been enhanced by collecting these cases for many years. The bulk of our knowledge of mediastinal lymph nodes, however, comes from anatomic studies. Lymph node anatomy varies from patient to patient in terms of the number of nodes that may be found in any given chain and to a lesser degree in their position. In general, this text follows the nomenclature of Rouvière with minor modifications, but it is recognized that there is variability in the nomenclature used by different anatomists. The following list describes the key mediastinal lymph node chains and the distribution of nodes within them according to the work of Rouvière.[31]

Anterior Mediastinal or Prevascular Nodes

1. On the right, nodes lie in front of the superior vena cava and the right innominate vein, along the distribution of the phrenic nerve or the border of the thymus.
2. Nodes on the left are along the main pulmonary artery (the ductus node) and ascend along the distri-

bution of the phrenic and vagus nerves, in front of and along the superior border of the aortic arch, and anterolateral to the common carotid artery. Some nodes may be placed more medially in front of the thymus.

3. A transverse chain of nodes or lymphatic trunks along the left innominate vein connects the two ascending anterior mediastinal chains and the right paratracheal chain.

Peritracheobronchial Nodes

1. The *right paratracheal chain* ascends anterolateral to the trachea, behind the superior vena cava and the right innominate vein. The lowest node of this chain is the azygos node. It is large and almost always extends as low as the arch of the azygos vein. The highest node is posteriorly and laterally placed, below the right subclavian artery.

2. The *left paratracheal chain* ascends posterolateral to the trachea, along the distribution of the left recurrent nerve, medial and posterior to the anterior portions of the aortic arch and the left subclavian artery. These nodes are usually small.

3. The *bifurcation nodes* (intertracheobronchial nodes, or subcarinal nodes) are located beneath the trachea and the main bronchi cephalad to the inferior pulmonary veins. The largest node of the group occupies the subcarinal space and extends to the right, with smaller nodes adjacent. Nodes under the left main bronchus are also smaller. Inconstantly, small nodes may be found in front of (pretracheal) or behind (retrotracheal) the carina or the lower trachea acting as stations uniting bifurcation nodes with paratracheal nodes (usually the right).

4. Rouvière does not have a classification of nodes designated as "hilar." I believe that the *nodes of the pulmonary roots,* as designated by Rouvière, comprise at least a portion of the nodes that are radiographically considered as "hilar," with some interlobar and lobar nodes providing the rest. The mediastinal pleura is reflected over vessels and main bronchi as they pass from the mediastinum into the lungs. When traction is placed on the lung, the nodes of the pulmonary roots are found located on the mediastinal side of these pleural reflections. They are grouped as anterior, posterior, superior, and inferior according to their position relative to the main bronchi. They are characterized by variability in position and number. A node of the left suprabronchial group is related to the left recurrent nerve, and when abnormal may be a cause of left recurrent nerve paralysis.

5. *Nodes of the pulmonary ligament* are located below the inferior pulmonary veins, more often on the left than the right. According to Rouvière, in some specimens they may not be found on either side.

Posterior Mediastinal Nodes. These nodes extend along the lateral borders of the esophagus caudally from the level of the inferior pulmonary veins. Some may be found between the esophagus and the aorta, and sometimes nodes may be found in front of the esophagus on the diaphragm and behind the aorta near the diaphragm.

Intrapulmonary Nodes. The *interlobar nodes* are those generally situated at the angles of branching of major bronchi, arteries, or veins. Some of these nodes are also found centrally in the interlobar fissures. The *lobar nodes* are located at the angle of branching of lobar bronchi into segmental bronchi. *Subpleural nodes* are sometimes found on perilobular, subpleural lymphatics at lobular junctions.

Parietal Intrathoracic Nodes

1. The *posterior parietal nodes* are located along the intercostal spaces (posterior and lateral intercostal nodes) and on the lateral and anterior surfaces of the vertebral column (juxtavertebral nodes). The latter are more numerous along the lower half of the thoracic spine.

2. The *diaphragmatic nodes* (pericardiac nodes) are located along the diaphragm anterior to the pericardium and more laterally at the location of the phrenic nerve. On the right side the lateral pericardiac nodes (juxtaphrenic nodes) are relatively constant and frequently found in front of the inferior vena cava and the phrenic nerve. On the left side these nodes are inconstant.

3. The *internal mammary nodes* (anterior parietal nodes) are located alongside the sternum behind the intercostal spaces and costal cartilages along the internal mammary vessels. They are more commonly found, and more numerous, superiorly than inferiorly.

Proposed American Thoracic Society Definitions of Nodal Stations

Analysis of 5-year survivors in a few series of patients with carcinoma of the lung raised the question of whether patients with limited mediastinal node metastases should be classified as having resectable rather than unresectable disease (see Ch. 6). In 1981 the Board of Directors of the American Thoracic Society (ATS) called attention to the lack of a commonly accepted nomenclature that would permit localization of lymph nodes to a specific anatomic site in the mediastinum. This deficiency was considered to be a hindrance to strict comparison of various data banks for study of the staging of lung cancer.

TABLE 7-1. ATS Definition of Lymph Node Locations to be Used in Evaluating Lymph Node Metastases From Lung Cancer[34]

X	Supraclavicular nodes
2R	Right upper paratracheal (suprainnominate) nodes: nodes to the right of the midline of the trachea between the intersection of the caudal margin of the innominate artery with the trachea, and the apex of the lung. (Includes highest right mediastinal node.) (Radiologists may use the same caudal margin as in 2L.)
2L	Left upper paratracheal (supra-aortic) nodes: nodes to the left of the midline of the trachea between the top of the aortic arch and the apex of the lung. (Includes highest left mediastinal node.)
4R	Right lower paratracheal nodes: nodes to the right of the midline of the trachea between the cephalic border of the azygos vein and the intersection of the caudal margin of the brachiocephalic artery with the right side of the trachea. (Includes some pretracheal and paracaval nodes.) (Radiologists may use the same cephalic margin as in 4L.)
4L	Left lower paratracheal nodes: nodes to the left of the midline of the trachea between the top of the aortic arch and the level of the carina, medial to the ligamentum arteriosum. (Includes some pretracheal nodes.)
5	Aortopulmonary nodes: subaortic and para-aortic nodes, lateral to the ligamentum arteriosum or the aorta or left pulmonary artery, proximal to the first branch of the LPA.
6	Anterior mediastinal nodes: nodes anterior to the ascending aorta or the innominate artery. (Includes some pretracheal and preaortic nodes.)
7	Subcarinal nodes: nodes arising caudal to the carina of the trachea but not associated with the lower lobe bronchi or arteries within the lung.
8	Paraesophageal nodes: nodes dorsal to the posterior wall of the trachea and to the right or left of the midline of the esophagus. (Includes retrotracheal, but not subcarinal nodes.)
9	Right or left pulmonary ligament nodes: nodes within the right or left pulmonary ligament.
10R	Right tracheobronchial nodes: nodes to the right of the midline of the trachea from the level of the cephalic border of the azygos vein to the origin of the right upper lobe bronchus.
10L	Left peribronchial nodes: nodes to the left of the midline of the trachea between the carina and the left upper lobe bronchus, medial to the ligamentum arteriosum.
11	Intrapulmonary nodes: nodes removed in the right or left lung specimen plus those distal to the main stem bronchi or secondary carina. (Includes interlobar, lobar, and segmental nodes.)

Note: (A) Generally, anterior thoracostomy is required to sample nodes in stations 5 and 6 because they are not accessible by mediastinoscopy.

(B) On CT nodal stations 4R and 10R are separated by the azygos vein; 4L and 10L are separated by the tracheal carina.

A committee of the ATS developed a system for the precise designation of lymph node stations in relationship to anatomic structures identifiable by mediastinoscopy, CT scans, chest roentgenograms, and tomograms Table 7-1 lists the recommended anatomic definitions of nodal stations to be used in evaluating the localization of lymph node metastases from lung cancer.

These nodal stations are comparable to those that Rouvière groups as peritracheobronchial and prevascular, but they do not include all the parietal intrathoracic nodes.

LYMPHADENOPATHY

In day-to-day practice the mediastinal abnormality most commonly seen, aside from cardiovascular disorders, is lymphadenopathy. In fact, when classifying mediastinal abnormalities we can consider an important group to be composed of those disorders that manifest with lymphadenopathy. Common causes of mediastinal lymphadenopathy are the following:

1. Hodgkin's disease and non-Hodgkin's lymphoma,[6,7,10] the leukemias, and less common entities that mimic lymphoma such as malignant histiocytosis and angioimmunoblastic lymphadenopathy[20]
2. Metastases from a variety of intrathoracic or extrathoracic primary neoplasms
3. Noninfectious granulomatous disease, including sarcoid, certain of the pneumoconioses (e.g., silicosis, berylliosis), uncommonly eosinophilic granuloma, and rarely Wegener's granulomatosis
4. Infectious granulomatous disease (e.g., tuberculosis, atypical mycobacterioses, histoplasmosis, coccidioidomycosis, cryptococcosis, blastomycosis)
5. Other.

The first four groups account for the vast majority (an estimated 95 percent) of cases of mediastinal lymphadenopathy.

Hilar lymphadenopathy may or may not also be present or may be more conspicuous than the mediastinal components of adenopathy. In some cases, especially of metastases or infectious granulomatous disease, hilar lymphadenopathy may be present without mediastinal adenopathy. Pulmonary components of disease may or may not be visible in any of these entities at the time the lymphadenopathy is first detected.

Hilar and mediastinal lymphadenopathy due to tuberculosis, histoplasmosis, coccidioidomycosis, and other infectious granulomatous diseases is the least common of the four common groups. However, these causes are more common in my experience than all the entities in the group labeled "Other". Furthermore, they represent treatable conditions that may escape appropriate clinical consideration when the adenopathy is not associated with visible pulmonary disease. Their inclusion in the radiologic differential diagnosis is therefore important.

The "Other" group consists of a much longer list of causes that will account for the remaining minority of cases. Table 7-2 lists these entities. Although some are not uncommon (e.g., myeloma, drug abuse, *Mycoplasma* pneumonia), their association with detectable mediastinal or hilar adenopathy revealed by imaging studies is uncommon. Others are frequently associated with mediastinal or hilar adenopathy but the disease itself is uncommon or rare in North America (e.g., anthrax, plague pneumonia).

Lymphadenopathy Associated With AIDS

Mediastinal or hilar adenopathy should not simply be accepted as part of the generalized lymphadenopathy so common in patients with AIDS or related syndromes. Patients with AIDS may have mediastinal or hilar lymphadenopathy due to infections with cryptococcus or typical or atypical mycobacteria in spite of the fact that a granulomatous tissue response to these organisms is not likely in these patients. AIDS patients may also have involvement of mediastinal and hilar nodes by Kaposi's sarcoma, Hodgkin's disease, or non-Hodgkin's lymphoma.

Lymphatic Drainage of the Lung

Figure 1 is a flow diagram of lymphatic pathways from various lung regions to mediastinal and hilar lymph node stations as well as pathways between nodal stations. Notice that portions of most lung zones have lymphatic channels that pass directly to mediastinal lymph nodes as well as channels draining to intermediate interlobar or hilar nodes. Lymphatic channels from these intermediate stations drain to mediastinal nodes directly or by a series of cascades through intervening stations. The lymphatic drainage of the lung is variable. Figure 1 is constructed from data provided by anatomical studies,[31] that define pathways that are theoretically possible. Studies performed by surgeons, pathologists, and radiologists were used to define likelihood in terms of involvement actually found in pathologic specimens.[12,21,22,26] You can understand how these data are hard to come by and probably are seriously biased. Reliance on autopsy data leads to a bias in favor of advanced disease. Reliance on surgical data also produces a biased selection of cases —presurgical confirmation of lymphadenopathy will strongly favor exploration of only those cases in whom a curative resection is considered feasible; when contralateral nodal metastases are confirmed by mediastinoscopy, scalene node biopsy, or parasternal incisional biopsy, surgical resection is rarely attempted.

TABLE 7-2. Causes of Mediastinal Lymphadenopathy

Usual Causes

Hodgkin's disease, non-Hodgkin's lymphoma, leukemias, and lymphoma-like variants

Metastases from intrathoracic or extrathoracic primary neoplasms

Noninfectious granulomatous disease

Infectious granulomatous disease. In patients with AIDS, the organisms responsible for this group of diseases may not evoke a granulomatous response in the enlarged lymph nodes.

Other Causes

Infections
  Mononucleosis and other viral pneumonias
  Mycoplasma pneumonia
  Lung abscess
  Chronic infections (e.g., in patients with mucoviscidosis or chronic indolent pneumonia peripheral to bronchial obstruction)
  Unusual pneumonias
    Anthrax
    Plague
    Tularemia
    Brucellosis

Plasma cell dyscrasias
  Myeloma
  Waldenström's macroglobulinemia
  Heavy chain disease

Allergies
  Analeptic drugs
  Intravenous drug abuse
  Asthma (?)
  Hypersensitivity pneumonitis

Benign changes
  Hyperplastic lymphadenopathy[19]
  Hamartomatous lymphadenopathy[1]

Parasites (e.g., tropical eosinophilia)

Amyloidosis

Connective tissue diseases (?)

Recognition of Abnormal Contours in Key Areas

The diagnosis of mediastinal lymphadenopathy from chest films depends on recognition of abnormal mediastinal contours. This, of course, requires an understanding of the spectrum of appearances of normal mediastinal contours. The concept of increased density of an absorber is also valuable in this analysis, but because of its subjective nature it virtually cannot be learned from words. Examples can serve to illustrate the use of the concept in evaluating the mediastinum.

Gross departures from normal require less skill to recognize, but minimal contour changes can be extremely difficult to recognize or to accept when seen. Earlier chest films for comparison are invaluable in permitting recognition of subtle changes. It is a mistake to undertake the critical evaluation of the mediastinum without comparing the present films with older ones available for comparison whenever that is feasible.

Because of the relative frequency of involvement of the azygos node of the right paratracheal chain and the ductus nodes and para-aortic nodes of the left prevascular chain, a few key anatomic regions are especially critical in assessment of mediastinal lymphadenopathy.

The Right Paratracheal Region

Any convexity (toward the lung) that begins and ends above the right tracheobronchial angle and that cannot clearly be ascribed to the azygos vein must be suspect as abnormal.

The azygos node occupies a pocket between the right anterolateral tracheal wall and the posteromedial wall of the superior vena cava (see Fig. 7-9E). The azygos vein passes around the lower part of the node on its way to the posterior wall of the superior vena cava above the level of the right upper lobe bronchus. When the azygos node enlarges, it may displace the azygos vein, the superior vena cava, or the mediastinal pleura laterally. These displacements result in a focal lateral bulge of the mediastinal pleural reflection above the takeoff of the right upper lobe bronchus (Fig. 7-11). Sometimes you have to decide whether you are looking at an enlarged azygos node or an enlarged azygos vein. Usually the distinction can be made by comparing films made with the patient supine with those made with the patient upright. The azygos vein shows appreciable reduction in size in the upright position compared to the supine. Also, if the patient can perform and sustain a Valsalva maneuver for more than 10 seconds, the azygos vein will show a reduction in size, on films or at fluoroscopy, compared to its size before the maneuver. The node changes little with these maneuvers.

When there is a large paratracheal pocket in which the azygos node can remain without displacing the marginal pleura of the mediastinum, an enlarged azygos node may not be detectable on chest film (see Fig. 7-17).

Thickening of the Right Paratracheal Soft Tissues

When several nodes in the right paratracheal chain are enlarged and extend cephalad from the azygos node, the right paratracheal stripe is replaced by a wide band of soft tissue. This is a result of the right upper lobe being displaced from the right tracheal wall by a chain of enlarged lymph nodes (Fig. 7-12).

The Spurious "Dilated Ascending Aorta"

The vena cava forms part of the border for the supracardiac segment of the right side of the mediastinum and may present an edge that is slightly convex toward the right lung. When the ascending aorta becomes considerably dilated or tortuous, it may present an edge that is also border forming on the right side of the mediastinum. At times, two edges may thus be seen superimposed. However, it is important to determine that any edge you are ascribing to the ascending aorta has an arc that supports that analysis. The curvature should be one that by extrapolation should extend from the level of the aortic valve to the transverse portion of the aortic arch. If the arc seen does not meet that expectation, or if comparison with previous films shows that it is a new image or a clear increase in tissue density in the area in question, the likelihood that it is an abnormal mass should be evaluated by further studies (Figs. 7-13 and 7-14).

The Aortic Arch and the Left Subclavian Artery

The pleural reflection over the transverse portion of the aortic arch and the takeoff of the left subclavian artery commonly presents a well-defined image on PA chest films. When nodes of the left prevascular chain enlarge, they displace the left mediastinal pleura away from the great vessels. As the nodes enlarge further, the sharp lung interface with these vessels becomes distorted and then lost as the pleura is moved further from them by the enlarging nodes (Figs. 7-15 to 7-17).

The Aortopulmonic Window

Any edge convex to the left that is projected between the level of the aortic arch and the left pulmonary artery must be suspected of being abnormal. Furthermore, a change from a concave contour toward the left lung to a straightened contour on subsequent films is also suspect.

The space between the aortic arch and the left pulmonary artery is often called the aortopulmonic window.

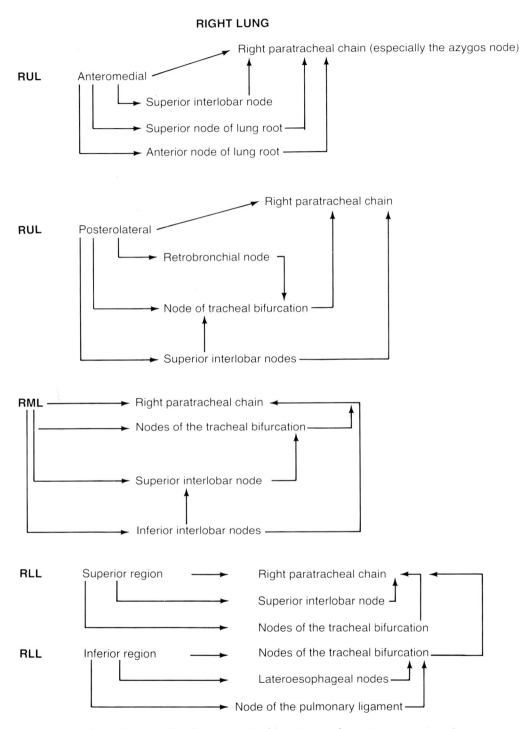

Fig. 1. Possible direct and indirect lymphatic pathways from the lungs to various lymph node chains. *, Nodes of the tracheal bifurcation drain to the azygos node and hence to the right paratracheal chain. (RUL, right upper lobe, etc.) *(Figure continues.)*

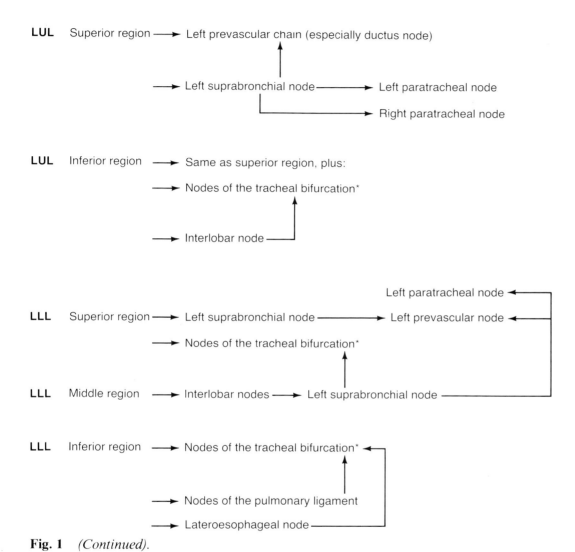

Fig. 1 *(Continued).*

The ductus node (or nodes) sits on top of the pulmonary artery, anterior to the ligamentum arteriosum and relatively close to the mediastinal pleura. Although these nodes are the lowest of the left prevascular chain, they are analogous to the azygos node of the right paratracheal chain in importance.

When the mediastinal pleura bridging these structures presents a sufficient tangent to be recognized on frontal films, it may be seen as an edge that is concave toward the left lung, or straight but inclined like the sloping side of a tent (Figs. 7-4A, 7-18, and 7-19). It should not be convex toward the lung (Figs. 7-20 and 7-21). When a previous film shows this edge to be concave, and a subsequent film shows it straight, that is abnormal. Thus, a contour that is still within the *spectrum* of normal may actually be *abnormal* when it represents a change from a previous state.

Films made in slight degrees of rotation away from the true PA projection may show a change in the relative sharpness of mediastinal-lung interfaces or cause them not to be seen. Thus, mediastinal masses may become recognizable on films of slight obliquity (while appearing equivocal or obscure on true PA projection) because they have longer tangents projected in profile. However, slight rotation does not convert normal contours into abnormal contours.

Normal mediastinal margins may be projected as convex contours on films made at expiration or in the lordotic projection. Therefore, those films should not be used for critical assessment of the mediastinum. Films made with the patient supine are also unsuitable for critical assessment as to the presence or absence of a mediastinal mass. Both false-negative and false-positive assessments can result from misinterpretation of increased width of the superior mediastinum caused by blood vessel distension when the patient is supine.

A convex contour along the left side of the mediastinum beginning caudal to the level of the left main bronchus can be normal even though it continues cephalad above the level of the bronchus. This convexity is often exaggerated in patients with an enlarged pulmonary artery due to pulmonary hypertension.

Subcarinal Lymphadenopathy

When subcarinal nodes enlarge, they displace lung away from (a) the posterior and medial wall of the bronchus intermedius, (b) the superior margin of the superior pulmonary vein, and (c) the azygoesophageal recess interface. The margins of these structures are then not seen on radiographic study (Fig. 7-22). Frequently, the loss of these images is accompanied by an increase in the radiodensity of the subcarinal region. This increased radiodensity is usually more easily recognized on the right side. On the lateral view, the image of the posterior wall of the bronchus intermedius[32] is often effaced by soft tissue masses that extend caudally in the subcarinal space. Subcarinal adenopathy can be confused with right hilar adenopathy on a lateral view of the chest.

Although subcarinal adenopathy can frequently be deduced from well-exposed PA and lateral views of the chest, it is much easier to appreciate its presence on tomography, CT scans, or MRI scans, and small subcarinal masses may only be detected with these modalities (see Fig. 7-9 and 7-10). Esophagography can be used to study the subcarinal space, but subcarinal adenopathy usually has to be quite large before it significantly distorts the esophagus, which may be off to the left of the adenopathy.

An increase of the angle between the right and left main bronchi may also be a sign indicating the presence of a subcarinal mass. Because of the sizeable variation of this angle in the normal individual, its use in the assessment of subcarinal adenopathy is limited, and other manifestations of subcarinal mass are usually apparent.

Elevation of the left main bronchus has been used as a classic sign of left atrial enlargement, but subcarinal masses can cause similar elevation. Increased tissue density of the subcarinal region is also a radiographic sign of

mass, but density gradients in the mediastinum are very easily overlooked or misinterpreted when there are no "edges" of mass visible for corroboration.

Other Sites and Other Examples

Figures 7-23 through 7-29 illustrate a variety of changes in mediastinal contours produced by adenopathy in the regions discussed above as well as in the posterior mediastinal, paravertebral, internal mammary, and diaphragmatic lymph node groups. In Hodgkin's disease, non-Hodgkin's lymphoma, and some leukemias, the thymus may also be involved (Fig. 7-29).

Other Imaging Techniques for Demonstrating Lymphadenopathy

Fluoroscopy, esophagography, tomography, and pneumomediastinography have all been used to demonstrate mediastinal adenopathy but generally are not as effective as CT or MRI. Of course, esophagography should be used to examine those patients whose signs and symptoms or chest radiographs indicate that the esophagus may be intrinsically involved in the disease process, but that is a different matter from using esophagography to search for occult adenopathy.

Lymph Node Size as a Criterion for the Presence of Metastases

CT provides a remarkable opportunity to locate mediastinal lymph nodes, but one cannot distinguish non-calcified normal from abnormal nodes except by size.[11,13,14,30] Size is an imperfect criterion since small or normal-sized nodes may contain microscopic metastatic foci, whereas nodes in excess of 2 cm in diameter have occasionally been found to be free of metastases even though they are in the drainage path of a malignant primary neoplasm (see Ch. 6). Benign reactive hyperplasia can cause lymph node enlargement that is grossly indistinguishable from metastases on imaging studies.

In general I use the following guidelines:

1. Locate lymph nodes in relation to anatomic landmarks and measure them as accurately as is feasible. Note their location, size, and number. Measurements of nodes on transverse sections, do not represent the greatest dimension, which usually is that of cephalocaudad length. The latter, however, is not measured accurately using the transverse (axial) CT format.

2. Some studies[13,14,30] have used the measurement of the short transverse axis of lymph nodes, or their area, in the transverse plane to establish criteria for normal. This data indicate that if nodes of 1.0 cm diameter, in the short axis, are considered to be the upper limit of normal, there will be a small false negative rate, but a moderate false positive one. Thus, sensitivity will be high.

 a. In the region of the azygos node (right tracheobronchial), the ductus node (aortic-pulmonic window), or the subcarinal nodes, dimensions greater than 1.0 cm can be normal. Therefore, in these zones the presence of lymph nodes between 1.0 and 1.5 cm in diameter does increase the level of uncertainty when they are the only suspect nodes in the entire mediastinal examination.

 b. In the high paratracheal and prevascular regions, most normal nodes will be 7 mm or less in short transverse axis diameter, but a minority can reach 1 cm.[11,14]

3. Clusters of unusual numbers of nodes in any location (that is, more than five or six nodes per slice) are noted but are of indeterminate significance when they are small.

4. Nodes over 1.5 cm in short transverse axis diameter are considered abnormal in any location in the mediastinum. Biopsy of the node or nodes is recommended, however, before any definitive treatment is *withheld* based on the *assumption* that the suspect node is positive for neoplasm. Some of these nodes will be enlarged simply as the result of reactive hyperplasia or extreme upper limits of normal.

5. When several large nodes (over 1.5 cm in diameter) are seen in any mediastinal position they will almost always be abnormal.

 a. In patients whose clinical and radiographic findings indicate the presence of a chronic or relapsing infection (e.g., peripheral to a partially obstructing bronchial neoplasm), it is best *not to assume* that enlarged nodes in the drainage path are metastases, since chronic relapsing infection can cause lymphadenopathy. Biopsy of these nodes is required to make the distinction (see Ch. 6).

No present rules in use will eliminate false-negative and false-positive errors from the analysis of mediastinal adenopathy, but, if you call nodes under 1 cm in short transverse axis diameter positive you will increase your false-positive rate markedly while decreasing your false-negative rate very little. If you do not call nodes over 1.5 cm positive you will decrease your accuracy and sig-

nificantly increase your false-negative rate.[13,14,30] Using these limits does not contradict our knowing that nodes under 1 cm in diameter may be positive whereas nodes over 1.5 cm in diameter may be involved with benign reactive changes rather than metastases. At present, however, we have no noninvasive tools to permit recognition of these exceptions. Gallium scanning is used with varying degrees of enthusiasm to evaluate mediastinal lymphadenopathy, but cannot distinguish neoplasm from inflammatory changes in lymph nodes with enough certainty to obviate the need for biopsy when such distinction is critical to patient management.

At present, MRI suffers in comparison to CT in that small juxtaposed nodes may be mistaken for a single enlarged node because of the poorer spatial resolution of some MRI techniques, and precise distinction between normal and abnormal size nodes on MR images has not been clearly established. It is probably not wise to apply the criteria derived from CT studies of lymph node size directly to MRI studies.[35]

Knowledge of the presence or absence of enlarged mediastinal lymph nodes in conjunction with other pertinent clinical data, can be used to plan diagnostic biopsy and therapeutic surgical approaches that minimize the need to rely on presumption as to whether or not the nodes contain tumor cells.

It is interesting that patients who undergo surgery for pulmonary malignancies have mediastinal lymph nodes, whether positive or negative, that are almost always retrievable from the right superior mediastinum, the aortopulmonic window, the subcarinal region, and near the inferior pulmonary ligament, whereas nodes are not always found higher in the left superior mediastinum.[21]

The foregoing discussion has been concerned with the detection and assessment of non-calcified lymphadenopathy. Calcified lymphadenopathy is discussed in Chapter 8.

If lymphadenopathy were the only pathologic process to contend with in the mediastinum, the challenge would still be sufficient. In fact, however, lesions involving the blood vessels, nerves, thymus, thyroid, esophagus, and heart, as well as primary neoplasms or cysts, may present as mediastinal masses that can mimic lymphadenopathy (see Ch. 8).

SUMMARY

1. Mediastinal contours vary considerably from individual to individual, but certain recurrent patterns can be used to create a spectrum of normal.

2. Comparison with earlier films whenever possible is especially helpful in detecting minimal departures from normal. The abnormal "lives" within the normal spectrum. A change from a previous appearance may be the first clue to an abnormality even though the overall appearance of the mediastinum is still within the normal spectrum.

3. Anatomic studies of intrathoracic lymph nodes have defined a series of lymph node chains or groups whose names[31] are indicative of their position: anterior mediastinal or prevascular, peritracheobronchial, posterior mediastinal, parietal, and intrapulmonary. Each group has subsets.

4. Mediastinal masses are recognized on chest films when they have achieved sufficient size to distort mediastinal contours against adjacent lung or, less commonly, to distort mediastinal contents. Some regions are more commonly involved than others:

   a. Any convexity (toward the lung) that begins and ends above the right tracheobronchial angle and cannot clearly be attributed to the azygos vein is likely to be abnormal. (A very tortuous brachiocephalic artery can cause such a convexity but is still considered abnormal.)

   b. Any convex edge that is projected between the level of the aortic arch and the left pulmonary artery must be suspected of being abnormal.

   c. Distortion of the image of the transverse portion of the aortic arch and the origin of the left subclavian artery is also suspect.

   d. Other zones also have predictable contour changes as a result of adenopathy but are less commonly involved or more difficult to evaluate on chest films.

5. CT and MRI studies are more sensitive than chest films in detecting mediastinal or hilar lymphadenopathy or other masses.

   a. The criteria for considering lymph nodes abnormal on CT or MRI are principally based on size. There are no absolutes; if, on CT studies, you call nodes under 1.0 cm in short axis diameter abnormal you will have a high false-positive rate; if you do not call nodes over 1.5 cm abnormal you will have a high false-negative rate. Enlarged nodes should be biopsied whenever determination of their histopathology is critical to choosing between treatment alternatives.

   b. Imaging criteria do not permit distinction among the various causes of noncalcified lymphadenopathy.

6. The differential diagnosis of mediastinal and hilar lymphadenopathy is extensive, but the vast majority of cases will occur within the first four of these five categories:

1. Lymphomas, leukemias, and variants thereof
2. Metastases from either intrathoracic or extrathoracic primary neoplasms
3. Noninfectious granulomatous disease, especially sarcoid and silicosis
4. Infectious granulomatous disease (e.g., tuberculosis, atypical mycobacteriosis, histoplasmosis, coccidioidomycosis, and cryptococcosis)
5. A miscellaneous group accounting for a large number of causes of low incidence (Table 7-2).

BIBLIOGRAPHY

1. Abell MR: Lymphoid hamartoma. Radiol Clin North Am 6:15, 1968
2. Aronberg DJ, Peterson RR, Glazer HS, Sagel SS: The superior sinus of the pericardium: CT appearance. Radiology 153:489, 1984
3. Axel L, Kressel HY, Thickman D, et al: NMR imaging of the chest at 0.12T: Initial clinical experience with a resistive magnet. AJR 141:1157, 1983
4. Blank N, Castellino RA: Patterns of pleural reflections of the left superior mediastinum: normal anatomy and distortions produced by adenopathy. Radiology 102:585, 1972
5. Blank N, Castellino RA: Mediastinal lymphadenopathy. Semin Roentgenol 12:215, 1977
6. Blank N, Castellino RA: Intrathoracic manifestations of the malignant lymphomas and leukemias. Semin Roentgenol 15:227, 1980
7. Castellino RA, Blank N: Adenopathy of the cardiophrenic angle (diaphragmatic) lymph nodes. Am J Roentgenol 114:509, 1972
8. Cho CS, Blank N, Castellino RA: CT evaluation of cardiophrenic angle lymph nodes in patients with malignant lymphoma. AJR 143:19, 1984
9. Felson B: Chest Roentgenology p. 419. WB Saunders Co, Philadelphia, 1973
10. Filly R, Blank N, Castellino RA: Radiographic distribution of intrathoracic disease in previously untreated patients with Hodgkin's disease and non-Hodgkin's lymphoma. Radiology 120:277, 1976
11. Genereux GP: Normal mediastinal lymph node size and number: CT and anatomic study. AJR 142:1095, 1984
12. Gladnikoff H: A radiographic study of the mediastinum in health and pulmonary carcinoma. Acta Radiol, suppl., 73, 1948
13. Glazer GM, Orringer MB, Gross BH, Quint LE: The mediastinum in non-small cell lung cancer: CT surgical correction. AJR 142:1101, 1984

14. Glazer GM, Gross BH, Quint LE, et al: Normal mediastinal lymph nodes: number and size according to American Thoracic Society Mapping. AJR 144:261, 1985

15. Heelan RT, Martini N, Wescott JW, et al: Carcinomatous involvement of the hilum and mediastinum: computed tomographic and magnetic resonance evaluation. Radiology 156:111, 1985

16. Heitzman ER, Scrivani JV, Martino J, et al: The azygos vein and its pleural reflections. I. Normal roentgen anatomy. Radiology 101:249, 1971

17. Heitzman ER, Scrivani JV, Martino J, et al: II. Applications in the radiological diagnosis of mediastinal abnormality. Radiology 101:259, 1971

18. Keats TE, Lipscomb GE, Betts CS III: Mensuration of the arch of the azygos vein and its application to the study of cardiopulmonary disease. Radiology 90:990, 1968

19. Keller AR, Hochholzer L, Castleman B: Hyaline-vascular and plasma-cell types of giant lymph node hyperplasia of the mediastinum and other locations. Cancer 29:670, 1972

20. Limpert J, MacMahon H, Variakojis D: Angioimmunoblastic lymphadenopathy: clinical and radiological features. Radiology 152:27, 1984

21. Martini N, Flehinger BJ, Zaman MB: Prospective study of 445 lung carcinomas with mediastinal lymph node metastases. J Thorac Cardiovasc Surg 80:390, 1980

22. McCort JJ, Robbins LL: Roentgen diagnosis of intrathoracic lymph node metastases in carcinoma of the lung. Radiology 57:339, 1951

23. McDonald CJ, Castellino RA, Blank N: The aortic "nipple." The left superior intercostal vein. Radiology 96:553, 1970

24. Mintzer RA, Malave SR, Neiman HL, et al: Computed vs. conventional tomography in evaluation of primary and secondary pulmonary neoplasms. Radiology 132:653, 1979

25. Naidich DP, Zerhouni EA, Siegelman SS: Computed Tomography of the Thorax. p. 13; 37–40. Raven Press, New York, 1984

26. Nohl HC: The Spread of Carcinoma of the Bronchus. Year Book Medical Publishers, Chicago, 1962

27. Osborne DR, Korobkin M, Ravin CE, et al: Comparison of plain radiography, conventional tomography, and computed tomography in detecting intrathoracic lymph node metastases from lung carcinoma. Radiology 142:157, 1982

28. Proto AV, Simmons JD, Zylak CJ: The anterior junction anatomy. CRC Crit Rev Diagn Imaging 19:111, 1983

29. Proto AV: Mediastinal anatomy: emphasis on conventional images with anatomic and computed tomographic correlations. J Thorac Imaging 2:1, 1987

30. Quint LE, Glazer GM, Orringer MB, et al: Mediastinal lymph node detection and sizing at CT and autopsy. AJR 147:469, 1986

31. Rouvière H: Anatomy of the Human Lymphatic System. Edwards Brothers, Ann Arbor, MI, 1938

32. Schnur MJ, Winkler B, Austin JHM: Widening of the posterior wall of the bronchus intermedius: a sign on lateral chest radiographs of congestive heart failure, lymph node enlargement, and neoplastic infiltration. Radiology 139:551, 1981

33. Shapeero LG, Blank N, Young SW: Contrast enhancement in mediastinal and cervical lymph nodes. J Comput Assist Tomogr 7:242, 1983

34. Tsi GM, Friedman PJ, Peters RM, et al: Clinical staging of primary lung cancer. Official statement of the American Thoracic Society. Am Rev Respir Dis 127:659, 1983

35. Webb WR, Jensen BG, Sollito R, et al: Bronchogenic carcinoma; staging with MR compared with staging with CT and surgery. Radiology 156:117, 1985

Atlas

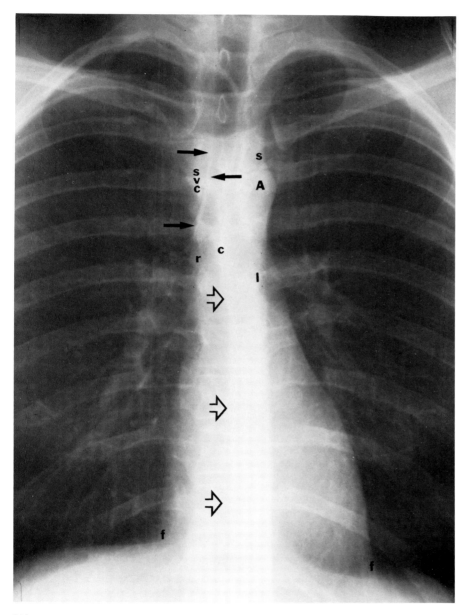

Key

A. Aortic knob
s. Left subclavian artery
r. Right main bronchus
l. Left main bronchus
c. Tracheal carina
svc. Superior vena cava

(A)

Fig. 7-1.   Radiographic Anatomy of the Mediastinum: Anteroposterior View

(A) Coned view of a heavily exposed film of the chest illustrates some details of mediastinal anatomy that will be referred to frequently. **(B,C,D)** Selected tomographic cuts of the same man emphasizing anatomic details. The CT scans in Figure 7-2 (from another patient) show these anatomic details in the axial plane. *(Figure continues.)*

Aortic Knob. The posterior turn of the transverse portion of the aortic arch ordinarily forms part of the border against the mediastinal pleura-lung interface on the left and presents as the so-called aortic knob (A).

This image varies considerably from patient to patient. In infants and children it may not be at all distinct. In patients whose aortas are dilated or tortuous from any cause, this arch may be very prominent. In patients with abundant mediastinal fat only a small segment of the lateral edge of the aortic knob may be seen to interface with the lung, or the mediastinal fat may displace the mediastinal pleura so that it actually passes tangential to or slightly lateral to the aortic arch. Calcific bands and crescents are commonly seen in the aortic arch in adults as a sign of atherosclerosis.

Left Subclavian Artery. The pleural reflection over the left subclavian artery (S) is border forming from the level of the aortic arch cephalad. It presents an arc that is usually concave toward the lung, although the degree of concavity varies considerably. It passes up toward the apex of the chest. In some individuals a segment of this border may appear double because of projection of lung against a more anterior portion of the supra-aortic anterior mediastinal pleura lateral to mediastinal fat.

Main Bronchi and Right Tracheobronchial Angle. The right (r) and left (l) main bronchi can be seen beyond the tracheal carina (c), which is obscured in this person by a superimposed vertebral spinous process. The "r" is also positioned medial to the orifice of the right upper lobe bronchus. The angle made by the junction of the superior wall of the right main bronchus and the right lateral wall of the trachea is called the right tracheobronchial angle (RTBA).

The main bronchi appear as darker gray tubes with fairly parallel walls. Centrally they may not be visible on high-contrast, low-kilovoltage, or underexposed films. Sometimes they are more easily recognized if you hold the film oblique to your line of vision.

Azygos Vein. The azygos vein (z in Fig. B) presents an elliptical image of varying size adjacent to the right side of the trachea at or above the RTBA. It may vary in width from imperceptible (as in Fig. A) to an extreme of 9 mm (measured from the inside wall of the trachea to the outer edge of the vein) in normal individuals. The azygos vein contains more blood and becomes wider when the patient is supine than when the subject is erect. The image is a projection of the arch of the azygos vein as it passes anteriorly (from a prespinal position) lateral to the trachea to empty into the superior vena cava (SVC). The azygos vein image is seen in at least 80 percent of PA chest films using modern technique.

Right Paratracheal Band. In the majority of patients (approximately 80 percent) the right lateral wall of the trachea may be seen as a band of soft tissue 1 to 4 mm thick, passing cephalad from the level of the RTBA. This is called the right paratracheal band (horizontal, staggered arrows in Fig. A). It is seen because air in the trachea provides one contrast interface while air in the lung adjacent to its lateral wall provides another. If fat in the mediastinum, or enlarged right paratracheal lymph nodes, (see Fig. 7-12) or any other type of mass or fluid (e.g., hemorrhage) moves the lung interface away from the outer trachea wall, a thick band of soft tissue may become evident alongside the tracheal air column.

Since the right tracheal wall is not seen as a distinct image in all normal individuals, its absence cannot be assumed to be abnormal.

Superior Vena Cava. The pleural reflection over the lateral edge of the SVC is border forming along the right mediastinum above the level of the right atrium. In some individuals it presents a very distinct interface tangential to the beam and is seen as a sharp image on the radiograph. In others, however, the tangent is apparently not long enough to produce a sharp image, and an ill-defined edge or no edge at all may be seen. In some, only segments of the edge of the SVC may be seen (see Fig. 7-5). The shape is variable within a narrow range (see Fig. 7-6). Do not confuse the SVC with a thickened right paratracheal band. In Fig. A the SVC presents an image that is difficult to see, in part, because it is projected so close to the image of the spine. In Fig. B the edge of the SVC can be seen (in bright light) between the white arrows.

Azygoesophageal Recess Interface (Azygoesophageal Stripe). In Fig. A there is a distinct change in gray tone (from darker on the patient's right to lighter on the left) over the thoracic spine from the level of the tracheal carina caudally. This interface represents the junction between the right lung and the mediastinum anterior to the vertebral column. It is referred to as the azygoesophageal recess interface (or stripe; open arrows) because in many individuals either the azygos vein or the esophagus or both are located just to the left of this pleural reflection. The azygoesophageal recess interface is seen in approximately 50 percent of PA chest films,[29] although not always in its entirety.

Occasionally images of spinous processes of thoracic vertebrae may line up and produce a spurious azygoesophageal stripe, or they may contribute to its conspicuity by their added density. Air in the esophagus may commonly be seen to the left of the recess interface, but less often than the pleural reflection itself is seen. *(Figure continues.)*

(B) Tomogram at a level just anterior to the thoracic spine. The azygoesophageal recess interface (dotted line) has a curve that is gently convex to the right at the level of the confluence of the pulmonary veins of the right lung (V). Beginning caudal to the tracheal carina (c), the edge becomes concave toward the right and can be followed cephalad to the image of the azygos vein (z) above the RTBA. The tomogram is made with the patient supine; hence the increased size of the azygos vein compared to its size on the upright chest film. In addition, the SVC is more distended, and its right lateral margin is seen continuing cephalad (between the white arrows) from the level of the azygos vein.

Posterior Junction Line. A thin band of soft tissue is superimposed on the tracheal air column (staggered arrows in Fig. B). It is continuous with arcs of lung-soft tissue interfaces that pass cephalad along the medial aspects of both apices (highest arrows). This is the posterior junction line, and it marks the adjacent boundaries of the right and left lung in front of the upper thoracic spine. On the plain-film image (Fig. A) you can see a curved, thin band shadow (unmarked) superimposed on the spine extending from the upper right corner of T2 to the lower left corner of T3. This is the plain-film counterpart of the posterior, prespinal junction line seen in Fig. B. Some portion of the posterior junction line can be seen in approximately 40 percent of PA chest films.[29]

(C) Tomogram at a level just behind the manubrium (M) and the sternum.
Anterior Junction Line. The anterosuperior portions of both lungs form an interface at this level, and the pleural surfaces between them constitute the anterior junction line (arrows). This thin band of apposed pleural layers may be seen on the plain chest film in about 25 percent of cases.[29] The technique must be optimum, the subject must not be heavy set, and the image must be searched for. Cephalad to the anterior junction line the retromanubrial soft tissues have arcs that interface with the anterosuperior aspects of both lungs. You cannot see the anterior junction line in Fig. A, but you can deduce where it should be.

The anterior junction line is frequently seen on CT scans as a sheet of pleura that passes obliquely forward from the mediastinum to the anterior chest wall so that its anterior end is to the left of its posterior end (see Fig. 7-2C). *(Figure continues.)*

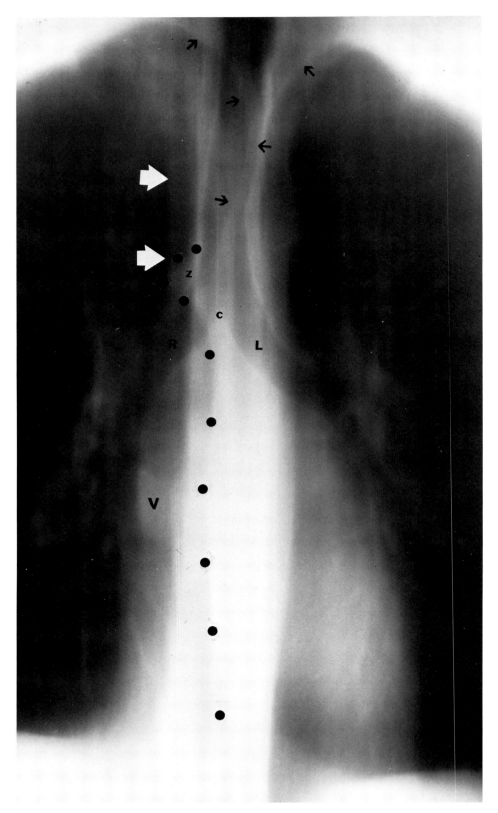

(B)

Fig. 7-1. *(Continued).*

Key

z. Azygos vein
r. Right main bronchus
l. Left main bronchus

c. Tracheal carina
v. Confluence of pulmonary vein

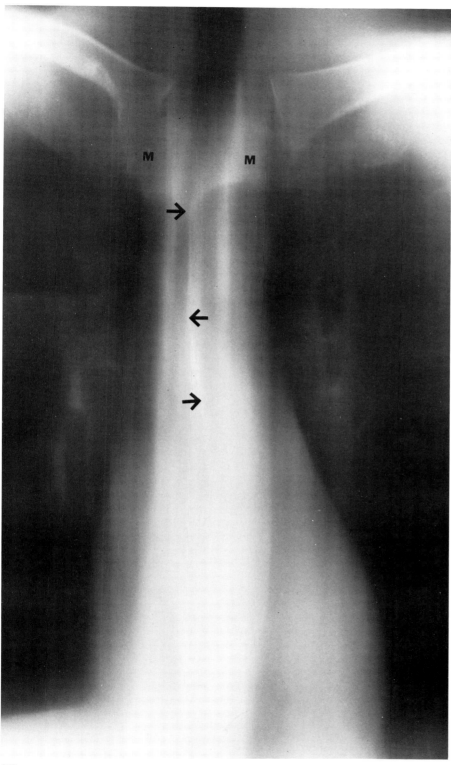

(C)

Fig. 7-1. *(Continued).*

Key

M. Manibrium

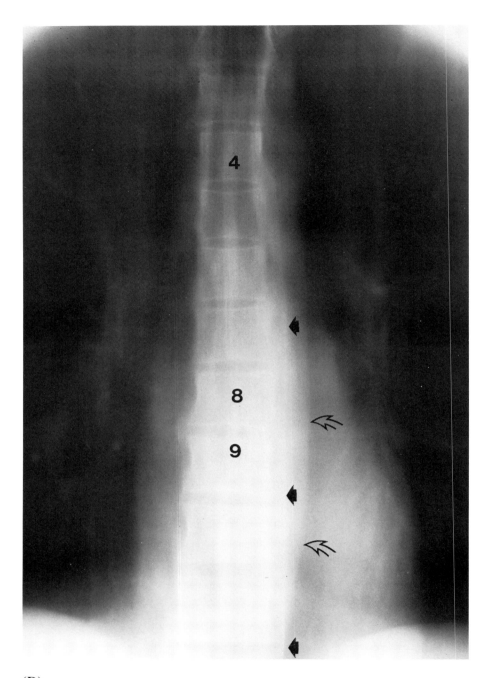

(D)

Fig. 7-1. *(Continued).* **(D)** Posterior tomogram.

Paravertebral Stripe. The vertebral bodies are in focus, but the out-of-focus carrythrough images of their spinous processes line up to form a pseudo-band shadow passing roughly down the middle of the vertebral column. On the left side there is a paravertebral stripe of soft tissue (short arrows) extending from the lower margin of the film (lowest black arrow) in a uniform manner up to the level of T4 (4) where it curves medially to disappear at the margin of the vertebra. The left paravertebral stripe is seen on fewer than half of all PA chest films, and a right paravertebral stripe is seen even less often.

To the left of the paravertebral stripe you see the left margin of the descending aorta (open arrows). It has an arc that is gently convex toward the left lung. It is the interface with the left lung that permits the descending aorta to be seen at all. If you go back to Fig. A, you will see that the distinction between the

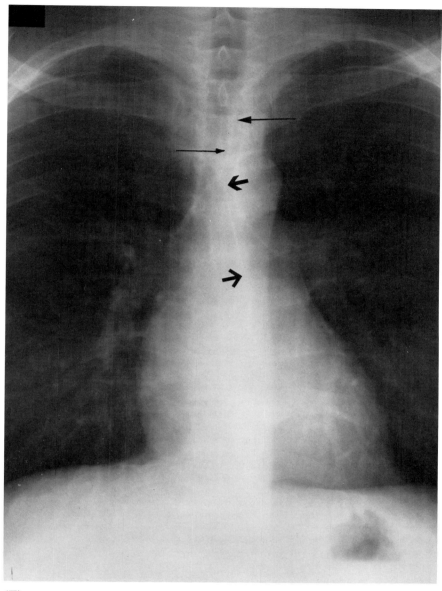

(E)

left paravertebral stripe and the descending aorta is not clear. In patients whose descending aorta is more dilated or tortuous and impresses against the left lung, the distinction is made more easily. However, in those patients whose descending aorta is located in front of the spine, "buried" in the mediastinum, the edges of the descending aorta may not be seen at all.

On the right side of Fig. D there is a bulge of soft tissues at the T8–T9 interspace due to a laterally bulging intervertebral disc. Bulging intervertebral discs or vertebral spurs may be seen on plain films when they are prominent. They are not seen on the left side when the descending aorta is located alongside the vertebrae, but when the descending aorta is prespinal in location, bulging discs and associated osteophytes may also be seen on the left.

Cardiophrenic Angles. The areas between the heart borders and the diaphragm are commonly designated the cardiophrenic angles. Frequently there is a fat pad, (f) which can vary markedly in size, in this location. Commonly the left fat pad is larger than the right.

(E) Coned view of a heavily exposed film shows both the anterior junction line (thick arrows) and the posterior junction line (thin arrows).

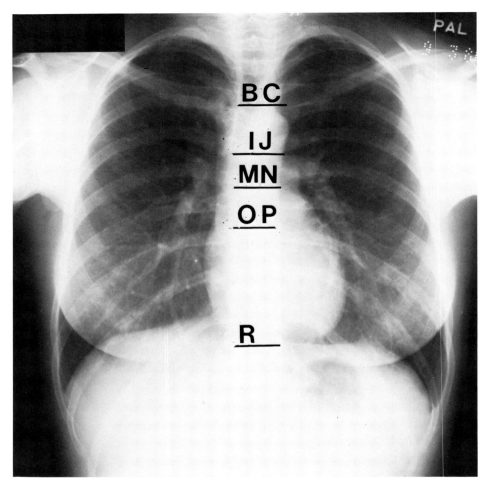

(A)

Fig. 7-2. CT Examination of the Mediastinum

This series of CT scans emphasizes some important features of mediastinal anatomy and relates them to appearances on chest films. CT scans are done with the patient supine, whereas chest films are taken, when possible, with the patient erect. Usually there is an increase in mediastinal width and some alteration of contour when the patient is supine. These changes must be considered when comparing chest films made with the patient upright to those made with the patient supine. Nevertheless, those structures that are border forming in the normal individual remain so whether the patient is erect or supine, and the correlation of anatomy between chest films and CT scans thus remains valid.

The scans in each pair were taken at the same level in the chest. The lefthand scans were all filmed at a gray scale that optimally displays mediastinal structures, whereas the righthand scans were photographed at a gray scale that shows pulmonary details.

(A) PA chest film showing the approximate level of some of the scans. Letters indicate level of corresponding CT scans. The other CT scans are intercalated in alphabetical order. (Before actual scanning, a CT scout view is made. The portions of the body to be examined — chest, abdomen, pelvis, etc. — are moved through the scanner on a moving tabletop, and a digital image is made. Each level scanned is then accurately annotated on that image).

Note. The centimeter scale for the CT scans shown in this and other chapters has usually been cropped off of the display. A rough estimate of the size of any lesion can be obtained by comparison with the transverse diameter of the trachea and assuming an average value of 2.0 centimeters for that measurement. *(Figure continues.)*

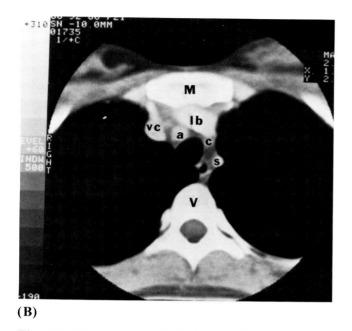

(B)

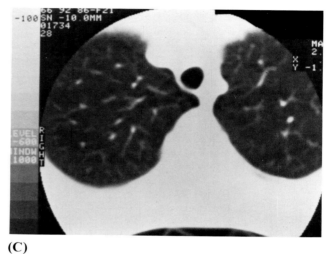

(C)

Fig. 7-2. *(Continued).* **(B,C)** Scans taken at the level of the manubrium (M). The left subclavian artery (s) protrudes into adjacent lung, and you can see why the mediastinal pleura along its lateral margin would produce a sharp edge image above the aortic arch. Fat (gray-black) is located medial to the left subclavian artery, and posteromedially there is a small, oval, black zone caused by air in the esophagus. Anteriorly the mediastinal pleura is reflected over the left carotid artery (c) and then the left brachiocephalic vein (lb). This vein is quite wide in this patient and is seen passing anterior to the right brachiocephalic artery (a), in its usual position.

The superior vena cava (vc) is border forming on the right. A portion of the right brachiocephalic vein is seen near its junction with the anterior aspect of the SVC. The medial end of the left brachiocephalic vein is caudal to its lateral end, as would be expected from the usual oblique course of this vein, and therefore the medial portion of this vein is not seen until the next scan, made 1 cm caudally. (Actually the SVC is not formed until the junction of the right and left brachiocephalic veins.)

A small band of fat separates the right and left lungs behind the esophagus anterior to the spine (V). This constitutes a segment of the posterior junction line or band.

Notice that the image filmed with mediastinal window settings (Fig. B) shows the trachea as having no right lateral wall, whereas when lung window settings are used (Fig. C) this wall is clearly seen. You can see how it is possible to change the apparent size of many structures by varying the window and level settings used to view them. To measure the true dimensions of an anatomic structure or of a lesion, it is necessary to make the measurements at a window level setting that is halfway between the CT number of the part to be measured and the CT number of the surrounding tissues. *(Figure continues.)*

Fig. 7-2. *(Continued).* **(D)** CT scan at a level 1 cm caudal to that in Figs. B and C. The medial portion of the left brachiocephalic vein (lb) can now be seen. This vein is rather wide in this patient, but all of the vessels in this scan are seen to enhance following the intravenous injection of contrast material. (The small white square marks the left subclavian artery.)

Notice again the width of the soft tissues that separate the right and left lungs in front of the spine.

(E) CT scan at the level of the aortic arch (AA), which is seen as a sausage-like structure along the left side of the trachea. The superior vena cava (vc) is seen adjacent to the right anterior extremity of the aortic arch, and the conjoint image of the aortic arch and the SVC resembles an elephant seal. The space anterior to the trachea between the images of the aortic arch and the SVC, called the paratracheal pocket (dot), is filled with fat.

After puberty the normal thymus seldom accounts for any confusing image on chest films, but on CT a normal thymus may be seen in adults as a bilobed, more or less triangular mass anterior to the ascending aorta and the aortic arch. Normal measurements for the thymus as seen on CT scan have been defined.[25] In many adults a discrete bilobed thymus is not seen on CT; rather there are islands of residual thymic tissue seen in fat, which has replaced much of the gland.

Immediately in front of the thoracic spine, along the left posterolateral aspects of the trachea, you can see a small amount of air (small, black, round area) in the esophagus. This can also be seen in Fig. D, and even more air in the esophagus can be seen on Fig. B, where the esophagus is posteromedial to the subclavian artery. Notice the close relation of the prevertebral, retrotracheal recess of the right lung to the esophagus (arrow).

The mediastinal pleural reflection over the anterior ends of both lungs — the anterior junction line — is seen as a thin strand between the aortic arch and the sternum(s). Cephalad (see Fig. D), the pleural boundaries comprising the anterior junction line diverge to follow the margins of the right and left lungs behind the manubrium and may be seen on some chest films as V-shaped edges superimposed on or projecting slightly lateral to the manubrium (Figs. 7-1C and E).

(F) Lung window settings portray the anterior junction line wider than it is on the image at mediastinal window settings, and once again the right lateral tracheal wall is seen. *(Figure continues.)*

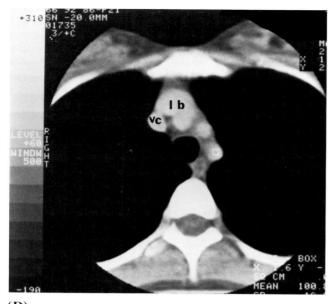

(D)

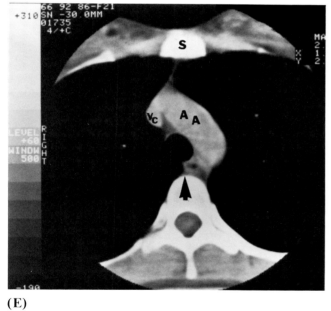

(E)

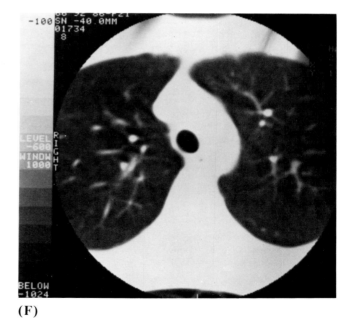

(F)

Fig. 7-2. *(Continued).*

Fig. 7-2. *(Continued).* **(G,H)** Scans taken approximately 1 cm caudal to that in Fig. F. **(G)** The rounded opacity anterior to the airway represents the ascending aorta (A), with the SVC intimately associated with its right lateral wall. The impingement of the ascending aorta on the SVC is unusual. Anterolateral to the vertebrae you can see the descending thoracic aorta (a). Between the ascending and the descending thoracic aorta there is a low-density area consisting of fat in the aortopulmonic window, plus small lymph nodes and partial-volume effects of the aortic arch itself. The thickness of tissues included in this slice is 10 mm. Partial-volume effect occurs when only part of a structure is included in the total thickness of a slice, so that the resulting image is a product of averaging the tissue density of the structure with other tissue densities above or below it in the same slice thickness.

The esophagus is seen just anterior to the vertebra, and no air is visible in its lumen. Notice the changing shape of the airway, indicating that we are near the region of its bifurcation into the right and left main bronchi.

(H) The caudal continuation of the anterior junction line is seen as a thin band (arrow). When there is little intervening fat the image is linear, when there is moderate intervening fat a bandlike image results, and when there is abundant mediastinal fat neither a line nor a band image is seen. The anterior junction line has an oblique course between the region of the ascending aorta and the sternum, with the ventral end usually located to the left of the dorsal end. If you rotated the image so as to simulate a patient in the left anterior oblique projection, you could see how the beam would traverse the full depth of the anterior junction line. Thus, the anterior junction line often is clearly and easily seen on the left anterior oblique projection of the chest. In addition, the caudal end of the anterior junction line is usually to the left of its cephalic end (Fig. 7-1C and E). Occasionally the anterior junction assumes a near-vertical course, and uncommonly its ventral end is to the right rather than the left of its dorsal end.

(I,J) Scans taken 1 cm caudal to Figs. G and H. **(I)** The carina of the trachea and the right and left main bronchi are shown. The soft tissue images along the left side of the image of the ascending aorta (A) are due to partial-volume effect of the pulmonary outflow tract. The descending thoracic aorta (a) is located along the left anterolateral aspects of the vertebra. The esophagus is seen medial to the descending thoracic aorta. There is a small, rounded opacity seen in intimate association with the right anterolateral aspect of the vertebra alongside the esohagus; this is the image of the prespinal portion of the azygos vein (open arrow).

(J) At lung window settings you can see the right upper lobe bronchus extending laterally from the right main bronchus. The tracheal carina is seen as a thin band between the right and left main bronchi. *(Figure continues.)*

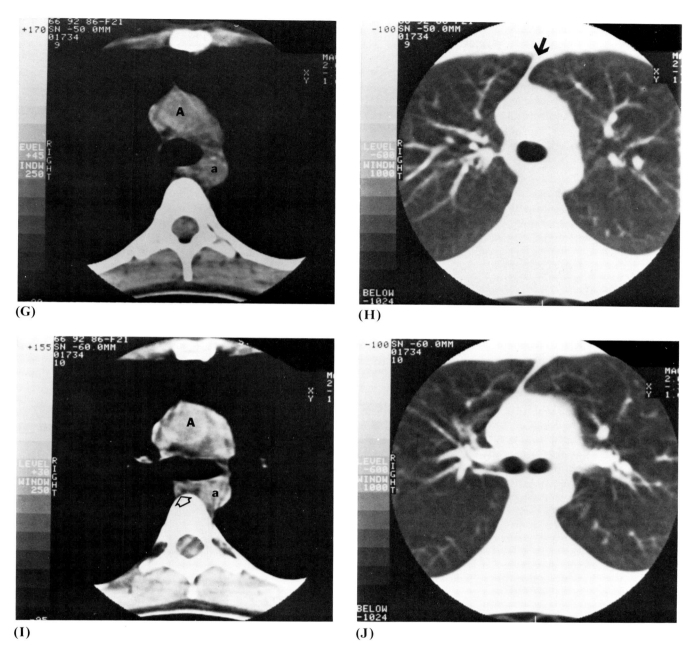

(G)

(H)

(I)

(J)

Fig. 7-2. *(Continued).*

Fig. 7-2. *(Continued).* **(K,L)** Scans taken 1 cm caudal to Figs. I and J. **(K)** The superior vena cava (vc) just above the level of the cavoatrial junction is border forming on the right side of the mediastinum, whereas the main pulmonary artery (pa) is border forming on the left. The azygos vein (small black rectangle) is seen as a small, rounded density anterior to the thoracic vertebra with a very sharp mediastinal pleural reflection along its right lateral aspect. This is a segment of the pleural reflection (arrow) of the azygoesophageal recess. Notice that it extends cephalad and can be seen on Fig. I. There is a similar sharp mediastinal pleural reflection superiorly on Figs. B, D, and E, which are at a level above the azygos vein. The arch of the azygos vein is seen as a partial-volume structure along the right side of the airway on Fig. G where it adds to the thickness of the right tracheal wall as seen on Fig. H.

(L) The airways at this level are the origin of the bronchus intermedius on the right (arrow) and the lower end of the left main bronchus on the left. A small, black, round structure among the left hilar vessels is a cross section of the apicoposterior segmental bronchus of the left upper lobe. Notice that lung is closely approximated to the dorsal margin of the right bronchus intermedius.

(M,N) Scans taken 1 cm caudal to Figs. K and L. **(M)** The top of the right atrium (ra) is border-forming along the right side of the cardiomediastinal silhouette. The pulmonary artery and the pulmonary outflow tract (P) are still border forming on the left. A partial image of the right pulmonary artery (rpa) crosses to the right, anterior to the airway, and enters the hilum after passing dorsal to the SVC. The root of the aorta (A) is visible in the center of the image. The descending thoracic aorta (a) is readily identified along the left anterolateral aspects of the vertebra. There is a small amount of fat between the right side of the descending thoracic aorta and the azygos vein (dot), which is located immediately in front of the vertebral body. Again you can see the sharp mediastinal pleural reflection along the right side of the azygos vein outlining this segment of the azygoesophageal recess. The esohagus (e) is seen as a rounded opacity anterior to the small fat pad that separates the descending thoracic aorta and the azygos vein.

(N) On images made at lung window settings you can see the cross section of the bronchus intermedius on the right. On the left side the left upper lobe bronchus and the origin of the lingular bronchus are seen. The ball-like density posterior to the left upper lobe bronchus is an image of a portion of the left pulmonary artery (lpa). The small soft tissue mound anterior to the left upper lobe bronchus here and on some of the more cephalad cuts is a portion of the left superior pulmonary vein. The anterior junction line appears as though it is a continuation of the pleural reflection over the right atrium. *(Figure continues.)*

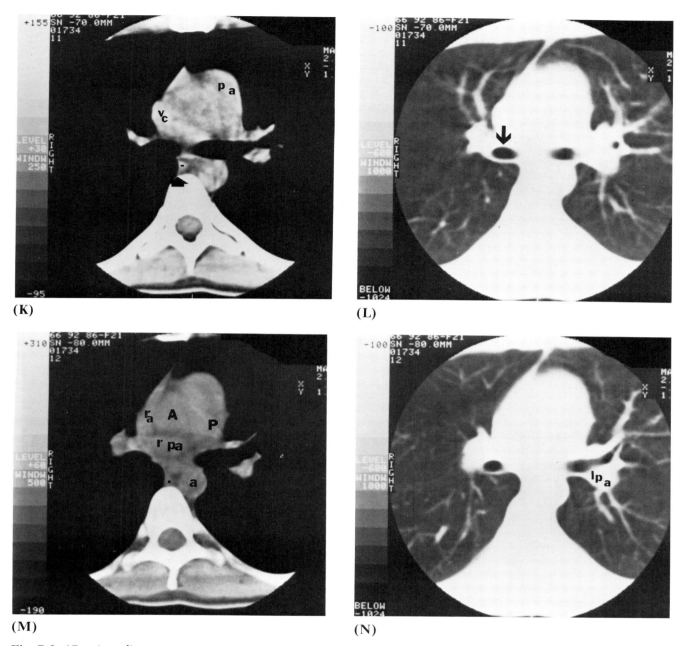

(K)

(L)

(M)

(N)

Fig. 7-2. *(Continued).*

Fig. 7-2. *(Continued).* **(O,P)** Scans taken approximately 2 cm caudal to Figs. M and N. **(O)** The pleural reflection over the azygoesophageal recess is still seen as a sharp image anterior to the vertebra, but the esophagus itself and even the azygos vein are not seen as distinct images.

(P) Cross sections of the right and left lower lobe bronchi are seen with their adjacent vascular bundles. Large veins are also seen coursing to the left atrium. The lungs are separated from each other by the interposed heart and mediastinal contents. Caudally the pleural boundaries of the anterior junction line diverge over the retrosternal, or bare areas, of the heart (arrows) and adjacent pericardial fat pads.

The level of this divergence is quite variable. In patients with large-volume lungs (e.g., those with emphysema), the anterior junction line may extend almost to the diaphragm.

(Q) Slice taken approximately 8 cm caudal to Figs. O and P. Portions of the right and left hemidiaphragms are included. The blackness posterior to the diaphragmatic expanses represents lung in the caudal portions of the hemithorax. The large oval low-density area seen just beneath the diaphragm posteriorly on the right side is the image of the intrahepatic portion of the inferior vena cava. The esophagus (e) is seen immediately anterior to the descending thoracic aorta (a) which is now seen to lie anterior to the thoracic vertebra rather than along its left lateral aspect. The aorta in this position may abut the pleural reflection of the azygoesophageal recess and constitute the left boundary of the recess at this level.

(R) Scan taken 3 cm caudal to Fig. Q. It is included primarily to show the posterior aspects of both lungs caudal to the diaphragmatic domes. The lungs appear as dark black crescents (small square) at these window and level settings. The image of the spleen (S) is seen under the left hemidiaphragm. Low-density foci in the liver (L) are due to nonopacified vessels. A mixture of gas and fluid is seen in the stomach (st) between the images of the liver and the spleen.

These scans can be referred to when comparisons with mediastinal abnormalities are indicated on subsequent CT scans in this chapter.

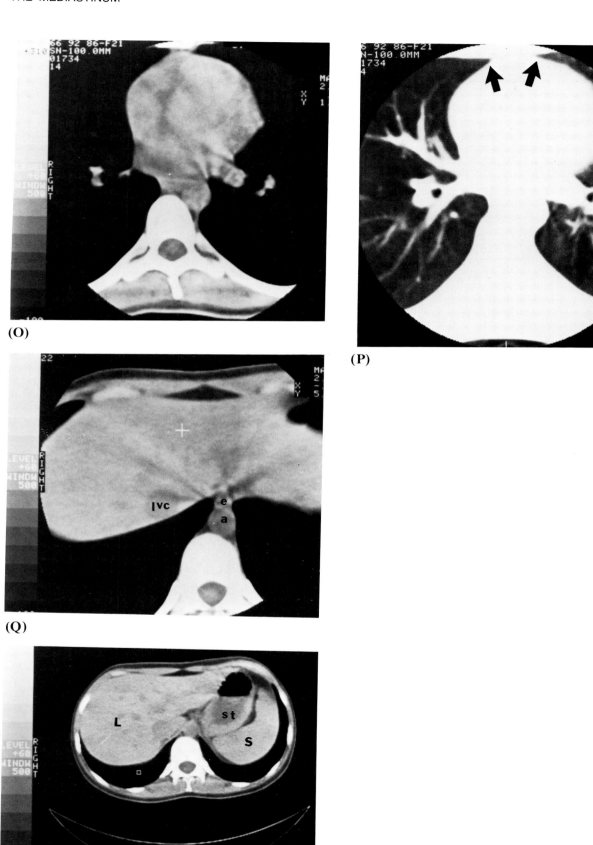

(O)

(P)

(Q)

(R)

Fig. 7-2. *(Continued).*

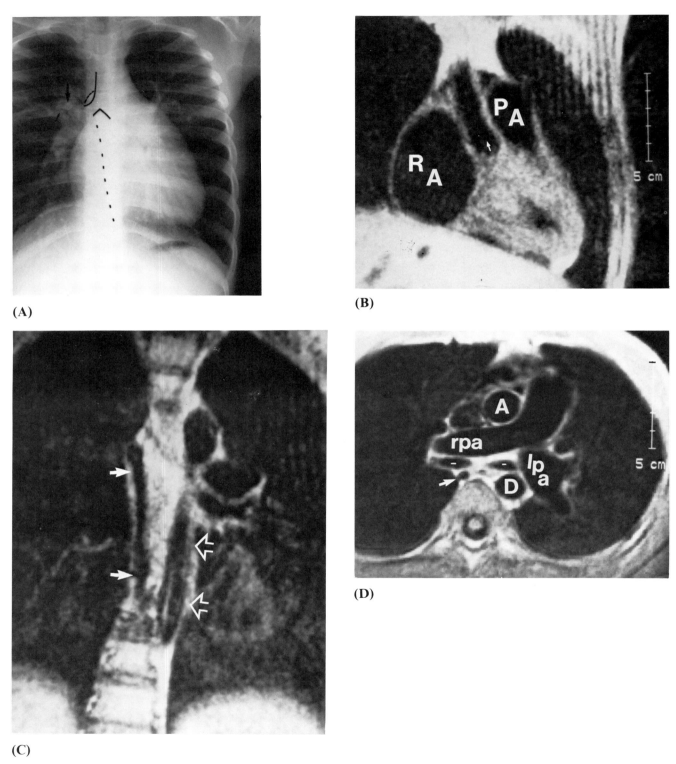

(A)

(B)

(C)

(D)

Fig. 7-3. *(Figure continues.)*

Fig. 7-3. Azygos Vein and Other Vessels on MRI Scans

(A) AP view of the chest of a child with an interatrial septal defect. The right atrial margin is seen as a long smooth arc to the right of the spine. Dashed lines mark the azygoesophageal recess interface. The inverted "v" marks the tracheal carina, and the "j" marks the right wall of the trachea and the upper edge of the right main bronchus at its origin. The azygos vein is outlined to the right of the lower trachea and the right tracheobronchial angle. A vertical arrow indicates a large branch of the pulmonary artery seen end-on in the right hilum.

(B) MRI scan in an anterior coronal plane through the heart at a level that demonstrates the right atrium (RA) best. It provides a graphic correlation with the chest film. Moving blood creates a signal void on MRI scans, which is recorded as black on the gray scale chosen for filming here. Hence the cavity of the RA is seen as a large, black ovoid. The ascending aorta is seen as a black tube (small arrow) to the left of the right atrium, and the pulmonary artery (PA) is seen as a black, pear-shaped structure to the left of the ascending aorta. This is not its true shape but is the appearance of the knuckle of a curved tube after its top edge has been cut off.

The lungs are also shown as black images, and the mottled gray-white vertical bands and dashes that pervade the image are artifacts.

(C) MRI scan in a posterior coronal plane through the region of the azygos vein. The vein is seen as a black tube passing from the left lower corner of the spine obliquely cephalad toward the right tracheobronchial angle (solid white arrows). It corresponds very well to the path of the dashed line in Fig. A that was used to mark the azygoesohageal recess interface.

A portion of the descending aorta (open arrows) is seen as a black ellipse to the left of the spine.

(D) MRI scan in axial cross section just caudal to the tracheal carina (below the inverted "v" shown in Fig. A). At this level the azygos vein (small arrow) is seen along the right anterolateral aspect of the vertebra. The esophagus is identified by a small, black oval in areolar tissue (white) anterior to the vertebra, and the descending aorta (D) is seen along the left side of the vertebra. You can see how a coronal slice through the middle of the lumen of the azygos vein at this level would also pass through the anterior third of the lumen of the descending aorta as in Fig. C.

Because of the variable positions of the azygos vein and the aorta in reference to the thoracic spine, these precise relationships would vary from patient to patient and with the cephalocaudal level at which the axial slice was obtained. (A, ascending aorta; RPA, right pulmonary artery; LPA, left pulmonary artery, short bars in bronchus intermedius on the right and main bronchus on the left.) *(Figure continues.)*

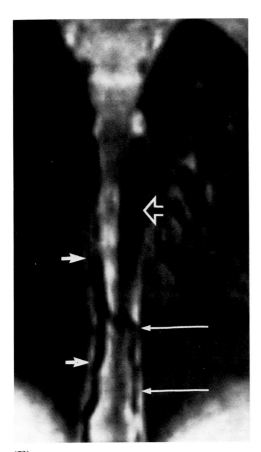

Fig. 7-3 *(Continued).* **(E)** MRI scan in a posterior coronal plane through the azygos vein, the hemiazygos vein, and the descending aorta. This image from a different patient shows the azygos vein (short arrows) ascending along the right side of the vertebral column. The hemiazygos vein (long arrows) ascends on the left and crosses over to join the azygos vein. The descending aorta (open arrow) is partly included in this section. *(Figure continues.)*

(E)

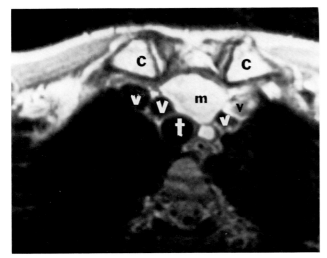

(F)

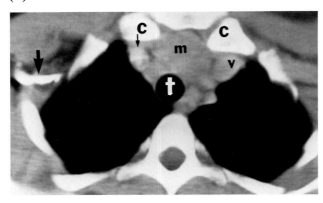

(G)

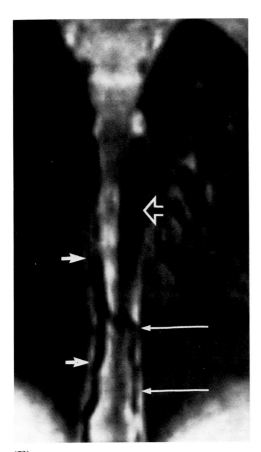

(H)

(F-H) Retromanubrial Mass Shown on MR and CT.

Fig. 7-3. *(Continued).* Axial (F)/MR slice at the level of the medial ends of the clavicles (c). The MR unit had a magnet with a strength of 1.5 Tesla. A spin echo pulse sequence of TR 2400 : TE 30 was used so that the image is neither T1 nor T2-weighted but contains elements of both. This image is dependent upon the proton density of the tissues studied.

A 2.5 cm × 3.5 cm retrosternal mass (m) is easily distinguished from the vessels (v) which surround it and from the trachea (t) along its right posterolateral aspect.

(G) Cut from a CT scan at approximately the same level as the MR scan of Fig. F. The gray scale image of the retrosternal mass (m) is much closer to that of the vessels which surround it. However, a small amount of contrast material (small vertical arrow) is seen in the right brachiocephalic vein and a higher concentration of contrast material is seen in the right axillary vein (larger vertical arrow). The left brachiocephalic vein (black v) contains very little contract material and its gray scale is quite similar to that of the retrosternal mass. Even on the MRI study (Fig. F) the lumen of the left brachiocephalic vein (v) is not as black as the lumina of the vessels on the right side of the mass due to a flow phenomena which is discussed in the references pertaining to the MRI section of Ch. 2.

Compare the anatomy of the retromanubrial region in Figs. F and G with the appearance of this region on Fig. 2B and C. This region, just above the anterior junction line, varies in size—due to differences in amounts of fat, thymic remnant, and size of branch vessels which occupy this space. A fairly large mass can be located behind the manubrium and defy recognition on a PA view of the chest. Until the mass becomes large enough to cause lateral bulging of the mediasternal pleural reflections in the retromanubrial space, these lesions may be extraordinarily difficult to recognize on chest films.

(H) A coronal MR image of the same patient. It shows the mass (m) cradled between the right and left brachiocephalic veins above the level of the vena cava (small black square) and the aorta (small o). (The small horizontal bar marks a coronal section through the pulmonary artery and T, a segment of trachea.)

Although the cephalocaudad dimensions of the mass (5 + cm) could also be calculated from stacked cuts made in the axial plane, it is displayed more graphically in the coronal plane. The pulse sequences for the coronal image were TR 800 : TE 25. At 1.5 Tesla, these produce a T1-weighted image. The signal intensity (brightness) of the mass (m) is less than on the axial image of Fig. F made with different imaging parameters. It is clearly distinguished from fat.

Notice that fat in the subcutaneous tissues, the intermuscular planes, and in the marrow spaces, has a high signal intensity (on the white end of the gray scale) on these MR images. On CT (Fig. G), however, the low density of the subcutaneous fat is displayed on the near-black end of the gray scale.

Fig. 7-4. **(A) Common Variations in the Contours of the Left Mediastinum on the PA Chest Film**

This series of diagrams shows the configuration of the mediastinal pleural reflections along the left side of the mediastinum. The data are based on 278 subjects with no known mediastinal disease. The relative incidence of these variants is as follows: I, 23 percent; II, 8 percent; III, 5 percent; IVa, 14 percent; IVb, 2 percent; V, 48 percent; Ao-LPA, 38 percent. Since Ao-LPA may be seen with other patterns of the group, these numbers add to more than 100 percent. However, the numbers are much less important than the simple recognition that all of these variations do occur.

Diagrams I through IVb represent the common variations in shape of this segment of the left mediastinal border. In the region of the main pulmonary artery and the left pulmonary artery (pa), the mediastinal pleural reflection may show a pronounced convexity to the left (I and II) and still be within normal limits. However, between the level of the aortic arch (A) and the left pulmonary artery the mediastinal pleural reflection should be either concave toward the left lung as in diagram I or straight as in diagram IVa. Any convex edge contour that is projected toward the left lung between the level of the aortic arch and the left pulmonary artery should be suspected to be abnormal. The conversion of a once concave contour to a flat contour must also be looked on with a high degree of suspicion.

Diagram III shows the lateral margin of an elongated and dilated descending thoracic aorta that is projected lateral to the anterior mediastinal pleural reflection under consideration. The descending thoracic aorta, however, is in an entirely different plane; therefore, it does not influence the shape of this pleural reflection. It is important not to mistake the contours of a dilated descending aorta, which can be considerably more convex toward the lung than is depicted here, for the anterior mediastinal reflection.

Diagram IVb shows the mediastinal pleural reflection passing tangential to the transverse portion of the aortic arch. This occurs in people who have abundant mediastinal fat. In some people this edge can actually project lateral to the image of the aortic knob, which is in a more posterior plane.

Fewer than half of the study group showed a sharp interface between the top of the left pulmonary artery and the transverse portion of the aortic arch (diagram Ao-LPA). This reflection may also be concave toward the left lung or straight but should not be convex toward the left lung.

The mediastinal pleural reflection which passes cephalad above the aortic arch is adjacent to the left subclavian artery (ls in diagram I). In some subjects this pleural reflection may present a double edge. One is the mediastinal pleural reflection over the left subclavian artery, whereas the other is due to a mediastinal pleural reflection over fat or the common carotid artery, which is more anteriorly located in the mediastinum at this same level. The second edge is usually medial to that of the left subclavian artery. This anterior mediastinal pleural reflection can be thought of as the supra-aortic segment of the left anterior mediastinal pleura.

Note: The trachea and main bronchi are outlined with dash marks. The right side of the trachea is shown, but the details of the anatomy of the right side of the mediastinum are not shown on these diagrams. (From Blank and Castellino,[4] with permission.)

(B) Variations in Position of the Left Superior Intercostal Vein

This series of diagrams is based on a study of a group of normal volunteers and patients with known or suspected chest disease. The image of the left superior intercostal vein (arrow) is seen on chest films and supine tomograms in fewer than 10 percent of adults. It is important to recognize it as an anatomic structure in order to avoid mistaking it for a mediastinal abnormality, particularly lymphadenopathy, which can also occur in this region.

Just as the azygos vein (z) responds to changes in intrathoracic pressure or changes in the patient's posture from upright to supine, so does the left superior intercostal vein.

In this illustration the left superior intercostal vein is depicted as a small, nipple-like projection adjacent to the aortic arch. Most commonly it is situated along the lateral convexity of the aortic knob, but it can also be seen more cephalad and medially about the aortic knob. (From McDonald et al.,[23] with permission.) *(Figure continues.)*

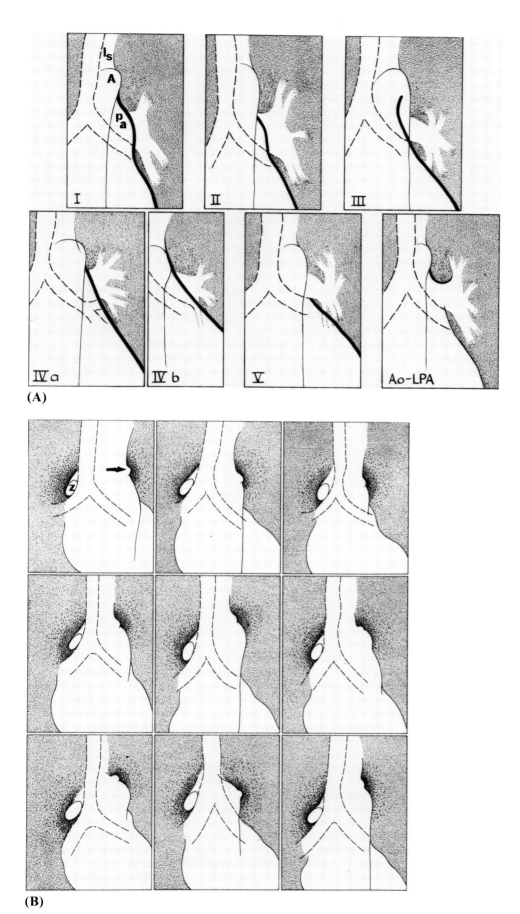

(A)

(B)

Fig. 7-4. *(Continued).*

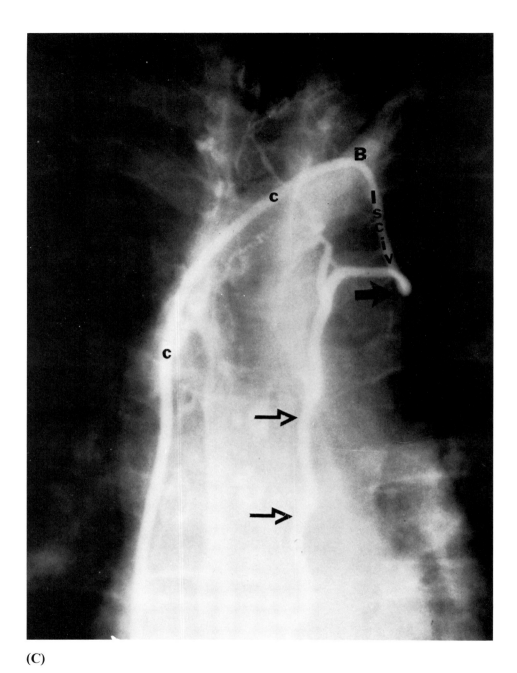

(C)

Fig. 7-4. *(Continued).* **(C) Angiographic Study of the Left Superior Intercostal Vein**

A catheter (c) has been passed from below through the right atrium and the superior vena cava into the left brachiocephalic vein (B). The injected contrast agent fills the left superior intercostal vein (lsicv, solid arrow), which communicates with the accessory hemiazygos vein (open arrows) posteriorly. Intercostal veins 2, 3, and 4 (not filled) empty into the LSICV, which then passes around the aortic knob (horizontal vessel above black arrow) to enter the left brachiocephalic vein anteriorly and superiorly (B).

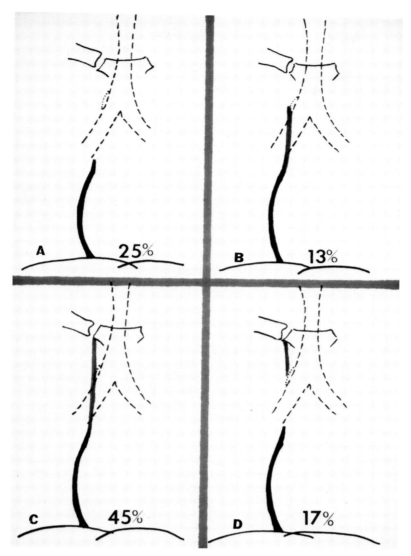

Fig. 7-5. Common Variations in the Cephalocaudad Extent of the Sharp Interface Between the Right Side of the Mediastinum and the Adjacent Lung

This series of diagrams is based on an analysis of approximately 275 normal chest films. The major airways are shown as dashed lines. The mediastinal pleura along the right side of the mediastinum is shown as a solid line where it appeared sharply defined and as a void where it appeared indistinct or so poorly defined that one could dispute its presence.

(A) In 25 percent of the group there was a sharp interface between the right heart border and the adjacent lung, but no sharp mediastinal interface was seen cephalad from the right heart border. The mediastinal interface in this cephalad region is undoubtedly present but does not project a sufficient tangent to produce an easily recognized image.

(B) In 13 percent of subjects the right mediastinal pleural reflection appeared sharp up to the level of the right tracheobronchial angle.

(C) In 45 percent of the group the right mediastinal interface was seen as a sharp edge from the diaphragm to approximately the level of the manubrium.

(D) In 17 percent of the subjects the right mediastinal pleural interface appeared sharply defined above the right main bronchus and below the bronchus intermedius, but there was a segment in between that was indistinct or not visible.

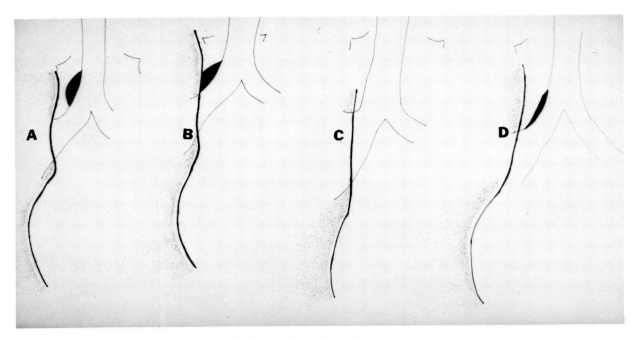

Fig. 7-6. Contours of the Right Mediastinum-Lung Interface

These line drawings show the contours of the right mediastinal pleural reflection when it is seen as a continuous, sharp interface. **(A,B)** The pleural reflection may be convex toward the right lung over part of its course, but the convexity begins well below the level of the right tracheobronchial angle. Usually this is the mediastinal pleural reflection over the SVC, but occasionally it may be a pleural reflection over a dilated ascending aorta. Above the level of the azygos vein the pleural reflection frequently deviates laterally in an arc or as a straight edge. This is the pleural reflection over the right brachiocephalic vein (right innominate vein). The contour of this segment may be slightly concave toward the right lung, or it may have an oblique course with a flat contour.

(C) The mediastinal pleural reflection cephalad to the right heart border may be flat in relationship to the right lung and near-vertical in its course. **(D)** Alternatively, there may be a slight concavity toward the right lung or a slight obliquity.

The edge of the azygos vein is shown in black. There is some variation in the relationship of the pleural reflection over the SVC and the lateral margin of the azygos vein as seen in Figs. A to D. The azygos vein is not seen in everyone (Fig. C).

The edge of the azygos vein may appear as a short arc that is convex toward the right lung, but otherwise there are no convex edges that both begin and end above the right tracheobronchial angle in this normal population. (N. Blank and R.A. Castellino, unpublished data.)

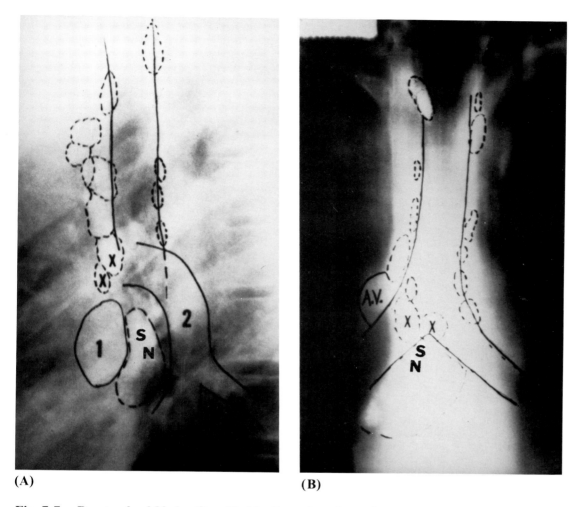

(A)   (B)

Fig. 7-7. Paratracheal Nodes Opacified by Lymphangiography

(A,B) Coned lateral and PA views, respectively, of the mediastinum of a young man who had had a lymphangiogram as part of a diagnostic workup for malignant lymphoma. An unusual number of mediastinal nodes were fortuitously filled with contrast material.

The opacified nodes have been enhanced with dashed outlines to augment their reproduction. The largest nodes are located in the right paratracheal chain along the right anterolateral side of the trachea. Smaller nodes along the left posterolateral aspects of the trachea correspond to nodes in the left paratracheal chain. Pretracheal or precarinal nodes (X) are also filled.

Subcarinal nodes (SN) are shown as a group that is projected behind the bulk of the right hilum (1) and anterior to the descending limb of the left pulmonary artery (2) on the lateral view. On the AP view they project beneath the tracheal carina and extend more to the right than to the left. On the right side they frequently reach the level of the inferior pulmonary veins. The subcarinal nodes are also designated as intertracheobronchial nodes.

The right and left prevascular node chains (not shown) are more anterior than the paratracheal chains. On the right they are anterior to the SVC whereas on the left they are distributed from the pulmonary artery, cephalad along the margins of the aorta, in the distribution of the phrenic and vagus nerves. (From Blank and Castellino,[5] with permission.)

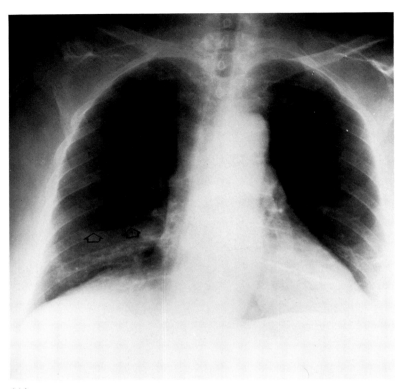

(A)

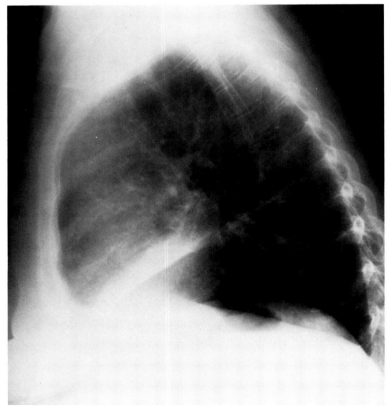

(B)

Fig. 7-8. Abnormal Mediastinum Due to Lipomatosis and Adenopathy

(A,B) PA and lateral views, respectively, of the chest of a woman who presented with classic signs and symptoms of Cushing's disease. The superior mediastinum is abnormally wide. In a patient with Cushing's disease such a finding is likely due to fat deposition.

There is also reduction in volume and partial consolidation of the right middle lobe. Open arrows identify the minor interlobar fissure. There was no clinical evidence to suggest pneumonia. The combination of radiographic and clinical findings raises the question of a paraneoplastic syndrome consequent to an undifferentiated carcinoma of the lung, which could explain all of the abnormalities.

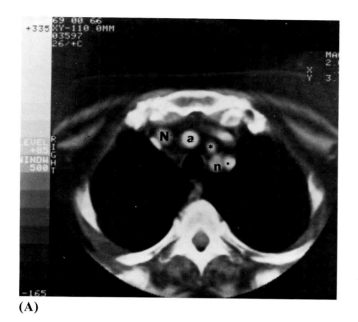

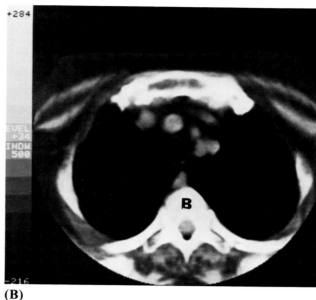

(A)   **(B)**

Fig. 7-9.   **Mediastinal Lipomatosis and Lymphadenopathy in the Right and Left Paratracheal, Right Prevascular, and Subcarinal Lymph Node Groups**

(A – F). Selected CT scans of the woman shown in Fig. 7-8.

(A) CT scan at the level of the manubrium. The patient had been given contrast material via an arm vein. Between the trachea and the left subclavian artery (dot) there is a slightly darker gray, oval image of an enlarged left paratracheal lymph node (n). The carotid artery (asterisk) is seen anterior to this node. The lymph node has a darker gray image than either the sublcavian or the carotid artery, because the latter have been opacified by intravenously administered contrast material.

Although lymph nodes, particularly abnormal ones, may show some enhancement following intravenous injection of contrast agents, they almost never enhance to the same degree as patent vessels in the bolus phase of injection.

A cross section of the right brachiocephalic artery (a) is seen anterior to the lumen of the trachea, and portions of opacified right and left brachiocephalic veins are seen more laterally. Medial to the slender image of the opacified right brachiocephalic vein there is another, darker gray oval due to an abnormally large right prevascular lymph node (N). All these images are buried in an unusually large amount of mediastinal fat (dark gray). The fat at these window and level settings is almost as black as the lungs.

(B) CT scan at the same level as Fig. B before the injection of contrast. The distinction between the abnormal right prevascular lymph node and the adjacent slender image of the right brachiocephalic vein could be missed, and the abnormal node could be misidentified as a normal vein.

This demonstrates the value of using intravenous contrast material, whenever feasible, during CT examination of the mediastinum. However, a useful examination can still be obtained if contrast use is contraindicated, when a thorough understanding of the anatomic relationships between mediastinal vessels and mediastinal lymph node chains has been attained and when there is sufficient fat in the mediastinum to serve as a contrast medium. Most adults have adequate mediastinal fat for CT diagnostic purposes, but children and infants often do not. MRI studies may prove more valuable in the examination of the mediastinum than CT when there is little mediastinal fat and the use of intravenous contrast agents is contraindicated for any reason. *(Figure continues.)*

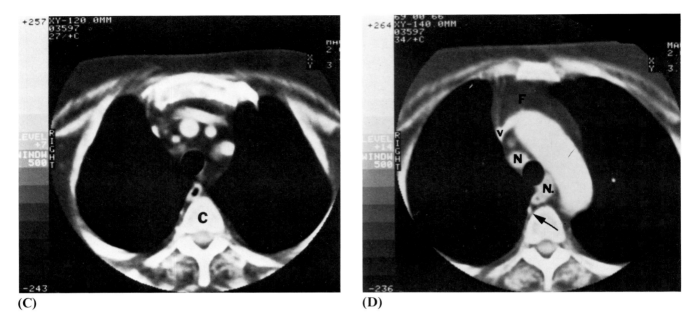

(C)   **(D)**

Fig. 7-9. *(Continued).*   **(C)** CT scan 1.0 cm caudal to Figs. A and B. The opacified left brachiocephalic vein crosses anterior to the left carotid artery and the larger brachiocephalic artery. Dark gray oval images of lymph nodes are seen in the right and left paratracheal and right prevascular chains. The esophagus is easily identified along the right anterolateral margin of the vertebra by a collection of air (black) within it. The mediastinal fat is abundant and provides sharp contrast with the vessels and nodes which it surrounds. The fat at this gray scale is near black (compare with the subcutaneous fat of the anterior chest wall).

   (D) CT scan at a level 3 cm caudal to Fig. A. The transverse portion of the aortic arch, opacified by contrast material, is the dominant image in this portion of the mediastinum. The superior vena cava (v) is in its usual position. In the fat between the right anterolateral aspects of the trachea and the svc (the paratracheal pocket) are two rounded structures. The larger of these (N) appears quite dense. This is an abnormal right paratracheal lymph node, whose image has become enhanced by the intravenously administered contrast material. Notice that it is more dense than the nodes that are seen in the more cephalad Fig. A. In the fat anterior to this lymph node there is a smaller, less opacified right paratracheal node.

   An enlarged left paratracheal node (N.) is seen along the left posterolateral margin of the trachea. The esophagus, posteromedial to the left paratracheal node, contains a small central collection of air, which is seen as a darker gray region in its middle.

   The small, dense, elliptical shadow along the right anterior aspects of the vertebra (arrow) is a cross section of the right superior intercostal vein. It descends caudally in this position and joins the azygos vein as the latter turns anteriorly to become the azygos arch, which empties into the svc. The position of the right superior intercostal vein, above the level of the azygos arch, is analogous to the position of the azygos vein below the level of the azygos arch.

   Mediastinal pleura forms sharp borders against the mediastinal fat (F). *(Figure continues.)*

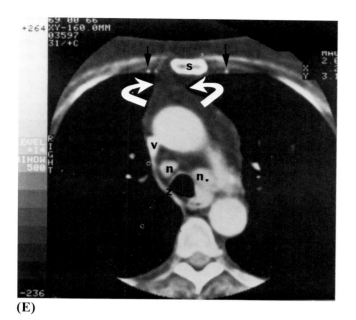
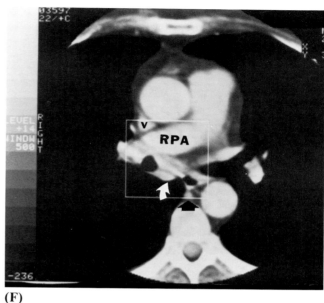

(E)   **(F)**

Fig. 7-9. *(Continued).* **(E)** CT scan at a level 2 cm caudal to Fig. D. The transverse portion of the arch of the azygos vein (z) passes from a prespinal location around the right side of the trachea to enter into the superior vena cava (v). There is a bean-shaped, partially opacified azygos node (n) in the fat medial to the azygos arch. There is also an abnormally large left paratracheal node (n.).

Cross-sectional images of opacified internal mammary vessels (straight arrows) are seen on either side of the sternum (s). The light gray band between the ascending and the descending aorta is a partial-volume image of the left pulmonary artery. Fat (curved arrows) prevents juxtaposition of the right and left lungs behind the sternum so that an anterior junction band rather than a line is the result.

(F) CT scan 3 cm caudal to Fig. E. A square demarcates a key portion of this image. The right pulmonary artery (RPA) crosses the mediastinum anterior to the airways and posterior to the superior vena cava (v). The black, oval, cross-sectional image of the bronchus intermedius is seen behind the distal right pulmonary artery. Abnormal soft tissue (white arrow) medial to the bronchus intermedius produces a posterior bulge into the lung of the azygoesophageal recess. The medial pleural boundary of the recess, however, is not distorted because the mass is not large enough to move the lung completely out of the recess. Anterior to the azygos vein (short black arrow), the esophagus has a rounded collection of air in its lumen. The sharp margin along the right side of the azygos vein and the esophagus is produced by the pleural boundary of the lung in the azygoesophageal recess. The mediastinal fat is lighter gray at these window level settings than it is on A–D.

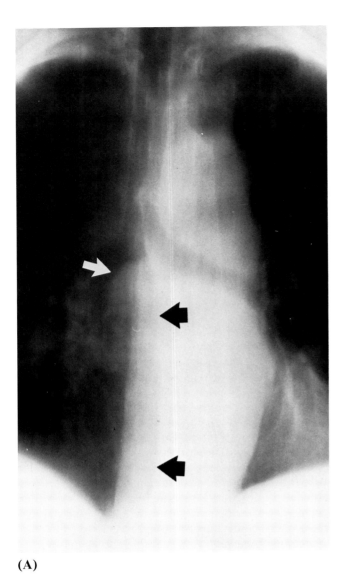

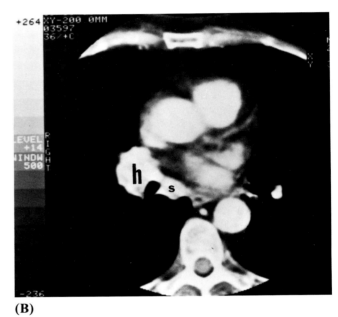

(A)   **(B)**

Fig. 7-10.   Preserved Image of the Azygoesophageal Recess Interface in the Presence of a Subcarinal Mass

(A) Coned portion of a tomogram of the same patient in Figs. 7-8 and 7-9. A well-defined edge (black arrows) extends from the level of the diaphragm cephalad beyond the level of the tracheal carina. This represents the azygoesophageal interface. A soft tissue mass is present under the right mainstem bronchus and medial to the bronchus intermedius (white arrow). This conforms to the subcarinal mass seen on the CT scan in Fig. 7-9D. The left paraspinal stripe is well defined on this scan, and the bowed left lateral margin of the descending thoracic aorta is also well shown.

(B) CT scan showing the subcarinal mass (s) impinging upon and flattening the medial wall of the bronchus intermedius (black hole between s and h). A large right hilar mass (h) also impinges on the bronchus intermedius laterally.

The cross section of the azygos vein anterior to the vertebra and the air-containing section of the esophagus anterior to the vein are medial to the azygoesophageal recess of the right lung. The recess is preserved, despite the presence of subcarinal adenopathy, and hence the azygoesophageal interface can still be seen in the subcarinal region on the tomogram in Fig. A.

There is no good reason to perform mediastinal tomography and CT on the same patient unless the examinations are part of a study to compare the relative merits of the imaging modalities.

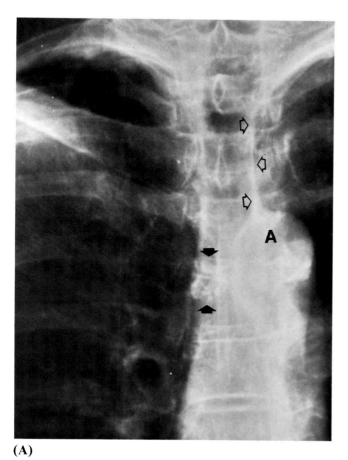

(A)

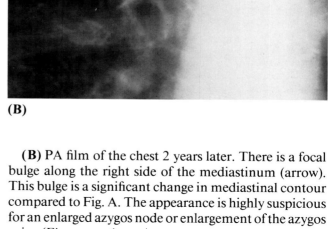

(B)

Fig. 7-11. Azygos Node Enlargement

(A) Coned view of the mediastinum shows calcification in the lower nodes of the right paratracheal chain. The calcification is seen as small, irregular foci of increased brightness (between black arrows). Incidentally, you can see a thin posterior junction line (open arrows) extending cephalad from the aortic arch (A). A small (5 mm) nodule is present in the right apex above the clavicle.

(B) PA film of the chest 2 years later. There is a focal bulge along the right side of the mediastinum (arrow). This bulge is a significant change in mediastinal contour compared to Fig. A. The appearance is highly suspicious for an enlarged azygos node or enlargement of the azygos vein. *(Figure continues.)*

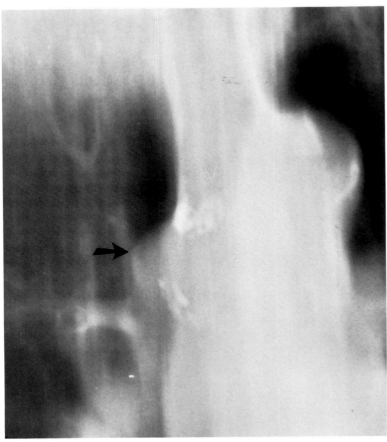

(C)

Fig. 7-11. *(Continued).* **(C)** Tomogram of the mediastinum. There is a small mass along the right tracheobronchial angle. There is no significant change in size of the mass between the films made with the patient upright (Fig. B) and supine (Fig. C), allowing for magnification in Fig. C, which was made at a shorter targetfilm distance. The location and behavior of the mass are consistent with adenopathy in the right paratracheal lymph nodes. In addition to the soft tissue components of this adenopathy there are clusters of calcification along its superior and inferior aspects. (Compare the density of the calcification in these marginal nodes to that of the calcific plaques in the aortic arch.)

If the earliest film (Fig. A) were not available, one could accept the adenopathy seen in Figs. B and C as calcified residuals of tuberculosis or histoplasmosis. From Fig. A, however, it is clear that the noncalcified component of lymphadenopathy is new. One would not expect this sequence on the basis of infectious granulomatous disease alone.

The likelihood that metastatic neoplasm had caused this lymph node to become enlarged was strongly considered in this patient with meningeal carcinosis from an unknown primary.

The 6- or 7-mm nodule in the right apex remained stable over the 2-year interval between Figs. A and B and probably represents a residual of the infectious granulomatous disease (tuberculosis) responsible for the calcified right paratracheal nodes originally.

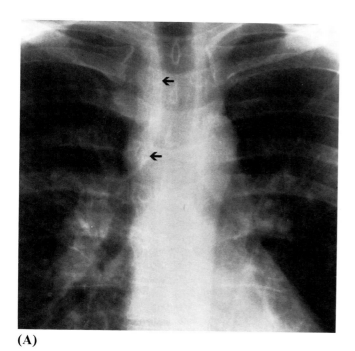

(A)

**Fig. 7-12. (A–C) Right Paratracheal Lymphade-
nopathy**

Chest films of a 41-year-old man who had noted the
waxing and waning of bilateral groin adenopathy for
approximately 1 year. Four weeks before the first film
(Fig. A) was taken he noticed the presence of a right neck
mass. A biopsy from the right supraclavicular region
showed nodular mixed lymphoma.

(A) A characteristic appearance of widening of the
paratracheal soft tissues due to lymphadenopathy in the
right paratracheal chain (arrows). The wall of the trachea
may be seen in approximately 80 percent of normal
chest radiographs, and it rarely measures as much as
4 mm in thickness. Measured above the level of the
azygos vein, the tracheal wall is usually on the order of 2
to 3 mm in thickness.

In addition to the abnormal right paratracheal stripe
notice the size and contours of the right hilum (long
arrows).

(B) Film made approximately 9 months after Fig. A.
The patient had received chemotherapy. There is considerable reduction in the width of the right paratracheal
stripe (arrows) as well as a decrease in the size of the right
hilum.

(C) Film made approximately 2 months after Fig. B.
There is further reduction in the width of the right paratracheal stripe. It is now within the limits of normal.
There has been further reduction in the size of the right
hilum. The series of short arcs lateral to the interlobar
branch of the right pulmonary artery in Fig. A (long
arrows) is now gone. The right paratracheal and hilar
adenopathy has resolved with chemotherapy. (From
Blank and Castellino,[6] with permission.)

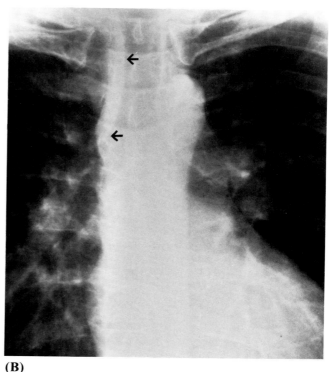

(B)

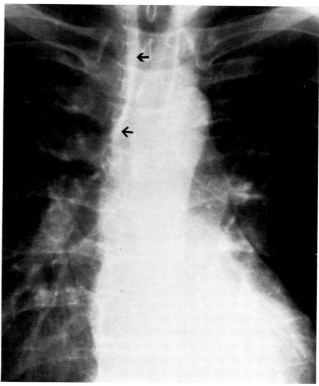

(C)

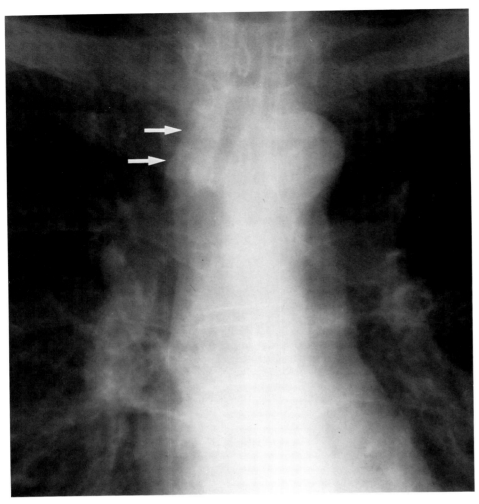

(D)

Fig. 7-12. (D) Right Paratracheal Adenopathy Due to Coccidioidomycosis

This man from Asia had recently traveled through parts of California where coccidioidomycosis is endemic. He developed symptoms of malaise and low-grade fever. A chest film showed evidence of right paratracheal and right hilar adenopathy.

The band of soft tissue extending cephalad along the right side of the trachea from the right tracheobronchial angle is abnormally wide and is readily distinguished from the margins of the SVC, which are projected lateral to it. The upper and lower right hilar structures have short convex arcs that are suspicious for hilar lymphadenopathy.

A right paratracheal node was removed at mediastinoscopy, and organisms of *Coccidiodes immitis* were found in the node.

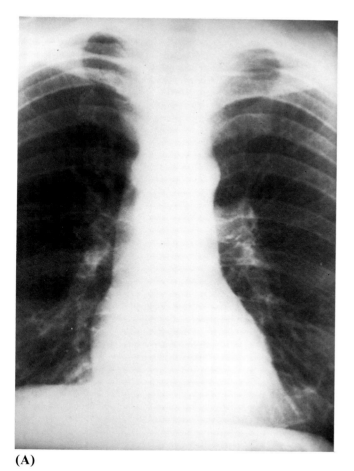

(A)

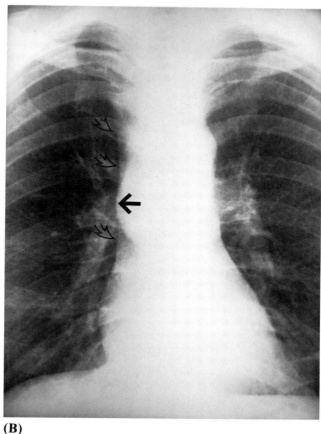

(B)

Fig. 7-13. Anterior Mediastinal Mass Simulating a Dilated Ascending Aorta

(A,B) Coned views of PA chest films made several months apart of a young man who has Hodgkin's disease. Compare the contours of the right side of the mediastinum. In Fig. B there is a pronounced edge (black arrow) that is convex toward the right lung. This was not present on the earlier film (Fig A). Although a markedly dilated ascending aorta could cause a similar contour, the radius of the arc is too short. It would also be most unusual for an aortic abnormality of this magnitude to develop in a young man over a few months' time unless he had suffered a dissecting aneurysm. The margins of the SVC and the brachiocephalic vein (open arrows in B) are unaffected by this new mass, indicating that it is in a different plane.

(C) Lateral view shows that the mass (arrow) is anterior in the retrosternal region. It is due to recurrent Hodgkin's disease, probably in the thymus. Because its edges are so poorly defined on the lateral view, it is more difficult to recognize than it is on the PA view (Fig. B).

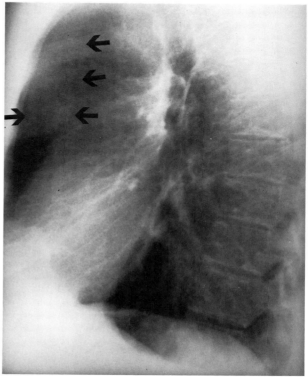

(C)

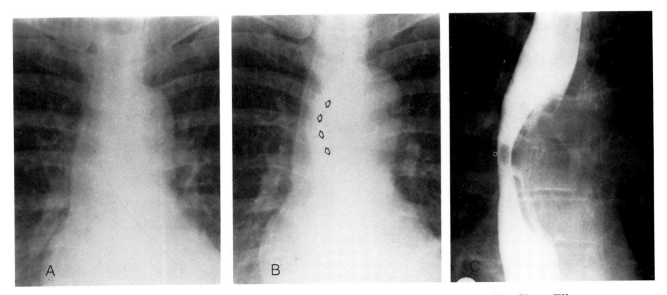

Fig. 7-14. Posterior Mediastinal Mass Simulating a Dilated Ascending Aorta on PA Chest Film

(A – C) Coned views of the mediastinum of a woman with malignant lymphoma. In Fig. B there is an edge image that is convex toward the right, similar to that seen in Fig. 7-13B, but in this case it is not border forming. Nevertheless, for it to be seen as a distinct edge it must interface with lung in a plane separate from that of the SVC. There also has been an overall increase in the radiodensity of this portion of the mediastinum when compared with Fig. A.

Fig. C shows deviation of the esophagus by this new mass. This represents lymphadenopathy involving the posterior mediastinal paraesophageal lymph nodes. Although its appearance on PA view (Fig. B) resembles the mass seen in Fig. 7-13B, these masses are in entirely different coronal planes. (From Blank and Castellino,[5] with permission.)

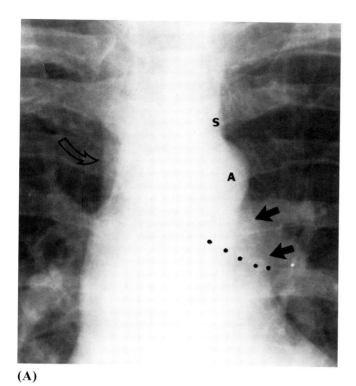

(A)

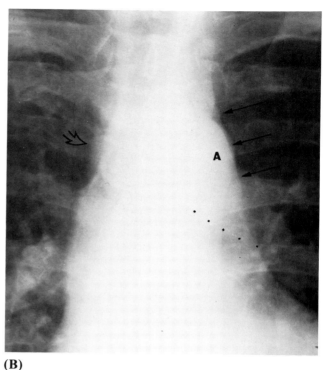

(B)

Fig. 7-15. Recurrent Lymphoma in the Left Prevascular Lymph Nodes Displacing the Mediastinal Pleura Away From the Aortic Arch

(A) Coned view of the mediastinum of a man who had surveillance films taken following treatment for nodular mixed lymphoma (NML). The posterior portion of the aortic arch (the aortic knob, A) has a well-defined, sharp interface with adjacent lung. The pleural reflection over the left subclavian artery (S) extends cephalad from the aortic arch. The upper edge of the left main bronchus is outlined with dots. The anterior mediastinal pleural reflection over the region of the pulmonary artery is seen faintly between the heavy black arrows, and it is normal.

(B) Film taken approximately 6 months later. A sharp mediastinal pleural reflection (thin arrows) passes nearly tangential to the aortic arch (A). Only a small portion of the posterior turn of the aortic arch (middle arrow) is projected lateral to this pleural reflection. The pleural reflection has an oblique straight edge that is neither concave nor convex toward the left lung. The appearance of this pleural reflection is within the spectrum of normal, and if this were the only film available it would be regarded as such. However, since it represents a distinct change from the earlier film, it is now considered suspect for recurrent lymphadenopathy displacing the mediastinal pleura to the left. Gross deposition of fat in the mediastinum could cause a similar change but would be unlikely to occur in 6 months in a patient who had not been receiving steroids or who had not become morbidly obese in that interval.

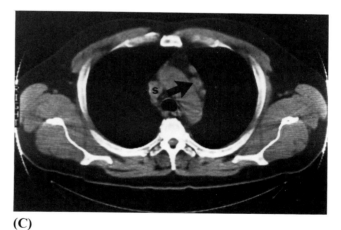

(C)

The right side of the mediastinum—the edge of the SVC (open arrows)—and the appearance of the right tracheal wall are normal and unchanged from Fig. A.

(C) CT scan shows three masses—large lymph nodes—in the fat (black) to the left of the aortic arch. The largest node is in the middle (arrow). The mediastinal pleural reflection is displaced laterally from the aorta by the abnormal lymph nodes of the left prevascular chain. This displacement accounts for the changes seen in Fig. B.

Notice that the paratracheal pocket, between the images of the SVC (s) and the aortic arch, contains fat and a small, barely visible (normal-sized) right paratracheal lymph node.

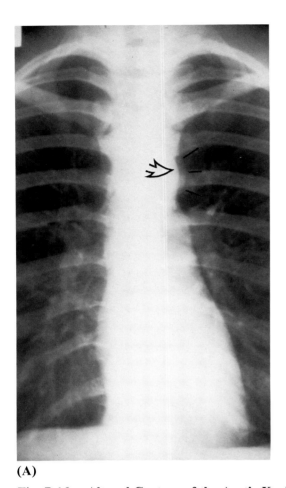

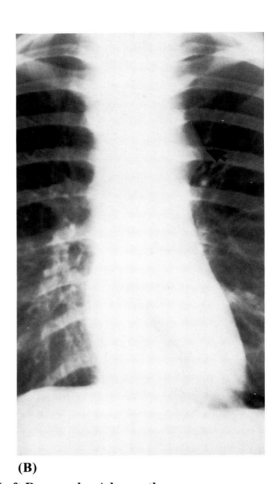

(A)   **(B)**

Fig. 7-16.   Altered Contour of the Aortic Knob Due to Left Prevascular Adenopathy

PA views of the chest of a young woman who was suffering from malaise and fevers of undetermined origin. The films were taken approximately 1 month apart.

(A) An arc of soft tissue (black bars) is projected to the left of the aortic knob (open arrow).

(B) There is effacement of the aortic knob by a mass, which could be mistaken for an abnormal aorta were the previous films not available for comparison. An aortic dissection could produce the altered contour seen in this film, but the history is not at all supportive. A CT scan or MRI study would serve to remove all doubt.

On a lateral view (not shown) there was increased soft tissue density in the mediastinum, but no edge contour changes were seen as they are on the PA view.

The patient was proven to have a non-Hodgkin's lymphoma, and the mediastinal contour changes seen in Fig. B are produced by enlargement of left prevascular lymph nodes. As the left prevascular nodes located anterior and along the margin of the transverse portion of the aortic arch enlarge, they distort and displace the para-aortic mediastinal pleura (and the left lung). When these nodes are very large, even the contours of the posterior turn of the arch (the aortic knob) become effaced.

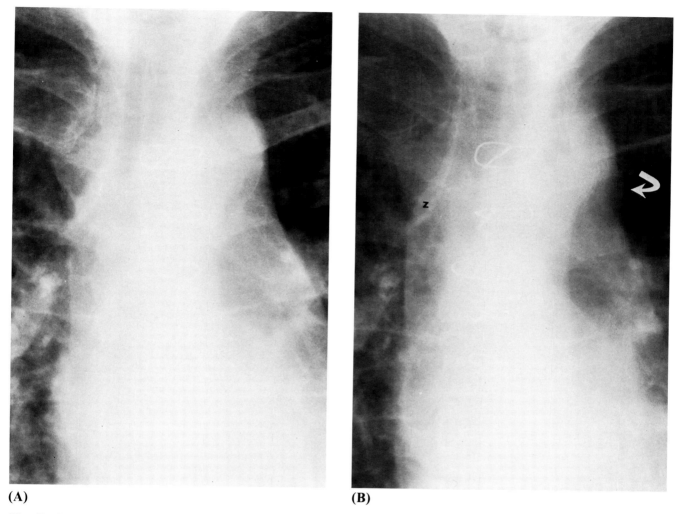

(A)   **(B)**

Fig. 7-17.   Adenopathy of Left Prevascular Nodes Adjacent to the Aortic Arch Plus a Large Azygos Node Demonstrated by CT but Not Visible on Chest Film

(A,B) Coned PA views of the upper mediastinum of a cardiac transplant recipient on August 2 (Fig. A) and on September 9 (Fig. B). The mediastinal pleural boundaries can be compared even though the films are technically different. The pleural reflection adjacent to the aortic arch on September 9 has a convex bulge to the left (arrow) that was not present on August 2. In a patient who is on long-term immunosuppressive therapy, this change raises the question of the development of mediastinal lymphadenopathy caused by a malignant lymphoma. This diagnosis was subsequently proven. *(Figure continues.)*

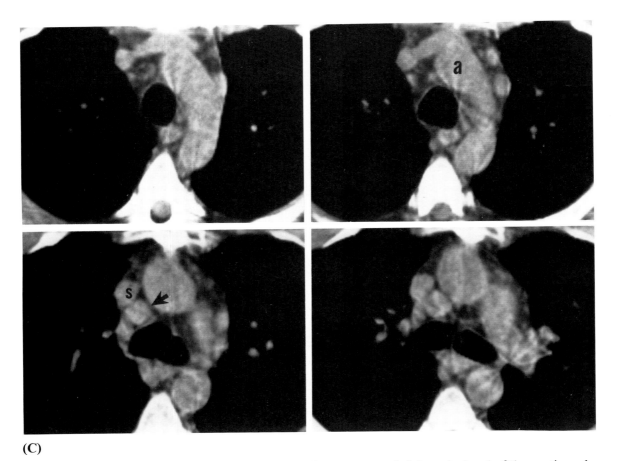

(C)

Fig. 7-17. *(Continued).* **(C)** Series of CT scans. The scan at top left is at the level of the aortic arch, whereas the top right scan is at a level that just shaves the bottom of the aortic arch. There are two moderately enlarged lymph nodes in mediastinal fat to the left of the ascending aorta (a). The distortion of the mediastinal pleura against the lateral aspect of these enlarged nodes produces the bulge of the mediastinal contour seen in Fig. B.

The scan at bottom left is at the bifurcation of the trachea. The azygos vein passes anteriorly from its posterior prespinal position and then above the right main bronchus to enter the SVC (s). In the paratracheal pocket, there is a moderately enlarged azygos node (arrow). The bottom right scan includes the anterior portion of the azygos vein and its junction with the SVC. The enlarged azygos node remains visible.

Notice that there is no evidence of azygos adenopathy on the chest films, even in retrospect. The azygos vein (z in Fig. B) and the right paratracheal stripe appear normal.

The CT scans help to understand this: (a) Above the azygos vein level the lung is adjacent to the right tracheal wall; thus the paratracheal stripe should not appear thickened on the PA chest film, and it does not. On CT scan the azygos vein is not displaced by the large azygos node, nor is the SVC displaced or distorted. The enlarged node remains within the fat-containing pocket bordered by the SVC, the ascending aorta, and the airway. It would not be recognized on chest films until large enough to distort the mediastinal pleura over the right side of the mediastinum or, as may occasionally be the case, to distort the lower portions of the anterior wall of the trachea and become visible on a lateral view. Thus, it is possible for significant right paratracheal adenopathy to be present, in spite of a chest film that appears normal, when there is a spacious right paratracheal pocket in which the adenopathy can hide.

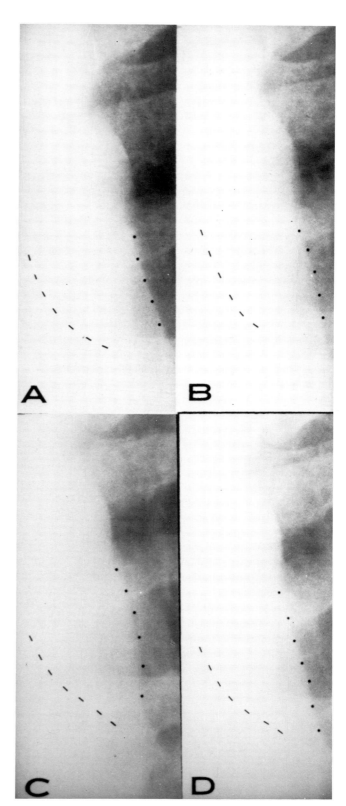

Fig. 7-18. **Change in Left Mediastinal Contour by Enlarged Nodes in the Caudal End of the Left Prevascular Chain**

Series of coned views of the left side of the mediastinum of a woman who developed recurrent Hodgkin's disease. Dotted lines mark the mediastinal pleura between the level of the aortic arch and the left mainstem bronchus (dashed lines). This is the pleural reflection over the aortopulmonic window. The caudal nodes of the left prevascular chain, particularly the ductus node, are located medial to this pleural reflection.

(A) In this film, this pleural reflection is relatively straight. Although its course is oblique, it is neither concave nor convex toward the left lung. It is normal.

(B) The pleural reflection has become convex toward the left lung. This change is subtle, but it is all that is needed to indicate that there is a mediastinal mass present in this region. This finding, however, is easily overlooked or misinterpreted.

(C) The convex contour toward the left lung has become more pronounced. This change indicates further growth of the mass, which in this case is due to enlargement of the left prevascular nodes by recurrent Hodgkin's disease.

(D) The situation after the patient had received treatment. The mediastinal pleura has returned toward a normal configuration.

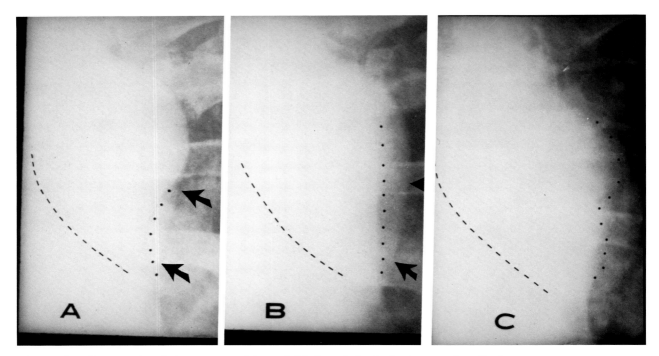

Fig. 7-19.   Progressive Enlargement of Lymph Nodes of the Left Prevascular Chain

In this patient the descending thoracic aorta (arrows) is projected lateral to the left anterior mediastinal pleural reflection and should not be mistaken for that reflection.

(A) Coned view of the mediastinum at a time when no mediastinal mass was apparent.

(B) The mediastinal pleural reflection, which had been slightly concave toward the left lung in Fig. A (dotted lines), has now shifted laterally and is nearly vertical in its course. If we had only the film in Fig. B we could not be certain that the mediastinum is abnormal. It is the *change* between Figs. A and B that is convincing. Fat in the mediastinum could cause an appearance similar to that in Fig. B. The change in contour between Figs. A and B over a short time would be highly unlikely to be due to deposition of mediastinal fat in a patient who has not been on high-dose steroids or has not become noticeably obese.

Note that the length of the segment of descending aorta seen in Fig. B is longer than that in Fig. A because of a slight difference in projection, yet its contour is not changed.

(C) Radiograph made a short time after Fig. B. There has been further distortion of the anterior mediastinal pleural reflection, which has become more convex toward the left lung. There is also lobulation of this mediastinal contour. Even the descending limb of the aortic knob is distorted. This distortion is due to the progressive enlargement of lymph nodes of the left prevascular chain involved with malignant lymphoma.

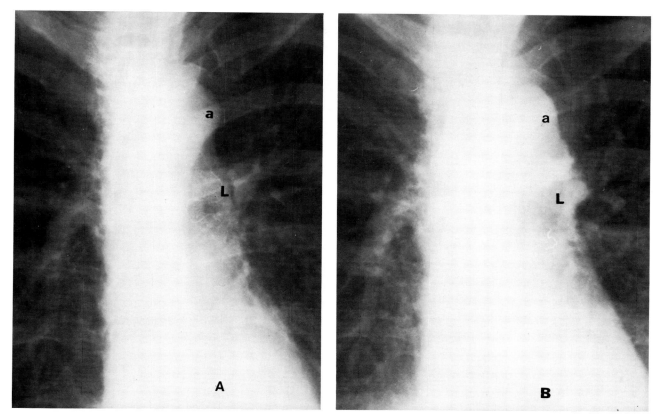

Fig. 7-20. Left Prevascular Adenopathy Due to Metastatic Breast Carcinoma

(A,B) Coned views of the mediastinum of a woman who has carcinoma of the breast. Fig. A is from an earlier chest film obtained to compare with the current examination (Fig. B).

There has been a striking change in the appearance of the mediastinal contours between the aortic arch (a) and the left pulmonary artery (L). In Fig. A these contours are normal. In Fig. B, a mass has distorted the mediastinal contour so that the concave arc between the arch and the pulmonary artery has become convex and lobulated. The mediastinal pleural reflection intersects with the aortic knob at a higher level in Fig. B than in Fig. A.

This is a clear indication of the presence of a growing mass, which in this case is a metastasis from the breast carcinoma causing adenopathy of the ductus node and left prevascular nodes.

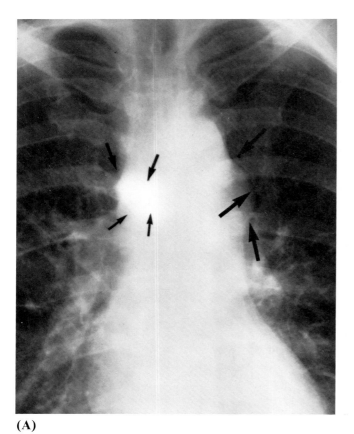

(A)

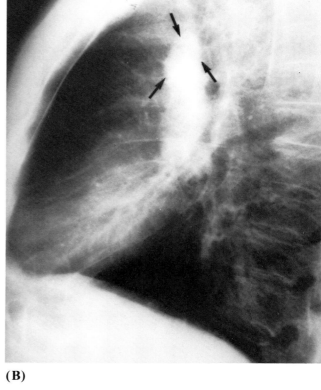

(B)

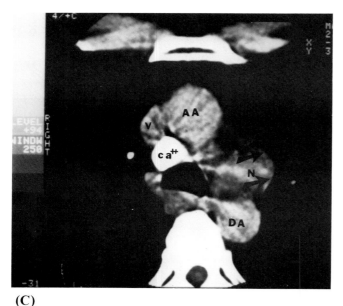

(C)

Fig. 7-21. Adenopathy of the Ductus Node(s) and Calcification of the Azygos Node

(A) The mediastinal plural reflection between the aortic arch and the left pulmonary artery has a pronounced convex contour to the left (large arrows). This contour is abnormal. A large, calcified azygos node is present as well (small arrows).

(B) Lateral view shows the relationship of the calcified azygos node (arrows) to the anterior wall of the airway. The mass in the region of the ductus nodes on the left side, however, is not clearly seen because it is projected en face.

(C) CT scan at a level just beneath the transverse portion of the aortic arch. On the left there is a mediastinal mass (N) located between the ascending (AA) and descending (DA) limbs of the thoracic aorta. The mediastinal pleura (arrows) deviates around the mass, which accounts for the abnormality seen on the PA view. This is a characteristic location for the ductus node of the left prevascular chain. In this patient it is markedly enlarged because of involvement by malignant lymphoma. (Compare its size to that of the adjacent airway.)

The densely calcified azygos node (ca++) is easily seen in the right paratracheal pocket. Densely calcified mediastinal or hilar lymph nodes generally are evidence of infectious granulomatous disease, most commonly tuberculosis or histoplasmosis, of remote onset. Frequently patients have no knowledge of ever having been ill with these infections. This case also illustrates that benign calcified nodes can coexist with malignant lymph nodes in the same mediastinum and even sometimes in the same lymph node chain (see Fig. 7-11).

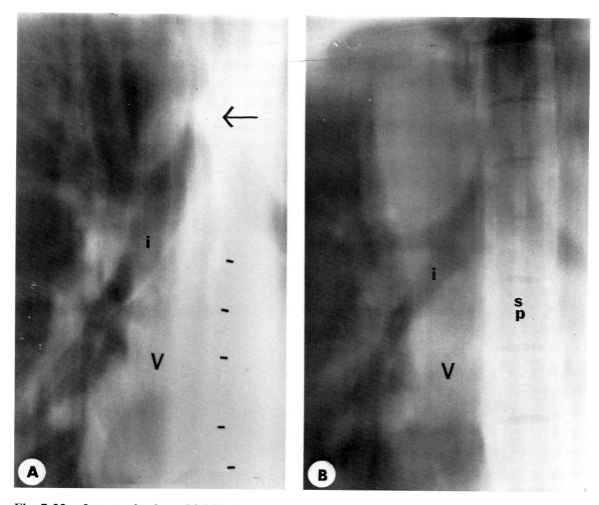

Fig. 7-22. Intertracheobronchial Nodes

(A,B) Selected tomograms from two patients, one of whom had subcarinal lymphadenopathy whereas the other did not. The arrow points to the image of the azygos vein as it crosses to the right behind the airway and then is projected as an oval soft tissue image in the right tracheobronchial angle as it comes anteriorly. (i, bronchus intermedius; v, confluence of pulmonary veins as they enter the left atrium.)

(A) The azygoesophageal interface is visible (dash marks) against adjacent lung in the azygoesophageal recess. The superior aspect of the venous confluence and the entrance of the superior pulmonary vein into the venous confluence are visible because of lung with which it interfaces. The thin medial wall (a white line) of the bronchus intermedius is visible because of air in its lumen and lung or mediastinal fat against a portion of its outside wall.

(B) An obvious mass in the right paratracheal region impinges upon and depresses the right upper lobe bronchus. In the subcarinal region, the superior aspect of the venous confluence and the superior margin of the entering superior pulmonary vein are not seen. The thin wall of the bronchus intermedius is not seen. A subcarinal mass has displaced lung from the usual interfaces with these structures; hence they are no longer visible. These features indicating the presence of a subcarinal mass can also be seen on chest films that are of good technical quality. The tomograms, however serve better for illustrations.

The out-of-focus spinous processes (sp) of the thoracic vertebrae line up and simulate an azygoesophageal stripe but do not precisely mimic one.

(From Blank and Castellino,[5] with permission.)

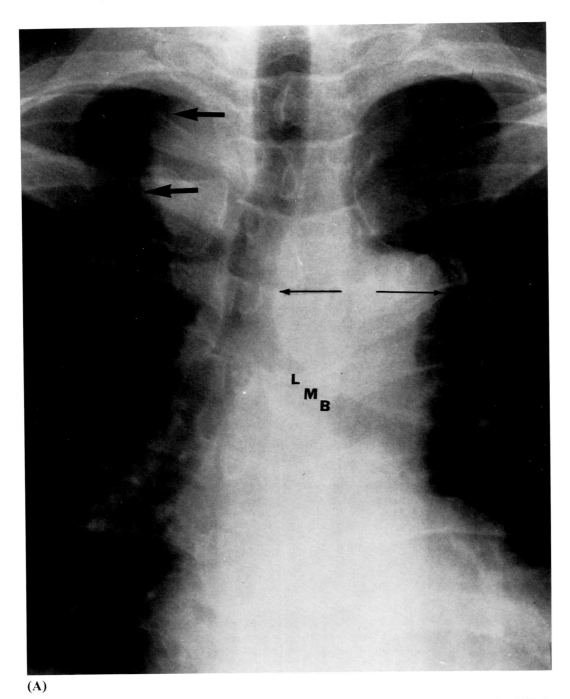

(A)

Fig. 7-23. Adenopathy of a Left Suprabronchial Node and High Right Paratracheal Nodes

This patient has a carcinoma of the esophagogastric junction.

(A) The distance between the air column of the trachea and the lateral edge of the aortic arch (bidirectional arrows) is abnormal. The aortic arch per se appears neither enlarged nor aneurysmal. There also is a high right paratracheal mass (short arrows). What accounts for the separation of the airway from the aortic arch? *(Figure continues.)*

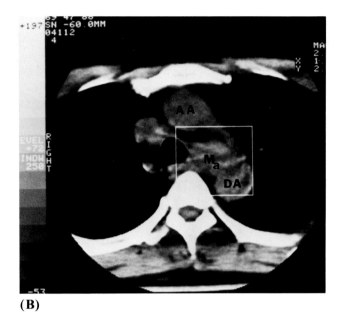
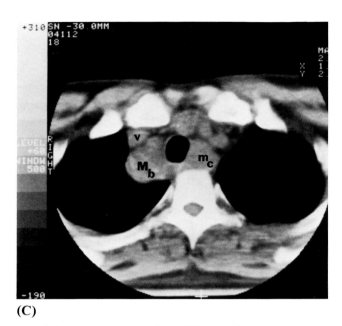

(B) **(C)**

Fig. 7-23. *(Continued).* **(B)** CT scan at the level of the bottom of the transverse portion of the aortic arch shows a large mass (Ma) displacing the trachea away from the aortic arch. The trachea is displaced considerably to the right of the midline. The location of the mass conforms to that of the left suprabronchial node. It accounts for the rightward displacement of the trachea seen on the PA chest film and for the stretched appearance of the left main bronchus (LMB in Fig. A). Notice that it does not distort the left anterior mediastinal pleura reflection as would enlarged ductus nodes.

Adenopathy of the left suprabronchial node may be responsible for vocal cord paralysis, as it involves the recurrent laryngeal nerve, which passes under the aortic arch. (AA, ascending aorta; DA, descending aorta.)

(C) CT scan at the level of the clavicular heads shows the high right paratracheal mass (Mb) dorsal to the right brachiocephalic vein (v). There is also a high left paratracheal adenopathy (mc) dorsal to the carotid artery and the left subclavian artery. These are presumptive lymph node metastases from the patient's carcinoma of the esophagogastric junction.

Fig. 7-24. Paraesophageal (Posterior Mediastinal) Lymphadenopathy From Carcinoma of the Prostate

(A,B) Coned PA views of the mediastinum of a man who was undergoing routine surveillance following treatment for carcinoma of the prostate. Fig. B was made 16 months after Fig. A. A mass, which is projected in the left paraspinal region, has an edge convex toward the left lung (short bars). It is not seen in Fig. A.

(C) Spot film obtained at fluoroscopy further locates this mass (short bars).

(D) The impression (arrow) of this mass on the barium-filled esohagus (E) is clearly shown. This mass was due to metastasis from the patient's carcinoma of the prostate. It is located in the paraesophageal (posterior mediastinal) lymph node chain.

A small mass in a retrocardiac position may escape detection if misinterpreted as the transverse process of a vertebra or as a venous confluence. On the other hand, it is also possible to mistake a transverse process or a venous confluence for an abnormal mass unless great care is used in the assessment of this region (see Fig. 8-3). (From Blank and Castellino,[5] with permission.)

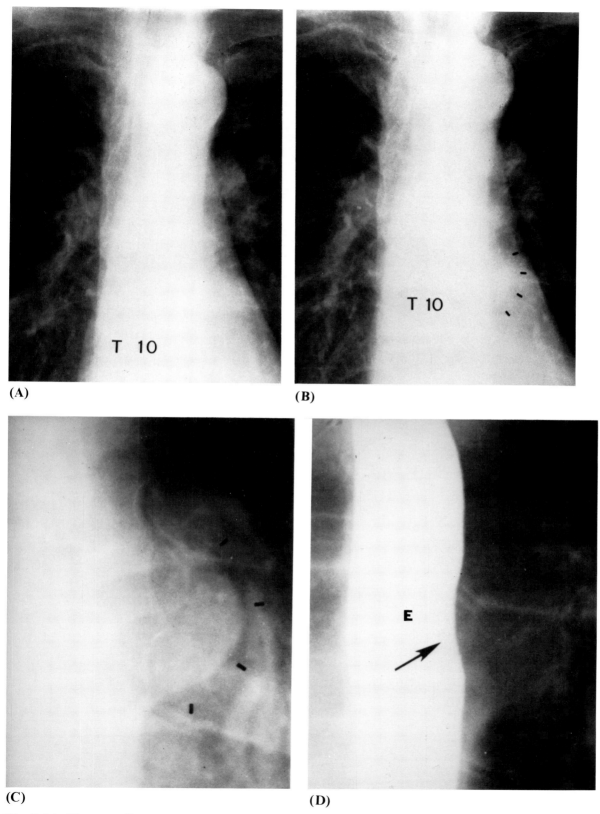

(A)

(B)

T 10

T 10

(C)

(D)

E

Fig. 7-24. *(Continued).*

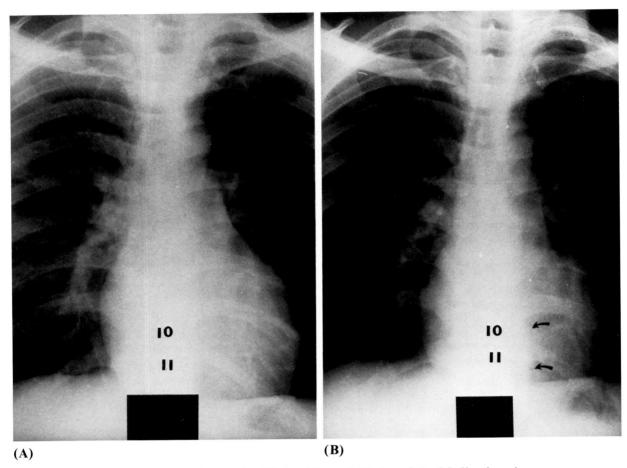

(A)   **(B)**

Fig. 7-25. Paraspinal Lymphadenopathy (Parietal Lymph Nodes of the Mediastinum)

(A,B) Coned views of the chest of a man who had Hodgkin's disease. The films were taken 3 months apart. The later examination (Fig. B) shows a bulge of the paraspinal stripe to the left of T10–T11. Although the finding is subtle, it is clearly a change from the appearance on the earlier films. This is an example of paraspinal lymphadenopathy due to malignant lymphoma. There are no other signs of recurrent adenopathy elsewhere in the mediastinum.

Notice the resemblance of this lesion to the focal bulge produced by the dilated hemiazygos vein in Fig. 8-35. There are many other causes of paravertebral masses, such as hematomas associated with vertebral fracture, inflammatory masses associated with osteomyelitis, neurogenic tumors, duplication cysts, extramedullary hematopoiesis, and, commonly, hypertrophic vertebral spurs. Hiatal hernias, herniation of fat through Bochdalek foramina, and rarely lipomatosis may also account for paravertebral masses. Attention to the history, physical findings, laboratory data, and chest film analysis permits an appropriate ordering of the differential diagnosis, but definitive diagnosis requires specific examinations: CT or MRI to show fatty or vascular lesions, angiography to show vascular lesions, gastrointestinal examination to demonstrate herniations of gut, or biopsy.

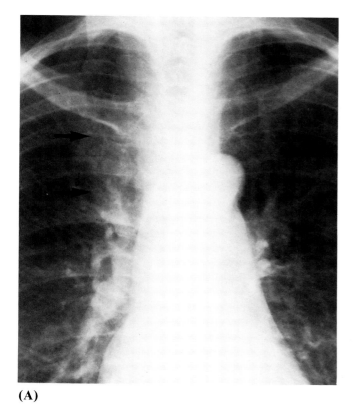

(A)

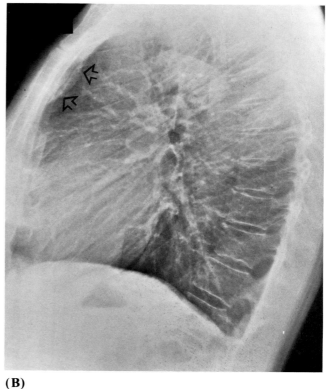

(B)

Fig. 7-26.   Internal Mammary Lymphadenopathy (Parietal Lymph Nodes of the Mediastinum)

(A) Lateral view of the chest of a woman with nodular lymphoma, poorly differentiated. A soft tissue mound behind the upper sternum (arrows) has a sharply defined posterior margin that is convex toward the lung. This region of the chest can be very difficult to evaluate because there may be slight undulations of the pleural reflections over the costal cartilages that mimic parasternal or retrosternal masses. In addition, slight differences in rotation off of true lateral cause significant differences in the projection of parasternal and retrosternal soft tissues. Erroneous assessments as to whether a finding is new or old, or increased or decreased in size, can result when the films being compared are not of the same projection.

In this case you can see that the lesion extends over *two* anterior rib ends and therefore could not be explained on the basis of a fortuitous projection of undulating pleural reflections over costal cartilage.

(B) PA view. The only clue we have to the presence of this lesion is a slight increase in radiodensity in the paramediastinal portions of the right upper hemithorax (arrows). (Compare the relative densities of the right and left sides). This is a weak signal because the retrosternal mass is small and has no edges tangential to the beam on a PA projection. Internal mammary lymphadenopathy may have this appearance on routine chest films. *(Figure continues.)*

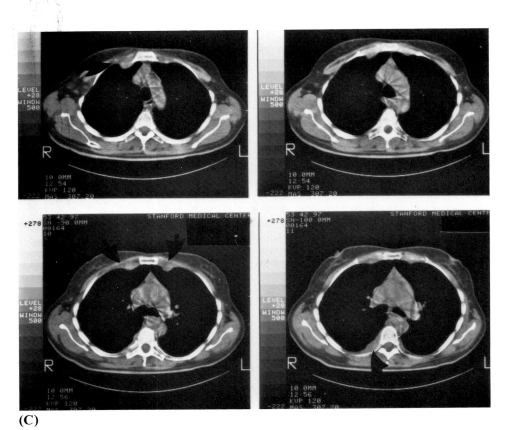

(C)

Fig. 7-26. *(Continued).* **(C)** Series of four CT scans at levels extending from above the aortic arch (upper left) to below the carina of the trachea (lower right). On the upper left scan there is a soft tissue mass against the right anterior chest wall lateral to the sternum (arrow). It has a sharp edge that is convex toward the lung. This corresponds to the mass (internal mammary lymphadenopathy) seen on the lateral view of the chest and to the area of increased tissue density seen on the PA view. On the lower left scan there is another mass located to the left of the sternum. You can understand how this small mass might not be recognized on the lateral view because it is superimposed so precisely on the lesion from the other side (arrows). Furthermore, since the left-sided mass is small and situated in the axial plane of the left pulmonary artery, it does not add enough of an increment absorber in the x-ray beam path to be recognized on the PA view of the chest.

On the scan at lower right there is a paravertebral soft tissue mound on the patient's right, consistent with ex-

trapleural involvement by lymphoma (arrow). On the lateral view of the chest there is no signal that permits recognition of this lesion. Notice from its configuration on the CT scan that it would have no significant tangent parallel to the beam on the lateral view. On an AP view that was penetrated well enough to show the spine, it might have been recognized, but even that is uncertain because of its orientation to the beam. A left anterior or right posterior oblique view, however, would place its interface with lung in tangent and show a good image.

Although it is important to recognize internal mammary lymphadenopathy, care must be used on CT scan interpretation to avoid confusion with benign protrusions of pleura over exuberant cartilage of the anterior first ribs, which occurs in some people. This can be accomplished by comparing narrow-window images with wide-window images. (Reprinted from Shapeero L, Blank N, Young F: The mediastinum in Hodgkin's and non-Hodgkin's lymphoma. J Thorac Imaging 2:66–71, 1987, with permission of Aspen Publishers, Inc.)

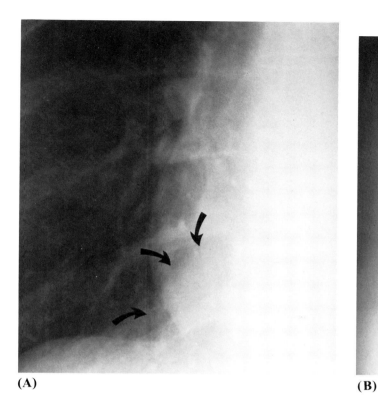

(A)

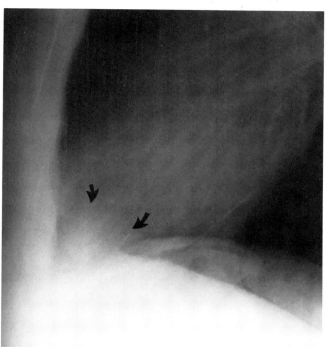

(B)

Fig. 7-27. Cardiophrenic Angle Lymphadenopathy

(A) Coned view of the right base of a man who had diffuse histiocytic lymphoma of the tongue. A subtle zone of increased tissue density is superimposed on the right heart and extends slightly lateral to it (arrows). It is not unusual for fat pads or pleural reflections over the inferior vena cava to present in this fashion. However, adenopathy of the diaphragmatic lymph nodes can present in an identical manner.

(B) Lateral view shows this poorly marginated zone of increased tissue density anteroinferiorly (arrows). Either fat or diaphragmatic lymph nodes can be present at this site and produce this image.

(C) CT scan shows an enlarged diaphragmatic lymph node (n) adjacent to the pericardium over the right heart just above the diaphragm. A small portion of the dome of the right diaphragm (D) is shown at this level. (IVC, inferior vena cava.)

After chemotherapy there was complete resolution of this lymphadenopathy on both follow-up chest films and CT scan.

It is unusual for the diaphragmatic nodes to be the only sign of involvement of the mediastinum by lymphoma or metastases from a variety of neoplasms. When

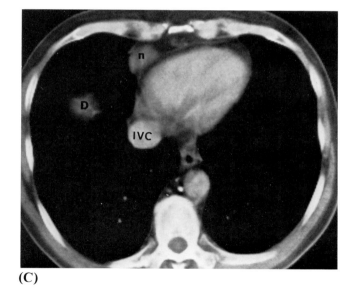

(C)

that occurs, however, it can present a difficult diagnostic problem, since on chest films cardiophrenic angle adenopathy on either side is often indistinguishable from the more ubiquitous pericardial fat pads (see Fig. 7-28). (From Cho et al.,[8] with permission.)

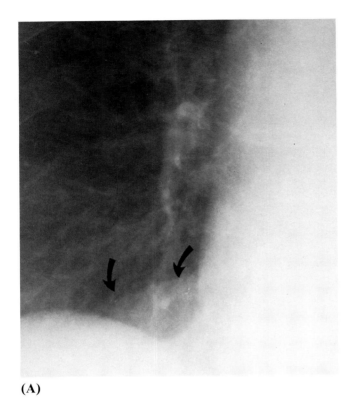

(A)

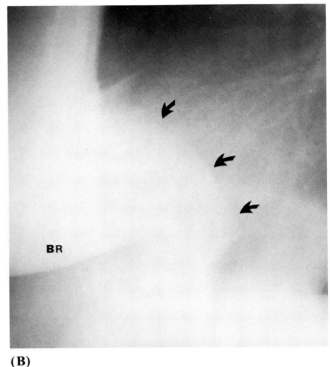

(B)

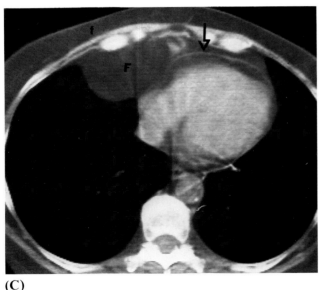

(C)

Fig. 7-28. Fat Pad in the Cardiophrenic Angle

(A) Coned view of the right base of a woman who has left hilar adenopathy (not shown) from a carcinoma of the lung. There is a soft tissue mound (arrows) in the right cardiophrenic angle.

(B) On lateral view the mound is seen anteriorly (arrows). The soft tissues of the breast (BR) are seen further anteriorly.

(C) On CT scan a very large fat pad (F) is present in the right cardiophrenic angle. Compare its density to that of the subcutaneous fat of the chest wall (f), and to the density of the enlarged node in Fig. 7-27C.

The pericardium anterior to the heart (open arrow) is seen as a 1- to 2-mm curved line between the epicardial fat behind it and the pericardial fat in front.

Although cardiophrenic angle fat pads, enlarged nodes, cysts, and other masses cannot be distinguished from one another on plain films, CT scans or MRI studies usually permit ready distinction. The filming technique for this CT image was chosen to display fat as lighter gray than on many other previous CT illustrations in order to enhance the display.

In daily practice, cardiophrenic angle opacities seen on chest films are ordinarily accepted as fat pads without further investigation, but in patients with Hodgkin's disease, non-Hodgkin's lymphoma, or with other primary neoplasms, CT scan is used to make the necessary distinction from lymphadenopathy. Of course, changes in the size or contours of cardiophrenic angle opacities on serial films would also prompt further diagnostic study, since enlarging lymph nodes are more likely to account for *changes* in the appearance of cardiophrenic angle opacities.

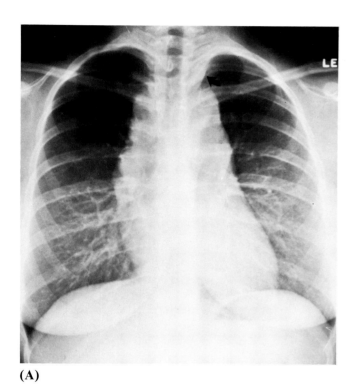

(A)

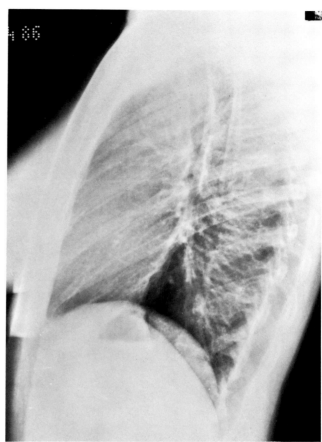

(B)

Fig. 7-29. Permeating Mediastinal Masses (Thymic Involvement)

(A) PA view of a young woman with Hodgkin's disease. A mediastinal mass extends from the thoracic inlet to the base of the heart. The margins of the mass blend with the right and left heart borders so well that it is not possible to tell the precise caudal extent of the mass. Above the left clavicle there is also evidence of an extrapleural, posterior, paraspinal extension of the tumor (arrow).

(B) Lateral view. The edges of the mass are not seen because they are not tangential to the beam. However, the anterior portion of the mediastinum from the thoracic inlet almost to the diaphragm shows a uniform increase in soft tissue density. Ordinarily the right and left lungs are in contact anterior to the upper and middle portions of the mediastinum and would be seen as a darker gray zone than is present here.

(C) CT scan at the level of the top of the aortic arch (A). The arch and the superior vena cava (v) are opacified from intravenous injection of a contrast agent. They are surrounded by a mottled, inhomogeneous mass (M) that permeates the mediastinum anteriorly and surrounds the great vessels.

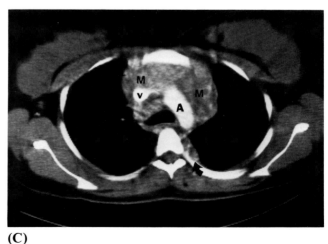

(C)

The aortic arch is effaced on the chest film because the mediastinal mass displaces lung entirely away from it. The left-sided, posterior paravertebral, extrapleural extension of tumor (arrow) corresponds to the extrapleural component seen on the PA chest film. *(Figure continues.)*

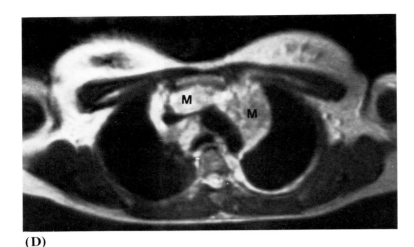

(D)

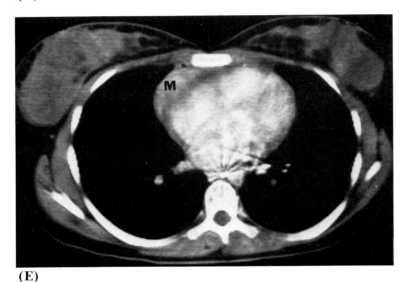

(E)

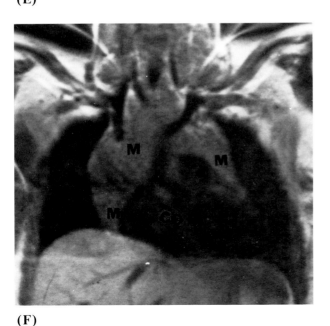

(F)

Fig. 7-29. *(Continued).* **(D)** MRI scan at approximately the same level as Fig. C. Under these imaging conditions the aortic arch, the SVC, and the trachea appear black. The mediastinal mass components, however, appear light gray to near-white. Fat also appears light gray to near-white. By varying the pulse sequences so that T_1- and T_2-weighted images are obtained, distinctions between fat and non-fat masses can be made.

(E) CT scan above the diaphragm but well below the tracheal carina. Portions of the inferior pulmonary veins are seen as they course to the left atrium. Abnormal soft tissue (M) represents a caudal paracardiac extension of the mass, which is seen blending with the right heart border on the PA chest film.

(F) MRI scan in the coronal plane; images of the great vessels and the cardiac chambers (COR) are black. A mass begins at the thoracic inlet, encompasses the great vessels, and extends caudally to the diaphragm on the right and to the pulmonary outflow tract on the left (M).

This mass is in the distribution of the thymus, and this appearance is that of thymic involvement by Hodgkin's disease. The display of the distribution of this mass in the coronal plane is graphic and aids in determining the caudal limits of radiation treatment portals.

8

Evaluation of the Hila and Mediastinal Tumors, Aneurysms, Vascular Anomalies

EVALUATION OF HILAR ABNORMALITIES

Evaluation of the hila is difficult because there is such a wide spectrum of normal variation. Attempts to formulate absolute measurements result in upper limits of normal that include too many abnormal cases to be of practical use. In addition, size alone is not the determinant of normality; there are also contour changes and density differences to consider.

Neophytes have a difficult time evaluating hila. In particular, they have a pronounced tendency to call normal hila abnormal, especially the left. Although I have no data to support my belief, I think experienced observers err more on the side of mistaking the subtly abnormal hila for normal rather than vice versa.

Right Hilum Landmarks

Assessment of the hila is aided by relating hilar structures to constant anatomic landmarks.

Right Interlobar Artery

Find the right main bronchus and follow it to its division into the right upper lobe bronchus and the bronchus intermedius. The interlobar or descending branch of the right pulmonary artery passes into the hilum anterior to the bronchus and turns caudally. Beyond this point it gives off branches that mainly supply the segments of the right middle and right lower lobes. The trunk of the interlobar artery passes caudally anterolateral to the bronchus intermedius and the right lower lobe bronchus. On a PA view the vessel is projected along the lateral aspects of these bronchi and has an obliquely vertical course (Fig. 8-1).

On the lateral view the bulk of the right hilar vessels is projected anterior to the major airways (Fig. 8-2). The major trunk to the right lower lobe then courses posteriorly as it passes caudally.

Truncus Anterior

The truncus anterior branch of the right pulmonary artery supplies tributaries mainly to the right upper lobe. It divides from the right pulmonary artery while still in the mediastinum. The origin of the truncus anterior is not seen on chest films. It is a water-density absorber, branching from another water-density absorber while passing through an airless space, the mediastinum, that also behaves as a water-density absorber. Hence, at its origin there is no natural contrast to permit its recognition as a discrete entity. The truncus anterior becomes visible on chest films as it passes into surrounding lung at the level of the right upper lobe bronchus, and it adds very little bulk to the radiographic right hilum (Fig. 8-1B).

On CT scan, fat in the mediastinum serves as a surrounding contrast material that permits the right pulmonary artery to be seen (see Fig. 7-9F), and on MRI scan (see Fig. 7-3D) there is a negative signal because of flowing blood in the vessels themselves.

Right Superior Pulmonary Vein

The superior pulmonary vein forms from tributaries of the right upper lobe segmental veins and passes anterior to the interlobar branch of the right pulmonary artery en route to the left atrium (Fig. 8-1D). It thus makes a major contribution to the bulk of the right hilum on plain films and on tomograms. When the vein is prominent or engorged, as in the event of left heart failure, it can have a convex lateral margin and appear to be an abnormal mass at the site where it crosses the interlobar artery.

Right Inferior Pulmonary Veins

The inferior pulmonary veins pass toward the left atrium below the horizontal course of the interlobar artery and do not make a contribution to those structures that make up the right hilum radiographically (Fig. 8-1D). However, the confluence of the right inferior pulmonary veins at the left atrium can frequently be seen as a right retrocardiac, paraspinal, "half-moon" image, especially on films or tomograms made with the patient supine (see Fig. 7-1A). This venous confluence can also be seen on routine PA chest films (Fig. 8-3A). This image is easily mistaken for an abnormal mass, but the error is avoided by recognizing the inferior pulmonary vein tributaries joining this structure. Rarely, the opposite occurs; that is, a true retrocardiac mass can be mistaken for the confluence of veins (Fig. 8-3B and C). If there are doubts from chest film appearances, they can be resolved by tomograms, fluoroscopy, or CT or MRI scans, which demonstrate this anatomy well.

Left Hilum Landmarks

First find the left main and upper lobe bronchi (Fig. 8-4). The left pulmonary artery passes from front to back over the left upper lobe bronchus; hence it is higher in position than the interlobar branch of the right pulmonary artery, which comprises a major bulk of the right hilum (Fig. 8-5). In addition, the left pulmonary artery has not yet divided at this level; thus, it can produce a rather formidable elliptical or ball-like "mass" on frontal

view. I call this "the medical student's tumor," because it is a structure that students frequently identify as an abnormal mass. With modest experience the left pulmonary artery is readily recognized because of its intimate relationship to the left upper lobe bronchus. Its bulk is variable, but it can produce an image with a diameter up to approximately 3.0 cm measured from the edge of the bronchus to the upper edge of the artery against adjacent lung. After the left pulmonary artery arches over the bronchus it passes caudally posterolateral to the left lower lobe bronchus. Hence, on PA views the descending branch is seen in close relation to the lateral aspects of the lower lobe bronchus, whereas on a lateral view it passes obliquely caudally along the posterior aspect of the lower lobe bronchus.

Left Superior Pulmonary Vein

The left superior pulmonary vein passes anterolateral to and then under the left pulmonary artery and usually does not cause confusion with an abnormal mass as the right sometimes does (Fig. 8-4C).

Left Inferior Pulmonary Veins

The confluence of the inferior pulmonary veins on the left is usually slightly cephalad of that on the right, but these veins also course toward the left atrium well below any possible confusing shadows of the central portions of the left pulmonary hilum.

Signs of Hilar Mass

Short, Sharp Arcs or Encased Airways

The hila are composed of individual trunks of vessels and bronchi, and there are vessel branches projected over the hila from lung both in front and behind. Since hilar structures are all surrounded by air-filled lung, they are recognizable as separate images. Thus, the image we call the "hilum" on a radiograph has individual components that can be recognized rather than lumped together. Pulmonary vessels that are traced from the lung periphery backward into their respective hila should appear to gradually increase in caliber in a logical fashion.

When short, sharp, convex arcs of soft tissue density are seen along the proximal course of vessels and cannot be explained as being due to other superimposed vessels, consider the possibility of lymphadenopathy (Fig. 8-6). Similarly, on a lateral view, if you encounter short, sharp arcs that are convex anteriorly or posteriorly along the proximal course of hilar vessels, consider the possibility of lymphadenopathy (Fig. 8-7). If you see major bronchi that appear to be entirely surrounded by soft tissue densities, consider the possibility of lymphadenopathy; arteries accompany bronchi but do not completely encase them. Enlarged lymph nodes can and do (Fig. 8-8). However, very large pulmonary vessels that occur in patients with pulmonary hypertension or left-to-right shunts may be confused with lymphadenopathy (see Ch. 9).

The most difficult decision to make about a hilum is to decide whether it is normal or abnormal. The grossly abnormal hilum presents the least difficulty, and the clearly normal hilum is usually not difficult to assess with modest experience, but that leaves a considerable group of "in-betweens." Judgment is then based on experience in evaluating the hila of large numbers of people of different ages, different body builds, and with different conditions known to effect hilar anatomy such as emphysema or bronchitis, pulmonary hypertension, segmental resection, atelectasis, postirradiation reaction, congestive heart failure, and pulmonary embolism.

As for the mediastinum, hilar evaluation is considerably more reliable when there are previous chest radiographs for comparison, particularly if the comparison films are several months or years old.

Increased Density

The concept of increaed density of a hilum is important but not easy to learn except through practice. Since the radiographic hilum is composed of vessels that extend into surrounding lung, any mass or masses that displace lung from the vessels will cause the hilum to become more radiodense by changing the air-water ratio of hilar constituents. The problem is, more dense than what? The answer is, more dense than it was before the mass or masses developed. How can we determine that with precision? If no previous films of comparable technique are available, we cannot. We can use the opposite hilum for comparison only to a limited extent. First of all, it, too, may be involved with the abnormality (e.g., adenopathy) and thus be of no use as an internal standard of normal tissue density. Second, the anatomy of the two hila is sufficiently different that, centrally, their densities may be different even when they are normal. The solution is to develop an abstract mental image of normal hilar density. With practice and attention to detail, not only can you do that, but you can modulate the abstraction based upon a judgment of the overall radiographic technique used. However, as in the evaluation of any subjective variable, the error rate can be high.

The Abnormal Hilum

Once we have decided a hilum is abnormal, we have to determine:

1. Is it an isolated abnormality, or is the opposite hilum abnormal as well?
2. Is the mediastinum abnormal?
3. Is the lung normal or abnormal? If there is a pulmonary lesion, is it:
   a. Focal and ipsilateral?
   b. Multifocal and unilateral or bilateral?
   c. Diffuse?
4. Is the abnormality due to a soft tissue mass; to abnormal, enlarged, unusual, or anomalous vessels; or to diminished vessels?

There are four principal causes of abnormal hila:

1. *Adenopathy.* The many causes of hilar adenopathy are essentially the same as the causes of mediastinal adenopathy discussed earlier. Adenopathy may be present in either one or both hila. Mediastinal adenopathy may or may not be present concurrently.
2. *Mass lesion* due to primary neoplasm originating in a major bronchus and invading adjacent lung. Such lesions will almost always be unilateral, due to bronchogenic carcinoma, uncommonly to carcinoid tumor or bronchial gland carcinoma, and rarely to metastasis to a bronchus from an extrapulmonary primary site.
3. *Abnormal vessels*
   a. Large
      (1) Due to pulmonary hypertension secondary to chronic obstructive airway disease or to primary pulmonary hypertension, Eisenmenger's physiology, or multiple pulmonary emboli.
      (2) Left-to-right cardiac shunts
      (3) Anomalies
      (4) Stuffed with thrombus or neoplasm (rare)
      (5) Pulmonary artery aneurysm (rare)
      (6) Idiopathic (rare)
   b. Small
      (1) Anomalies
      (2) Prior surgery
      (3) Decreased blood flow consequent to severe pulmonary disease in a lung during childhood (e.g., Swyer-James snydrome)
      (4) Obstructed by embolus or clot proximally, rarely by tumor
4. *Distortion* (iatrogenic or due to pulmonary disease)
   a. Prior surgery
   b. Radiation reaction when the hila are included in treatment portals
   c. Acute or chronic disease that contracts lung volume (atelectasis) and displaces or distorts hilar vessels.

Fortunately, abnormal hilar vessels are rarely isolated findings, but are usually seen in patients with acquired or congenital heart or pulmonary disease. In most cases, there are signs and symptoms or past history to alert you to the right choice. For some, the radiographic appearances may be characteristic enough to prompt inclusion of the correct diagnosis in your analysis, even in those few patients who are without classic symptoms.

The differential diagnosis of unilateral hilar enlargement is not significantly different from that of bilateral hilar enlargement except that primary bronchogenic carcinoma is not a serious consideration in bilateral hilar involvement. When there is bilateral hilar enlargement due to bronchogenic carcinoma, it is the nodal metastases that are responsible rather than the primary neoplasm alone.

Ordinarily the patient's age, past history, and clinical signs and symptoms will strongly influence the rank-order of your differential diagnosis. Other radiographic findings may also play a decisive role.

Calcification in Lymph Nodes

Calcification in hilar or mediastinal lymph nodes usually is evidence of previous infection due to tuberculosis or histoplasmosis and less commonly due to the other infectious granulomatous diseases. Node calcification may also result from silicosis or sarcoidosis, in which case the calcium may show a peripheral "eggshell" distribution. Other reported but uncommon causes of eggshell calcification of lymph nodes include post irradiation changes of Hodgkin's disease, blastomycosis, scleroderma, and amyloidosis.[13]

Problems may arise when partly calcified lymph nodes or adjacent noncalcified lymph nodes become involved with metastases. Since the assumption is made that calcified nodes are benign, it is easy to miss metastases that are also present. Older films for comparison, however, make it possible to recognize that a change has occurred and this prompts further investigation (see Fig. 7-11). (See also Ref. 23, Ch. 6 re lymph node calcification in bronchoalveolar carcinoma.)

Hilar Imaging Studies

Tomograms of the hila are very helpful because they permit examination of segments of the hila free from superimposed images of adjacent vessels. They are very useful in distinguishing normal or abnormal vessels from lymphadenopathy as a cause of hilar lesions. They can be performed in AP, oblique, and lateral projections when necessary to clarify questionable appearances. CT and MRI examinations of the hila (Fig. 8-9) are also of great help in the evaluation of otherwise indeterminate

findings.[38,39] Rapid-sequence filming after bolus injection of intravenous contrast material may be required on CT scans to separate vascular from nonvascular hilar components. MRI scans are also effective in hilar evaluation and may become the method of choice. None of these techniques, however, achieves perfect sensitivity or specificity, nor do they eliminate observer error.

Although pulmonary vein varix might be considered in a discussion of hilar vascular abnormalities, this rare lesion usually presents more caudally. Pulmonary vein varix most commonly presents as a nodule or small mass in the lung just proximal to the entrance of a pulmonary vein branch into the left atrium. Frequently other clinical and radiographic findings of pulmonary venous hypertension are also present. Confirmation of the venous nature of the lesion depends on angiography or CT contrast studies, and MRI examination would also be capable of making the determination.

In general, hilar abnormalities may be found in conjunction with mediastinal abnormalities (e.g., lymphadenopathy), cardiovascular abnormalities (e.g., congenital or acquired heart disease), or lung disease (e.g., bronchogenic carcinoma, infectious and noninfectious granulomatous disease). However, there are many cases in which the hilar abnormality is the most compelling or even the only chest film evidence that disease is present at all (see Fig. 8-7).

MEDIASTINAL TUMORS, ANEURYSMS, AND VASCULAR ANOMALIES

Nonlymphomatous Primary Tumors of the Mediastinum

Primary tumors in the mediastinum may occur as either solid or cystic masses. They may be grouped as:

1. Thymomas, thymic cysts, thymolipomas, and other thymic neoplasms
2. Germinal cell tumors
3. Neurogenic tumors
4. Pericardial cysts, duplication and bronchogenic cysts, neurenteric cysts, and meningoceles
5. Intrathoracic thyroid masses
6. Mesenchymal tumors including blood and lymph vessel neoplasms.

Thymoma

Although thymomas are relatively uncommon neoplasms, they are the most common primary tumor found anteriorly in the mediastinum.[4] Thymomas are most often solid but occasionally may be cystic. They may be either benign or malignant, and it is often difficult to make the distinction by any means. The prognosis is based primarily on whether the neoplasm is invasive, or encapsulated and noninvasive. However, certain cell types have a worse prognosis than others, independent of invasiveness.[37] Estimates are that 25 to 30 percent of thymomas behave as locally malignant tumors, and that up to 50 percent of patients who have thymomas also have myasthenia gravis, whereas only 9 to 15 percent of patients with myasthenia gravis have thymomas.[10]

Other syndromes that have been reported to be associated with mediastinal thymomas include aregenerative erythrocytic anemia or red cell hypoplasia and acquired hypogammaglobulinemia.[9] Some patients have been reported to have Cushing-like syndromes, but that is more likely a manifestation of carcinoid tumors of the thymus than of thymomas.[5,31] The histopathology of thymic carcinoid is similar to that of oat cell carcinoma. Thymomas may be found at any age, but peak incidence is in the middle years and thymomas are rare in the young.

In patients who do not have myasthenia gravis, the majority of thymomas are discovered as incidental findings on chest films. Other patients may have symptoms of chest pain, pleural effusion, or cough. Instances of superior vena cava obstruction and pericardial effusion have also been reported.

Thymomas may occur anywhere in the mediastinum between the thoracic inlet and the diaphragm (Fig. 8-10). They are commonly located anteriorly at the base of the heart[9] at approximately the level of the cavoatrial junction on the right, or at the level of the pulmonary artery on the left (Fig. 8-11). Calcification has been reported in thymomas and about the periphery of thymic cysts, but is uncommon.

If the mass seen on imaging studies does not have a relatively sharp interface with lung, but seems to be extending into the lung with short tentacles or linear extensions, presumption favors a malignant lesion. Likewise, when thymomas are large and extend to both the right and left sides of the mediastinum, they are more likely to be malignant than benign[9] (except in the case of thymolipoma).

Distant metastases are rare, however, and malignant thymomas usually do their damage by local invasion. They spread to the pleura and may be responsible for extensive pleural masses and effusion, which may mimic mesothelioma. The pleural implants may become manifest many years after the primary thymoma has been removed or otherwise treated.

The search for a thymoma in a patient with myasthenia gravis and a negative or equivocal chest film is done most efficiently by CT scan.[10] The examination is sensitive, but false-positives may result from confusing a normal thymus in adults for thymoma. Whether or not MRI scans are more specific is as yet unknown.

Thymolipoma

Thymolipomas are rare tumors of the thymus that may occur at any age. When small they are indistinguishable from thymomas. However, these tumors are often not found until they are huge, extend from thoracic inlet to diaphragm, and nearly surround the heart.[36] In spite of their size they are invariably benign. On chest films these large tumors may appear to be part of the heart and erroneously invoke a diagnosis of cardiomegaly. CT, MRI, and ultrasonography all permit distinction of the tumor from the heart, but CT and MRI provide an added increment in that they permit recognition of a large fatty tumor with interspersed soft tissue densities (of thymic tissue).

Germinal Cell Tumors

Germinal cell tumors of the mediastinum include dermoid cysts and adult teratomas, teratocarcinomas, choriocarcinomas, seminomas, endodermal sinus tumors (yolk sac tumors), and embryonal carcinomas. Teratomas are the most common of the group, and approximately half of all patients who have benign teratomas will be asymptomatic[19] (Fig. 8-12). Others will complain of such symptoms as pain and dyspnea. In some series the male-female ratio is as high as 2:1, whereas in others the incidence is equal. The patient's age may vary from infancy to advanced middle age, with the average patient being in the third decade of life. The lesions may be solid or cystic or mixed and can vary from 2 to 15 cm in size. Gross calcification may be visible in a minority of these lesions but is not a distinguishing feature between benign and malignant teratomas. Uncommonly a tooth or bone will be seen in a dermoid cyst.

The malignant teratomas are more often found in the male.[17] Patients with mediastinal seminomas and choriocarcinomas are almost invariably males, and gynecomastia and positive tests for pregnancy are frequently found in males with choriocarcinoma. The age range is approximately the same as for those patients who have benign teratomas. Most patients with malignant teratomas have symptoms such as chest pain or dyspnea.

Whereas the benign teratomas can usually be removed in toto, seldom is it possible to completely resect any of the malignant germ cell neoplasms. They are commonly found to permeate the mediastinum and may involve bronchi, arteries, and veins. Before the advent of modern chemotherapy the majority of these patients died within a year of diagnosis, but the prognosis now is improved.

Neurogenic Tumors

Tumors of nerves, such as neurolemmoma (schwannomas), may rarely present as mediastinal masses along the distribution of the vagus[1] and phrenic nerves (Fig. 8-13). More commonly, neurogenic tumors such as neurolemmomas and neurofibromas are found in the posterior periphery of the mediastinum where more nerves are located[1,4,30] (Fig. 8-14). Likewise, sympathetic and parasympathetic nerve tissue "lives" in the posterior parietal portions of the mediastinum, and ganglioneuromas (Fig. 8-15) and neuroblastomas as well as pheochromocytomas and paragangliomas will also be found there. The aortic bodies located along the distribution of the great vessels contain paraganglionic cells, and paragangliomas may therefore arise in this part of the mediastinum as well. However, paragangliomas and pheochromocytomas are rare in the chest.[30]

Some of the neurogenic tumors may reach great size before the patient presents for medical attention, and some may be malignant (Fig. 8-16). The tumors are usually rounded, elongated, or lobulated, and the edge that interfaces with lung is usually well defined when seen tangentially. Tumors of the sympathetic ganglia — ganglioneuromas and neuroblastomas — may be partially calcified and are usually found in children. Neurogenic tumors occurring alongside the spine may cause local pressure changes such as erosion of vertebal bodies or pedicles, enlargement of intervertebral foramina, and erosion and displacement of adjacent ribs. The tumors themselves may extend into the spinal canal to varying degrees and myelography is useful in assessing such extension. In cases of neurofibromatosis the tumors may be multiple and extend throughout the mediastinum. Nevertheless, a *solitary* paraspinal intrathoracic mass in a patient with known neurofibromatosis is more likely to be an intrathoracic meningocele than a neurofibroma.[1]

Many of the neurogenic tumors would be correctly designated as paravertebral rather than mediastinal neoplasms. So long as their location is clearly identified with reference to adjacent anatomic structures, the name applied to the space becomes less important. Occasionally a neurolemmoma may present as a rounded extrapleural mass in the extreme apex of the chest (see Fig. 6-23). One surface presents a convexity toward the adjacent lung whereas the other blends with and becomes indistinguishable from the extrapleural soft tissues. A (rare) apical meningocele may precisely mimic an apical neurolemmoma.

The fact that a tumor mass is located in a posterior paravertebral position is no guarantee that it is of neurogenic origin. Other neoplasms such as those of muscle or pleura or even lung may also be located there (Fig. 8-17). Inflammatory masses and aortic aneurysms may also be located paravertebrally.

Cysts of the Mediastinum

Pericardial Cysts

Pericardial cysts are most commonly found in the cardiophrenic angles. They are more common on the right than on the left. Usually they have a smooth, although sometimes lobulated, contour (Fig. 8-18). They are rounded or oval in shape, but occasionally the superior aspect may have a pointed appearance on a lateral view where it extends into the region of the major interlobar fissure. The majority of these cysts are seen to be in contact with both the diaphragm and the anterior chest wall on a lateral view. A small minority are located more superiorly in the mediastinum. These do not touch the diaphragm but are usually within a few centimeters of it and clearly interface with the pericardium. In a very small number of cases the cysts appear to be superior to the pericardium. These cystic lesions may rarely show rim calcification. They are invariably benign, and there have been no reports of malignant change.

On fluoroscopy, pericardial cysts have been noted to change in shape when they communicate with the pericardium. However, only a small number (fewer than 10 percent) have been shown to have visible communication with the pericardial sac at the time of surgery.

The majority of the patients have no symptoms. As many as 20 percent, however, have complained of chest pain, and uncommonly there may be symptoms of cough, paroxysmal atrial tachycardia, pneumothorax, hemoptysis, and fever. Pericardial cysts have varied from a few centimeters to over 15 cm in size. Pericardial cysts may be found from childhood to old age, with the majority of cases occurring in the third and fourth decades.[18]

Bronchogenic Cysts

Bronchogenic cysts may occur anywhere in the chest but most commonly are located in the subcarinal region of the mediastinum.[25] These lesions are also benign, although they may recur if incompletely removed.

Bronchogenic cysts occur from childhood through adulthood and only rarely communicate with an airway (see Fig. 8-3). Duplication cysts or gastroenteric cysts are identical in radiologic appearance to bronchogenic cysts but histopathologically possess a different type of lining. Rarely do they occur in the paraspinal regions.

Gastroenteric Cysts

Gastroenteric cysts may communicate with the gastrointestinal tract, particularly the esophagus. In contrast to bronchogenic cysts, gastroenteric cysts are usually located above the level of the carina.

Thoracic Duct and Neurenteric Cysts

Thoracic duct cysts may occur and communicate with the thoracic duct, but they are extremely rare. Neurenteric cysts are also rare congenital lesions that are connected by a stalk to the meninges, the spinal cord, or a vertebra and occasionally to the gastrointestinal tract via a stalk penetrating the diaphragm. When there is open communication between the cyst and the gastrointestinal tract, or an airway, the cyst may contain air, which can be seen on a chest film. The diagnosis may be suggested when a mediastinal mass is seen in conjunction with anomalies of the lower cervical or thoracic spine such as cleft vertebra, widened neural canal, spina bifida, or hemivertebra.[41] The spinal defect may be located cephalad to the cyst itself. Neurological symptoms and intraspinal lesions may or may not also be present.

Thymic Cysts

Thymic cysts occur in the same locations that thymomas ordinarily do and on plain films would be indistinguishable from thymomas. However, on CT or MRI studies their cystic nature is usually appreciated.

Cystic lesions may occur in the thymus of patients with Hodgkin's disease, either at the time of initial diagnosis or following mediastinal irradiation, and they can cause confusion with recurrent lymphadenopathy or thymic permeation by Hodgkin's disease.[2,20] CT scans may indicate the cystic nature of these lesions but do not exclude the possibility of Hodgkin's disease in the cyst wall (Fig. 8-19). Meningoceles and meningomyeloceles may also present as intrathoracic paraspinal masses.

Pancreatic Pseudocysts

Pancreatic pseudocysts may herniate into the chest through various diaphragmatic foramina. Although usually located low in the chest, they have no other distinguishing features. CT scans that include the upper abdomen may provide clues to the presence of chronic pancreatitis, such as calcifications in the pancreas.

Echinococcal Cysts

Echinococcal cysts may occur anywhere in the mediastinum, but the disease is rare in the United States, with the possible exception of Alaska.

Distinguishing Between Cystic and Solid Mediastinal Masses

Chest roentgenograms do not permit one to distinguish between solid and cystic masses of the mediastinum or paravertebral regions. However, CT and MRI scans very frequently will permit such a distinction because of differences in the tissue characteristics of solid and cystic lesions. When intravenous contrast material is used in the course of CT examination, there is also a demonstrable difference in the enhancement of cystic and solid masses due to differences in blood supply.

At times the CT numbers (Hounsfield units) of a cystic lesion may be much higher than would be expected for serous liquids. In such cases the cyst may have a high protein content or may be hemorrhagic or contain blood breakdown products.[22,24] However, only the cyst wall has a true blood supply, and so there will be negligible enhancement of the lesion when scans done before intravenous contrast are compared with those made following bolus injection of contrast. However, it is also important to know how the computer in your CT scanner changes the Hounsfield units of nonenhancing tissues adjacent to or surrounded by structures that do enhance after contrast injection.

Schwannomas are low in density, may not show enhancement of CT numbers after intravenous contrast injection, and thus may mimic cysts in their behavior.[1] A nonenhancing lesion could also be a very necrotic tumor or inflammatory mass rather than a cyst, but seldom are tumors completely necrotic. On the other hand, a mass that enhances well after intravenous contrast injection cannot be a simple cyst.

Calcification of the rim of the lesion is more likely with cystic than with solid tumors but can also be seen with aortic and rare pulmonary artery aneurysms.

Ultrasound examination is also effective in distinguishing cystic from solid masses in the mediastinum, provided the lesion is situated so that no lung is interposed between the lesion and the chest wall. Gas in the lung interposed between the ultrasound transducer on the chest wall and the mediastinal lesion makes the technique ineffective.

Intrathoracic Thyroid

In the majority of cases of intrathoracic thyroid, the mass arises anteriorly and extends into the mediastinum in front of the trachea. In a minority of cases (about 20 percent) the mass originates from a lower pole of the thyroid and passes caudally into the mediastinum posterior to the trachea on the right side (Fig. 8-20).

When intrathoracic thyroid is due to a functioning goiter, the diagnosis may be established by radionuclide scan. CT examinations also show these lesions well.[3] Intrathoracic thyroid almost always displaces or deforms the trachea in either the PA or the lateral view, or both, whereas tortuous great vessels, most notably the right brachiocephalic (innominate) artery, which also may appear as a mass below the thoracic inlet, do not displace the trachea (see Fig. 8-33).

Rarely, primary mediastinal goiter may occur and show no connection with the thyroid in the neck. Calcifications may be present in both benign and malignant thyroid masses.

Although parathyroid adenomas may occur in the mediastinum, they are seldom recognizable as masses on plain chest films. They can be difficult to image by any technique when they are small but have been identified successfully, but not invariably, on CT scans. However, ectopic parathyroid adenomas often appear similar to mediastinal lymph nodes or remnants of thymic tissues.[24]

Vascular Neoplasms

Hemangiomas and lymphangiomas are rare primary tumors of the mediastinum. When phleboliths are visible, a correct diagnosis can be made. Otherwise, these tumors have no features distinguishing them from other neoplasms that primarily occur anteriorly. They may be lobulated and commonly are asymptomatic or cause disturbances by pressure on neighboring structures. They may insinuate themselves throughout the mediastinum.[8,26] Other primary vascular neoplasms do occur in the mediastinum but are very rare.

Other Masses

Omental fat may herniate into the mediastinum and not be recognized as fat on plain films, but instead may appear as a nonspecific soft tissue mass. However, fat is readily distinguished from other tissue on CT and MRI scans. Rarely, abdominal viscera may herniate into the mediastinum and present a difficult diagnostic challenge, but one usually resolved by CT or gastrointestinal contrast studies (Fig. 8-21).

There are other causes of mediastinal masses, such as extramedullary hematopoiesis and hematomas. Mesenchymal tissue tumors occur, but these are uncommon.[4]

Think of any and every tissue that occurs in the mediastinum, and sooner or later you will find a report of a benign or malignant neoplasm of that tissue substrate.

Whereas good history and laboratory data may permit prediction of a hematoma or extramedullary hematopoiesis as the cause of a mass, there are no findings that permit accurate prediction of the histopathologic nature of the more uncommon neoplasms of the mediastinum, except for the identification of phleboliths in some hemangiomas or lymphangiomas.

Lesions of the Esophagus

Intrinsic lesions of the esophagus are studied best by meticulous fluoroscopy (usually using barium as contrast agent), by endoscopy, or by both modalities. The accuracy of CT in staging esophageal cancer is controversial.[29]

Obstructing lesions and disorders of esophageal motility, either neoplastic, inflammatory, or neuromuscular, may cause esophageal dilatation, which may appear as a distended air- and fluid-filled esophagus on either the PA or the lateral view of the chest or both (Fig. 8-22). The most marked dilatation is associated with achalasia. A diverticulum of the upper or the distal esophagus may be projected laterally over the lung and simulate a cavitary or mass lesion of lung.

Hiatus hernia is relatively common and may become large enough to be seen as a masslike image in the retrocardiac, supradiaphragmatic region when devoid of air (see Fig. 8-14). When a hiatus hernia contains air it is readily recognized; when in doubt, confirmation is obtained by barium swallow examination under fluoroscopy.

Carcinoma of the esophagus may metastasize to the mediastinal lymph nodes, which can become detectable on chest films or CT[29] or MRI scans, but the accuracy for detecting regional nodal metastastes from esophageal cancer is not high. A leiomyoma of the esophagus may become large enough to be seen as a mass on a chest film, and so may a duplication cyst.

Sometimes the esophagus can be seen against the posterior wall of the trachea on the lateral view of the chest. When there is thickening of the esophageal wall or retention of fluid—often consequent to chronic partial obstruction from either benign or malignant lesions—the combined images of the posterior tracheal wall and the thickened esophagus (Fig. 8-22) are seen as a posterior tracheal stripe of abnormal width.[33] Apparent thickening of the posterior wall of the trachea (greater than 4.0 mm) is one of the known radiographic signs of esophageal disease. However, confirmation by other examination, (e.g., esophagram) should always be obtained. The posterior tracheal wall is not always clearly defined on lateral chest films, and rotation off the true lateral projection will affect its apparent width as will other mediastinal abnormalities.

Contrast studies of the esophagus are useful to demonstrate esophageal displacement caused by anomalies of the great vessels (see Fig. 8-31). Large posterior mediastinal or subcarinal adenopathies may also distort, displace, or invade the esophagus (see Fig. 7-14).

The Trachea

After the age of 30 years the tracheal width on a frontal view (coronal plane) is on the order of 17 to 18 mm (range 11 to 26 mm), and 19 to 20 mm (range 11 to 30 mm) in the AP (sagittal plane) dimension.[25] In adults, the caliber of the trachea in the sagittal plane exceeds that in the coronal plane by about 1.0 mm in males and less than 1.0 mm in females. In patients with obstructive airways disease, however, the trachea may assume a saber-sheath shape, with the coronal diameter less than two-thirds that of the sagittal.[12]

Primary tumors of the trachea are quite rare and may be benign or malignant. The majority of the benign lesions, such as fibromas, papillomas, hemangiomas, and cartilaginous tumors, are found in children. Malignant tumors may be primary or, rarely, metastatic (Figs. 8-23 and 8-24). Direct extension to the trachea from laryngeal, thyroid, pulmonary, or esophageal neoplasms may also occur. Any type of mediastinal mass and a variety of congenital vascular rings or slings can distort the trachea. Symptoms and signs include dyspnea, hemoptysis, cough, wheezing, dysphagia, change in voice, stridor, air trapping, and pneumonia.

Tracheal stenosis following prolonged or traumatic intubation or occurring as a complication of trauma or tracheostomy may cause mild to severe air flow obstruction. Surgical correction may be required to restore adequate function for ordinary physical activity.

Narrowing of the trachea may occur from other causes such as tracheopathia osteoplastica, fibrosing mediastinitis, or relapsing polychondritis.[16] Dilatation of the trachea (tracheobronchomegaly) is a rare condition, as is congenital tracheomalacia.

Injury to the trachea from trauma, intubation, or even severe chronic cough may also cause dysfunction similar to that of tracheomalacia. Under conditions of maximum expiratory flow (e.g., during coughing the increased compliance of the malacic tracheal wall can produce functional stenosis, which acts as a flow-limiting segment.

Extensive calcification of tracheal and bronchial cartilages may be seen with advanced age in women.

Mediastinal Fat

Fat may be profusely deposited throughout the mediastinum, particularly in patients receiving long-term, high-dose steroid treatment and to a lesser extent in those who are obese. Voluminous fat in the mediastinum is not clearly distinguishable from masses of more ominous nature on chest films (Fig. 8-25). CT and MRI scans, however, make it relatively easy to distinguish between fat and nonfatty masses in the mediastinum.

Many people have prominent fat pads at the cardiophrenic angles. Large masses of cardiophrenic angle fat have been removed surgically because their true nature was not recognized prior to surgery. The name "lipoma" has been applied to such masses, but they may only be exaggerations of ordinary fat pads.

CT is ideal for distinguishing between cardiophrenic angle lymphadenopathy and prominent fat pads (see Figs. 7-27 and 7-28). Even better, CT can show lymph nodes within fat pads. This distinction is a great help in evaluating patients with Hodgkin's disease and non-Hodgkin's lymphoma. Recognition of involvement of pericardiac diaphragmatic lymph nodes in these patients is important so that radiation treatment portals can be planned appropriately. Neither plain chest films nor tomograms permit a reliable distinction between fat pads and diaphragmatic lymphadenopathy.[7]

Pneumomediastinum

Air in the mediastinum is frequently recognized as lucent streaks, which may be seen on both PA and lateral views. In adults there is often associated air in the soft tissues of the neck, whereas in infants air in the neck is unusual. (see Ch. 3 for a discussion of pneumomediastinum.)

Pericardial Effusion

Epicardial fat is often recognizable on the lateral view of the chest, or more easily on fluoroscopy, as a radiolucent stripe along the ventricular margins of the heart. The pericardium, which is normally thin (Fig. 8-26), can then be seen as a stripe of water density sandwiched between the epicardial fat and the mediastinal fat anterior and inferior to the pericardium.

Pericardial effusion causes a widening of the space between the epicardial and pericardial fat (Fig. 8-27), which are boundary markers for the pericardial space. During fluoroscopy you can position these markers tangential to the beam. When a pericardial effusion is present you can see a distinctive, active pulsation of the epicardial fat (corresponding to cardiac pulsation) even though the outer margins of the fluid-filled pericardial sac quiver or undulate in a severely damped fashion. This combination distinguishes pericardial effusion from other causes of an enlarged cardiomediastinal silhouette, but decreased amplitude of marginal pulsation by itself does not distinguish between myocardial dysfunction and pericardial effusion.

The widening of the pericardial sac between the epicardial and pericardial fat markers can also be seen on chest films when these fat planes are projected tangentially. This fortunate projection must not occur in many cases of pericardial effusion to judge from the numerous instances of pericardial effusion being diagnosed by echocardiography while remaining unrecognizable on concurrent chest films. Therefore, when the sign of a widened pericardial space is present it is very useful, but its absence, when epicardial fat is not visible, is of no use in ruling out pericardial effusion.

Ultrasonographic examination has replaced most other imaging methods for detecting pericardial effusion because of its ease of use, reliability, and absence of associated morbidity. CT scans and MRI studies can also detect pericardial effusion when these examinations are done for other purposes. Experience with ultrasonographic studies and CT examinations indicates that pericardial effusion is more common than is anticipated from clinical and radiographic examination alone. Small-volume pericardial effusion that is not acute may not cause detectable physiologic disturbance or alteration of cardiomediastinal silhouette beyond those expected on the basis of other causes of an apparently enlarged heart.

When pericardial effusion is voluminous, an erroneous diagnosis of cardiac enlargement may be made on the basis of chest film appearances. The contours of the cardiomediastinal silhouette may resemble a water bag and prompt the correct assessment, but in general the mediastinal configurations in pericardial effusion lack specificity.

Constrictive pericarditis per se cannot usually be diagnosed from chest films. The secondary effects of raised systemic venous pressure may prompt further investigation, however, and pericardial thickening is readily displayed on CT scans. The radiographic diagnosis of constrictive pericarditis is facilitated when calcific plaques are seen in the pericardium of a patient whose clinical signs and symptoms are indicative of constrictive pericarditis.

Mediastinitis

Mediastinitis due to spontaneous acute bacterial or viral infection must be infrequent or underdiagnosed. Most acute mediastinitis I have seen has occurred fol-

lowing esophageal rupture, usually after retching and vomiting, or has been iatrogenic or, rarely, post-traumatic. In the absence of mediastinal air there are few radiographic clues to prompt the diagnosis. Simultaneous pneumothorax may be present, but it is a nonspecific sign. Mediastinitis may also occur as an infection after penetrating trauma or after chest or cardiac surgery.

Chronic mediastinitis may occur from granulomatous infection such as tuberculous or histoplasmosis, and fibrosing mediastinitis may occur as an idiopathic condition. Rarely, obstruction of the superior vena cava, pulmonary arteries, veins, or airways may occur as the result of chronic fibrosing mediastinitis.[32,40]

Vascular Lesions

Dilatation, elongation, and tortuosity of the thoracic aorta are common changes associated with age, atherosclerosis, or hypertension. Beginning students often interpret these contour changes as being due to mediastinal tumor. This is particularly true when the ascending aorta is primarily involved, as in patients with systemic hypertension, aortic valve lesions, syphilitic aortitis, and, much less commonly, Marfan's syndrome. A variety of other vascular abnormalities cause deformities of mediastinal and paravertebral contours that may closely resemble changes produced by lymphadenopathy.[6]

Aortic Aneurysms

Frequently, patients who present with an aneurysm of the aorta can be distinguished on the basis of clinical signs and symptoms from those presenting with lymphadenopathy or other masses. There will be many instances, however, where such distinction cannot be made.

Radiographically, aortic aneurysms present as masses closely associated with the aorta but indistinguishable from nonvascular masses on the basis of plain-film appearances. Rarely, an aneurysm may arise from the inferior aspect of the aortic arch and present as a mass extending into the left lung. It is important to recognize these aneurysms in order to avoid surgical disaster (Fig. 8-28). Unfortunately, determining the presence or absence of pulsations fluoroscopically does not permit a distinction between aneurysm and neoplasm. The critical distinction between aortic aneurysm and other mediastinal mass can be made by angiography, which also provides accurate anatomic detail for planning a surgical approach to the aneurysm. CT scanning before and after intravenous administration of contrast material is suitable as a less invasive diagnostic approach in many cases (Fig. 8-28).

Dissecting aneurysms of the aorta may be mistaken for nonvascular masses, and metastatic or lymphomatous lymph node masses, intimately associated with the ascending aorta, may mimic dissection.

Frequently, extensive calcific plaque formation simplifies the diagnosis of aortic ectasia and elongation by outlining large segments of the aortic wall. Occasionally, separation of a calcific plaque from the aortic wall margin is seen on chest films and makes the tentative diagnosis of aortic dissection possible. CT and MRI scans are very useful in confirming or excluding the diagnosis of aortic dissection suspected from plain-film findings or from signs and symptoms. However, CT does not provide reliable evidence of the patency of key branch vessels that is so critical to surgical planning. Therefore, aortography is still the preferred imaging study in acute cases of aortic dissection (Fig. 8-29). CT scans remain very useful for follow-up studies. To avoid false-positive and false-negative diagnoses of aortic dissection on CT it is important that the examination be performed and interpreted meticulously. Certain computer-generated artifacts can mimic aortic dissection.[11,14]

Whether MRI studies (Fig. 8-30) are capable of replacing preoperative angiography is as yet undetermined. If the accuracy of MRI studies in the diagnosis of aortic aneurysm remains high, then MRI is likely to replace CT in establishing this diagnosis.

Aortic Arch Anomalies and Variants

Anomalies of the aortic arch,[34,35] such as right aortic arch, the rare double aortic arch, or aberrant right subclavian artery, may cause no symptoms (Fig. 8-31). They often, however, have characteristic radiographic appearances especially when the esophagus is filled with barium and studied fluoroscopically and radiographically. Thus, simply thinking of these possibilities at the appropriate time may allow for analysis without the need of angiography.

Coarctation of the aorta (Fig. 8-32) can usually be recognized when accompanied by rib notching, but changes in aortic contours can be erroneously ascribed to nonvascular masses when the rib notching is absent, subtle, or missed. Poststenotic dilatation of the descending aorta may be mistaken for a posterior mediastinal mass. This may also be true of patients with pseudocoarctation who have dilatation of the arch and often of the proximal subclavian artery as well. Since there is no pressure gradient across the buckled section, there is also no collateral circulation and no rib notching. Tortuosity of the right brachiocephalic (innominate) artery can also be mistaken for a mediastinal mass (Fig. 8-33).

Enlarged Pulmonary Arteries

Idiopathic dilatation of the pulmonary artery, aneurysms of the pulmonary artery, and dilatation of pulmo-

nary arteries secondary to cardiac or pulmonary disease may cause radiographic changes that can be mistaken for lymphadenopathy, but usually there are clinical signs and symptoms that alert one to the distinction (see Ch. 9).

Distended Veins

Dilated intrathoracic veins may also produce contour alterations that can be mistaken for neoplastic masses.[6] Total anomalous pulmonary venous return may cause gross alteration of mediastinal contours. Persistent left superior vena cava or a left vertical vein may be unrecognizable on plain films, but occasionally may cause widening of the superior mediastinum that is visible on PA chest films in asymptomatic individuals (Fig. 8-34). The diagnosis usually can be either ruled out or confirmed by intravenous injection of contrast or by the somewhat less traumatic isotope angiographic technique. CT and MRI are other ways to confirm the diagnosis of suspected left superior vena cava. Persistent left superior vena cava in association with a variety of congenital heart lesions is ordinarily not a diagnostic dilemma since it is elucidated in the ordinary course of the investigation. The same is true of the presence of a left vertical vein in association with congenital heart and vessel anomalies.

Dilatation of the superior vena cava may occur with any condition that interferes with right atrial filling or that causes increased flow through the vena cava.[23,27] The commonest cause of superior vena cava dilation, of course, is congestive heart failure (see Ch. 9). Superior vena cava dilatation causes the mediastinum to appear wide, especially when films are made at short target-film distances with the patient supine (and often in poor inspiration). In fact, even the normal mediastinum can show disconcerting widening on supine films made at short target-film distances in persons of mesomorphic body habitus and in the obese. It is not safe to make a diagnosis of mediastinal adenopathy based on such widening alone unless there are earlier films, in the same position, available for comparison, or the degree of widening exceeds the extremes of normal.

Any condition that leads to dilatation of the azygos or the hemiazygos vein or the left superior intercostal venous system can cause mediastinal contour changes mimicking tumor masses or adenopathy.[6,21] This is true not only of the right tracheobronchial angle region, where one expects to see the azygos vein, but also along with paravertebral and para-aortic distribution of these veins (Fig. 8-35).

Inadvertent ligation of an azygos continuation of the inferior vena cava, which represents the main source of venous return from the lower half of the body to the heart, can be disastrous (Fig. 8-36). Determination of azygos vein size is a useful and important aspect of mediastinal analysis. In most adults the azygos vein will be 8 mm or less in greatest diameter when measured on chest films made at a target-film distance of 6 feet with the patient upright. (The measurement is made from the edge of the tracheal air column to the lateral edge of the azygos vein image at its widest point, and thus the tracheal wall and the pleural reflection over the azygos vein are included in the measurement). Measurements up to 9 to 10 mm in width, however, can be acceptable as normal, particularly in large subjects when there is no clinical reason to suspect abnormalities of pressure or flow in the azygos system. On films made with the patient supine an azygos width of 14 mm can be normal, although in some patients it may be a reflection of slightly raised venous pressure.[28] An increase in circulating blood volume in pregnant women may be associated with temporary physiologic enlargement of the azygos vein, and measurements up to 15 mm may be acceptable.[15] When the azygos vein exceeds these limits, careful clinical assessment of the possibilities of increased systemic venous pressure or chronic increase of flow volume in the azygos system should be made. Another possible explanation is that the image in question is not that of the azygos vein itself but rather that of a small but abnormal mediastinal mass, usually adenopathy of the azygos node.

In this chapter only a few examples of abnormalities of the aorta and great vessels and the veins of the mediastinum have been used to show how they can mimic other types of mediastinal mass. Many more vascular lesions involving mediastinal vessels[35] could be included, but a more thorough discussion of even the most common mediastinal vessel abnormalities would require another chapter of equal length.

SUMMARY

1. Evaluation of the hila is difficult. False-positive and false-negative evaluations are common.
   a. The distinction between large vessels and large lymph nodes is simplified when earlier films are available and used for comparison.
   b. Short, sharp, arclike edges, distinct from vessel margins, are strong indications of hilar masses.
   c. CT and MRI studies are very helpful in analyzing the hila and often show lesions that are not apparent on plain films. Tomography is also useful but is becoming a lost art.
   d. The differential diagnosis of hilar adenopathy is much the same as for mediastinal adenopathy.
2. Primary tumors (neoplasms and cysts) usually present as solitary masses in the mediastinum but occasionally have polylobulated contours that can

mimic adenopathy. Thymoma is the commonest primary tumor of the anterior mediastinum.
3. Neurogenic tumors occur where nerve tissue is most heavily concentrated: in the paravertebral regions and much less commonly along the distribution of the vagus and phrenic nerves.
4. Mediastinal cysts cannot be distinguished from solid tissue masses on chest films, but CT and MRI studies often can provide sufficient evidence to make the distinction. Ultrasound may also be effective when the lesions are against the chest wall.
5. A dilated, distended esophagus may appear as a mediastinal mass. When visible, a fluid level is often a clue to the correct interpretation.
6. Primary and metastatic tumors of the trachea are rare, are easily overlooked, and cause symptoms that can be confused with those of chronic obstructive pulmonary disease or asthma.
7. Mediastinal lipomatosis occurs in patients who have been on long-term steroid treatment (or have Cushing's disease); occasionally it is idiopathic or an accompaniment of obesity. Lipomatosis can be distinguished from other causes of mediastinal mass by CT or MRI.
8. Herniation of abdominal viscera or omental fat may also present as a mediastinal mass. Rarely, pancreatic pseudocyst may extend into the mediastinum.
9. Pericardial effusion may be present with or without signs of gross cardiac enlargement. Small, acute effusions may cause tamponade whereas large, slowly accumulating effusions may or may not.
10. Vessel abnormalities (e.g., extreme tortuosity, dilatation, aneurysm, or anomaly) may produce mediastinal contour changes resembling those of adenopathy. Distinctions can be made by CT, MRI, or angiography.

BIBLIOGRAPHY

1. Aughenbaugh GL: Thoracic manifestations of neurocutaneous diseases. Radiol Clin North Am 22:741, 1984
2. Baron RL, Sagel SS, Baglan RJ: Thymic cysts following radiation therapy for Hodgkin's disease. Radiology 141:593, 1981
3. Bashist B, Ellis K, Gold RP: Computed tomography of intrathoracic goiters. AJR 140:455, 1983
4. Benjamin SP, McCormack LJ, Effler DB, et al: Primary tumors of the mediastinum. Chest 62:297, 1972
5. Brown LR, Aughenbaugh GL, Wick MR, et al: Roentgenologic diagnosis of primary corticotropin-producing carcinoid tumors of the mediastinum. Radiology 142:143, 1982

6. Castellino RA, Blank N, Adams D: Dilated azygos and hemiazygos veins presenting as paravertebral intrathoracic masses. N Engl J Med 278:1087, 1968

7. Castellino RA, Blank N, Hoppe R: Contributions of chest CT scanning in the initial staging evaluation of newly diagnosed Hodgkin's disease. Radiology 103:603, 1986

8. Davis JM, Mark GJ, Greene R: Benign blood vascular tumors of the mediastinum. Radiology 126:581, 1978

9. Ellis K, Gregg HG: Thymomas-roentgen considerations. AJR 91:105, 1964

10. Fon GT, Bein ME, Mancuso AA: Computed tomography of the mediastinum in myasthenia gravis. Radiology 142:135, 1982

11. Godwin JD, Breiman RS, Speckman JM: Problems and pitfalls in the evaluation of thoracic aortic dissection by computed tomography. J Comput Assist Tomogr 6:750, 1982

12. Greene R: "Saber-sheath" trachea: relation to chronic obstructive pulmonary disease. AJR 130:441, 1978

13. Gross BH, Schneider HJ, Proto AV: Eggshell calcification of lymph nodes: an update. AJR 135:1265, 1980

14. Heiberg E, Wolverson M, Sundaram M, et al: CT findings in thoracic aorta dissection. AJR 136:13, 1981

15. Keats TE, Lipscomb GE, Betts CS III: Mensuration of the arch of the azygos vein and its application to the study of cardiopulmonary disease. Radiology 90:990, 1968

16. Kilman WJ: Narrowing of the airway in relapsing polychondritis. Radiology 126:373, 1979

17. Knapp RH, Hurt RD, Payne SW, et al: Malignant germ cell tumors of the mediastinum. J Thorac Cardiovasc Surg 89:82, 1985

18. LeRoux BT: Pericardial coelomic cysts. Thorax 14:27, 1959

19. Lewis BD, Hurt RD, Payne SW, et al: Benign teratomas of the mediastinum. J Thorac Cardiovasc Surg 86:727, 1983

20. Lindfors KK, Meyer JE, Detrick CJ, et al: Thymic cysts in mediastinal Hodgkin's disease. Radiology 156:37, 1985

21. McDonald CJ, Castellino RA, Blank N: The aortic "nipple." The left superior intercostal vein. Radiology 96:533, 1970

22. Mendelson DS, Rose JS, Efremidis SC, et al: Bronchogenic cysts with high CT numbers. AJR 140:463, 1983

23. Milne ENC, Pistolesi M, Miniati M: The vascular pedicle of the heart and the vena azygos. Part 1: the normal subject. Radiol 152:1, 1984

24. Naidich DP, Zerhouni EA, Siegelman SS: Computed Tomography of the Thorax. Raven Press, New York, 1984

25. Paré JAP, Fraser RG: Synopsis of Diseases of the Chest. p. 20. WB Saunders Co, Philadelphia, 1983

26. Pilla TJ, Wolverson MK, Sundaraman M: CT evaluation of cystic lymphangiomas of the mediastinum. Radiology 144:841, 1982

27. Pistolesi M, Milne ENC, Miniati M, et al: The vascular pedicle of the heart and the vena azygos. Part II: acquired heart disease. Radiology 152:9,1984

28. Preger L, Hooper TJ, Steinbach HL, et al: Width of azygos vein related to central venous pressure. Radiology 93:521, 1969

29. Quint LE, Glazer GM, Orringer MB, et al: Esophageal carcinoma: CT findings. Radiology 155:171, 1985

30. Reed JC, Hallet KIK, Feigin DS: Neural tumors of the thorax: subject review from the AFIP. Radiology 126:9, 1978

31. Rosai J, Higa E: Mediastinal endocrine neoplasm of probable thymic origin, related to carcinoid tumor. Clinicopathologic study of 8 cases. Cancer 29:1061, 1972

32. Schowengerdt CG, Seyemoto R, Main FB: Granulomatous and fibrotic mediastinitis. A review and analysis of 180 cases. J Thorac Cardiovasc Surg 57:365, 1969

33. Shields JB, Holtz S: The retrotracheal space. Radiology 120:19, 1976

34. Shuford WH, Sybers RG, Edwards FK: The three types of right aortic arch. Am J Roentgenol 109:67, 1970

35. Stewart JR, Kincaid OW, Edwards JE: An Atlas of Vascular Rings and Related Malformations of the Aortic Arch System. Charles C Thomas, Springfield, IL, 1964

36. Teplick G, Nedwich A, Haskin ME: Roentgenographic features of thymolipoma. Am J Roentgenol 117:873, 1973

37. Verley JM, Hollman KH: Thymoma: a comparative study of clinical stage, histologic features, and survival in 200 cases. Cancer 55:1074, 1985

38. Webb WR, Glazier G, Gamsu G: Computed tomography of the normal pulmonary hilum. J Comput Assist Tomogr 5:476, 1981

39. Webb WR, Glazier G, Gamsu G: Computed tomography of the normal pulmonary hilum. J Comput Assist Tomogr 5:485, 1981

40. Weinstein JB, Aronberg DJ, Sagel SS: CT of fibrosing mediastinitis: findings and their utility. AJR 141:247, 1983

41. Wilson CS: Neurenteric cyst of the mediastinum. AJR 107:641, 1969

Atlas

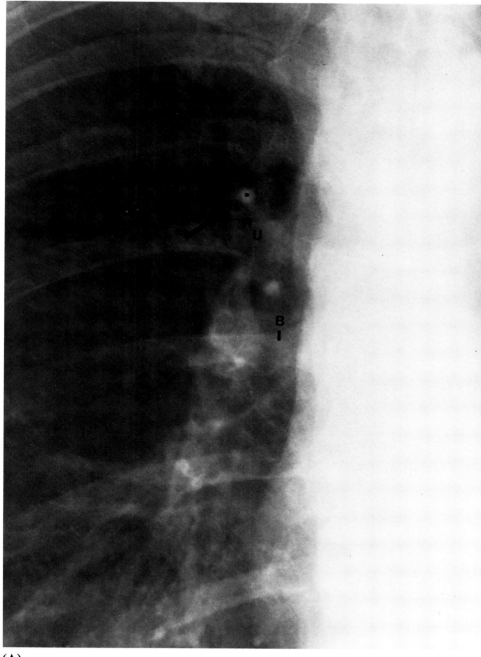

(A)

Fig. 8-1. Vessels of the Right Hilum

(A) Coned view of the right hilum and parahilar portions of the right lung. *(Figure continues.)*

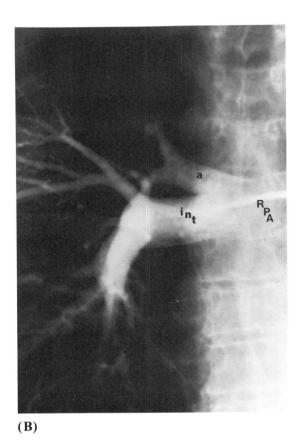

(B)

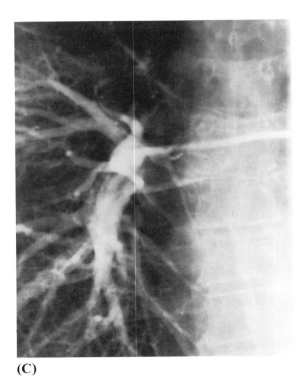

(C)

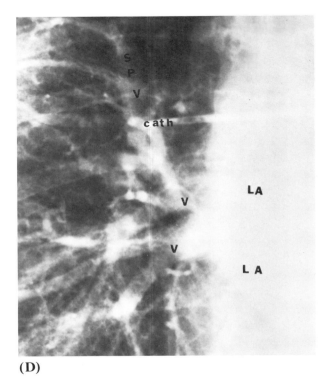

(D)

Fig. 8-1. *(Continued).* **(B)** Pulmonary arteriogram shows a catheter in the right pulmonary artery (RPA). Contrast material fills the anterior (a) and interlobar (int) branches of the RPA. The RPA bifurcates into these branches while still in the mediastinum, and the branches enter the lung separately. Here only a few peripheral branches are filled. A small dot identifies an anterior branch that is already well into the lung. Since it is seen end-on, it is easy to identify on the PA view of the chest as well as on the angiogram. In Fig. A a thin arrow denotes the ring of a branch of the right upper lobe bronchus (RU) seen end-on.

The bulk of the right hilum seen on the PA chest film (Fig. A) consists of the interlobar trunk of the RPA, which is projected lateral to the bronchus intermedius (BI).

(C) Another view later in the course of the pulmonary arteriogram. Injection had been made directly into the interlobar trunk, so that the anterior trunk is no longer seen. There is more peripheral filling of the branches of the interlobar trunk.

(D) Venous phase of the anteriogram. Large veins (V) have a near-horizontal course as they approach the venous confluence before entering the left atrium (LA). The right superior pulmonary vein (SPV) is not filled well, but it can be seen as it passes obliquely caudally from the right upper lobe to the venous confluence. The injection catheter (cath) remains in the interlobar artery, which the SPV has to cross before it reaches the left atrium. It crosses anteriorly.

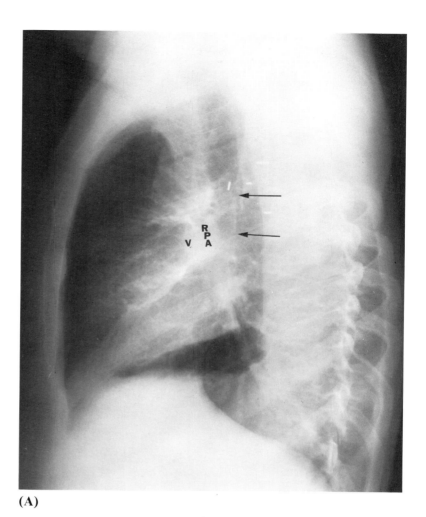

(A)

Fig. 8-2. The Right Hilum After Left Pneumonectomy

(A) Lateral view. This patient has had a left pneumonectomy. All of the vessels visible therefore must be those of the right hilum and lung. The bulk of the right hilum, predominantly the interlobar branch of the right pulmonary artery (RPA) with the right superior pulmonary vein (V) along its anterior margin, is located anterior to the major airways. When the left lung and its vessels are gone there are no large hilar vessels projected posterior to the major airways. Arrows point to the back wall of the right main bronchus at the takeoff of the upper lobe bronchus and the continuous back wall of the bronchus intermedius. This is easily seen because the images of the left hilum are not present to interfere.

(B) PA view. The right hilar vessels are difficult to assess because of the marked shift to the left. The classic findings of a left pneumonectomy are present: (1) near-opacification of the left hemithorax with marked shift of the heart and mediastinal structures to the left; (2) a fairly well defined zone of increased lucency to the left of T5–T7, representing herniation of a portion of the right lung across the anterior mediastinum into the left hemithorax; (3) partial resection of the left fifth rib; and (4) effacement of the images in the left hemithorax except medially, where herniated right lung provides a short segment interface.

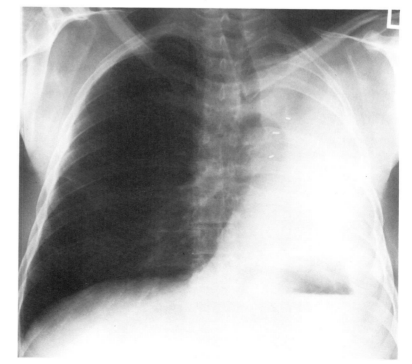

(B)

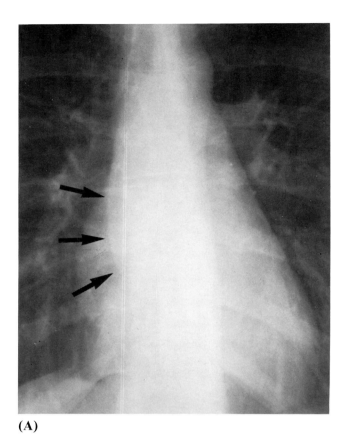

(A)

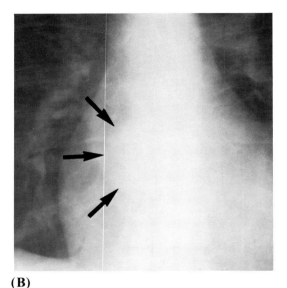

(B)

Fig. 8-3. Bronchogenic Cyst Simulating Venous Confluence

(A) Coned view of a chest showing a characteristic appearance of the venous confluence of the right pulmonary veins (arrows) superimposed on the right heart.

The venous confluence has features that resemble the lesion shown in Fig. B. However, the edge of the lesion seen in Fig. B has an arc with a smaller radius. In both cases pulmonary veins course toward the retrocardiac image. The distinction between this normal venous confluence and the mass seen in Fig. B is extremely difficult to make on a chest film. Unless some element of clinical history prompts further examination, such lesions may go undetected. Fortunately, small mass lesions that simulate a normal pulmonary venous confluence are rare.

(B) PA film shows a sharply circumscribed mass behind the right side of the heart (arrows).

(C) Lateral view. Only a short segment of the margin of the mass is visible, and that is easily mistaken for a pulmonary vein (arrows).

This 40-year-old man had a 1-year history of retrosternal fullness and dysphagia only after ingesting large vitamin pills. Because of retrosternal discomfort he presented himself at the emergency room of a local hospital. An EKG was normal.

An esophagram (not shown) demonstrated that the mass was intimately related to the esophagus. CT scan (not shown) showed a water-density mass with a thick, irregular wall. The wall had a slight enhancement after intravenous contrast injection.

The lesion was removed. It was a foregut cyst with ciliated bronchial epithelium, bronchial glands, and hyaline cartilage in its wall. Bronchogenic cysts may occur almost anywhere in the chest. Commonly, however, they occur in a subcarinal position.

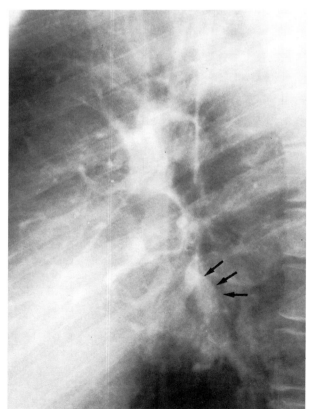

(C)

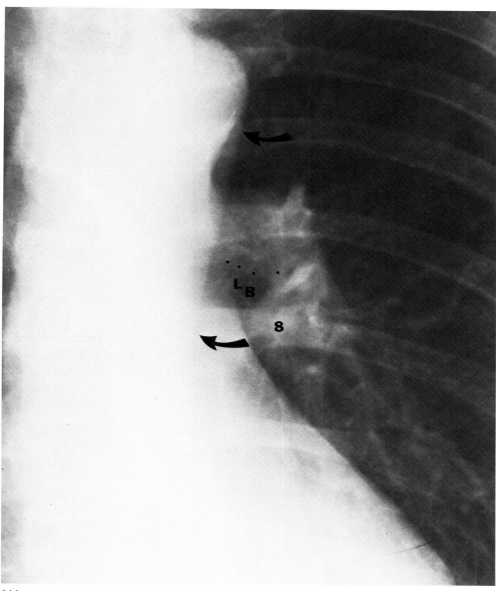

(A)

Fig. 8-4. Vessels of the Left Hilum

(A) Coned view of the left hilum and parahilar portions of the lung. Dots are placed on the upper edges of the left main and upper lobe bronchi. The air column of the distal left main bronchus (LB) appears to have a flattened and truncated inferior margin because of projection of the posteromedial end of the left eighth rib (8) on the air column.

Curved arrows mark the lateral edge of the moderately ectatic descending thoracic aorta, which is obscured caudally because of the technique used for this reproduction. *(Figure continues.)*

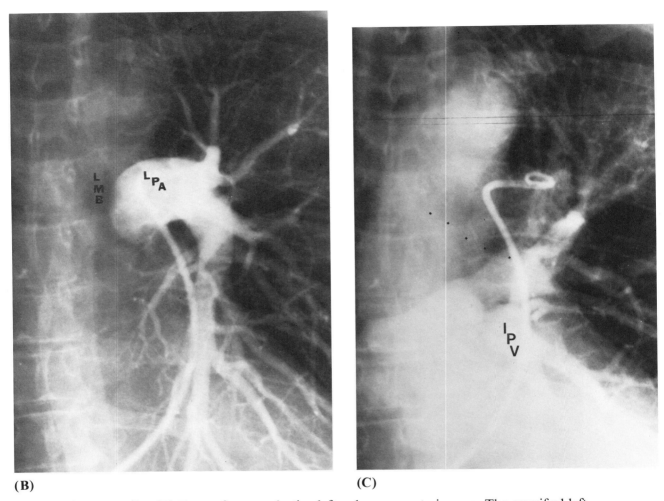

(B)   **(C)**

Fig. 8-4. *(Continued).*   **(B)** Frame from a selective left pulmonary arteriogram. The opacified left pulmonary artery (LPA) corresponds to the soft tissue opacity projected above the left main (LMB) and upper lobe bronchus in Fig. A. The vessel branches, which pass caudally into the left lower lobe, are superimposed on the heart. In PA chest films that are properly exposed these vessels should be visible. Unfortunately, the technique used for the reproduction of Fig. A does not permit these vessels to be seen.

   (C) Frame from the venous phase of the arteriogram. The upper lobe veins course obliquely from the upper lung zone and cross (anteriorly) the major arterial trunk as they approach the left atrium. They are superimposed on the bulk of the left pulmonary artery and thus do not present conspicuous hilar images on the PA chest film. The inferior pulmonary veins (IPV) become confluent and enter the left atrium well below the left main bronchus.

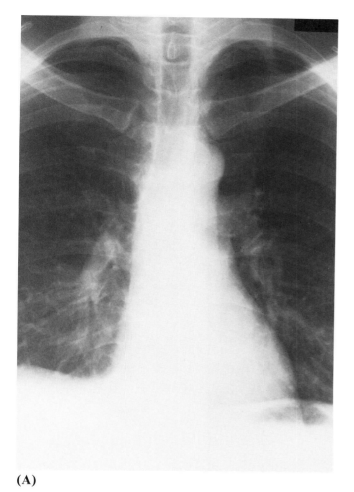

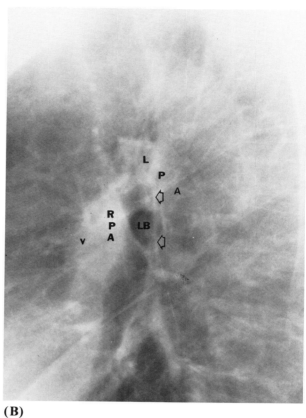

(A)   (B)

Fig. 8-5.   The Left Hilum After Right Pneumonectomy

(A,B) Coned views of the hilar regions of the chest of a man before he underwent a right pneumonectomy. **(C,D)** Comparable views taken after the pneumonectomy. There has been little shift of the heart and mediastinal shadows to the opaque right side, which permits better evaluation of the left hilum. In Fig. A, the bulk of the left hilum is projected cephalad of the bulk of the right hilum, as is usual.

In comparing lateral views (Figs. B and D) before and after pneumonectomy, notice that the bulk of soft tissue anterior to the major airways consists of the right interlobar pulmonary artery (RPA) and the superior pulmonary vein (V). They are no longer visible in Fig. D following right pneumonectomy. Conspicuous large branch vessels anterior to the airway in Fig. D represent both arterial and venous branches of the left lung. *(Figure continues.)*

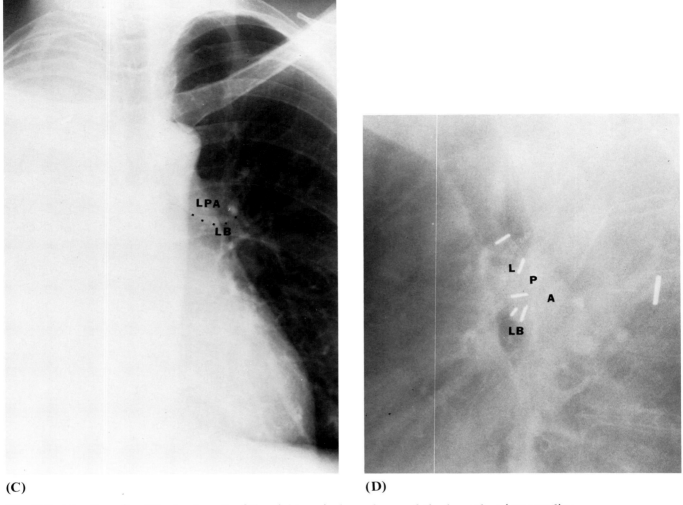

(C)   **(D)**

Fig. 8-5. *(Continued).* The back wall of the right main bronchus and the bronchus intermedius, visible in Fig. B (open arrows), is no longer seen in Fig. D. The sharp upper edge of the left upper lobe bronchus (LB), which is seen in Fig. B, is also present in Fig. D but is partially hidden by clips, which are superimposed from the right side. The bulk of the left pulmonary artery (LPA) remains visible above and behind the image of the left upper lobe bronchus in both Fig. B and Fig. D.

There is an overall loss of detail of the vessels of the left lung in Fig. D compared to Fig. B. The tissues occupying the opaque right hemithorax act as a filter that not only absorbs but also scatters x-rays so that the definition of fine structures is impaired.

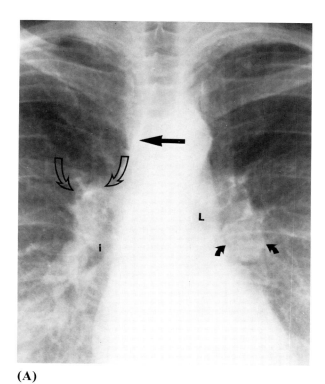

(A)

Fig. 8-6. Bilateral Hilar Adenopathy With Hidden Azygos Adenopathy

(A) Coned PA view of the hila and mediastinum of a woman with recurrent Hodgkin's disease. The lower portions of the left hilum (curved black arrows) have a ball-like configuration. Its lateral and inferior margins present arcs unassociated with any branch vessels. Those vessels that emanate from its inferolateral corner bear no relationship to the size of the small mass and are in another plane. The left main bronchus (L) is identified just proximal to the origin of the left upper lobe bronchus.

There is also adenopathy in the right hilum, but this is subtle. The bronchus intermedius (i) serves as a landmark for evaluating the right hilum. The right hilum has a slightly lobulated contour with a small defile in its lateral aspect (lateral to the bronchus intermedius). There is also an unusual rounding off of its superior aspect (open arrows).

The straight arrow points to the region of the azygos vein and right paratracheal stripe. The right paratracheal stripe is of normal thickness, and neither the azygos vein nor the azygos node appears enlarged.

(B) Magnified view of a CT scan at the level of the aortic arch (AA). The superior vena cava (sv) and the azygos vein (azv) are shown well. The azygos vein passes from its prespinal position around the right side of the lower trachea to enter the vena cava. The soft tissue mass medial to the azygos vein is an enlarged lymph node (N). Since it does not displace lung away from the right

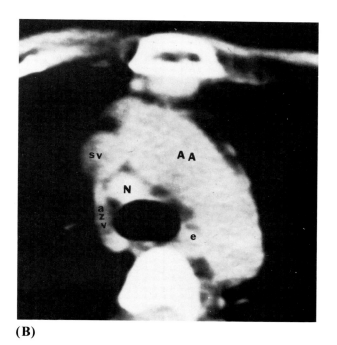

(B)

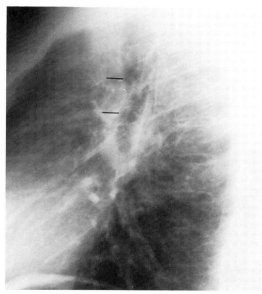

(C)

wall of the trachea, nor does it displace or extend lateral to the azygos vein, its presence is undetected on the PA chest film (e, esophagus). The airway (black) is wide at this level because it is branching into main bronchi.

An enlarged azygos node can hide in the paratracheal pocket of fat medial to the azygos vein and not produce any sign of its presence on PA chest films. (Courtesy of Anton Pogany, M.D., Oakland, California.)

(C) On lateral chest film the slight indistinctness of the anterior wall of the airway (the portion that extends between the two straight line markers) might be considered a marker for the presence of this azygos lymph node, but it is a subtle, easily overlooked signal.

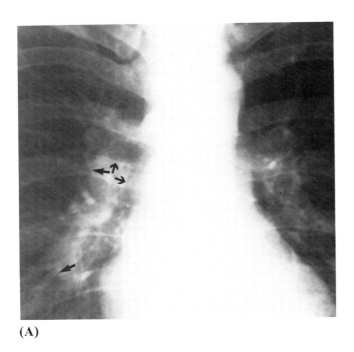

(A)

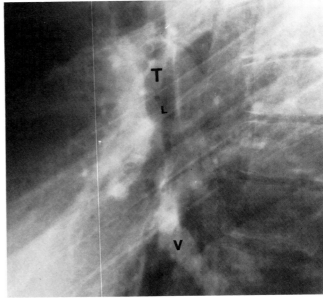

(B)

Fig. 8-7. (A–F) Hilar Adenopathy Due to Sarcoidal Granulomas

(A–C) Films of the chest of a 28-year-old man who had been successfully treated for a carcinoma of the testicle. He returned for a follow-up visit.

(A) An abnormal amount of soft tissue is seen in the right hilum. There are short, sharp, arclike interfaces between the right hilum and adjacent lung (lateral arrows). The undersurface of the right upper lobe bronchus (vertical arrow) and the lateral surface of the bronchus intermedius (horizontal arrow) are seen sharply because the angle between them has become filled by soft tissue, which contrasts with air in the bronchi and has a short, sharp lateral edge convex toward the adjacent lung.

Inferiorly in the right hilum there are very short, sharp, soft tissue arcs projecting between vessels. These abnormalities, due to right hilar lymphadenopathy, are relatively subtle, but changes of even lesser magnitude can be appreciated when old films are used to make comparisons.

The left hilum is normal.

(B,C) Coned lateral views of the hila taken approximately 6 months apart. In the interval there has been a marked increase in the amount of soft tissue, which is projected anterior to the lower trachea and the main bronchi (L, orifice of the left upper lobe bronchus; T, the approximate level of origin of the right upper lobe bronchus). There is a lobulated, elongated succession of nodal masses (N in Fig. C), which are more sharply defined anteriorly than posteriorly. They extend caudally to the level of an inferior pulmonary vein (V). Fig. C is slightly magnified compared to Fig. B). *(Figure continues.)*

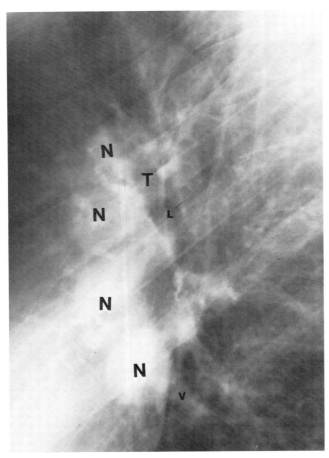

(C)

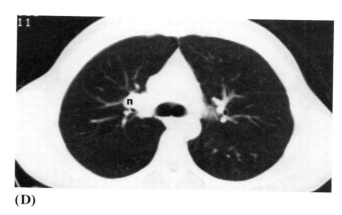

(D)

Fig. 8-7. *(Continued).* **(D)** CT scan at the level of the tracheal carina. There is a lobulated soft tissue mass in the right hilum (n).

(E) CT slice at the level of the right middle lobe bronchus. An enlarged lymph node (n) lies between the middle lobe bronchi (gray branching structures anteromedial to the node) and the black, oval image of the bronchus intermedius.

(F) CT scan at the level of the inferior pulmonary vein. An enlarged lymph node (n) is seen as a mass anterior to a branch of the right inferior pulmonary vein. This corresponds to the enlarged lymph node seen in this region on the PA and lateral views of the chest.

The left hilum appeared normal on the CT scan, as did the mediastinum. The patient had no other signs of recurrent neoplasm and no symptoms. Right hilar nodes were biopsied at thoracotomy and showed only noncaseating granulomas consistent with sarcoid.

This case illustrates two important points: (1) It is good practice to document at least the first recurrence of a malignant disease by obtaining tissue for histopathologic confirmation rather than assuming that new abnormalities are due to spread of the original neoplasm. (2) You can rank-order a differential diagnosis based on all available data, but that does not imply that all but one diagnosis are eliminated from serious consideration.

Unilateral hilar lymphadenopathy is unusual as the sole manifestation of sarcoidosis. More commonly there is bilateral hilar and right paratracheal lymphadenopathy (Fig. G). However, prevascular (anterior mediastinal), posterior mediastinal, and paravertebral adenopathy may also be seen in some cases. *(Figure continues.)*

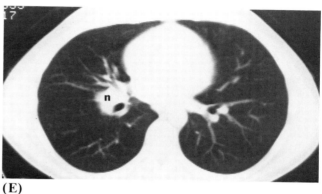

(E)

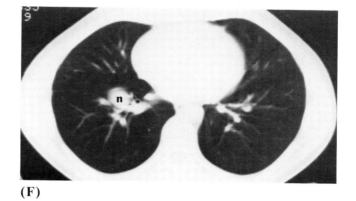

(F)

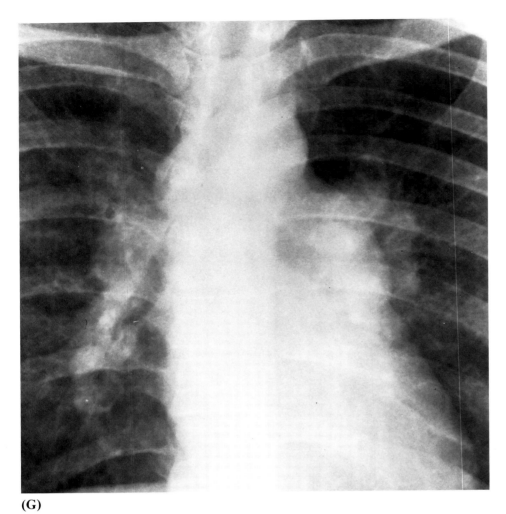

(G)

Fig. 8-7. *(Continued).* **(G) Characteristic Distribution of Lymphadenopathy in a Patient With Sarcoidosis**

Coned view from a different patient shows the typical or characteristic distribution of lymphadenopathy in patients with sarcoidosis. There is prominent right paratracheal and bilateral hilar lymphadenopathy. Although the distribution is characteristic, it is not diagnostic in that not all patients with sarcoid have this distribution, and in some patients with this distribution the adenopathy may be due to malignant lymphoma, metastases, or even infectious granulomatous disease. However, in a totally asymptomatic patient with no known primary neoplasm, this distribution of adenopathy warrants giving sarcoidosis first rank in the differential diagnosis.

In a large cohort of patients with sarcoidosis this adenopathy may resolve within 2 years. Resolution is much more common in white patients than in black patients. In some, the adenopathy may persist and become associated with pulmonary lesions that become visible radiographically. (Biopsy-proven pulmonary involvement may be present even in the absence of radiographically visible pulmonary lesions.)

In a small cohort of patients with sarcoidosis the adenopathy may become chronic. After several years these chronically enlarged lymph nodes may calcify.

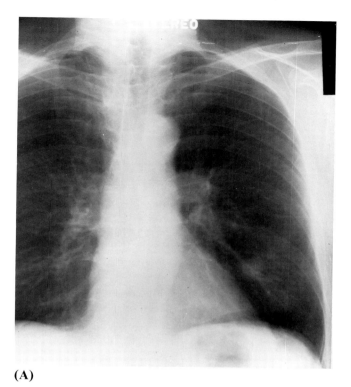

(A)

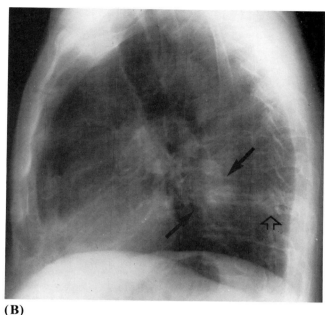

(B)

Fig. 8-8. Enlarged Lymph Nodes Surrounding Bronchi

(A,B) Coned PA and lateral views, respectively, of the chest of a man who has a small, cavitating carcinoma in the posterior aspects of the left lower lobe (open arrow on lateral view). The inferior portions of the left hilum appear abnormal on the lateral view (solid arrows). On the PA view the left hilum does not appear as abnormal as it does on either the lateral view or on the tomogram (Fig. C).

(C) Tomogram of the left hilum made with the patient in the left posterior oblique position; that is, the patient is lying on the tomographic table with his left side against the tabletop and his right side elevated off of the tabletop. Several small masses (n) due to adenopathy about the inferior portions of the left hilum are shown, and there is a rounded mass between the apicoposterior and anterior segmental branches of the left upper lobe bronchus; this mass is a large lymph node. The gray branches of the bronchi stand out because they are surrounded by the soft tissues of the enlarged lymph nodes, which also obliterate the images of the inferior pulmonary veins about the lower portions of the left hilum. The lower lobe bronchus is not seen because it is not within the plane of this cut. (P, left pulmonary artery; N, lymphadenopathy; u, upper division of the left upper lobe bronchus; l, lower division of the left upper lobe bronchus.

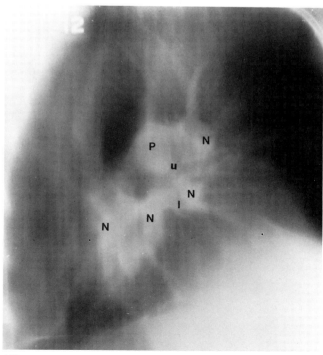

(C)

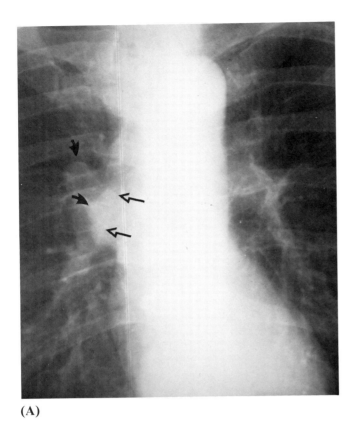

(A)

Fig. 8-9. Right Hilar Adenopathy on Chest Films, CT, and MRI

(A) The right hilum shows several rounded, arclike edges (solid arrows) that are not associated with branch vessels. There is also a double-density effect in the right hilum immediately adjacent to the lateral wall of the bronchus intermedius (open arrows). The double-density effect indicates that there are two soft tissue absorbers in different planes that are projected so that the edge of one is superimposed on the body of the other.

(B) Lateral view shows loss of detail of the right hilar structures as well as distortion, deformity, and enlargement of contours (black arrows). Note, incidentally, the exuberant spur formation bridging an intervertebral space (open arrow). *(Figure continues.)*

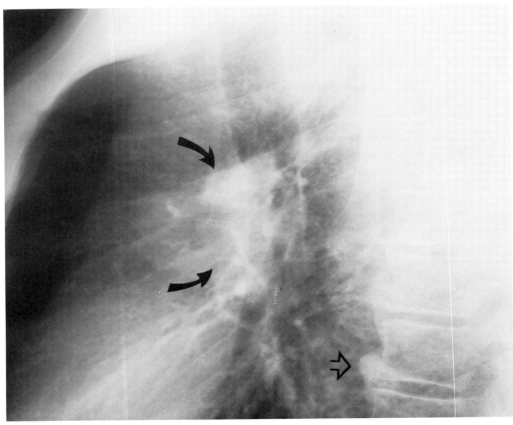

(B)

Fig. 8-9. *(Continued).* **(C)** Contrast-enhanced CT scan at a level just below the tracheal carina. Anterior to the carina the right pulmonary artery (rp) is seen. Laterally, it becomes lost in a mass (m) that has a lobulated contour extending from the anterior wall of the right mainstem bronchus forward to encompass the superior vena cava (v) and the right side of the ascending aorta (A). The polylobulated contour explains the double-density effect seen in the right hilum on the PA view. An x-ray beam passing from dorsal to ventral through this region would "see" a series of short tangents of hilar mass and adjacent lung, and thus allow superimposed edges to appear on the chest roentgenogram.

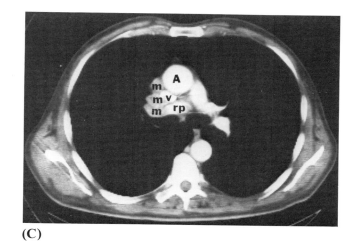

(C)

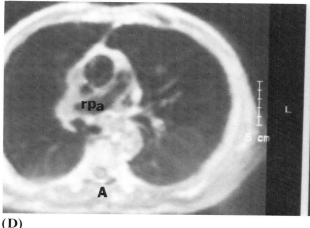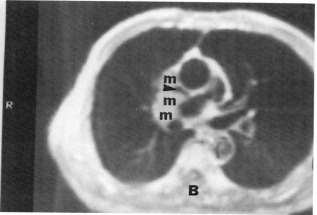

(D)

(D) Two consecutive scans from an MRI examination, just slightly caudal to the CT scan in Fig. C; more of the right pulmonary artery and less of the left pulmonary artery is seen. The magnet had a strength of 0.3 Tesla, and these images were obtained with a spin-echo pulse sequence that provided T1 weighting. In the lefthand scan the right pulmonary artery passes, from left to right, across the mediastinum posterior to the ascending aorta and the superior vena cava. Rapidly moving blood produces a signal void, which accounts for the vessel images appearing black. (Imaging artifacts are present in the descending thoracic aorta, along the left side of the spine, so that the lumen does not appear black.)

In the righthand scan the right pulmonary artery is still seen posterior to the slitlike lumen of the superior vena cava (arrowhead). The mass in the right hilum extends from the level of the bronchus intermedius anteriorly to the right side of the ascending aorta. The mass has a polylobulated lateral contour adjacent to the lung. Its appearance is very similar to that seen on CT (Fig. C). The right pulmonary artery is partially obstructed by the tumor mass, since even on scans on either side of those

shown, the lumen of the artery was never seen to have a normal caliber. The slitlike lumen of the superior vena cava indicates that there is also encroachment upon that vessel.

The anatomic display of the neoplasm on both the CT scan and the MRI scans is similar, but the MRI scans are made without the use of ionizing radiation, and the vessels are identified even without the use of intravenous contrast material.

Although unopacified vessels can be distinguished from other mediastinal contents by their position on CT scans, unopacified vessels are not as easily distinguished from abnormalities in the hila such as lymphadenopathy or neoplasm. Intravenous contrast material is used to increase the difference between the density of the hilar blood vessels and the enmeshed lymph node masses.

On the MRI scan, the fat anterior to the ascending aorta and along the left border of the left pulmonary artery is displayed as near-white, similar to the subcutaneous fat along the anterior chest wall. On the CT scan the subcutaneous fat is on the near-black portion of the gray scale.

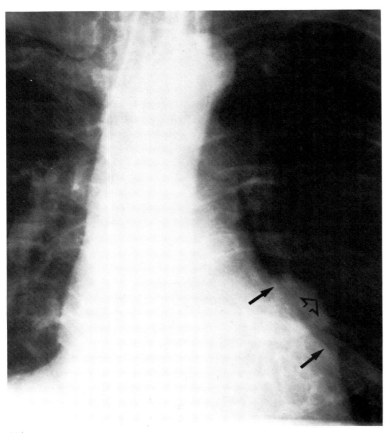

(A)

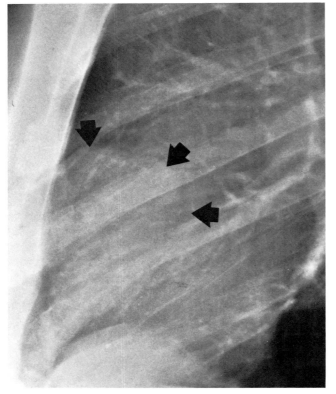

(B)

Fig. 8-10. Thymoma

(A,B) Coned views of the mediastinum of a 54-year-old asymptomatic man who had a routine chest film as part of a physical examination.

(A) PA view. The convex edge of a mass (open arrow) is seen adjacent to the left heart border (between black arrows). **(B)** Lateral view. The mass is seen superimposed on the heart in the low retrosternal region. The mass has a subtle polylobulated upper margin (arrows). *(Figure continues.)*

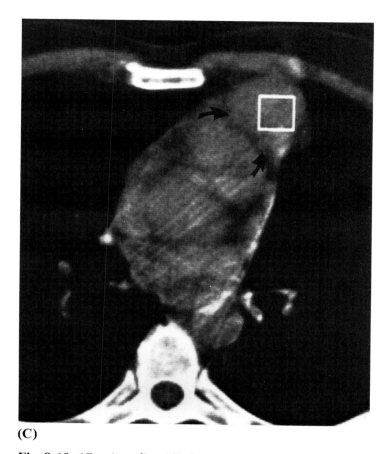

(C)

Fig. 8-10. *(Continued).* **(C)** CT scan. The mass is separated from the heart by a fat plane (arrows). The white box superimposed on the mass delineates a number of pixels for which the computer calculated an average Hounsfield number and its standard deviation.

A scan was made before the intravenous injection of contrast material, and a series of scans were made subsequent to the contrast injection. Hounsfield numbers increased by as much as 3 times on the postcontrast scans (not shown). This indicates that the lesion is a solid tumor with a blood supply rather than a cyst. The mass was removed and was a thymoma.

Notice the resemblance of this case to that in Fig. 8-18. The striking difference between them is in the increase in the Hounsfield number of the lesion following the administration of intravenous contrast material. This is important in distinguishing cystic from solid lesions because the Hounsfield numbers of some cysts, before the administration of contrast material, may be quite similar to those of solid masses if the cystic contents are not simply serous.

In addition to primary mediastinal tumors, any solid neoplasm metastatic to the heart or involving the pericardium or the caudal aspects of the mediastinum can present as a pericardiac mass—for example, lymphoma, malignant histiocytoma, and metastases from many primary sites. Large pericardial fat pads may not be distinguishable from other masses at the cardiophrenic angles on chest films, but fat is readily identified on CT or MRI examinations.

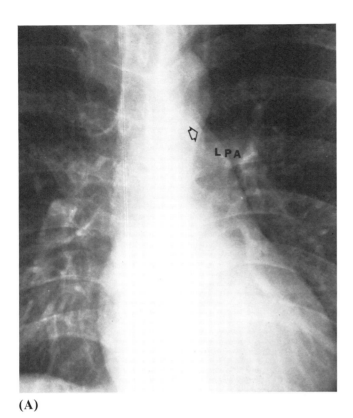

(A)

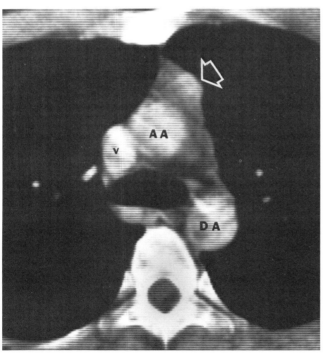

(B)

Fig. 8-11. Thymoma

Approximately 1 month before admission this 29-year-old man noted difficulty in keeping his eyes open, followed by diplopia, difficulty with chewing, and proximal upper extremity weakness, which seemed to be worse at the end of the day and early in the morning. A Tensilon test was positive.

(A) PA view shows a small mass (open arrow) projected just medial to the mediastinal pleural reflection over the left pulmonary artery (LPA). It is a subtle abnormality. Since the left edge of the mass is well defined, it must interface with adjacent lung on at least that surface. The fact that it can be seen entirely separate from the adjacent mediastinal pleura indicates that it is not in the same plane, but must either be anterior or posterior to it.

(B) CT scan at a level beneath the aortic arch. There is a small mass (arrow) that enhances with contrast material and causes a convex bulge of the mediastinal pleura to the left (arrow). This lesion projects anteriorly beneath the aortic arch. The ascending aorta (AA) is seen anterior to the airway, the descending aorta (DA) posterior to it, and fatty tissue and small lymph nodes are seen between them in the aorto-pulmonic window. This is precisely the level at which the small mass is seen on the PA chest film.

The patient had a thymectomy. A thymoma measuring 1.6 × 1.6 × 1.4 cm was removed, along with a thymus that showed thymic hyperplasia. The size of the thymus, of course, cannot be appreciated from only one scan in a series; rather one must use a series of stacked scans at known intervals in order to estimate the full extent of the thymus gland. Generally, however, histologic evidence of thymic hyperplasia cannot be predicted from the CT appearance of the thymus, whereas the presence of a thymoma can usually be predicted accurately. However, in a patient under the age of 25 years, a small thymoma may be difficult to diagnose because of the variable size of the thymus in the young.

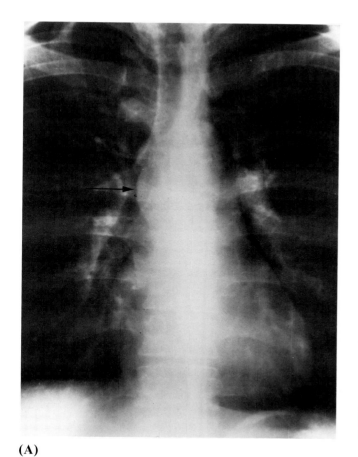

(A)

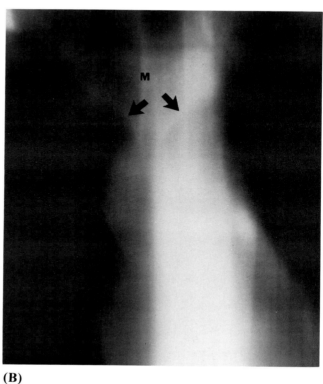

(B)

Fig. 8-12.   Thymic Seminoma

(A) PA chest film of an asymptomatic young man with a history of drug addiction. There is a pronounced bulge of the pleural reflection over the right side of the mediastinum, with a sharp edge that is convex to the right (arrow). The radius of this arc is too short to be accepted as the lateral margin of a dilated ascending aorta, and therefore we are dealing with either a mediastinal mass or an abnormality of the ascending aorta.

(B) Coned view of a tomogram. You can deduce its anterior location from the fact that the image of the manubrium (M) is only slightly out of focus and the medial edges of the retromanubrial portions of the right and left upper lobes (arrows) are coming together at the lower borders of the manubrium to form the anterior function line.

The lateral edge of the mediastinal mass is sharply defined by adjacent lung, but its medial margins are not distinguishable from other mediastinal tissues by the tomographic technique.

This mass is a thymic seminoma. From its radiographic appearances alone and from its position in the mediastinum it could not be distinguished from other lesions that can occur in the thymus, such as thymomas or thymic cysts, or even from other primary mediastinal tumors or other germ cell neoplasms or lymphoma.

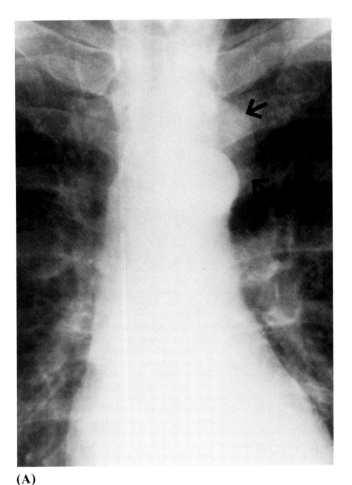

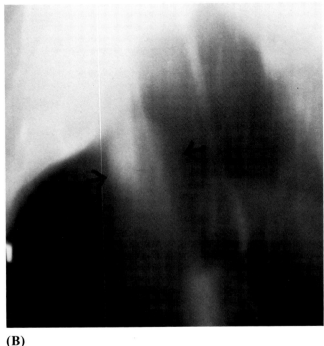

(A)   (B)

Fig. 8-13. Neurofibroma of the Vagus Nerve

This 43-year-old man had a history of shortness of breath and fatigue and equivocal evidence of a prior myocardial infarction. He also complained of pain in the left midclavicular line at the level of the anterior second and third interspaces. The pain usually occurred at night while he was in bed and radiated into his left infrascapular area.

(A) PA view shows the sharply defined lateral margin of a mass (arrows), which is projected over and above the image of the aortic arch. It does not efface the aortic knob (a posterior structure), and therefore we know the mass must be in a different plane. The lateral view of the chest (not shown) did demonstrate increased opacity in the region of the anterior portions of the aortic arch extending up into the thoracic inlet, but no discrete mass was seen.

(B) Tomogram showing well-defined posterior, anterior, and superior margins of an egg-shaped mass superimposed upon and projected superior to the anterior portions of the aortic arch. A 6 × 3 × 2 cm benign neurofibroma was removed from the vagus nerve.

Intrathoracic vagus nerve tumors are uncommon. Reportedly, symptoms are frequently absent or consist of vague chest pain or voice changes or a dry, nonproductive cough. Neurofibromatosis is frequently but not invariably present in these patients.

Although the lesion is localized well by tomography, CT or MRI would offer additional information to determine whether the lesion was cystic or solid.

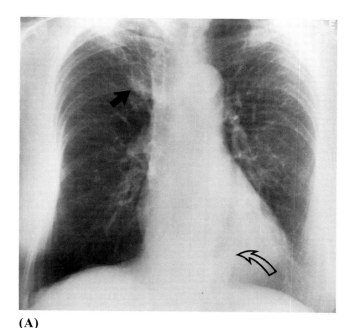

(A)

Fig. 8-14. Paravertebral Schwannom and Incidental Hiatus Hernia

This woman had a paravertebral mass that was first noted on chest films approximately 7 months before the present study. On follow-up examinations it appeared to have increased slightly in size. A needle aspirate revealed the mass to be a spindle cell tumor of probable neural origin. The patient had had several episodes of sharp right paraspinal pain at approximately the T6 level lasting 1 to 2 minutes and occurring several times a week for the past 3 months. The pain was acute in onset.

(A) PA film of the chest shows the fairly subtle edge (black arrow) of a mass on the right at the level of the posterior sixth interspace and the posterior seventh rib. The edge of another mass is seen lateral to the descending thoracic aorta and the thoracic spine at the left base (open arrow).

The darker gray tone over the right hemithorax in comparison to the left is due to a prior right mastectomy.

(B) Lateral view. A well-defined mass (n) is projected over the posterior elements of the spine. The central ray was centered slightly below this lesion for the PA view, and the beam is divergent (in spite of the use of a relatively small focal spot and a 6-foot target-film distance). The divergence of the beam and the considerable distance of the lesion from the film in the PA projection accounts for this lesion being projected slightly higher in relation to the aortic arch than on the lateral view.

In the retrocardiac region there is a localized gas shadow and an air-fluid level (arrow). On retrospective review of the PA film there is also a faint gas collection superimposed on the lower spine in the region of the mass medially at the left base. This appearance is characteristic of a hiatus hernia. Duplication cysts, which communicate with the airway, or a post-traumatic cyst may present a similar appearance; fortunately they are rare.

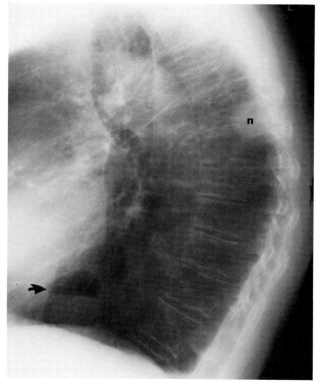

(B)

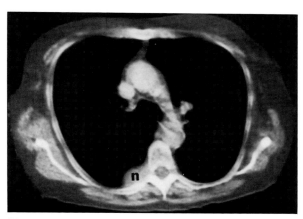

(C)

Hiatus hernias are common lesions in adults, and when they contain well-defined air-fluid levels they are relatively easy to recognize. However, when there is no air in the herniated portion of the stomach it is very difficult to distinguish it from any mass that might occur in the retrocardiac region. Esophagography is a definitive study for purposes of distinction.

(C) CT scan shows the right paravertebral mass (n) as it relates to the adjacent rib, the vertebra, and the intervertebral foramen. It does not show any extension into the neural canal. The mass was removed and proved to be a benign neurolemmoma (schwannoma). Its radiographic appearance and clinical manifestations are characteristic of this lesion, but that is not to say that they are specific or diagnostic.

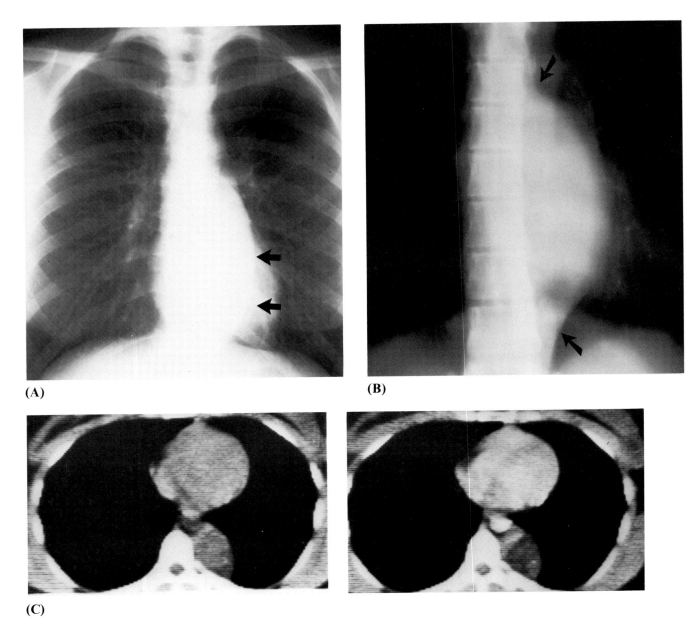

(A)

(B)

(C)

Fig. 8-15. Ganglioneuroma

(A) PA film of the chest of a 19-year-old woman who had a chest film as part of a routine physical examination. There is an elongated paraspinal mass on the left side (arrows), which on the lateral view (not shown) was located posteriorly.

(B) Tomogram cut confirms the paraspinous location of this elongated mass. The lateral margins of the mass have a sharp interface with adjacent lung. Medially there is no evidence of any erosive or destructive changes of the adjacent thoracic vertebrae seen. The superior and inferior obtuse margins of the mass (arrows) are characteristic of an extrapleural mass.

(C) CT scans were made at 1.0-cm intervals throughout the length of the lesion; only two are shown here. They graphically display the relationship of the neoplasm to the spine. They were useful in showing that nowhere was there evidence of extension into the neural canal, but they were not essential.

The tomograms showed the orientation of the mass in the coronal plan better than CT. The CT shows the relationship of the tumor to the spinal canal better than the tomograms. MRI is likely to replace both of those techniques in that it serves both purposes well.

The radiographic appearance of this mass is characteristic of a ganglioneuroma. These neoplasms are frequently large when first detected; they are frequently elongated and paraspinal and are commonly found in patients who have no symptoms.

The lesion was removed and had all the features of a ganglioneuroma.

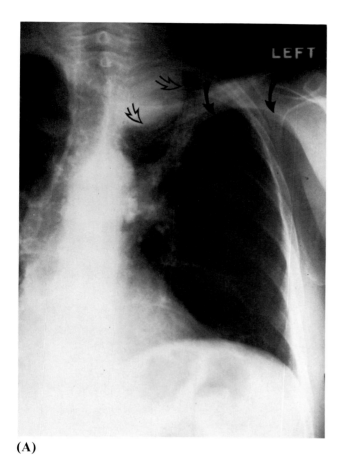

(A)

Fig. 8-16. Malignant Schwannoma and Occult Carcinoma

The patient is a 59-year-old woman who had a left mastectomy 26 years ago. She had postoperative radiation therapy and there was no evidence of recurrence. For the past 7 months, however, she had noted pain in her left shoulder, which radiated in the distribution of T1 and T2 and to the left arm. She also had a Horner's syndrome.

(A) PA view shows a well-defined mass occupying the medial portions of the left apex (open arrows). The left hilum is retracted upward. Calcified nodes are seen in the left hilum, and there is a fairly thick band of atelectasis extending into the left upper lobe from the left hilum. Soft tissue changes consequent to the radical mastectomy are seen extending from the chest wall to the left axilla (black arrows).

(B) MRI scan shows the mass (M) high in the apex of the left hemithorax. It encroaches upon the vertebrae of the upper thoracic spine as well as the intervertebral foramina.

(C) MRI scan through the adjacent spine. The mass does not reach the center of the spinal canal and does not displace or distort the spinal cord, which is shown dorsal to the vertebral bodies.

A CT scan was performed (not shown), and there was no evidence of bony invasion; however, both calcified and noncalcified nodes were seen in the mediastinum.

A 6 × 5 × 2.8 cm mass was removed from the left apex. It was associated with mature peripheral nerve as well as ganglion cells and on microscopic examination was interpreted to be a malignant schwannoma. In addition, nodes removed from the para-aortic area showed undifferentiated malignant neoplasm with no resemblance to either the patient's previous carcinoma of the breast or the malignant schwannoma of the left apex.

The origin of the neoplasm, which was metastatic to the nodes, remains conjectural, but in all likelihood it was from an undetected carcinoma of the lung, which may in turn have accounted for the segmental atelectasis seen in the left upper lobe. The latter, however, would not be an unusual manifestation of lung scarring following radiation treatment. Unfortunately, no earlier chest films were available for comparison to indicate whether the pulmonary parenchymal components were new or old. (Figs. B and C courtesy of Dr. Robert A. Clark, Walnut Creek, California.)

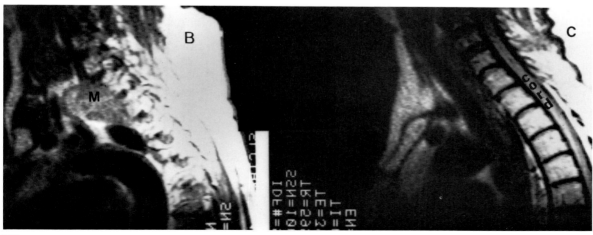

(B)

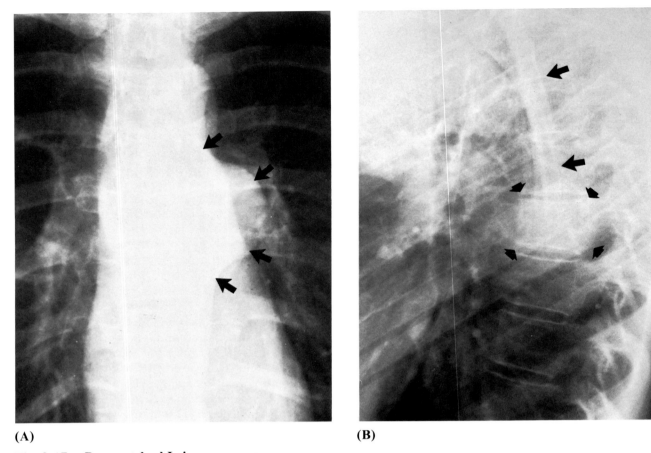

(A)   (B)

Fig. 8-17. Paravertebral Leiomyosarcoma

(A) PA view. This 33-year-old woman with mixed connective tissue disease had a 4-month history of thoracic pain. A mass is present to the left of the thoracic spine (arrows). The mass has smooth contours with tapered margins. Its appearance is characteristic of an extrapleural lesion. You can see the pleural reflection over the pulmonary artery segment of the cardiomediastinal silhouette right through the superimposed mass. This is a clear indication that the mass must be in a different plane.

(B) Lateral view. The lesion does not have sharp margins, because the portion that interfaces with adjacent lung is seen en face. Therefore, the lesion behaves only as an added absorber in the path of the x-ray beam and appears as an area of increased tissue density superimposed on the spine (short arrows). The anterior aspects of the scapula are also superimposed on the spine (long arrows) and should not be mistaken for an abnormality.

This lesion was a leiomyosarcoma. It is tempting to assume that all paraspinal masses are due to neurogenic tumors. In establishing a differential diagnosis it is important to consider all of the tissues that may be found in the compartment under consideration and to recognize that benign and malignant forms of neoplasms involving any of those tissues may occur.

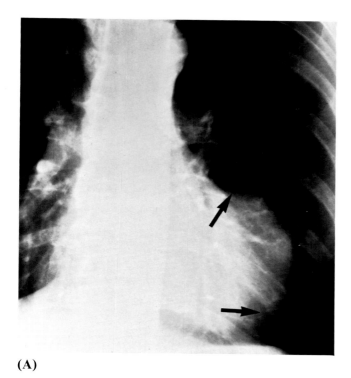

(A)

Fig. 8-18. Pericardial Cyst

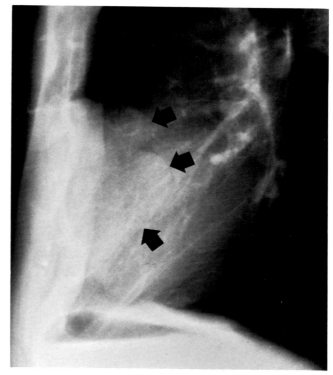

(B)

(A,B) Coned views of PA and lateral chest films, respectively, of a 58-year-old asymptomatic man. There is an abnormal lobulated contour over the left cardiac apex (between arrows). The lateral view shows a polylobulated contour of soft tissues, posterior to the lower sternum, superimposed on the heart (arrows). On the PA view the lesion is reminiscent of the changes that might be seen with a left ventricular aneurysm.

(C) CT scan. A discrete oval mass (M) is present anterior to the heart. CT scans following intravenous injection of contrast agent showed that over a period of time there was no significant change in the Hounsfield numbers of this lesion. This finding, in association with its relatively low Hounsfield number, indicated the presence of a cyst. The patient elected to have the lesion removed, and a pericardial cyst was found and removed at thoracotomy.

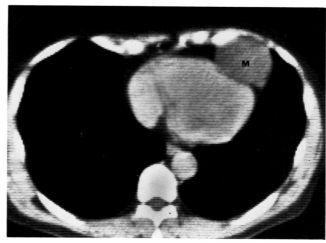

(C)

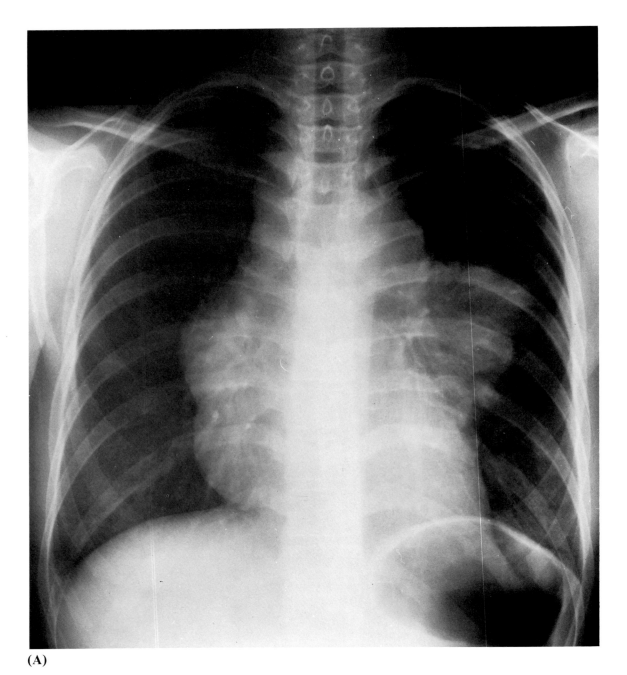

(A)

Fig. 8-19. Cystic Lesion of the Thymus After Radiotherapy of Mediastinal Hodgkin's Disease

(A) PA view. A large mediastinal mass extends from the thoracic inlet caudally over both hila and the cardiac margins so that its precise lower limit is not discernible. On a lateral view (not shown) the mass was located anteriorly, and the hila themselves appeared uninvolved. This distribution is not uncommon when there is extensive involvement of the thymus by Hodgkin's disease, as was the case in this woman. *(Figure continues.)*

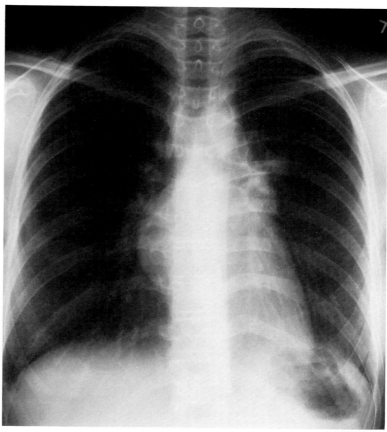

(B)

Fig. 8-19. *(Continued).* **(B)** Appearance of this patient's chest 17 months later, after treatment with radiation therapy and chemotherapy. There is a residual mass on the right that is inseparable from the right heart.

(C) CT scan coinciding with the chest film examination shown in Fig. B. There is a cystic mass with a well-defined wall impinging on the right heart. Cystic lesions in the thymus of patients with Hodgkin's disease may be seen both before and after treatment. They may fluctuate in size even though no active neoplasm is found on resection. However, from radiographic study alone it is not possible to determine whether or not viable neoplasm remains in the wall.

After further chemotherapy this cystic mass resolved, but there is no way of knowing if it would have resolved spontaneously had no further treatment been given. In other patients, cystic thymic masses remaining after treatment for Hodgkin's disease have been removed, and no viable neoplasm was found on histopathologic study.

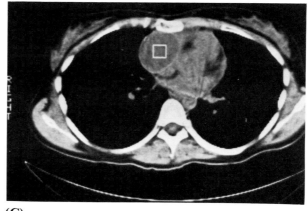

(C)

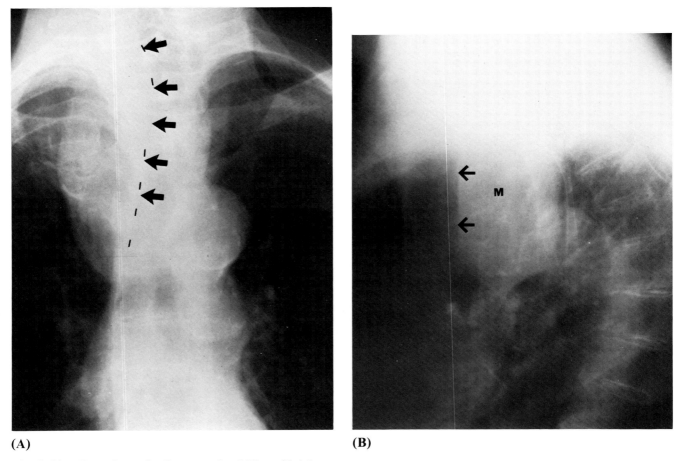

(A)   (B)

Fig. 8-20. Intrathoracic, Retrotracheal Thyroid Adenoma

(**A,B**) PA and lateral views of the chest of a woman who had been complaining of shortness of breath, dyspnea, and wheezing on exertion.

(**A**) On PA view the convex edge of a mass is seen in the medial aspects of the right upper chest. The arrows mark the right lateral wall of the trachea, which can barely be seen on this reproduction. The tracheal wall shows a moderate impression from the adjacent mass and a shift to the left away from the mass. The edge of the mass extends cephalad above the right clavicle. This indicates that it cannot be in the extreme retromanubrial portions of the mediastinum, but must be slightly farther back in order to maintain an interface with lung above the level of the clavicle.

(**B**) Lateral view shows that the mass (M) is retrotracheal. Arrows outline the posterior tracheal wall. The mass moves the lung away from the posterior wall of the trachea so that the retrotracheal space appears to be filled with soft tissue, and there is slight anterior bowing of the trachea. This lesion was removed and was a 12 × 6.8 cm colloid adenoma of the thyroid weighing 180 g.

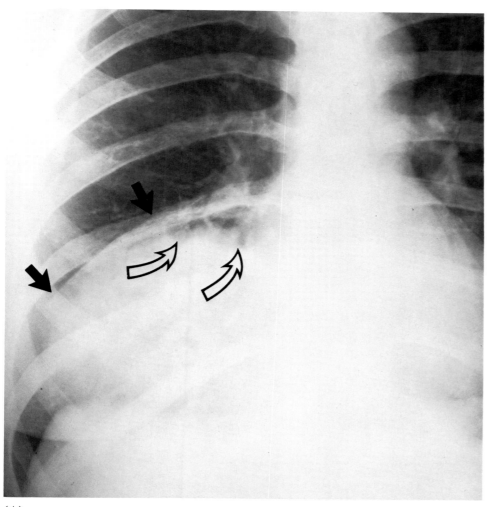

(A)

Fig. 8-21. Foramen of Morgagni Hernia

(A) PA view. There is a large mass adjacent to and effacing the right cardiac margin. It has a sharply defined superolateral margin (black arrows). Masses that commonly occur in this region include thymomas, pericardial cysts, and lipomas. However, in the superomedial aspects of this mass there are some rounded and irregular lucencies (open arrows). This finding would be unusual in any of the more common masses discussed. *(Figure continues.)*

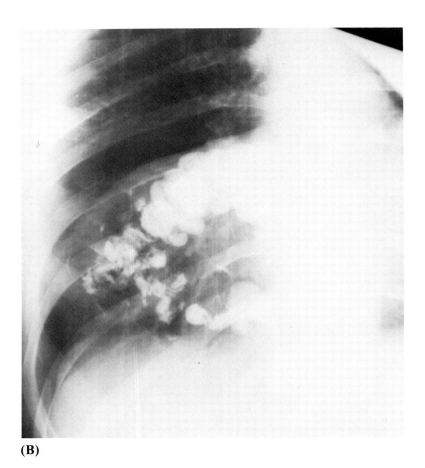

(B)

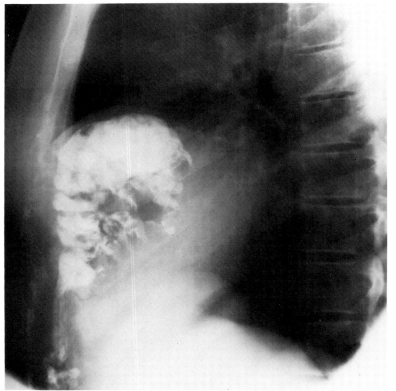

(C)

Fig. 8-21. *(Continued).* **(B,C)** A barium enema study shows that a large segment of colon has herniated through the diaphragm anteromedially. This is the characteristic location for herniation through the foramen of Morgagni. It may simulate a mediastinal or paramediastinal, mass although it is not truly a mediastinal lesion. At times, bowel and abdominal contents may actually herniate into the mediastinum itself, but that is far less common. Often there is a clue to herniation through the Morgagni foramen in that the transverse colon on chest films or films of the abdomen will have an unusually high position and will show a high point at the site of herniation. At other times, however, the herniation may not be at all apparent from plain-film studies, particularly when the bulk of the contents consists of herniated omental fat.

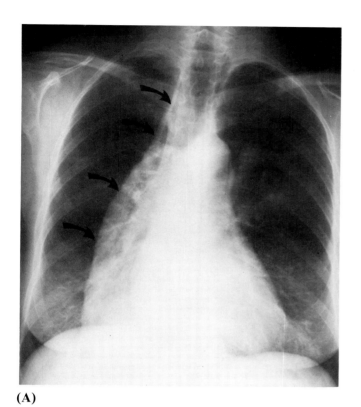

(A)

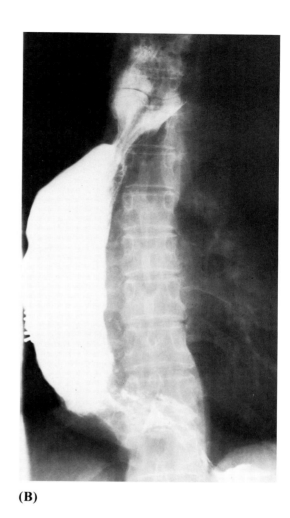

(B)

Fig. 8-22. Achalasia

(A) PA view of the chest of a woman known to have achalasia. The well-defined edge of a mass runs parallel to the cardiomediastinal silhouette from the level of the right diaphragm up to the level of the aortic arch. Above that a rather thick band of soft tissue extends cephalad to the neck (upper two arrows). This represents the thickened right lateral wall of the abnormal esophagus. The left lateral wall is not clearly defined. The fact that there is air in the upper portions of this distended esophagus makes it much easier to recognize it as esophagus. However, even if it were entirely full of food and fluid, and thus simulated a solid mass, the likelihood of its being esophagus would still be considered because there are very few mass lesions that extend from the neck all the way to the diaphragm unilaterally. A distended, tortuous esophagus is the most likely structure to be the cause of such an image.

The right heart border and mediastinal margins are seen to be independent of this superimposed mass, indicating that the mass is either quite far posterior or very far anterior in location.

(B) Esophagogram shows the barium-filled, dilated, tortuous esophagus characteristic of chronic obstruction such as occurs in patients with achalasia. *(Figure continues.)*

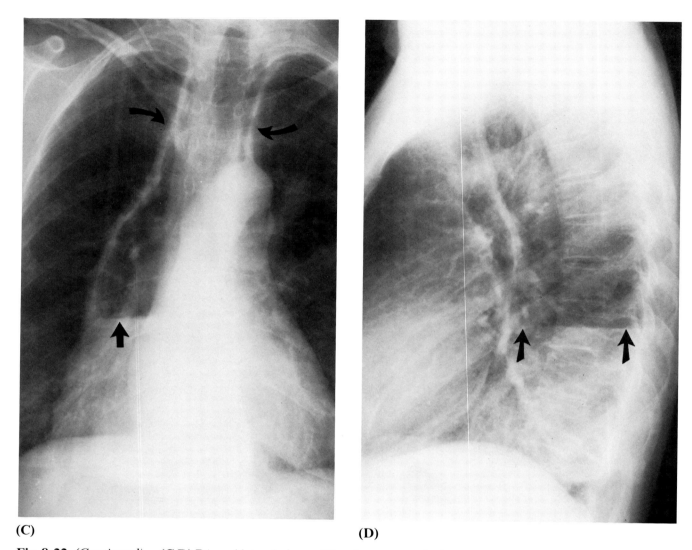

(C)   **(D)**

Fig. 8-22. *(Continued).*   **(C,D)** PA and lateral views of the chest, respectively, made when there was a large quantity of air and a moderate quantity of fluid in this abnormal esophagus (vertical arrows identify a long fluid level in Figs. C and D). The thickened esophageal walls are easily seen (curved arrows in Fig. C). The transverse diameter of this distended esophagus is more than twice that of the trachea, seen superimposed. On the lateral view, the posterior wall of the trachea appears thickened because it consists of not only the posterior wall of the trachea but also the thickened anterior wall of the abnormal esophagus.

Although achalasia is commonly the cause of massive dilatation of the esophagus, other esophageal abnormalities such as involvement by scleroderma or Chagas' disease may also cause gross dilatation. Dilatation may also accompany inflammatory strictures or neoplastic obstruction, but seldom does the esophagus reach such remarkable size from those causes.

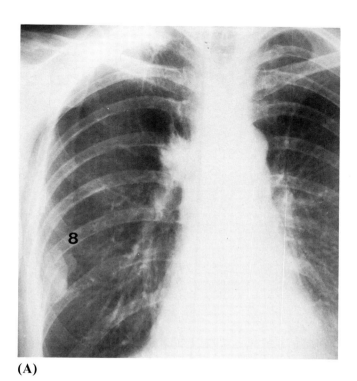

(A)

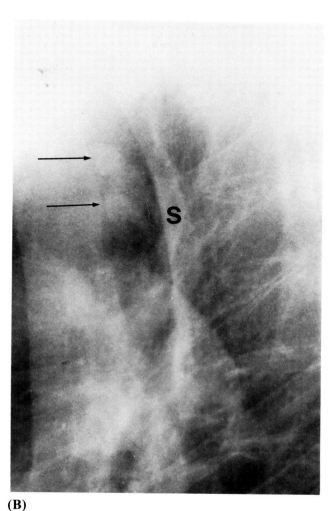

(B)

Fig. 8-23. Metastases to the Trachea

(A) PA chest film of a woman who has had a right mastectomy for carcinoma of the breast, followed by radiation therapy. There is characteristic alteration of the right axillary fold due to removal of the pectoralis muscles. The right hilum is retracted upward and distorted as a result of reduction in volume of the right upper lobe, and there are linear opacities extending from the hilum into the apex. There is also apical pleural thickening. These changes are characteristic of postirradiation reaction but are indistinguishable from those of chronic infection (e.g., tuberculosis).

There is a fracture of the right eighth rib (8) in the posterior axillary line. Adjacent opacities of soft tissue density have but one sharp margin, as is seen with pleural or extrapleural masses. This combination is common with metastatic lesions to the ribs or the chest wall. Hematomas adjacent to rib fractures can produce similar appearances, but the soft tissue components are usually not this large.

(B) Coned lateral view of the trachea shows clustered nodular opacities (arrows) in or superimposed on the trachea above the level of the aortic arch. The anterior margin of one scapula (S) is superimposed on the posterior tracheal wall. *(Figure continues.)*

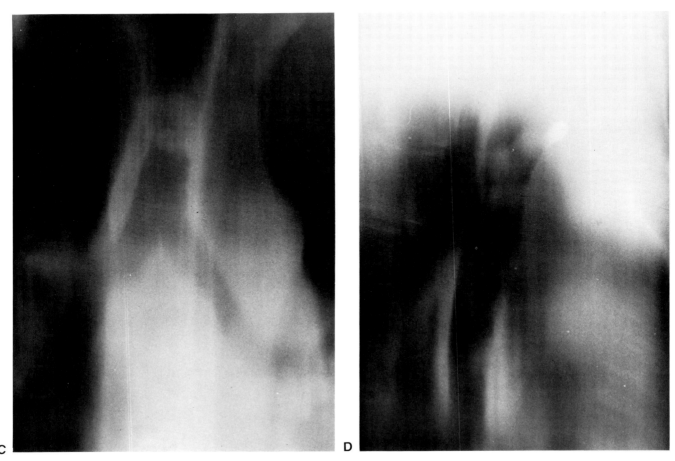

C   D

Fig. 8-23. *(Continued).* **(C,D)** Tomograms of the trachea (AP and lateral) show that the nodules arise from the tracheal wall and confirm that they are in the trachea rather than superimposed on it. They are metastases from the patient's breast carcinoma. Fig. D is oriented so that anterior is to your right (the opposite orientation to that of Fig. B).

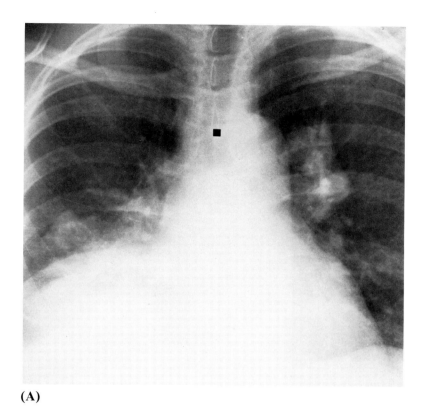

(A)

Fig. 8-24. Metastases to the Trachea

(A,B) PA and lateral views, respectively, of the chest of a woman with proven metastases to the lungs from breast carcinoma. There are numerous small masses in the hila and in the lung around the hila, and there is atelectasis of the basal segments of the right lower lobe. These metastases had been slowly increasing in size and number over several years. In spite of this, the patient had been functioning well. Just before having these films taken, however, she noted a sudden change in shortness of breath. *(Figure continues.)*

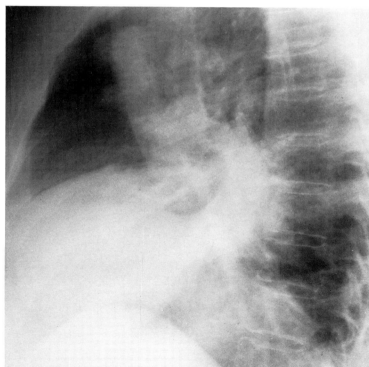

(B)

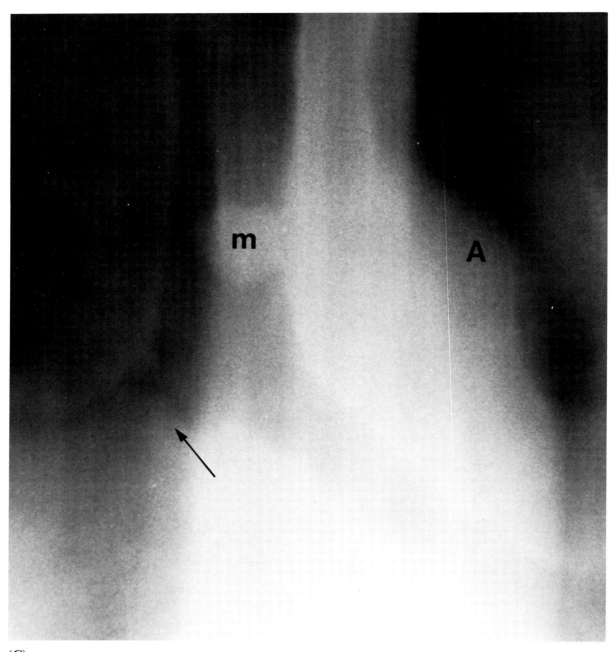

(C)

Fig. 8-24. *(Continued).* **(C)** Tomogram of the trachea and mainstem bronchi. A soft tissue mass (m) fills two-thirds of the lumen of the trachea at the level of the aortic arch (A). Another mass encroaches severely upon the takeoff of the right mainstem bronchus (arrow). When these lesions were resected via bronchoscopy, the patient had relief from her breathlessness even though extensive pulmonary metastases remained.

In retrospect, the polypoid lesion in the trachea can be identified on the PA view of the chest (square dot in center). The widening of the carina and the encroachment of neoplasm on the right mainstem bronchus can also be seen. On the lateral view (Fig. B), however, there are so many abnormalities in the lung and in the hila that you cannot determine which lesions are in the trachea as opposed to being superimposed on it. The tomogram makes the location of the lesions in the airway clear, CT or MRI would do the same. Tomography requires careful technique, but is less expensive than either CT or MRI for this limited purpose.

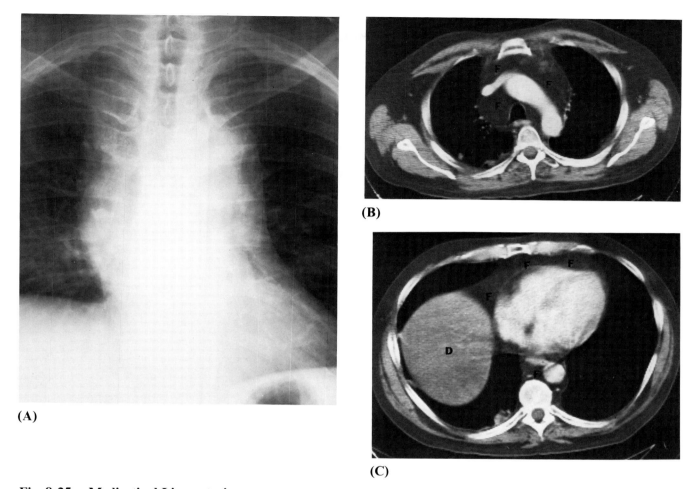

(A)

(B)

(C)

Fig. 8-25. Mediastinal Lipomatosis

This man had previously been treated for nodular sclerosing Hodgkin's disease. He later developed a cerebral granulomatous vasculitis for which he was treated with high-dose steroids.

(A) Coned view of the mediastinum, which is abnormally wide and has contours that are convex toward the lung on both sides. This appearance is worrisome for recurrence of the patient's Hodgkin's disease. However, the history of prolonged systemic steroid treatment makes mediastinal lipomatosis another likely cause of the abnormal appearance.

(B) CT scan through the aortic arch level. The left brachiocephalic vein is joining with the right to form the superior vena cava. A large amount of fat (F) distorts the mediastinal pleura and creates convex margins against the adjacent lung. A few small nodes are seen anteriorly on the left within this large fat store. The attenuation coefficient of fat is such that relatively high *negative* Hounsfield numbers (about − 100) are reached, and the resultant tissue display is of a darker gray than other soft tissues.

(C) CT scan at a lower level shows accumulations of fat adjacent to the vertebra and about the descending aorta as well as in the azygoesophageal recess anterior to the spine. Fat deposits in these regions may be much more voluminous than shown here and could be confused with paravertebral or posterior mediastinal masses on plain films.

Incidentally noted are irregular nodules in the pulmonary parenchyma adjacent to the pleural surfaces on the CT scans in Figs. B and C. In addition, large amounts of fat are seen anterior to and along the lateral aspects of the heart (D, right diaphragm dome).

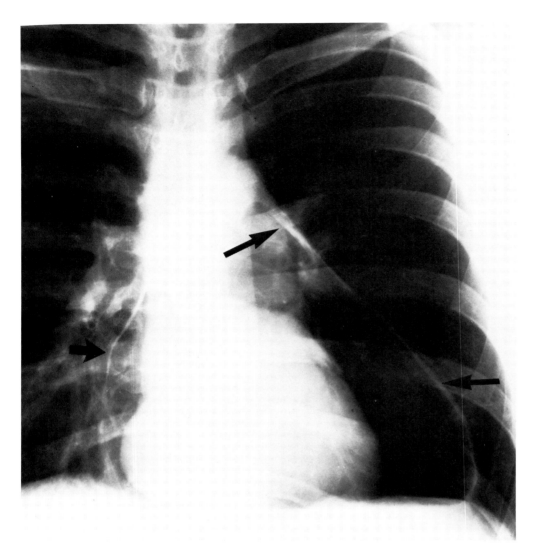

Fig. 8-26. Pneumopericardium

PA view of the chest of a 36-year-old man with nodular sclerosing Hodgkin's disease who had a therapeutic pericardiocentesis followed by installation of gas to define the inner margins of the pericardium. The pericardium should only be 1 to 2 mm thick. Along its upper portions it is thicker than normal (highest arrow). Along its right side and left lower aspects, however, it is of normal thickness (horizontal arrows).

This film mainly demonstrates the thickness and the anatomic limits of the pericardium. The pericardium reaches the level of the transverse portion of the aortic arch on the PA view, but does not extend above that level. The distinction between pneumopericardium and pneumomediastinum is seldom difficult because the streaks of air in the pneumomediastinum almost always extend above the level of the aortic arch and, in adults, often extend into the soft tissue planes of the neck.

Air in the pericardium will shift markedly in position between films made with the patient erect, supine, or in the left or right lateral decubitus positions, whereas the streaks of air in the mediastinal soft tissues (pneumomediastinum) show little shift with changes in patient position.

The pericardium can be stretched greatly by large amounts of pericardial fluid accumulated slowly over time. Notice how large a sac it appears to be after the fluid has been removed and replaced with gas. When fluid accumulates rapidly (e.g., with bleeding into the pericardium), cardiac tamponade can occur with relatively small amounts of fluid, as the pericardium does not stretch fast enough to avoid an increase in intrapericardial pressure, which in turn impairs cardiac filling.

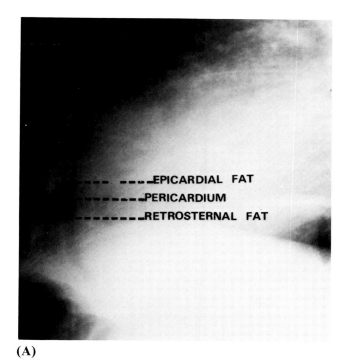

(A)

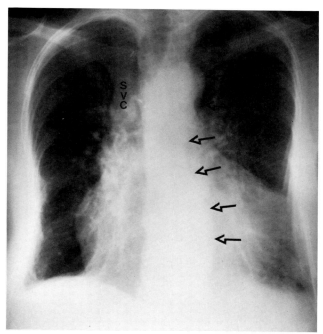

(B)

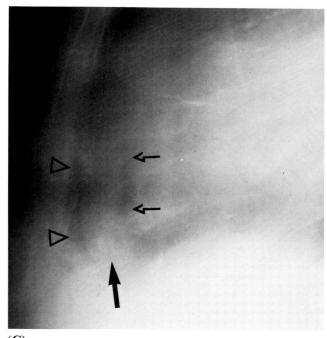

(C)

Fig. 8-27.   Pericardial Effusion

(A) Coned lateral view shows the normal relationships among the pericardium, the epicardial fat, and the retrosternal pericardial or epipericardial fat. (Courtesy of Dr. H. L. Abrams, Palo Alto, California.)

(B,C) PA and lateral views, respectively, of the chest of a woman with diffuse histiocytic lymphoma (DHL) who had a pericardial effusion. She also had an infiltrating ductal adenocarcinoma of the left breast, for which she underwent a mastectomy. Three hundred seventy cubic centimeters of hemorraghic pericardial effusion was removed and found to be positive for DHL on cytologic study.

(B) PA view of the chest shows cardiomegaly. The trachea is deviated to the right by a tortuous and ectatic aorta. The image of a meandering descending thoracic aorta is visible faintly (arrows). A distended superior vena cava (svc) bulges to the right.

The appearance of the cardiac enlargement is nonspecific; the distinction between pericardial effusion and enlargement from a diffuse myocarditis or myocardiopathy could not be made. Incidentally, the inward convexity of the middle and lower ribs in the axillary lines represents a variant of normal thoracic cage configuration.

(C) Coned lateral view of the retrosternal region. Posterior to the sternum a thick band of water-density tissue (vertical arrow) is sandwiched between darker gray bands along its posterior and anterior aspects. This is a characteristic appearance of a moderately large pericardial effusion. The dark gray band marking the posterior boundary (open arrows) of the pericardial effusion is due

to projection of fat in the epicardium. The gray band that marginates the effusion anteriorly (arrowheads) is due to fat in the outer aspects of the pericardium.

This configuration is a good sign of pericardial effusion, but it is not seen in all cases. It is worthwhile to look for, since pericardial effusion is not always appreciated clinically. Confirmation by echocardiography can be obtained. CT scans also show the pericardium well. *(Figure continues.)*

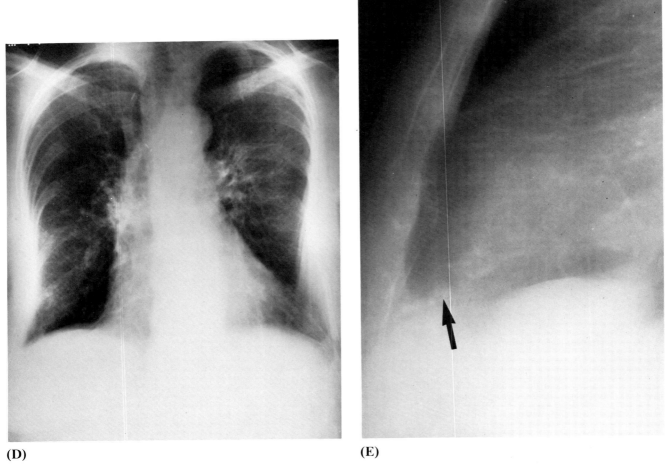

(D)   **(E)**

Fig. 8-27. *(Continued).* **(D,E)** PA and lateral views of the chest, respectively, after the patient had received additional chemotherapy for malignant lymphoma. There has been a marked decrease in the size of the cardiomediastinal silhouette and in the distension of the superior vena cava. On the lateral view there has been a striking decrease in the size of the water-density absorber (vertical arrow) projecting between the fat pads in the epicardium and in the pericardium, although it is still thicker than normal.

Incidentally, the fine white line of the posterior cortex of the xiphoid process projects over the anterior fat pad on the two lateral views.

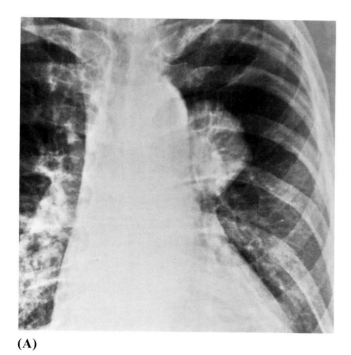

(A)

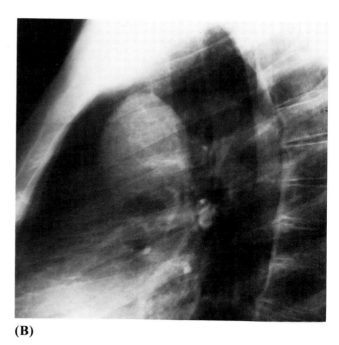

(B)

Fig. 8-28. Aortic Aneurysm

(A,B) PA and lateral views, respectively, of a man with an aneurysm of the aorta that masquerades as a left mediastinal or left anterior parahilar lung mass. Aneurysms that arise from the underside of the aortic arch can project in the left upper hemithorax as though they were pedunculated. These may be old, encapsulated post-traumatic pseudoaneurysms, or they may be aneurysms of the ductus arteriosus. Calcification may or may not be present in the wall.

(C) CT scan showing the aneurysm in relationship to the aortic arch. Calcification (irregular whitish plaques) is present in the arch but not in the aneurysm. The lumen of the aneurysm (L) fills with contrast material, but there is a thick, unopacified rind of thrombus (t), which might explain why intrinsic pulsations are seen so infrequently at fluoroscopy of aortic aneurysms.

If biopsy of these aneurysms is attempted at thoracotomy because their true nature is unknown, uncontrolled bleeding and death can occur.

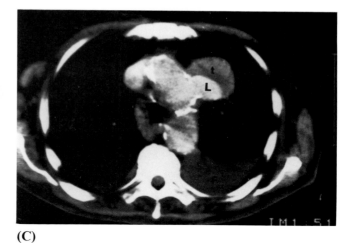

(C)

The mantle of pleural effusion (F) along the left posterior chest wall was, fortunately, unrelated to the aneurysm.

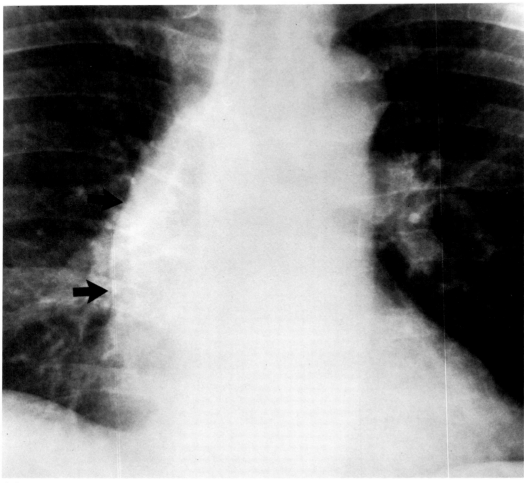

(A)

Fig. 8-29. Aortic Dissection

(A) PA chest view of a 58-year-old man who had a sudden onset of substernal pain radiating to the hips. Femoral pulses were decreased.

The size of the dilated ascending aorta is disproportionate to that of the descending aorta. A lateral view (not shown) confirmed that observation and showed no other masses. *(Figure continues.)*

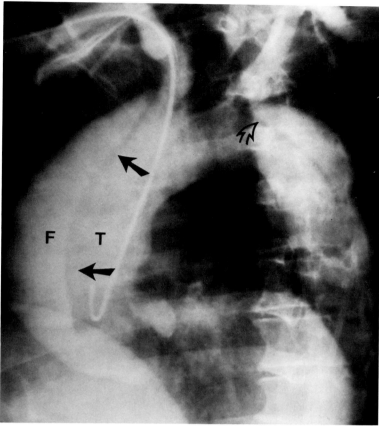

(B)

Fig. 8-29. *(Continued).* **(B)** Right posterior oblique view of an aortogram. A catheter was inserted into the aorta via the right femoral artery. Small test injections showed the catheter to be in the false lumen of a dissecting ascending aorta. That catheter was withdrawn and a second catheter introduced (via the right axillary artery) into the true aortic lumen above the aortic valve as shown here.

There is filling of the false lumen (F), with a lucent stripe (arrows) representing an intimal flap separating the false from the true lumen (T). This flap extends into the base of the right brachiocephalic artery. A second flap (open arrow) extends from the left subclavian artery around the arch into the descending aorta. Further filming showed the dissection extending all the way to the common iliac arteries.

(C) CT scan made after graft replacement of the ascending aorta shows persistence of the intimal flap in the nonreplaced aortic arch and filling of both true and false lumens. The flap is seen as a dark gray, linear image dividing the arch into two opacified channels.

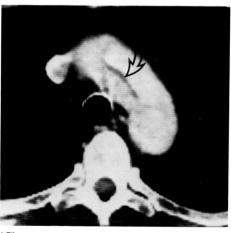

(C)

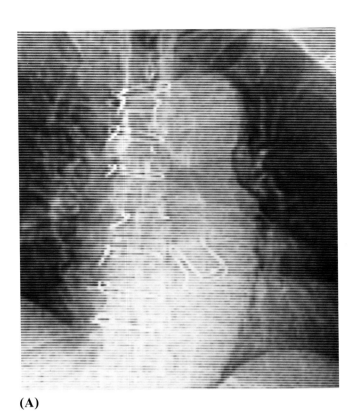

(A)

Fig. 8-30. Aortic Dissection on MRI

(A) Scout view of a patient who is having a CT scan to confirm a tentative diagnosis of dissecting aneurysm. Notice the marked dilatation of both the ascending and the descending thoracic aorta. A contrast agent was not injected because the patient had an allergy to the contrast material. The CT scan was inconclusive, and an MRI scan was performed.

(B) Nongated MRI image (TE 30 msec, TR 75 msec) through the level of the ascending aorta anteriorly and the descending aorta posteriorly, in the axial plane. A well-defined, curved, linear image of an intimal flap is seen in the ascending aorta. The channels on each side of the flap appear black because of the signal void produced by moving blood. This indicates that blood is flowing in both the true and the false channel. In the descending aorta, however, there is a marked signal produced by either slowly flowing blood or clot (c) in the false channel while the true channel (black) is compressed.

(C) MRI scan through the aortic arch in the axial plane. A long intimal flap is seen as a linear image between two channels. One channel consists only of rapidly flowing blood and is seen as the black image of signal void. This is the true channel. The false channel consists of a mixture of flowing blood (black signal void) and strong signal from slow flow or clot (c).

The MRI scan demonstrates that the aortic dissection involves the ascending aorta, the entire arch, and the descending thoracic aorta; the study is accomplished without the aid of any injected contrast material.

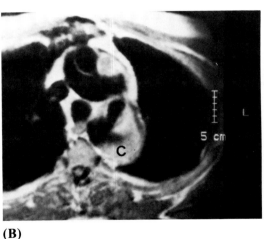

(B)

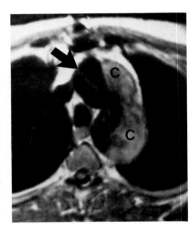

(C)

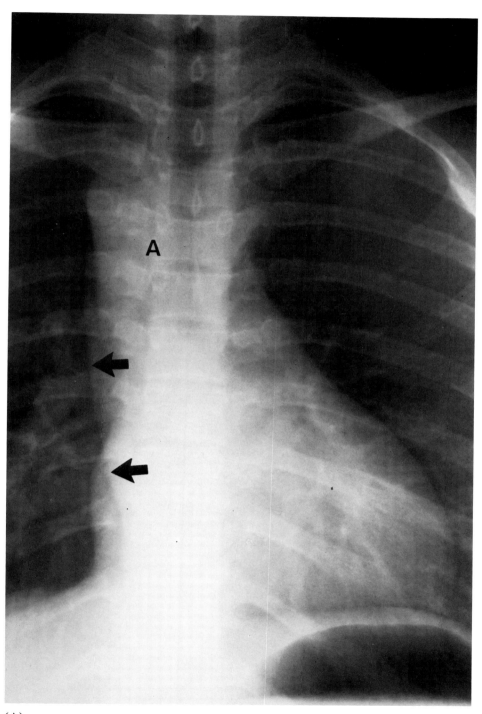

(A)

Fig. 8-31. Right Aortic Arch

This patient has a common type of right aortic arch that is discovered incidentally in patients who have no symptoms of chest or cardiac disease.

(A) PA view. The aortic arch (A) is on the right side of the trachea. The aorta descends on the right, and its lateral edge is outlined by arrows. The usual impression of the aortic arch on the left side of the trachea is absent in these patients and provides an important clue as to the nature of what otherwise appears to be a right superior mediastinal mass. *(Figure continues.)*

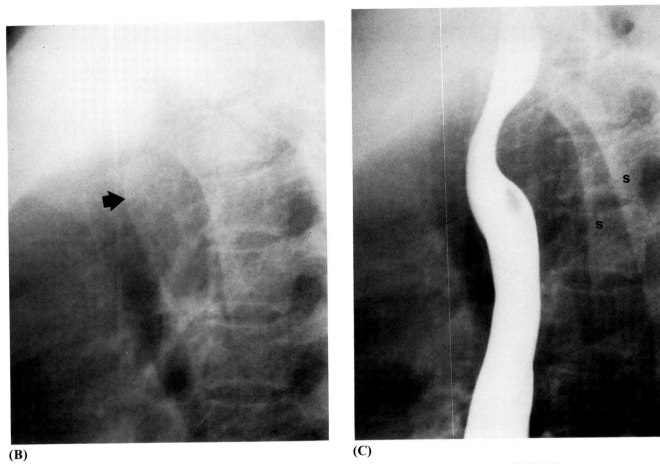

(B)

(C)

Fig. 8-31. *(Continued).* **(B,C)** Lateral views (Fig. C is an esophagogram). An aberrant left subclavian artery arises from a diverticulum (the diverticulum of Kommerell). The diverticulum accounts for the impression on the posterior wall of the trachea and the esophagus seen on Figs. B and C. The anterior margin of each scapula (S) is superimposed on the upper spine.

Sometimes a right aortic arch is associated with mirror-image branching of the great vessels, and these patients usually have associated cyanotic heart disease. A third, rare type of anomalous aortic arch may be associated with isolation of the left subclavian artery.[34]

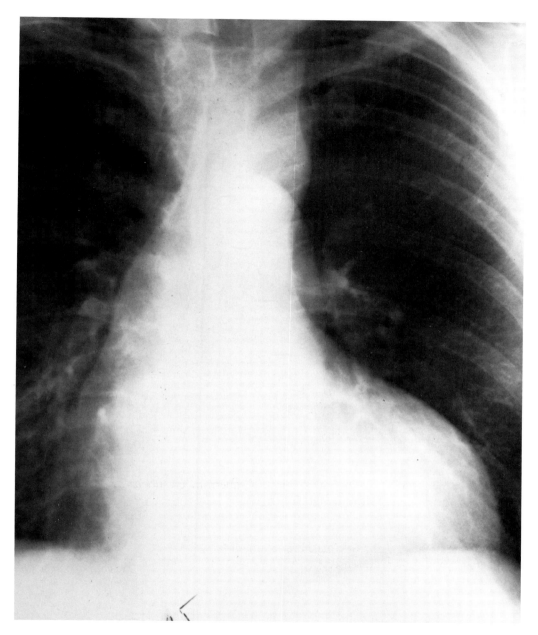

Fig. 8-32. Coarctation of the Aorta

Chest film of a 51-year-old robust man who had striking upper extremity hypertension. The mediastinal contours are abnormal because of a combination of severe coarctation of the aorta, dilatation of the left subclavian artery, and massive dilation of the collateral vessels. Rib notching present bilaterally, combined with the finding of upper extremity hypertension, is a powerful clue to the correct diagnosis. In young children, however, coarctation may not always be associated with easily recognized rib notching. Recall also that medial rib notching is common in normal people.

Uncorrected congenital aortic coarctation in a patient of this age is unusual, but the case is presented to emphasize how developmental or acquired abnormalities of mediastinal vessels can simulate nonvascular mediastinal masses on chest films. Modern imaging techniques, properly employed, can provide the data necessary to make the distinction.

Pseudocoarctation of the aorta is more common in this age group than is uncorrected true coarctation.

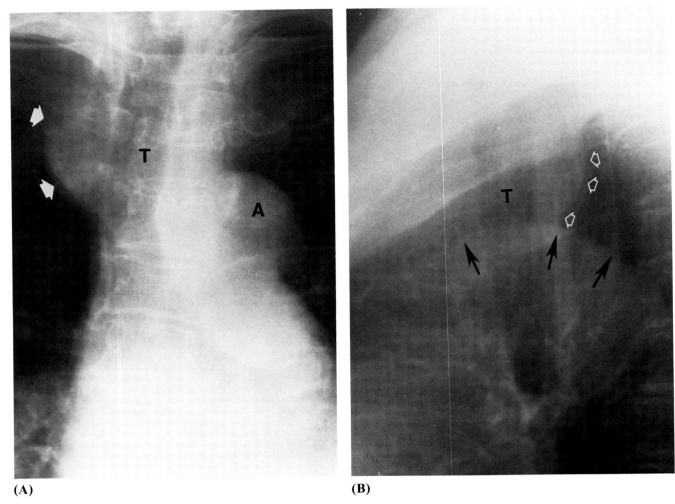

(A)   **(B)**

Fig. 8-33.   Tortuous Brachiocephalic Artery

(A) Coned view of the upper mediastinum and thoracic inlet of a man with a dilated, tortuous brachiocephalic (innominate) artery. The lateral margins of this vessel produce a sharp arc interface (arrows) with adjacent lung that is indistinguishable from that which could be produced by a similarly located mediastinal mass such as high right paratracheal adenopathy or substernal thyroid (see Fig. 8-20). (T, trachea; A, aortic arch.)

(B) Lateral view. The tortuous brachiocephalic artery is projected posterior to the trachea (T) and has an edge that is convex posteriorly at its interface with adjacent lung. The lower edge of this arc (lowest open arrow) stops precisely at the top of the aortic arch (black arrows).

The appearance of a dilated, tortuous brachiocephalic artery is rather characteristic, and often no further proof is needed when the plain-film findings, the patient's age, and the clinical situation are consistent.

Notice that on neither the PA nor the lateral view does the mass cause deviation of the trachea. A turn of the dilated right innominate artery may superimpose on the right side of the trachea and simulate focal impression on the wall, but it does not actually move the trachea. This is an important observation because tortuous great vessels do not displace the airway, whereas other mediastinal masses, especially thyroid masses, do so commonly. Aneurysms of the great vessels, however, may distort and displace adjacent structures including the trachea.

Angiography or, more simply, CT scans, using a good bolus of intravenous contrast material, can be used to prove that a tortuous brachiocephalic artery is the cause of a mediastinal mass. MRI scans should also prove useful in making this distinction. *(Figure continues.)*

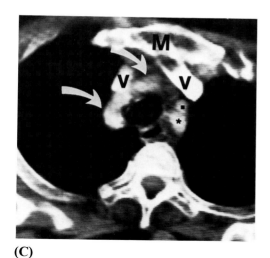

(C)

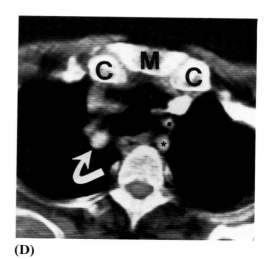

(D)

Fig. 8-33. *(Continued).* **(C)** Coned view of a CT scan at a level just above the aortic arch. The right and left brachiocephalic veins (V) are seen anteriorly. The left is only partly included on this scan, but on a scan made less than 1 cm caudally (not shown) it crosses over to join the right brachiocephalic vein to form the superior vena cava.

The brachiocephalic artery originates from the aortic arch anterior to the trachea (anterior arrow). When it is dilated and tortuous it curves laterally toward the right posterolateral aspect of the trachea (posterior arrow).

(D) CT scan taken 1 cm cephalad from C. The brachiocephalic artery is now seen end-on (arrow) where it turns to ascend in a cephalad direction (black star, left subclavian artery; black square, left common carotid artery; M, manubrium; C, clavicular head).

(E) Coned view from an arteriogram of another patient who also had extreme tortuosity of the brachiocephalic artery. Shortly after the artery originates from the aortic arch (A) it takes a sharp turn to the right (oblique arrow) and then a sharp turn cephalad, where it branches into the right subclavian and right common carotid arteries (curved arrow). The lateral margins of the second turn extend into the adjacent lung. This produces a sharp interface that accounts for the mass image seen on the PA chest film.

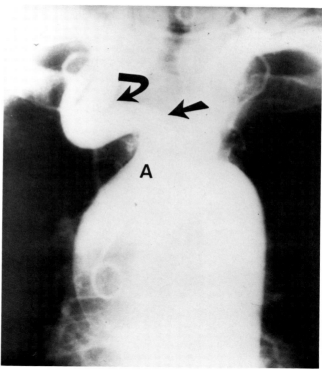

(E)

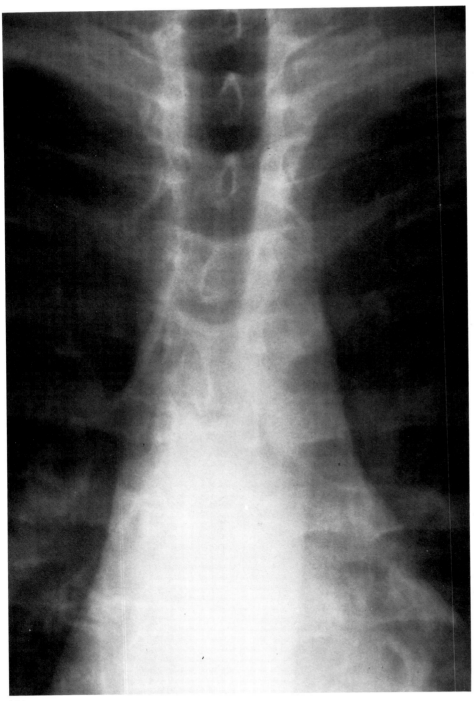

(A)

Fig. 8-34.   Left Superior Vena Cava

(A) Coned view of the mediastinum of a young man with newly diagnosed lymphoma. The mediastinum is within normal limits. The anterior pleural reflection along the left side of the mediastinum, however, passes tangential to the aortic arch. This configuration is part of the spectrum of normal, but in a young patient with lymphoma we would like to explore it further. If this contour were known to have changed from a previous appearance, we would be concerned about the presence of left prevascular adenopathy. Unfortunately, there are no older films for comparison. *(Figure continues.)*

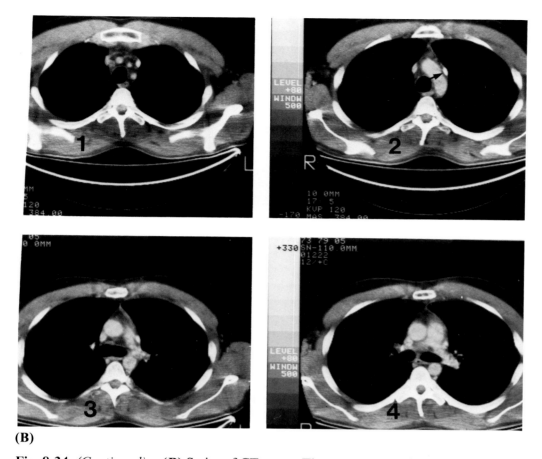

Fig. 8-34. *(Continued).* **(B)** Series of CT scans. The scan at top left is above the aortic arch. The rounded cross sections of the left subclavian and left carotid arteries are seen adjacent to the trachea. To the left of the carotid artery there is a dense elliptical structure within the mediastinal fat.

The top right scan shows a similar image along the left side of the aortic arch on a slightly more caudal plane (arrow).

On the bottom left scan the opacified structure is seen lateral to the left pulmonary artery; it is seen again slightly more caudally on the bottom right scan. This is the image of a persistent left superior vena cava (SVC) as it passes caudally from its cephalad origins to its termination in the coronary sinus of the heart. It is dense because it is opacified by contrast material injected via the left arm. Notice that a right SVC is also present, which is commonly the case. Although a left SVC may be present in people with congenital heart disease, this anomaly may also occur as an isolated finding in people with no signs or symptoms of cardiovascular disease of any sort. A left SVC may be a much larger vessel than is shown here. You can see, however, how the presence of a left SVC in this patient accounts for the projection of the mediastinal pleura tangential to the aortic knob.

A larger left SVC may be present without a right SVC, in which case the ascending aorta would be border forming on the right side of the mediastinum and appear as a prominent convex arc.

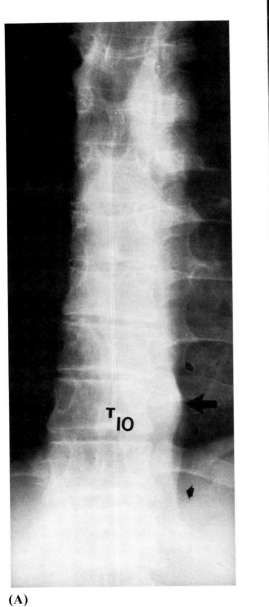

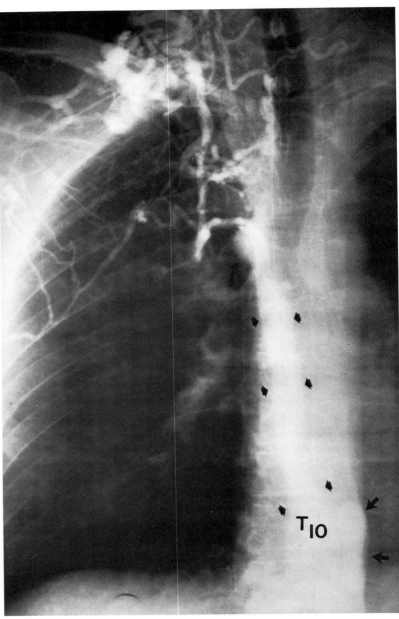

(A)   **(B)**

Fig. 8-35. Dilatation of the Hemiazygos Vein

(A) Overpenetrated view of the mediastinum shows a bulge (arrow) of the paraspinal stripe to the left of T10. Paravertebral adenopathy caused by malignant lymphomas or metastases from other primary neoplasms commonly account for these masses. However, enlargement of the azygos or the hemiazygos vein may also appear as a lobulated paravertebral mass when subjected to increased blood flow.

(B) Contrast study shows opacification of dilated azygos and hemiazygos veins (arrows), which act as collateral channels for venous return in this patient with superior vena cava obstruction. They are fed by a large number of smaller collateral vessels from the neck and shoulder girdle. The bulge to the left of T10 is produced by the cephalic end of the hemiazygos vein where it joins the azygos vein. The hemiazygos vein is opacified only faintly. (From Castellino et al.,[6] with permission.)

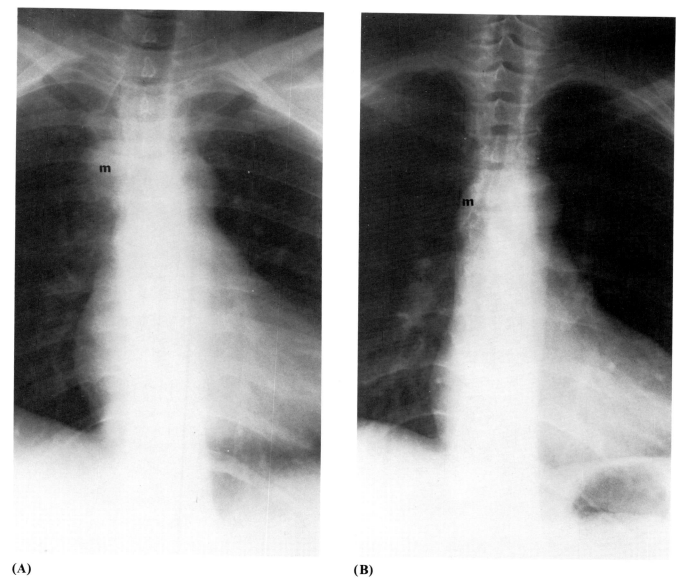

(A)   (B)

Fig. 8-36.   **Azygos Continuation of the Inferior Vena Cava**

(A) AP film of the chest made with the patient supine. (Courtesy of Dr. Martin Spellman, Fremont, California.)

(B) PA view of the chest made with the patient upright. There is a remarkable change in the size of the soft tissue "mass" (m in Figs. A and B) adjacent to the trachea above the origin of the right main bronchus. This change from the supine to the upright position is good evidence that the apparent mass is venous.

The vessel that "lives" in this region is the azygos vein. Why should the azygos vein be so large in a person who has no known cardiovascular difficulties or any evidence to suggest vena cava obstruction? *(Figure continues.)*

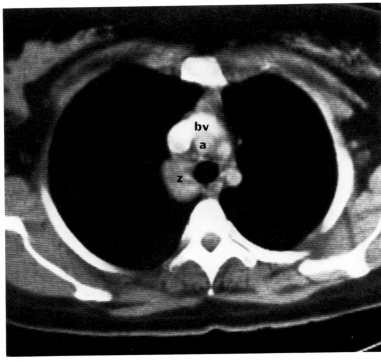

(C)

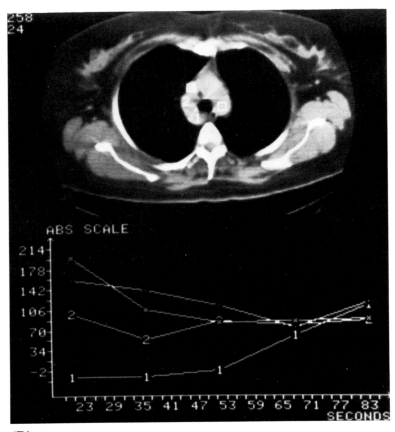

(D)

Fig. 8-36. *(Continued).* **(C)** CT scan at the level of the top of the aortic arch. Contrast material was injected as a bolus via a vein in the left arm, and a continuous rapid drip of contrast material was immediately begun at the end of the bolus. Intense enhancement of the left brachiocephalic vein (bv) is seen anterior to the right brachiocephalic artery (a). The sausage-shaped soft tissue density to the right of the trachea is the top of a dilated azygos vein (z), which at this time contains unopacified blood.

(D) CT scan made several seconds after Fig. C. It is illustrated with much less magnification. Contrast material is now in the great vessels and in the dilated azygos vein. On the graph below the scan, the number 1 refers to the Hounsfield numbers that were recorded from a cursor placed over the posterior aspect of the azygos vein at this level. The graph shows that the azygos vein enhances with contrast material much later than the other vessels that are included in this scan (represented by the other tracings on the graph). The blood has to enter the azygos vein from the lower half of the body, because this vein represents an azygos continuation of the inferior vena cava. This is a congenital variation in the development of the venous anatomy in the lower half of the body.

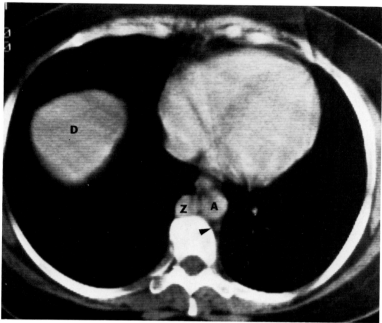

(E)

(E) CT scan at a level corresponding to the dome of the right diaphragm (D), which appears here as an island floating in a sea of black. The aorta (A) is seen along the left anterolateral aspects of the vertebra. The rounded structure to the right of the descending thoracic aorta is the enlarged azygos vein (Z). (The black cleft that seems to divide it is an artifact.)

Ordinarily, the azygos vein at this level would be a fraction of this size, but in this woman the azygos vein carries the entire venous return from the lower half of the body. It assumes a size almost equal to that of the descending thoracic aorta. The rounded opacity seen anterior to the aorta and the enlarged azygos vein is the esophagus. The hemiazygos vein (arrowhead) is a small, round opacity posterior to the descending aorta. Ordinarily, the azygos vein at this level, would be only slightly greater in size than the hemiazygos vein. In some patients the hemiazygos vein can also serve as a collateral channel and is then much larger.

It is important to recognize azygos vein continuation of the inferior vena cava, since inadvertant ligation would be disastrous. Also, an erroneous diagnosis of mediastinal mass or adenopathy is avoided.

(F) Contrast study shows a dilated azygos vein (arrows) in another patient. Its prevertebral and paravertebral course is poorly seen, but its arch is displayed well. As it empties into the superior vena cava, its caliber approaches that of the aorta. *(Figure continues.)*

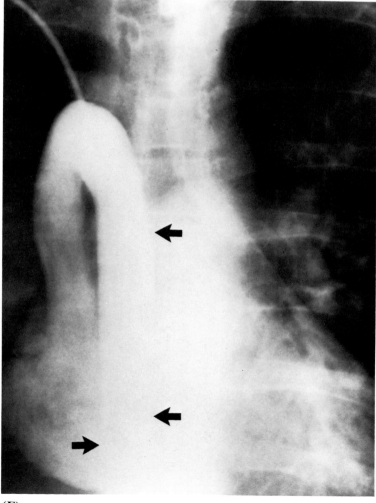

(F)

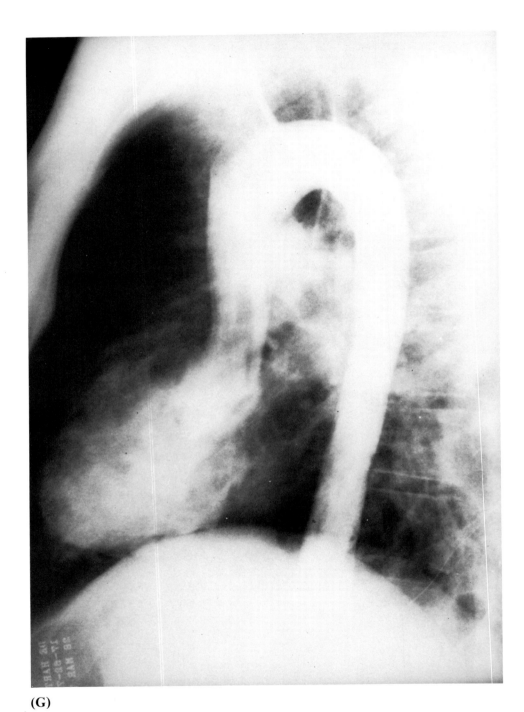

(G)

Fig. 8-36. *(Continued).* **(G)** Lateral view shows the entire intrathoracic course of the enlarged azygos vein. It simulates the aorta in its vertical course and its arch, but it empties into the superior vena cava.

9

Pulmonary Edema and Edema-Like Conditions; Pulmonary Embolism, and Infarction

PULMONARY EDEMA

Two broad classes of disorders account for the majority of cases of pulmonary edema. One class consists of those disorders in which there is an elevation of pulmonary capillary pressure, usually due to pulmonary venous hypertension, so that there is a net movement of fluid out of the microvasculature and into the tissues. The other class consists of those disorders that cause an increase in pulmonary capillary permeability. A third category, hypervolemic edema, may have components of both, compounded by a reduction in the colloid osmotic pressure of plasma. Combinations of these causes also occur.

Pulmonary lymphatics play an indispensable role in the clearance of fluid from the interstitium of the lung, and focal obstruction of lymphatic flow can result in localized edema.

Reductions in the colloid osmotic pressure of plasma per se are rarely severe enough, even in cases of severe hypoproteinemia from renal or liver failure, to cause pulmonary edema, but they contribute to the magnitude of the edema when other causes are operating. The pulmonary edema is more likely to occur at lower levels of left atrial pressure in patients with low levels of plasma protein.[32] In cases of acute intravenous fluid overload, however, low plasma colloid osmotic pressure may play a major role in the development of pulmonary edema.[37] In tertiary care hospitals, intravenous fluid overload may be the most common cause of pulmonary edema. The use of central venous catheters for pressure monitoring and to administer drugs, fluid, blood, and parenteral alimentation in patients with serious illnesses provides a setting in which fluid overload can easily occur. Physicians responsible for treating patients in the intensive care unit or during prolonged anesthesia are often faced with the choice of risking pulmonary edema from fluid overload or risking renal failure from low output.

Left heart failure from any cause is otherwise the most common antecedent of pulmonary edema. Arteriosclerotic cardiovascular disease, mitral valve disease, aortic valve disease, and myocarditis are among the more common causes.

A left atrial myxoma that intermittently obstructs the mitral valve can produce radiographic changes similar to those of mitral stenosis. Pulmonary veno-occlusive disease is a rare cause of pulmonary edema that may show striking, although nonspecific, radiographic changes of interstitial pulmonary edema.

A variety of congenital heart lesions[7] may cause obstructive changes resulting in pulmonary edema early in life. Anomalous pulmonary venous return may also cause pulmonary edema when there is elevated venous pressure from stenosis or compression of the anomalous vein.

Renal failure is another common cause of pulmonary edema, which often predominates in a central "butterfly" or "bat's-wing" distribution (Fig. 9-1). There is controversy as to whether or not left heart failure is also always present in such patients.

Many conditions are associated with an increase in pulmonary capillary permeability severe enough to result in pulmonary edema; in other conditions the pathogenesis of pulmonary edema is unknown, controversial, or idiosyncratic. Among these are aspiration of gastric juice of low pH, inhalation of smoke or irritant gases or chemicals (Fig. 9-2), narcotic abuse (particularly heroin), fat embolism, amniotic fluid embolism, ingestion of a variety of toxins, acute allergic reactions, chronic salicylate overdose, near-drowning, acute airway obstruction, and a variety of disorders that apparently produce a cascade of pathophysiologic changes resulting in the adult respiratory distress syndrome with a common factor of increased pulmonary capillary permeability. High-altitude sickness also manifests as pulmonary edema, by a mechanism that is incompletely understood. Patients with head trauma, seizures, brain tumors, and increased intracranial pressure or cerebral vascular insult may also develop pulmonary edema of uncertain cause. A variety of acute infections produce radiographic abnormalities that mimic pulmonary edema in either the interstitial or the alveolar flooding phase, and malignant lymphoma and certain metastases do likewise.

References 14, 26, and 32 are a few of the many worthwhile articles on the evolution of pulmonary edema.

The Radiographic Spectrum of Pulmonary Edema

The radiographic spectrum of pulmonary edema is surprisingly varied.

Pulmonary Venous Hypertension

Increase in the caliber of upper lobe vessels relative to lower lobe vessels is a radiographic sign of pulmonary venous hypertension, which may be an indication of left heart failure and thus a precursor of pulmonary edema. It is a common finding in patients with uncorrected mitral valve disease who have chronic elevation of left atrial pressure and at times associated chronic interstitial pulmonary edema (Fig. 9-3A to C).

Under normal conditions, the major vessels supplying the lower portions of the lung are of greater caliber than comparable-order vessels supplying the upper portions of the lung when the subject is erect. In the case of pulmonary venous hypertension there is an increase in the volume of blood flow to the upper lobes[13,30] and a diminution to the lower lobes, usually ascribed to an increase in lower lung zone interstitial tissue pressure or lower lung vasoconstriction from early edema.[36] The finding of relatively increased caliber of upper lung zone vessels may be obvious and easy to recognize, but there are times when even experienced observers disagree in this assessment. Earlier films are helpful for comparison if they were made at a time when the patient was not in left heart failure.

For the finding to be a valid sign of pulmonary venous hypertension, the chest films must be exposed while the patient is upright. When films are exposed with the patient supine, an equalization of flow to the upper and lower lung zones is to be expected even in the normal subject.

Other Conditions Influencing Vessel Caliber and Distribution

Impairment of lower lung zone blood flow due to basilar emphysema, chronic interstitial pneumonitis, or pulmonary emboli may also cause an increase of flow through upper zone vessels independent of left heart failure. Pulmonary vessels may be diminished in caliber and number in zones of impaired blood flow as a result of focal zones of emphysema or relatively hypoxic zones peripheral to partial bronchial obstruction, or peripheral to pulmonary emboli, thromboses, and rarely perivascular or intravascular tumor. Equalization of caliber of upper and lower zone vessels in the erect patient may be seen consequent to anemia, fever, hyperthyroidism, pregnancy, and other causes of high-output states as well as pulmonary arterial hypertension.

In certain conditions the major blood vessels throughout the lungs appear to be of increased caliber relative to normal. This is commonly seen in patients with left-to-right cardiac shunts (Fig. 9-3D and E) and may also be seen in some patients with pulmonary arterial hypertension from any cause (Fig. 9-3H and I). In pulmonary arterial hypertension, however, the central pulmonary arteries are often enlarged out of proportion to the peripheral branches[1] (Fig. 9-3F and G).

In assessing upper lobe vascular caliber it is also important to take pulmonary artery pressure into consideration. When pulmonary artery pressure is high, upper lobe venous distension may not occur even in cases of clearly established mitral stenosis.[22]

Loss of Sharp Vessel Margins

Often the earliest chest film finding in patients with pulmonary edema is loss of sharpness of the images of small peripheral vessels followed by engorgement of and loss of detail of hilar vessels (Fig. 9-4). As the edema progresses, vessels throughout the lung lose their relatively sharp margins and at the same time appear engorged. Vessels in the lower lung zones usually show more severe loss of image detail. The loss of vascular detail can be explained on the basis of increased fluid accumulating in the perivascular interstitial spaces and the air spaces and distorting the ordinary sharp interface between vessel and normal lung (Fig. 9-5).

Loss of vessel detail is a subjective determination. It is very helpful to have earlier films for comparison, but the films must be of comparably good quality. Respiratory motion, poor screen-film contact, inadequate level of inspiration, and other technical flaws can invalidate the study. However, one must avoid the trap of assuming that the changes in vessel clarity from film to film are due *only* to technical flaws rather than pulmonary pathology. In addition to technical flaws, other disease processes such as infection with *Pneumocystis carinii* or viruses or a variety of chronic interstitial diseases may produce equally convincing loss of small vessel detail and mimic other causes of pulmonary edema.

Septal Lines and Subpleural Fluid

Short, sharp linear images may appear in the lateral aspects of the lung bases on the PA view and in the retrosternal region on the lateral view as a result of edema fluid accumulating in interlobular septa and producing septal lines (Kerley-B lines; Fig. 9-5B). In addition, there may be longer similar, fine-line shadows in the middle and upper lung zones called A lines (Fig. 9-5C) and a reticular appearance called C lines. All of these images are produced by accumulation of edema fluid in the interlobular septa of the lung. Obstruction of pulmonary venous return or of lymph flow from the periphery of the lungs can also cause septal edema to become visible as septal lines. Edema fluid may also accumulate in peribronchial sheaths, causing a thickening of the peribronchial soft tissues most easily recognized when seen about bronchi projecting end-on, and often referred to as peribronchial cuffing.[6]

Fluid may also accumulate in subpleural positions along the lower chest wall (Fig. 9-5B) and along the distribution of the interlobar fissures. These subpleural fluid collections resemble those of true pleural effusions, but do not change location when films are exposed with the patient in the lateral decubitus position as free

pleural fluid does. On the other hand, in some patients there may be subpleural fluid collections as well as effusion in the pleural space.

Septal lines and subpleural fluid collections are manifestations of a predominantly interstitial phase of pulmonary edema. Frequently the diaphragm will be high, attesting to loss of lung compliance accompanying the pulmonary edema. The radiographic findings are important because there may be no, or few, auscultatory sounds to confirm the presence of pulmonary edema at this stage. Patients with chronic left heart failure, such as those with uncorrected mitral stenosis, may recognize few symptoms from interstitial pulmonary edema other than perhaps some dyspnea on exertion or a decrease in exercise tolerance.

There are other causes of septal lines, such as tumor cells in perilymphatic spaces in the case of lymphangitic metastases or interstitial deposition of dust-laden macrophages or fibrous tissue in cases of pneumoconioses. Do not count heavily on seeing septal lines (specifically, Kerley-B lines) in order to make a diagnosis of interstitial pulmonary edema. In fact, most of the cases of pulmonary edema seen daily will not have progressed to the stage of frank visibility of septal lines whereas others will have passed beyond into the stage of alveolar flooding. Patients with increased-permeability edema often do not show septal lines during the radiographic evolution of their edema (Figs. 9-2 and 9-6). Therefore, whereas septal lines are an important radiographic finding in the diagnosis of pulmonary edema, they are in no way a requisite, nor are septal lines always due to edema.

Alveolar Filling Phase

As pulmonary edema progresses to involve more and more of the alveolar spaces there is a further increase in the overall density of the involved lung, and there may be slight, moderate, or heavy confluent or patchy consolidation, often with visible air bronchograms. Clinical signs and symptoms in the conscious patient with heart failure are often classic—dyspnea, tachypnea, production of pinkish or blood-tinged frothy sputum, wheezing, and perhaps cyanosis, accompanied by orthopnea—leaving little doubt about the diagnosis. However, patients with noncardiogenic pulmonary edema may have similar alveolar flooding and similar signs and symptoms but no orthopnea (Fig. 9-6).

The radiographic signs of interstitial edema are usually lost within the more striking consolidations of the alveolar flooding phase of pulmonary edema. Mixtures of the interstitial phase and alveolar flooding phase may be present on the same roentgenogram in some patients.

ESTIMATION OF CARDIAC SIZE

Estimation of cardiac size and appraisal of mediastinal contours and width from radiographic appearances is critical in assessing patients with cardiogenic and noncardiogenic pulmonary edema. The size and shape of the cardiomediastinal silhouette is in part related to body habitus and the position of the diaphragm. Patients of mesomorphic or endomorphic somatotypes may have the diaphragm relatively high on full inspiration and may also have abundant mediastinal fat, which can exaggerate not only mediastinal width but cardiac size as well.

Cardiothoracic Ratio

There are several methods of measurement used to assess cardiac size, but the simplest is measurement of the cardiothoracic (CT) ratio on films exposed at a target-film distance of at least 6 feet with the patient erect. The greatest measurement from the right heart border to the midspine is added to the greatest measurement from the midspine to the left heart border, and the result is divided by the greatest distance between the inner margins of the right and left ribs at the lung bases (Fig. 9-7). It is important to exclude epicardial fat pads from measurements of cardiac size when the fat pads are large. Often they can be recognized because of an abrupt change in contour in the region of the fat pad, but sometimes they cannot.

There are problems in testing the accuracy of any system of cardiac size estimation based on chest film analysis, but in general a (CT) ratio of more than 50 percent (measured on upright PA chest films made at a 6-foot target-film distance) is useful in identifying cardiomegaly in a nonselected adult patient population.[20] A CT ratio of less than 50 percent is generally accepted as normal with reasonable accuracy. Increases or decreases in heart size compared to previous films must be considered in order to avoid false-negative results that will occur, because an abnormally large heart size for a given individual may still have a CT ratio below 50 percent. However, differences in the transverse diameter of the heart of 1½ cm can be seen normally (and at the extreme up to 2 cm) if one film is exposed during systole and the comparison film is exposed during diastole.[9] This possibility should be taken into account when assessing the significance of changes in heart size from film to film, since one ordinarily does not know in which phase of the cardiac cycle the films were exposed. Of course, heart size as seen on films made with the patient upright cannot be compared directly with heart size as seen on films

with the patient supine, nor can heart size as seen on films made in the AP projection be compared with heart size as seen on PA projections. The heart is farther from the film on the AP projection and therefore magnified compared to the PA projection. In addition, AP films (including supine films) are usually made at shorter target-film distances than are PA films, which are usually at a 6-foot target-film distance.

Pericardial effusion distending the pericardial sac can be misinterpreted as cardiomegaly, and rarely tumor surrounding the heart may also mimic cardiomegaly (Fig. 9-8).

When a supposedly enlarged heart is superimposed on both hila, beware that the image you are considering to be heart may be a combination of heart and a large pericardial effusion or hematoma. Mediastinal masses contiguous with the heart margins, particularly neoplasms involving the thymus such as thymomas or thymolipomas, or malignant lymphomas or germ cell tumors, can also be misinterpreted as cardiomegaly. A giant aneurysm of the aorta can also distort the cardiomediastinal silhouette so that its true nature may not be recognized on chest films alone.

The majority of patients with cardiogenic pulmonary edema will show an enlarged heart on chest films. Patients who have pulmonary edema due to acute heart failure following myocardial infarction or severe arrhythmia, however, may not show an enlarged heart even though the pulmonary edema is cardiogenic.

Assessment of Specific Cardiac Chamber Enlargement

Although estimation of cardiac enlargement from PA and lateral chest films is useful, assessment of specific chamber enlargement is much less reliable.[25]

In the past, the radiologic estimation of specific chamber enlargement was based on cardiac fluoroscopy (during which the esophagus was outlined by barium) augmented by radiographs in PA, lateral, and both oblique projections. The variables assessed or the accuracy of the assessments in determining specific chamber enlargement will not be discussed here. Estimates of relative chamber size from PA and lateral radiographs of the chest are necessarily subjective. Gross enlargement of the left ventricle is usually detectable. The posterior wall of the left ventricle constitutes the posterior margin of the cardiac image on the lateral view of the chest. Dilatation of the left ventricle is seen as posterior and caudal displacement of this heart margin. A numerical estimation of this displacement can be derived by relating the posterior heart border to the inferior vena cava and to the diaphragm (Fig. 9-7). On a PA view, estimation of left ventricular enlargement is often based on a rounding-off and downward and left lateral displacement of the cardiac apex. The estimation of left ventricular size from a PA view is less reliable than that derived from a lateral view.

False assessments of left ventricular enlargement based on the lateral view of the chest can result when there is rotation of the patient off of the true lateral projection (see Ch. 1) and when enlargement of the right ventricle displaces the left ventricle posteriorly.

Estimation of right ventricular enlargement on the lateral view of the chest is based on recognition of enlargement of the outflow tract, which encroaches on the lung anteriorly in the retrosternal space (see Fig. 9-3). The determination of enlargement of the right atrium on either the PA or the lateral view is, in my experience, the most difficult of all the chamber assessments. When it is extreme, however, there is a shift of the right heart border to the right and caudally, with a rounded inferior contour seen on PA view.

Dilatation of the left atrium is assessed by analyzing the relationship of the right side of the left atrium to the right heart border, and the relationship of the left side of the left atrium to the carina and left main bronchus (see Fig. 9-3B). The enlarged left atrium has an interface with lung behind the right heart and can be seen as a separate convex edge superimposed on the right side of the heart. It is projected in the same region as the normal pulmonary venous confluence, but presents a longer lateral arc. Extreme enlargement of the left atrium may cause its right edge to be projected lateral to the right heart border and stimulate right heart enlargement. Left atrium enlargement may also cause elevation of the left main bronchus.

On a lateral view the enlarged left atrium projects posteriorly beneath the level of the carina and may cause a posterior displacement of the left main bronchus. However, rotation of the lateral view off of the true lateral projection so that the left side is posterior to true lateral will also cause a posterior projection of the left main bronchus, which can be misinterpreted as caused by left atrial enlargement. Posterior displacement of the barium-outlined esophagus is another sign of left atrial enlargement (see Fig. 9-3B). An enlarged left atrial appendage may cause a convex bulge to be seen along the left cardiomediastinal border caudal to the left main bronchus and the pulmonary artery segment of the cardiac silhouette.

When precise estimation of specific chamber size is indicated for treatment planning, echocardiography or angiocardiographic examinations provide more accurate data. Hypertrophy of cardiac muscle without chamber dilatation cannot be assessed reliably from plain films.

Distention of the Superior Vena Cava or the Azygos Vein

Distention of the superior vena cava consequent to hypervolemia in patients with congestive heart failure, intravenous fluid overload, or renal failure can be recognized as widening of the superior mediastinum primarily to the right. The finding is more reliable as an estimate of hypervolemia when the chest films are made with the patient erect and when there are earlier chest films for comparison. The mediastinal widening will be present on films made with the patient supine but may be attributed to the normal effect of the supine position. A wide superior mediastinum is expected to be seen on chest films of supine endomorphs or mesomorphs even when congestive failure is not present.

You may find it convenient to use Milne's reference points[23] in measuring the width of the superior mediastinum: the distance between the intersection of the edge of the superior vena cava and the right upper lobe bronchus on the right side and the lateral margin of the left subclavian artery at its origin from the aorta on the left side (Fig. 9-7). Although there are other points one can use to measure mediastinal width, these are convenient and useful when comparing films of a given patient in order to estimate changes in circulating blood volume associated with congestive heart failure, uremia, fluid overload, and other hypervolemic states.

An increase in the size of the azygos vein (compared to films made before the onset of pulmonary edema, or above the acceptable transverse diameter of 8 or 9 mm on films made with the patient erect) may occur when there is increased pressure in the right heart due to congestive failure or even to acute pulmonary embolus or pulmonary arterial hypertension. An increase in flow through the azygos vein, from a variety of causes, will also cause an increase in its size (see Fig. 8-36).

On films made with the patient supine, the azygos vein may be as large as 14 mm in patients who have a normal central venous pressure.[28]

Distribution of Pulmonary Edema

Pulmonary edema is seldom uniformly distributed throughout the lungs except when it is severe. In patients who do not have associated obstructive lung disease the radiographic manifestations of pulmonary edema are usually more marked at the lung bases (see Fig. 9-5). Regardless of how much the middle and upper zones become involved, seldom does cardiogenic edema extend all the way to the apices.

Some patients, particularly those in renal failure (see Fig. 9-1), have a pronounced parahilar and central distribution of alveolar pulmonary edema. Patients who have pulmonary edema associated with central nervous system lesions and increased intracranial pressure may show upper lung zone predominance.

Patients with pulmonary edema due to hypersensitivity reactions may have interstitial edema or patchy or diffuse alveolar flooding on radiographs, with no signs of cardiomegaly or pulmonary venous hypertension. Clinically, these patients may have a history of sudden onset of severe dyspnea and a striking absence of orthopnea (see Fig. 9-6).

Frank pulmonary edema seldom presents a radiographic recognition problem when it is of a usual pattern. However, pulmonary edema may appear quite atypical in patients with underlying chronic lung disease[16] or occasionally in patients who have pulmonary edema associated with increased intracranial pressure. In patients with emphysematous lung, pulmonary edema will be seen only in those areas where pulmonary microvasculature is still present; hence, the more emphysematous areas are "spared," and the distribution of the edema may present unexpected patterns. Even in those areas where the edema is seen there may be cystic-appearing spaces or even a "pseudohoneycomb" appearance. If there is severe upper lung zone emphysema, the expected diversion of blood flow to upper zones due to pulmonary venous hypertension does not occur. If there is severe lower zone emphysema, blood flow will predominate in the upper lung zones, mimicking the distribution of pulmonary venous hypertension even though the latter is not present. When edematous changes occur only in the zones perfused best, radiographic appearances may mimic those of pneumonia.

Unilateral Pulmonary Edema

In the vast majority of instances of pulmonary edema the distribution is bilateral and frequently relatively symmetrical. In some patients, however, there is significant asymmetry, and uncommonly the edema is unilateral.[18]

Unilateral edema can occur in patients in whom the microvasculature of one lung is subject to high pressure while that of the other lung is not. Examples include iatrogenic systemic-to-pulmonary artery shunts such as the Blalock-Taussig and Potts' anastomoses. Conversely, a lung that is protected from high intravascular pressures, (e.g., by pulmonary artery branch stenoses) or that is underperfused because of loss of capillary bed (as in cases of extreme unilateral emphysema or unilateral bronchiolitis obliterans, as in Swyer-James syndrome) may not develop pulmonary edema under conditions in which the opposite lung does.

Unilateral obstruction of pulmonary venous return,

either congenital, postinflammatory, or secondary to obstruction by neoplasm, may also cause unilateral edema. Unilateral aspiration of gastric juice of low pH or other pulmonary irritants is another cause of edema in only one lung.

Unilateral pulmonary edema has also been reported following fairly rapid removal of large volumes of pleural fluid[35] or rapid removal of air from a large pneumothorax.[39] Patients in heart failure who lie on one side most of the time may also have edema predominantly in the dependent lung.

CONDITIONS THAT MAY PRODUCE EDEMA-LIKE PATTERNS

There are conditions that commonly produce radiographic patterns indistinguishable from those of pulmonary edema or that have zones of consolidation reminiscent of those associated with pulmonary edema, although atypical.

Infection

Some pulmonary infections, especially those afflicting patients with altered immunity, may present initially with a pulmonary edema-like pattern (see Ch. 5). Those most likely to do so are infections with *Pneumocystis carinii* or cytomegalovirus, or combinations of *Pneumocystis,* cytomegalovirus, *Toxoplasma,* and fungi simultaneously. Viral pneumonias due to varicella-zoster, measles, influenza, or adenoviruses may also present in this fashion, but they are less common. Considering the histopathology of an interstitial inflammatory cell infiltration combined with a proteinaceous or hemorrhagic exudate filling alveoli, the radiographic resemblance to pulmonary edema is not surprising. Miliary forms of tuberculosis, histoplasmosis, coccidioidomycosis, and other pathogenic fungi may also resemble pulmonary edema, but miliary involvement of the extreme apices and the extreme bases simultaneously is rare in pulmonary edema and common in miliary infections.

Almost any bacterial, fungal, viral, or parasitic infection can progress to a stage of bilateral lung involvement with extensive air space consolidation when the infection is uncontrolled. The majority, however, do not present with such radiographic appearances initially but instead show a progression on serial films from focal or multifocal lesions to diffuse disease. The progression can be extremely rapid — hours to days in some acute infections. As more effective antibiotics and chemotherapeutic agents have evolved, rapid progression is less common.

For example, before the advent of antituberculous drugs, tuberculous lesions could progress to involve both lungs so severely that bilateral consolidation resembling pulmonary edema occurred in some patients. Today such a condition would be rare in the United States or Europe in a host whose immunity was unimpaired.

Infections that may result in radiographic patterns that are similar to those of pulmonary edema are illustrated and discussed further in Chapter 5.

Pulmonary Hemorrhage

Patients with idiopathic pulmonary hemosiderosis (Fig. 9-9) or Goodpasture's syndrome (Fig. 9-10) may have bilateral pulmonary hemorrhage in the pulmonary edema pattern. Patients with systemic lupus erythematosus, Wegener's granulomatosis, other pulmonary capillaritis, vasculitis,[21,34] or hemolytic-uremic syndromes may also present with diffuse pulmonary hemorrhage, and patients with acute leukemia may do so as well. In adults suffering from acute leukemia, diffuse pulmonary hemorrhage may occur alone but is far less common than infection alone or infection along with hemorrhage as a cause of widespread pulmonary consolidation. None of the above conditions are common, but they occur with enough frequency that they should be considered as possibilities in a differential diagnosis. Although hemoptysis might be expected, it is not invariably present, particularly in children with idiopathic pulmonary hemosiderosis and adults with acute leukemia. The latter may have other indications of bleeding, however, such as petechiae or anemia and guaiac-positive stools, and the former may have hemosiderin-laden macrophages in gastric aspirates.

Although a tentative diagnosis of diffuse pulmonary hemorrhage can be made by correlating radiographic studies with clinical and laboratory data, the chest film findings are not specific and can be simulated by other causes of diffuse lung disease (Fig. 9-11).

Hypersensitivity Reactions

Pulmonary reactions may occur because of hypersensitivity to a variety of drugs, blood products, and inhaled antigens, and the chest film findings may resemble the alveolar flooding phase, the mixed phase, or the interstitial phase of pulmonary edema, depending on whether the patient is in the acute, subacute, or chronic phase of reaction and on the magnitude of the pulmonary reaction. Acute pulmonary hypersensitivity reactions (see Fig. 9-6) may manifest as pulmonary edema.

Distinctions between patients with cardiogenic pulmonary edema and those with hypersensitivity pulmonary edema are usually based on clinical and radiologic findings. Generally, patients with pulmonary edema from acute hypersensitivity reactions do not have enlarged hearts or dilatation of the superior vena cava or other signs of increased circulating blood volume, except by coincidence. On the contrary, these findings are common in patients with cardiogenic pulmonary edema.

Hypersensitivity pneumonitis due to inhaled organic dusts and adverse pulmonary reactions to therapeutic drugs are discussed in Chapter 10.

Neoplasms

Patients with bronchoalveolar cell carcinoma, Hodgkin's disease, or non-Hodgkin's lymphoma may develop bilateral consolidation in a distribution resembling pulmonary edema on chest films, but the clinical signs and symptoms do not resemble those of pulmonary edema. Uncommonly, but often enough to be troublesome, patients with malignant lymphoma may develop — within days — bilateral lung involvement that resembles the mixed or interstitial phase of pulmonary edema. More often they have clinical findings suggestive of infection rather than pulmonary edema per se, but because of the rapid onset, the chest film findings provoke consideration of pulmonary edema. The usual treatment for pulmonary edema does not alter the clinical or radiologic variables, however. Lung biopsy is often necessary to confirm the diagnosis of lymphomatous involvement of lung and to exclude infection.

Patients with lymphangitic spread of metastases may also have chest film findings consistent with the mixed pattern of pulmonary edema. In fact, when there has been no prior diagnosis of malignant neoplasm, and the patient is young, the correct diagnosis may have to await lung biopsy. This is especially so when the primary neoplasm is clinically silent, as can occur with some pancreatic, gastrointestinal, or breast neoplasms.

One of the features distinguishing pulmonary edema from conditions that may be confused with it — such as lymphangitic metastases, interstitial pneumonitis, or *Pneumocystis carinii* pneumonia — is the rapid radiographic clearance that can be observed on sequential radiographs when the patient responds to diuretics, fluid and salt restriction, or other treatment to correct left heart failure or fluid overload.

Diffuse neoplasm involving the lungs is illustrated and discussed further in Chapter 6.

Pulmonary Alveolar Proteinosis

Pulmonary alveolar proteinosis is an uncommon diffuse lung disease of unknown etiology that may resemble pulmonary edema radiographically. This disease is discussed in Chapter 10.

Adult Respiratory Distress Syndrome

Adult respiratory distress syndrome (ARDS) is a syndrome of severe respiratory insufficiency in which symptoms typically antedate radiographic abnormalities, but soon are accompanied by a radiographic pattern of extensive pulmonary edema. Frequent preceding events include shock, sepsis, severe trauma, drug intoxication, viral pneumonia, cardiopulmonary bypass, hypertransfusion, and a number of events that are commonly associated with acute pulmonary edema due to increased capillary permeability, such as oxygen toxicity, massive aspiration, and near-drowning. Disseminated intravascular coagulation is a common accompaniment or complication.[17] As in other causes of pulmonary edema such as smoke inhalation, there may be a lag period of several hours between the inciting event and onset of symptoms and the appearance of chest film evidence of pulmonary edema. The edema may be patchy at first and progress gradually over a few days to extensive inhomogeneous opacification of both lungs (Fig. 9-12). There may then be fluctuations in the radiographic appearance, but frequently there is an alarming, persistent, widespread consolidation lasting many days. Those patients fortunate enough to survive show slowly decreasing pulmonary abnormalities over many weeks with radiographic clearing lagging behind clinical improvement.

Others, not so fortunate, maintain a diffuse pattern of inhomogeneous pulmonary consolidation, often with air bronchograms visible and small, irregular opacities with focal zones of lucency mimicking honeycombing. At postmortem some of these foci are seen to be due to profound fibrosis of the interstitium causing a collapse of peripheral airways and airlessness deceptively like that seen with exudative alveolar filling. There may also be thromboses of small pulmonary vessels.

Increased capillary permeability is the hallmark of this disorder, accompanied by pulmonary edema, dyspnea, hypoxemia, and decreased pulmonary compliance. Increased heart size and other signs of congestive heart failure are usually not present initially. However, some patients can develop associated left heart failure, and all patients on prolonged steroids and ventilator therapy are subject to pulmonary infection with gram-negative organisms and ubiquitous fungi, which represent major complications. Complications of pulmonary infection or pulmonary infarction may be accompanied by pleural effusion, zones of intense consolidation, or foci of cavitation.

The pathologic changes associated with ARDS are more complicated than those of pulmonary edema alone. Even early in the course of the syndrome there is extensive damage to alveolar lining cells, and fibrin, platelet microemboli, and leukocytes may be found in capillaries. The pathophysiology of ARDS is complex.[17]

PULMONARY EMBOLISM AND PULMONARY INFARCTION

Embolism Without Infarction

Experiments on animals have shown that an embolus in a pulmonary artery branch does not lead to complete pulmonary infarction unless there is also interference with pulmonary venous return or the embolus is infected.[19] Humans also may suffer pulmonary emboli without showing any radiographic or pathologic evidence of associated pulmonary infarction. The radiographic diagnosis of pulmonary embolism is not possible when there are no correlative clinical signs, and the majority of these episodes are undiagnosed. Even when radiographic signs are present, the diagnosis is very difficult unless the clinical signs and symptoms are also known.

The radiographic signs of pulmonary embolism are easily overlooked or misunderstood and are quite nonspecific as isolated findings.[10] Reduction in lung volume may be seen as elevation of a hemidiaphragm without apparent cause. A focal zone of diminished vessels, presumably due to mechanical blockage of blood flow from an embolus lodged in the supplying branch vessel, can appear as a zone of increased radiolucency (Westermark's sign).[38] This zone of hypoperfusion is much more easily recognized in retrospect than in prospect. However, it is a valuable radiographic sign when interpreted correctly (Fig. 9-13C). The radiographic appearance of decreased perfusion of a lobe or lung may also be caused by bronchial obstruction, which usually can be distinguished on expiratory chest films by air trapping that causes the abnormal side to be even more radiolucent than the unobstructed side.

Increased caliber of proximal pulmonary arteries may also be a sign of pulmonary embolism when massive emboli stuff central pulmonary arterial branches.

On PA chest films made at 6 ft target-film distance, the widest diameter of the descending branch of the right pulmonary artery adjacent to the bronchus intermedius is 16 mm in men and 15 mm in women, and the widest diameter of the descending branch of the left pulmonary artery is also less than 17 mm. Measurements greater than these indicate enlargement.[1,5] Changes in caliber from earlier films may also be a strong sign of pulmonary embolism in an appropriate clinical setting. The finding in cases of pulmonary embolism may be transient, suggesting that the dilatation is due to incomplete obstruction of more peripheral vessels. When hilar vessels on both sides are enlarged, the finding is easily mistaken for changes of primary pulmonary hypertension or even erroneously ascribed to hilar lymphadenopathy (Fig. 9-14). In a study of patients with mitral stenosis, when the width of the descending branch of the right pulmonary artery measured 15 mm or more, there was an associated pulmonary hypertension of at least 25 mm Hg at rest.[29]

Sometimes, however, prominent central vessels will appear to have vanished when current films are compared with films made before the embolus occurred; this is presumably a result of obstruction of blood flow (Fig. 9-15).

Elevation of a hemidiaphragm may well be a sign of pulmonary embolism, but it is also a not-uncommon isolated finding of indeterminate cause. Linear shadows or bands of platelike or peripheral atelectasis may also be seen in patients with acute pulmonary emboli (Fig. 9-16), presumably as a result of bronchospasm. Linear or bandlike zones of lung scarring have also been implicated as residuals of previous pulmonary infarcts.[8] Identical images, however, may often be found as nonspecific changes in lungs of patients who have no clinical or laboratory indications or pathologic changes of pulmonary embolism.

Distention of the superior vena cava and of the azygos vein may be seen as a sign of increased right heart pressure secondary to pulmonary embolism. However, these findings may also be present in patients who have heart failure from other causes.

Interpretation of these chest film abnormalities is complicated, if not confounded, by the broad and often nonspecific clinical spectrum of pulmonary embolism. In the clinical setting of patients with cardiac disease, postoperative complications, obesity, estrogen therapy, postpartum respiratory symptoms, history of recent prolonged travel, peripheral venous thromboses, accelerated clotting mechanisms, stroke, and certain malignancies, these radiographic signs deserve special consideration.

Although pulmonary infarcts are uncommon in the upper lobes, pulmonary emboli are not. Pulmonary emboli in general are most often *not* followed by infarction.

Tumor emboli may cause widespread obstruction of pulmonary microvasculature accompanied by severe signs and symptoms of respiratory insufficiency without roentgenographic abnormalities.[4] The diagnosis, if given

clinical consideration, can be made from histopathologic study of transbronchial lung biopsies.

Pulmonary Infarction

When pulmonary infarction complicates pulmonary embolism, as it may often do in patients who are in heart failure at the time of the embolism, other radiographic abnormalities evolve. These include lobar, segmental, or subsegmental zones of consolidation or atelectasis with a major axis along a pleural surface (including the fissures), "Hampton's hump" (a zone of consolidation of variable size located in a costophrenic angle and having a centrally rounded configuration; see Fig. 9-13),[12] long bands of peripheral atelectasis,[2] or rarely a long band shadow due to a thrombosed pulmonary vessel. Unfortunately, none of these radiographic abnormalities are caused *only* by pulmonary embolism and infarction, and the diagnosis of pulmonary embolism with or without infarction can almost never be based on chest film findings alone. Infarcts may be of almost any shape or size, and they are usually but not always located in the lower lobes. They may be indistinguishable from pneumonia (Figs. 9-17 to 9-19). The fact that a zone of consolidation is seen to undergo significant resolution on follow-up films in only a few days does not exclude the possibility of pulmonary embolism as a cause. Intrapulmonary hemorrhage consequent to an embolus and incomplete infarction can cause a radiographic abnormality which may clear in only a few days. Complete infarcts, however, are slow to resolve and may leave scars in the form of band shadows or nodules or may clear completely.

Pleural Effusion Associated With Pulmonary Embolus

Pleural effusion, usually unilateral and small or moderately large, may be present with or without a detectable parenchymal abnormality (see Fig. 9-13). Whenever there is a clearly disproportionate volume of pleural fluid on one side of the chest in a patient with congestive heart failure, the possibility of pulmonary embolism and infarction as a contributing cause should be considered.

The pleural effusion is often present on the initial films or within 24 hours. Most commonly the fluid has characteristics of an exudate, but occasionally it may have those of a transudate. In cases of embolism without infarction the effusion may be small and last only a few days. In cases of infarction the fluid may persist for more than a week but does not increase in amount after 2 or 3 days.[3] The appearance of subpulmonic fluid may simulate an elevated diaphragm, from which it can be distinguished by obtaining films in the decubitus position.

Clinical Signs and Symptoms

The clinical spectrum of pulmonary embolism is broad. Signs and symptoms may be absent or negligible. Dyspnea, chest pain, cough, fever, tachypnea, hemoptysis, loss of consciousness, anxiety, tachycardia, and cyanosis are variable symptoms and signs. When the embolism is massive, there may be acute right heart failure. Left ventricular failure with acute pulmonary edema may follow, along with collapse due to low cardiac output. Laboratory findings include decreased PO_2 and elevated lactic dehydrogenase, serum glutamic-oxalocetic transferase, and bilirubin. The EKG may be normal or abnormal. None of the clinical or laboratory variables is definitive.

Other Diagnostic Methods

Diagnostic methods[11,24,27,31,33] include ventilation-perfusion scans and pulmonary arteriography for assessment of pulmonary emboli, and Doppler studies, impedance plethysmography, I^{121}-fibrinogen studies, and venography for the assessment of venous thrombosis.

A noninvasive method of diagnosing pulmonary embolism with a high degree of reliability remains an elusive yet important challenge for those working in the disciplines of pulmonary and cardiovascular medicine. Accurate diagnosis is important because effective medical and surgical treatments exist to prevent life-threatening recurrences. Yet the treatments themselves, whether consisting of anticoagulants alone, embolectomy, or venous interruption by ligation or filtering devices, are hazardous and difficult to defend in the absence of a definitive diagnosis.

Pulmonary angiography is accepted at present as the most reliable diagnostic technique. When the pulmonary angiogram includes the study of vessels selectively catheterized, accuracy is increased.[24] When clots are seen as filling defects protruding into the contrast column at a site of vascular obstruction, or as sausage-like filling defects surrounded by a deflected flow of contrast material (see Fig. 9-13), the studies are highly accurate. The accuracy of less striking findings, such as slow flow to segments of lung or the filling of tortuous peripheral vessels, is not as well documented. Reliance on these signs most likely results in false-positive diagnoses.

The accuracy of pulmonary angiography in assessing pulmonary embolism is difficult to test. However, there are data that indicate that those patients who were studied angiographically for a presumptive diagnosis of pulmonary embolism, and who had negative angiograms, did not suffer or die from recurrent embolic disease in the proportions expected from data derived from untreated patients with pulmonary embolic disease. It is emphasized that both selective and superselective catheterization techniques and multiple projections need to be used to classify a pulmonary angiogram as truly negative.[27]

Perfusion and ventilation lung scans using radioactive isotopes are frequently employed in the diagnostic workup for patients with suspected pulmonary embolism. Generally, when the perfusion scan is normal the diagnosis of pulmonary embolism is considered so unlikely that more invasive studies are seldom indicated. Clearly, the correlation depends on a correct interpretation of the isotope study, and as in the interpretation of any test, observer errors do occur. Reconsideration or a second interpretation can be sought whenever clinical findings warrant.

When ventilation-perfusion scans show more than one segmental or subsegmental zone of mismatch, the likelihood of pulmonary embolism as the cause is high. Whenever chest radiographs show no pulmonary abnormalities, segmental and subsegmental zones of ventilation-perfusion mismatch are most likely indicative of pulmonary embolism. However, perfusion defects per se and even zones of ventilation-perfusion mismatch can be caused by a variety of diseases and conditions other than pulmonary embolism, and much of the controversy about the efficacy of these studies arises from false-positive diagnoses. Patients with chronic obstructive lung disease, particularly emphysema, may suffer from both false-positive and false-negative ("low probability") diagnoses based on ventilation-perfusion lung scans. The more abnormal the lungs appear on chest films, the more questionable are the results of the isotope studies. Other conditions that cause vasculitis or pulmonary vascular lesions, such as collagen-vascular diseases, chronic scarring diseases, sarcoidosis, primary pulmonary hypertension or pulmonary hypertension from Eisenmenger's physiology, tumor emboli, or emboli of foreign material in intravenous drug abusers, can mimic the scintigraphic findings of pulmonary embolism. Therefore, these nuclear medicine studies should be interpreted in close correlation with cinical data and chest film findings.[31]

When chest films show pulmonary abnormalities such as zones of consolidation or atelectasis, abnormalities of ventilation-perfusion matching in these zones are nondiagnostic. Consolidation or atelectasis caused by pulmonary embolism cannot be distinguished reliably from other causes of these abnormalities such as pneumonia. However, if a zone of ventilation-perfusion mismatch is much larger than the zone of abnormality on the chest film, then the isotope study is more reliable as an indication of pulmonary embolus, or if zones of ventilation-perfusion mismatch occur in other areas where the radiographic appearance is normal, then the isotope study findings are more reliable.

The diagnosis of pulmonary embolism is a subject of controversy, but as more carefully controlled cooperative studies are performed, at least some of the issues should become more clear. Clinical studies indicate that deep venous thromboses of the legs or the pelvic veins are precursors of the majority of pulmonary emboli. Patients who are prone to develop peripheral venous stasis and subsequent thromboses include those with cardiac disease (especially myocardial infarction or congestive heart failure), those who have sustained fractures of the legs or pelvis, those who have had major surgical procedures, burn patients, postpartum women, patients with malignant neoplasms, and patients who have been at prolonged bed rest. The role of a hypercoagulable state in some or all of these patients is also under study. Advanced age and obesity are additional risk factors.

SUMMARY

1. Two broad classes of physiologic disorders can cause pulmonary edema: high pressure in the pulmonary microvascular bed, and increased alveolar capillary permeability. These are often cardiogenic and noncardiogenic in origin, respectively.
2. In cardiogenic pulmonary edema the heart is almost invariably enlarged, unless the failure is due to acute myocardial dysfunction e.g., secondary to infarction, severe arrhythmias, trauma.
3. Reduced plasma protein concentration may play a role in the development of pulmonary edema at lower elevations of left atrial pressure than would occur in patients with normal or elevated plasma protein concentrations.
4. Pulmonary lymphatics have a critical function in clearance of fluid from the pulmonary interstitium. Obstruction of pulmonary lymphatics may rarely cause pulmonary edema, which may be focal or unilateral.
5. On chest films made with the patient erect, the blood vessels to the lower lung zones are normally of larger caliber than those to the upper lung zones because of the influence of gravity on zonal blood flow.
   a. Zonal vessel caliber may appear relatively uniform when films are made with the patient supine, in high-output states, in the presence of left-to-right intracardiac shunts, or in some cases of pulmonary hypertension.
   b. Zonal changes in vessel caliber reflect changes in

blood flow and may be seen in cases of chronic heart failure, chronic lung disease, and disorders in which relatively hypoxic lung zones may occur.
6. The radiographic changes produced by pulmonary edema can be correlated with the pathogenesis.
   a. Cardiogenic pulmonary edema may be preceded by signs of pulmonary venous hypertension: increased caliber of upper zone vessels compared to lower zone vessels on films made with the patient upright.
   b. Interstitial pulmonary edema causes loss of sharp outlines of pulmonary vessels in the lung and in the hila, often followed by the appearance of a variety of septal lines and the accumulation of interstitial fluid adjacent to pleural surfaces. Decreased lung compliance may be recognized by the high position of the diaphragm at maximum inspiration.
   c. Alveolar flooding by pulmonary edema causes an increased density of lung, sometimes to the point of intense consolidation with visible air bronchograms.
7. The distribution of pulmonary edema can vary with the cause and the severity and even with the position in which the patient predominantly rests.
8. Lung abnormalities due to diffuse infection, lymphangitic spread of neoplasm, pulmonary hemorrhage, and chronic interstitial lung disease may produce radiographic abnormalities similar to those of pulmonary edema.
9. Increased capillary permeability is initially the main pathophysiologic disturbance of ARDS.
10. Pulmonary embolism and infarction remain difficult diagnostic problems in which both the clinical and radiographic abnormalities are nonspecific.
11. Radiographic abnormalities associated with pulmonary embolism include:
    a. No discernible abnormalities
    b. Pleural effusion with or without a visible parenchymal lesion
    c. A zone of hyperlucency not explained by air trapping or technical artifact
    d. Segmental or subsegmental zones of atelectasis or consolidation due to hemorrhage or infarction of lung (a Hampton's hump configuration occurs on occasion, but is still not specific)
    e. Increase in caliber of central pulmonary artery branches
    f. Loss or diminution of the image of a central pulmonary artery branch that was clearly visible on earlier films.
    g. Signs of hypoventilation such as a high diaphragm and bands of peripheral atelectasis.

12. Regarding the interpretation of ventilation-perfusion scintiscans, there is general agreement that:
    a. A normal perfusion scan excludes pulmonary embolism for practical purposes.
    b. Ventilation-perfusion scans showing two or more large perfusion defects and no ventilation defect in a patient with negative chest films indicate a high probability of pulmonary embolic disease as the cause.
    c. The reliability of findings in between these is debatable.
13. Pulmonary arteriography remains the accepted definitive examination to rule pulmonary emboli in or out, but its diagnostic accuracy is difficult to determine.
14. A universally applicable, specific test for pulmonary embolism has yet to be developed, but tests that are designed to detect clinically occult deep venous thromboses hold great promise for both diagnosis and planned prevention of pulmonary embolic disease.

BIBLIOGRAPHY

1. Abrams HL: Radiologic aspects of increased pulmonary artery pressure and flow. Stanford Med Bull 14:97, 1956
2. Baron MG: Fleischner lines and pulmonary emboli. Circulation 45:171, 1972
3. Bynum LJ, Wilson JE: Radiographic features of pleural effusions in pulmonary embolism. Am Rev Respir Dis 117:829, 1978
4. Chan CK, Hutcheon MA, Hyland RH, et al: Pulmonary tumor embolism: a critical review of clinical, imaging, and hemodynamic features. J Thorac Imaging 2:4, 1987
5. Chang CH, Davis WC: A roentgen sign of pulmonary infarction. Clin Radiol 16:141, 1965
6. Don C, Johnson R: The nature and significance of peribronchial cuffing in pulmonary edema. Radiology 125:577, 1977
7. Elliot LP, Schiebler GL: X-Ray Diagnosis of Congenital Heart Disease in Infants, Children and Adults. Charles C Thomas, Springfield, IL, 1979
8. Fleischner F, Hampton AO, Castleman B: Linear shadows in the lung (interlobar pleuritis, atelectasis and healed infarction). Am J Roentgenol 46:610, 1941
9. Gamill SL, Krebs C, Meyers P, et al: Cardiac measurements in systole and diastole. Radiology 94:115, 1970
10. Greenspan HR, Raven CE, Polansky SM, et al: Accuracy of the chest radiograph in diagnosis of pulmonary embolism. Invest Radiol 17:539, 1982
11. Hall RD, Hirsch J, Carter CJ, et al: Diagnostic value of ventilation-perfusion lung-scanning in patients with suspected pulmonary embolism. Chest 88:819, 1985
12. Hampton AO, Castleman B: Correlation of postmortem chest teleroentgenograms with autopsy findings. With special reference to pulmonary embolism and infarction. Am J Roentgenol 43:305, 1940
13. Harley H: The radiologic changes in pulmonary venous hypertension with special reference to the root shadows and lobular pattern. Br Heart J 23:75, 1961
14. Harris P, Heath D: The Human Pulmonary Circulation. Its Form and Function in Health and Disease. 2nd Ed. Churchill Livingstone, Edinburgh, 1977
15. Hoffman RB, Rigler LG: Evaluation of left ventricular enlargement in the lateral projection of the chest. Radiology 85:93, 1965
16. Hublitz UF, Shapiro JH: Atypical pulmonary patterns of congestive failure in chronic lung disease. Radiology 93:995, 1969
17. Iannuzzi M, Petty TL: The diagnosis, pathogenesis, and treatment of adult respiratory distress syndrome. J Thorac Imaging 1:1, 1986
18. Kalenoff L, Kruglik GD, Woodruff A: Unilateral pulmonary edema. Radiology 126:19, 1978
19. Karsner HT, Ash JE: Studies in infarction II: experimental bland infarction of the lung. J Med Res 27:205, 1912
20. Lusted LB, Keats TE: Atlas of Roentgenographic Measurement. 5th Ed. pp. 268–269. Year Book Medical Publishers, Chicago, 1985
21. Mark EJ, Ramirez JF: Pulmonary capillaritis and hemorrhage in patients with systemic vasculitis. Arch Pathol Lab Med 109:413, 1985
22. Milne ENC: Physiological interpretation of the plain radiograph in mitral stenosis, including a review of criteria for the radiological estimation of pulmonary arterial and venous pressures. Br J Radiol 36:902, 1963
23. Milne ENC, Pistolesi M, Minioti M, Giuntini C: The vascular pedicle of the heart and the vena azygos. Radiology 152:1, 1984
24. Moses DC, Silver TM, Bookstein JJ: The complementary roles of chest radiography, lung-scanning, and selective pulmonary arteriography in the diagnosis of pulmonary embolism. Circulation 49:179, 1974
25. Murphy ML, Blue LR, Thenabadu PN, et al: The reliability of the routine chest roentgenogram for

determination of heart size based on specific ventricular chamber evaluation at post mortem. Invest Radiol 20:21, 1985

26. Nobel WH: Pulmonary edema: a review. Can Anaesth Soc J 27:286, 1980
27. Novelline RA, Baltarowich OH, Christos A, et al: The clinical course of patients with suspected pulmonary embolism and a negative pulmonary arteriogram. Radiology 126:561, 1978
28. Preger L, Hooper TI, Steinbach HL, et al: Width of azygos vein related to central venous pressure. Radiology 93:521, 1969
29. Shwedel J, Escher D, Aaron R, et al: The roentgenologic diagnosis of pulmonary hypertension in mitral stenosis. Am Heart J 53:163, 1957
30. Simon M: The pulmonary vessels: their hemodynamic evaluation using routine radiographs. Radiol Clin North Am 1:363, 1963
31. Sostman HD, Rapoport S, Gottschalk A, et al: Imaging of pulmonary embolism. Invest Radiol 21:443, 1986
32. Staub NC: The pathogenesis of pulmonary edema.

Prog Cardiovasc Dis 23:53, 1980
33. Thickman D, Kressel HT, Axel L: Demonstration of pulmonary embolism by magnetic resonance imaging. AJR 142:921, 1984
34. Thomas HM III, Irwin RS: Classification of diffuse intrapulmonary hemorrhage (editorial). Chest 68:483, 1975
35. Trapnell DH, Thurston JTB: Unilateral pulmonary edema after pleural aspiration. Lancet 1:1367, 1970
36. West JB, Dollery CT, Heard BE: Increased pulmonary vascular resistance in the dependent zone of the isolated dog lung caused by perivascular edema. Circ Res 17:191, 1965
37. Wescott JL, Rudick MG: Cardiopulmonary effects of intravenous fluid overload: radiologic manifestations. Radiology 129:577, 1978
38. Westermark N: On the roentgen diagnosis of lung embolism. Acta Radiol 19:357, 1938
39. Ziskind MM, Weill H, George RA: Acute pulmonary edema following the treatment of spontaneous pneumothorax with excessive negative intra-pleural pressure. Am Rev Respir Dis 92:632, 1965

Atlas

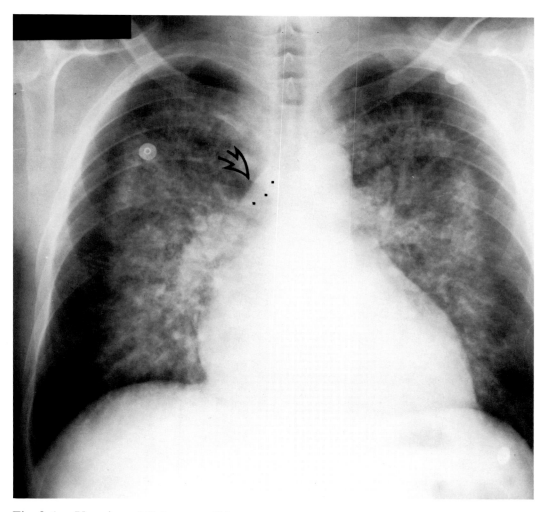

Fig. 9-1. Uremia and Pulmonary Edema

PA chest film of a young man who has been in and out of renal failure several times. There is an inhomogeneous bilateral consolidation in a classic "butterfly" distribution. The heart is moderately enlarged. The superior vena cava and the azygos vein (open arrow) are distended.

This distribution of parenchymal abnormalities is characteristic of pulmonary edema associated with uremia. That does not imply that this pattern only occurs in patients with uremia, or that all patients with uremia have this distribution of pulmonary edema. The precise reason for this striking distribution of the alveolar flooding phase of pulmonary edema is not understood.

The moderate cardiomegaly and the distended systemic veins attest to the presence of a large circulating blood volume, which is common in patients with renal failure.

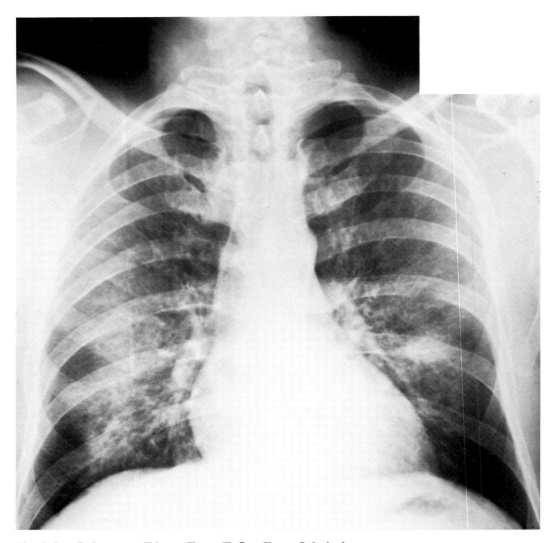

Fig. 9-2. Pulmonary Edema From Teflon Fume Inhalation

This 42-year-old man had stuck his head into an industrial oven (for inspection purposes), not realizing that there was some burning Teflon still left in the oven. Shortly after this incident he noted cough and difficulty breathing, which progressed over a short interval. He was brought to the hospital, and this chest film was made a few hours after the mishap.

Inhomogeneous mottled opacity is most marked in the central zone of each lung. The heart is not enlarged, and neither the superior vena cava nor the azygos vein is distended. These findings are characteristic of noncardiogenic pulmonary edema, which may occur after the inhalation of noxious gases or fumes. The clinical symptoms and the radiographic abnormalities cleared within a few days following treatment with intermittent positive-pressure breathing, bronchosol, O_2, and steroids.

Pulmonary edema due to increased capillary permeability may occur early after inhalation of toxic gases and may clear without apparent residuals. Some patients may also develop a late bronchiolitis obliterans with diffuse airway obstruction, manifest radiographically as pulmonary hyperexpansion with diminished peripheral vascularity.

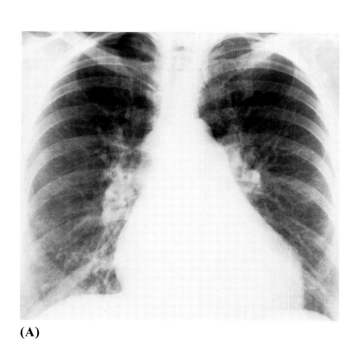

(A)

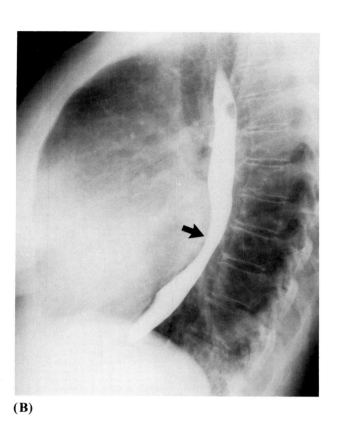

(B)

Fig. 9-3. **Pulmonary Vessel Patterns in Mitral Stenosis, Interatrial Septal Defect (Left-to-Right Shunt), Ventricular Septal Defect With Eisenmenger's Physiology, and Primary Pulmonary Hypertension**

(A,B) PA and lateral chest films, respectively, show the classic radiographic appearance of mitral stenosis. **(A)** Moderate generalized cardiac enlargement seen on the PA view. **(B)** The lateral view shows a characteristic sign of left atrium enlargement: a pronounced impression of the enlarged atrium on the barium-filled esophagus (arrow).

In addition, the anterior heart border extends high in the retrosternal position — a sign of right ventricular enlargement. The PA view shows large upper lobe vessels and small lower lobe vessels. The latter have lost their sharp outlines. Compare the sharpness of outline and the caliber of the vessels emanating from the upper portions of both hila with the appearance of the vessels in the lung adjacent to the right heart border. A similar appearance would be seen in the left lower lobe vessels, but on this reproduction they are obscured by the heart. The loss of definition of the lower lobe vessels is due to interstitial edema, which is common in patients with mitral stenosis, and reduced blood flow. The diversion of blood flow and the increased caliber of upper lobe vessels is also a reflection of chronically elevated end-diastolic left heart pressures and pulmonary venous hypertension. *(Figure continues.)*

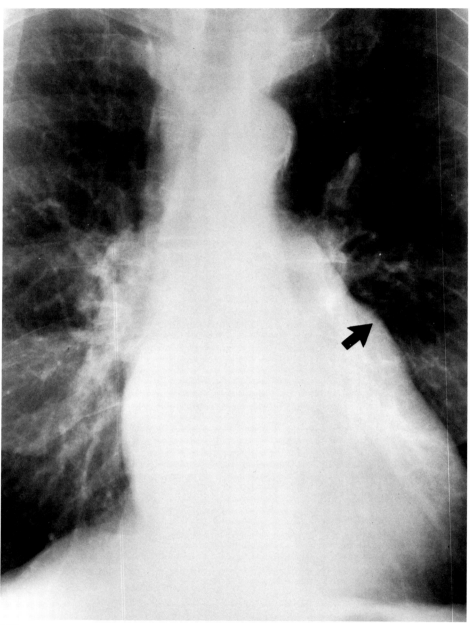

(C)

Fig. 9-3. *(Continued).* **(C)** PA view from another patient with mitral stenosis. The vessels emanating from the upper portions of both hila are relatively large in caliber compared to the vessels in the lower lung lateral to the right side of the heart. This patient shows another characteristic sign of mitral stenosis: a convexity of the left heart border (arrow), just below the pulmonary artery segment, due to enlargement of the left atrial appendage. Although the left atrium is also enlarged in the patient shown in Figs. A and B, the enlarged left atrial appendage does not present as a distinct convexity along the left heart border as it does in Fig. C. The enlarged left atrial appendage may cause only a straightening of the contour of the left heart rather than this focal convexity. Straightening of the left heart border may, however, also be seen in the normal individual. *(Figure continues.)*

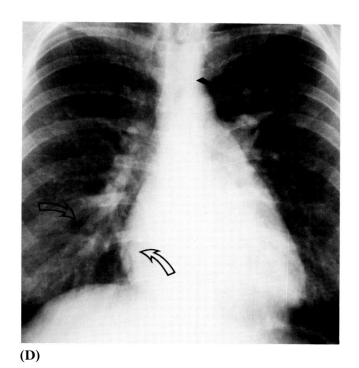

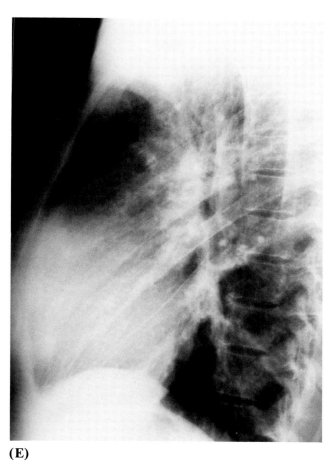

(D)   **(E)**

Fig. 9-3. *(Continued).* **(D,E)** PA and lateral views of a patient with a left-to-right shunt at the atrial level. Notice that the upper and lower lobe vessels are of increased caliber. Compare the size of the vessels emanating from the upper portions of the left hilum (between black arrows) with that of the vessels projecting medially in the right lower lung zone (between open arrows). The engorgement and increased caliber of these vessels is a reflection of increased pulmonary blood flow due to the left-to-right shunt.

There are many causes of increased pulmonary vascularity, but two broad classes account for most cases:

1. Congenital heart disease
   a. Most commonly left-to-right shunts due to atrial or ventricular septal defects or patent ductus arteriosus
   b. Uncommon anomalies such as total anomalous pulmonary venous return or transposition of the great vessels

2. High-output states
   a. Pregnancy
   b. Hyperthyroidism
   c. Paget's disease
   d. Various anemias
   e. Pickwickian obesity. *(Figure continues.)*

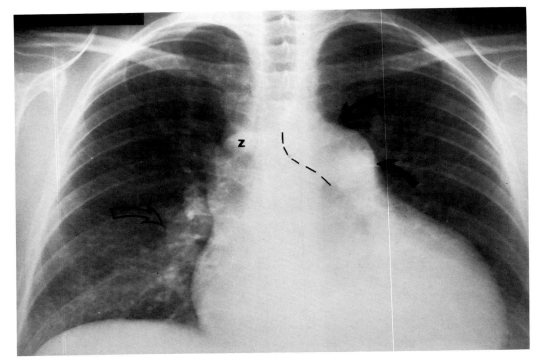

(F)

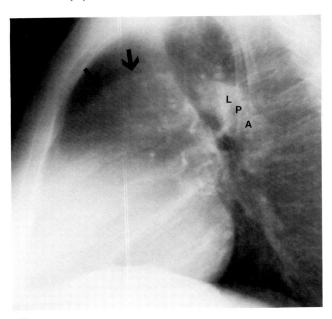

(G)

Fig. 9-3. *(Continued).* **(F,G)** PA and lateral views, respectively, of the chest of a woman with primary pulmonary hypertension. **(F)** PA view shows an enlarged heart. **(G)** Lateral view shows a high retrosternal position of the pulmonary outflow tract, (black arrows) which is a common sign of right ventricular enlargement.

On PA view, a markedly enlarged main pulmonary artery causes a pronounced convexity of the upper portions of the left cardiomediastinal border below the level of the aortic arch (between black arrows). The main pulmonary artery is so large that the aortic arch is diminutive in comparison. The aortic knob is seen as a barely recognizable image below the medial end of the left clavicle. The large main pulmonary artery is projected over the left pulmonary artery, which is seen as an area of increased radiodensity at the level of the lower black arrow. Dashed lines outline the upper margins of the left main bronchus.

On the right, the azygos vein (z) is enlarged. The mediastinal border between the right heart and the level of the azygos vein is convex to the right because of distension of the superior vena cava. The distension of the azygos vein and the vena cava are manifestations of increased right heart pressure.

Although the central pulmonary arteries are markedly enlarged (open arrow in Fig. F marks the interlobar right pulmonary artery), the peripheral pulmonary arteries are disproportionately small. This discordance of vessel caliber is a characteristic finding in pulmonary hypertension. The relatively even caliber of the peripheral vessels in the upper and lower lung zones is also a common finding. On the lateral view the main pulmonary artery shows a prominent arc where it interfaces with lung anteriorly (black arrows). The left pulmonary artery (LPA) is huge whereas the aortic arch is diminutive and presents no recognizable image in this view. *(Figure continues.)*

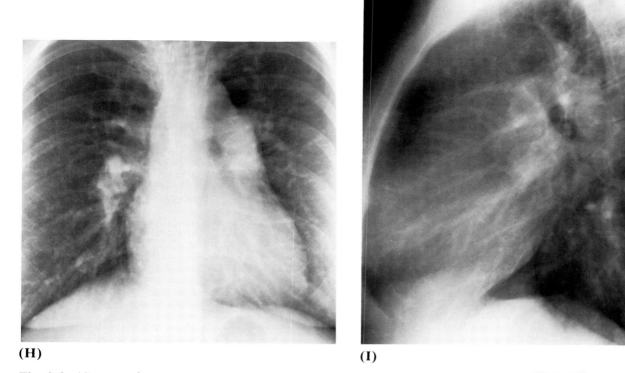

(H)

(I)

Fig. 9-3. *(Continued).* **(H,I)** PA and lateral films, respectively, of a patient with Eisenmenger's physiology from an uncorrected ventricular septal defect. The central vessels are larger than in the patient with the left-to-right shunt (Figs. D and E) and larger than the central pulmonary vessels in either of the patients with mitral valve disease (Figs. A to C). The vessels throughout both lungs are also large, as in the patient with the atrial septal defect. Furthermore, the caliber of the vessels in the upper lung zones is proportionately the same as that in the lower lung zones. Thus, this patient has large central vessels such as are seen in primary pulmonary hypertension, but rather than being disproportionately small the peripheral vessels are also larger than normal.

The series A to H illustrate the radiographic appearances of the pulmonary blood vessels as well as the mediastinal contours in patients with a variety of acquired and congenital cardiopulmonary defects. They are chosen because they display those abnormalities that are common in and characteristic of each entity. It is not always possible to make diagnostic distinctions on the basis of plain films, since some patients with Eisenmenger's physiology may show findings that are difficult to distinguish from those seen in patients with primary pulmonary hypertension, and vice versa. Furthermore, the characteristic diversion of blood flow to the upper lobes, which accounts for the increased upper lobe vessel caliber in patients with mitral valve disease, may also be seen in patients with other causes of left heart failure and with lung diseases that involve the lower lung zones more than the upper lung zones.

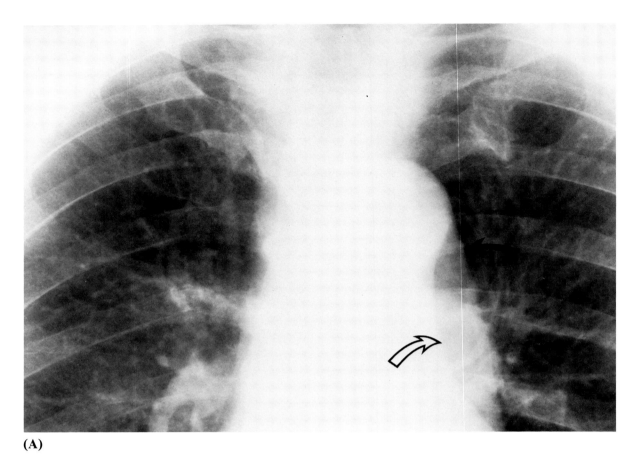

(A)

Fig. 9-4. Changes in the Appearance of Pulmonary Vessels With Left Heart Failure

Coned views of the upper lung zones of a man who has been in and out of left heart failure several times. These films are not sequential but are arranged to show progressive changes that may occur in the appearance of the upper lobe vessels and the parahilar lung as the severity of left heart failure increases.

(A) The upper zone vessels and the surrounding lung appear normal. The black arrow points to a segment of the descending thoracic aorta that is projected lateral to the anterior mediastinal pleural reflections (open arrow). The descending thoracic aorta, of course, is in a plane posterior to that of the anterior mediastinal pleural reflections. Separate edges are visible because each of these structures interfaces with adjacent lung.

(B) There is a considerable increase in caliber of the upper zone vessels and a decrease in the sharpness of detail of the hilar vessels. The black arrow again points to a segment of the descending thoracic aorta, which is more difficult to recognize in this projection, but should not be mistaken for displacement of the anterior mediastinal pleural reflection such as may occur with ductus adenopathy.

In addition to the changes in the pulmonary vessels there is an increase in width of the superior mediastinum. This is particularly noticeable in the region of the superior vena cava on the right side and the undivided portion of the pulmonary artery on the left side.

(C) Much further loss of detail of the vessels in the upper lung zones and in the hila is seen. There has also been a further increase in width of the superior mediastinum.

In Fig. B the loss of hilar detail is due to the presence of pulmonary edema, which at this stage is predominantly interstitial. Increasing width of the mediastinum is a reflection of an increased circulating blood volume. In Fig. C the pulmonary edema has progressed, and even the distended upper lobe vessels have lost their sharp interfaces with adjacent lung. The lung about the hila shows loss of detail of individual vessels as well as an overall increase in tissue density due to pulmonary edema. *(Figure continues.)*

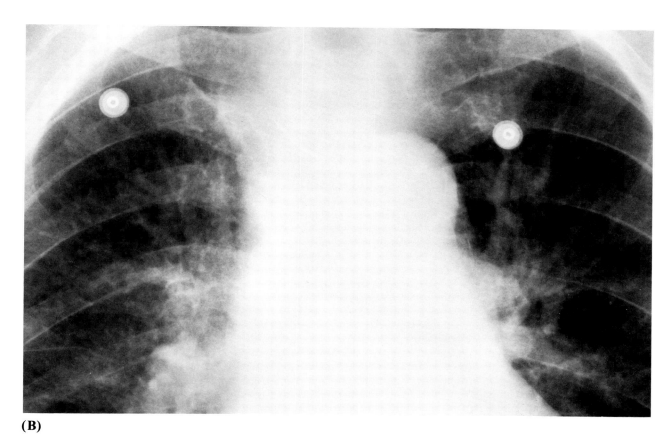

(B)

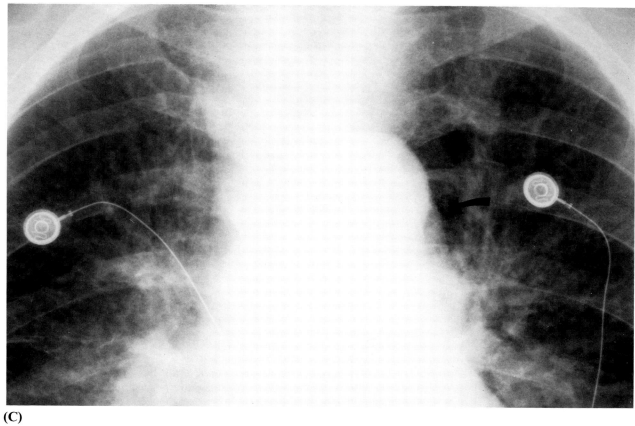

(C)

Fig. 9-4. *(Continued).*

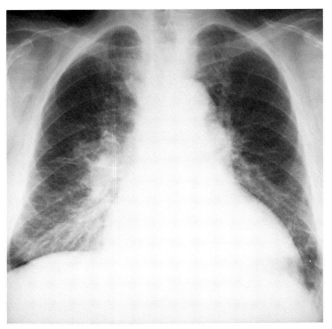

(A)

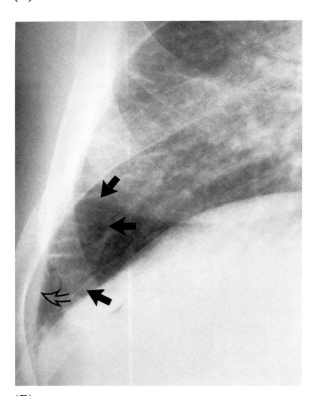

(B)

Fig. 9-5.   Interlobular Septal Lines (Kerley Lines) in Left Heart Failure

(A) PA film of a patient in left heart failure. The heart is enlarged, and the hilar and pulmonary vessels are engorged. There is marked loss of detail about the images of the perihilar vessels. The increased opacity of the lower

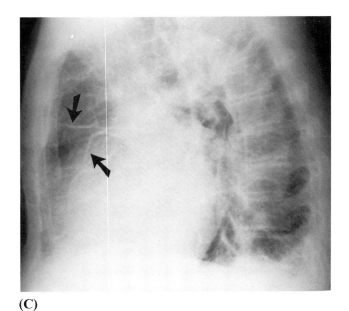

(C)

lung zones compared to the upper zones is due to pulmonary edema being more marked in the lower zones at this stage. The left hemidiaphragm appears unsharp in outline, consistent with the presence of pleural effusion. Without a lateral view, the presence of a small pleural effusion on either side is indeterminate. The ectatic descending aorta is not seen behind the heart because of the filming technique used.

(B) Coned view of the right lung base. Multiple short, nearly horizontal line images are seen in the zone of lung lateral to the black arrows. These are typical of interlobular septa distended by edema fluid in the interstitium of the lung. They are commonly known as Kerley-B lines. Also notice the gray band (open arrow) that separates the lung from the inner margins of the lowest lateral rib. This is a characteristic appearance of subpleural fluid, that is, fluid that is in the lung adjacent to the visceral pleura rather than in the pleural space itself. At times that distinction cannot be made without decubitus views.

Although septal lines are well-known signs of interstitial pulmonary edema, they may also be seen in patients with so-called lymphangitic spread of neoplasm and in patients with a variety of dust-induced diseases as a result of accumulation of abnormal cells in the interlobular septa. They may also be seen as part of the pulmonary abnormalities in other chronic lung diseases.

(C) Lateral view of the chest again shows the enlarged heart. The posterior gutters are obliterated, and the basal blood vessel images are lost within edematous lung. Anteriorly (arrows) there are long, thick septal lines (Kerley-A lines). Often, septal lines caused by edema fluid in interlobular septa are seen well in the anterior portions of the lung on a lateral view.

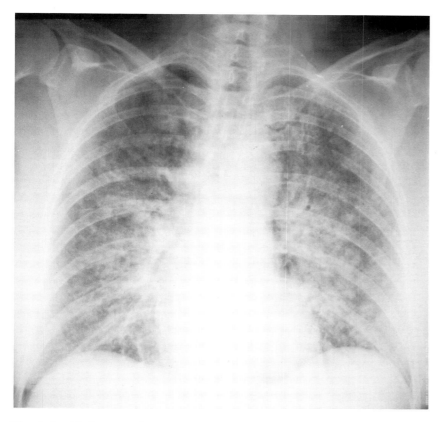

Fig. 9-6. Pulmonary Edema as an Acute Hypersensitivity Response to Blood Transfusion

This 65-year-old woman had a chest film made shortly after hip surgery when she developed signs and symptoms of pulmonary edema. She became hypotensive and was placed in the Trendelenburg position, in which she felt comfortable.

The film shows a characteristic appearance of pulmonary edema at the stage of alveolar flooding. There is mottled opacity in both lungs, which appears heaviest centrally. Along the periphery, the consolidation appears patchy and shows nodular foci measuring 1.0 cm or more and resembling acinar nodules. Notice, however, that her heart is not enlarged. The superior vena cava is distended, but the patient was supine when the film was made.

The patient's surgeon was concerned that she may have had an acute myocardial infarction. Pulmonary edema consequent to acute myocardial infarction can indeed present in this way radiographically while the heart is still not enlarged. However, a conscious patient with cardiogenic pulmonary edema would not be willing to lie flat, let alone feel comfortable in the Trendelenburg position.

During surgery this woman had received two units of blood. A transfusion reaction (hypersensitivity reaction) could cause this type of pulmonary edema by increasing capillary permeability.

The patient required intravenous fluids and pressor agents to maintain her blood pressure, and she was also treated with steroids and diphenhydramine (Benadryl). She responded promptly. Since patients with this type of pulmonary edema are depleting their intravascular volume by leaking fluid into the extravascular, extracellular spaces ("third-spacing"), it would be an error to treat them with diuretics and further reduce cardiac output.

Acute noncardiac pulmonary edema as a result of blood transfusion is thought to occur much more often than it is recognized or diagnosed. This syndrome can potentially develop in any recipient of a blood transfusion from a reaction between the leukoagglutinating and lymphocytotoxic antibodies of the donor and the leukocytes of the recipient. The reaction, which occurs within 4 hours after receiving the transfusion, is usually self-limited and consists of dyspnea, cough, fever, hypotension, and frequently an urticarial rash. Hypoxemia and diffuse pulmonary opacities are present in all affected patients. The pulmonary capillary wedge pressure is normal.

Fig. 9-7.   Measurement of the CT Ratio and Width of the Vascular Pedicle

(A) Measurement of the CT Ratio.   Line A is the distance from the estimated mid thoracic spine to the extreme right heart border. Line B is the distance from the estimated midthoracic spine to the extreme left heart border.

$$A + B = \text{transverse cardiac diameter}$$

The distance from the inner aspect of the ribs on the right side to a corresponding point on the left side across the widest part of the chest (usually just above the level of the diaphragm) is the transverse thoracic diameter (white arrows).

$$\frac{\text{Transverse cardiac diameter}}{\text{Transverse thoracic diameter}} = \text{CT ratio.}$$

The CT ratio is normally less than 50 percent in adults when measurements are taken from PA chest films made at a target-film distance of 6 feet with the patient upright.

Measurement of Vascular Pedicle Width (VPW).   Line a is the distance from the point where the image of the superior vena cava intersects the image of the upper wall of the right upper lobe bronchus to the estimated midthoracic spine. Line b is the distance from the image of the takeoff of the left subclavian artery from the aorta to the estimated midthoracic spine.

$$a + b = \text{VPW as defined by Milne et al.}^{[23]}$$

VPW is partially dependent on body habitus and varies with rotation off the true PA projection. VPW is appreciably greater in the supine than in the upright position. Although average measurements for different body types are given by Milne et al., the estimation of VPW is most useful when comparing different films of the same patient during the evolution and subsequent regression of hypervolemic states. Sequential comparisons serve as another monitor of relative circulating blood volume.

(B) Assessment of Left Ventricular Enlargement.   Left ventricular (LV) enlargement can be assessed using the criteria of Hoffman and Rigler.[15] The measurements are taken from a true right or left lateral view with a 6-foot target-film distance, made with the patient upright in deep inspiration.

Measurement A is the distance in centimeters that the posterior wall of the LV (long arrow) is projected behind the posterior margin of the inferior vena cava (IVC; arrowhead) at a level 2.0 cm cephalad from the intersection of the images of the IVC and the LV (horizontal arrow). The measurement is made on a plane parallel to the horizontal plane of the vertebrae.

Hoffman and Rigler found the mean for measurement A to be 1.15 cm and the standard deviation 0.47 cm. Using 1.8 cm as an upper limit of normal resulted in 11 percent false-positive and 19 percent false-negative predictions. (L, left diaphragm.)

Measurement B is the distance in centimeters that the intersection of the images of the IVC and the LV (horizontal arrow) is projected above the left diaphragm (vertical arrow). Using 0.75 cm as a lower limit of normal for this measurement resulted in 6 percent false-positive and 32 percent false-negative predictions.

The limitations of this method are that:

1. The intersection of IVC and the LV is not seen in approximately 20 percent of normal studies.
2. Marked deformities of the spine or the chest wall invalidate the use of these measurements.
3. Lung or pleural disease can obscure the region.
4. Enlargement of other chambers alters measurement B.
5. Rotation off of the true lateral projection causes spurious false-positive or false-negative values (see Ch. 2).

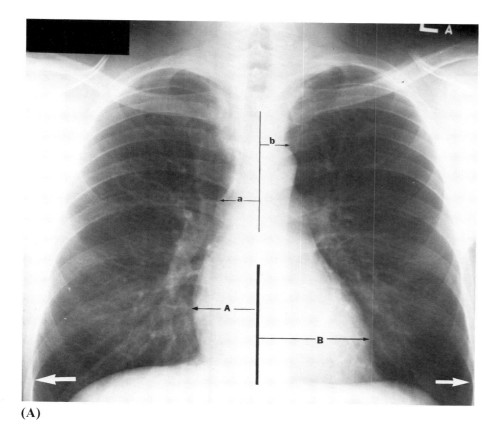

(A)

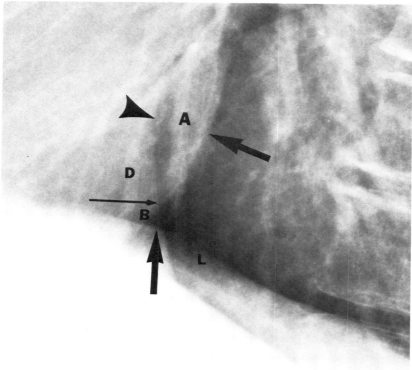

(B)

Fig. 9-7.

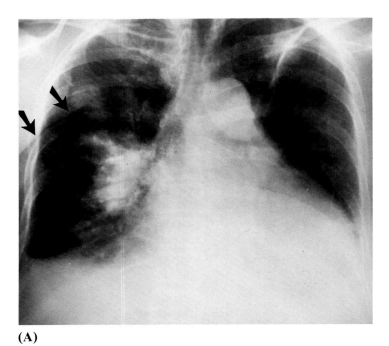

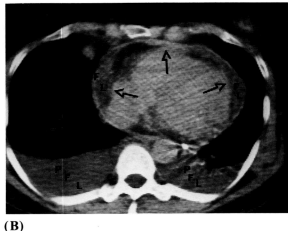

(A) **(B)**

Fig. 9-8. Enlargement of Cardiomediastinal Silhouette Due to Pericardial Effusion

(A) PA view of the chest of a woman who had had a right radical mastectomy for carcinoma of the breast. The characteristic alteration of the axillary fold seen following that operation is present on the right (arrows). A large mass is seen in the inferior portions of the right hilum, and there are irregularly margined nodules of varying size in both lungs due to metastases. A thick band image seen in the left upper lung zone is due to fibrosis from irradiation.

The heart is enlarged, and the left heart border extends almost to the chest wall. There is near-total opacification of the left retrocardiac region as a result of atelectasis and consolidation of the left lower lobe (notice the air bronchograms). There is also evidence of pleural effusion manifest by total loss of the left hemidiaphragm image and loss of the left costophrenic angle. The blunted right costophrenic angle is consistent with a pleural effusion on the right side as well.

(B) CT scan at a level just above the diaphragm. Arrows mark the margins of the heart, around which there is a mantle of pericardial fluid (FL). Pericardial effusion is a common cause of spurious cardiac enlargement on chest films or may be present in addition to cardiac enlargement. This patient underwent pericardiocentesis, and the pericardial fluid was positive for tumor cells.

Often pericardial effusion is the only radiographic manifestation of involvement of the pericardium by neoplasm, but there is no way to distinguish malignant from nonmalignant pericardial effusion on the basis of imaging studies alone. Occasionally, however, pericardial tumor nodules are large enough to be seen on CT scan.

Bilateral pleural effusions (PFL) are also present. The magnitude of pleural effusion seen on CT scan is often in excess of what would be predicted from the upright chest films (see also Fig. 8-27).

It is interesting that patients with bilateral pleural effusions from diverse causes often have evidence of excess pericardial fluid on echocardiography, and some have no chest film or clinical signs of pericardial effusion other than a slightly enlarged heart.

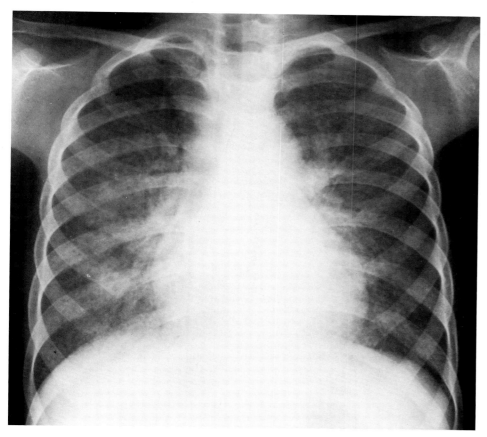

Fig. 9-9. Idiopathic Pulmonary Hemosiderosis

This young girl has a diagnosis of idiopathic pulmonary hemosiderosis (IPH). There is a mottled, granular opacification in both lungs with relative sparing of the periphery. Faint air bronchograms are present, and at the margins the consolidation has a coarsely nodular appearance.

The heart appears moderately enlarged, and there is distension of the superior vena cava. These findings are accentuated because the patient is supine, but they are also signs of the hypervolemia that is often present in patients who have profound anemia. Patients with IPH usually have a rather severe anemia, but not all have hemoptysis, especially those in the pediatric age group.

Although the appearance of the pulmonary abnormalities is characteristic of intrapulmonary hemorrhage, it is by no means specific. Alveolar flooding with blood can be precisely mimicked by alveolar flooding with edema fluid due to either cardiogenic or noncardiogenic edema or with fluid and cells from infection with a variety of microorganisms, especially *Pneumocystis carinii*.

It has been suggested that the diagnosis of IPH should be made only if immunofluorescent studies of lung biopsy specimens are negative; one should not simply rely on the absence of histopathologic changes of vasculitis. In addition, there should be no inflammation, necrosis, or granulomata in the pulmonary biopsy specimen, and no clinical evidence of renal or other organ involvement or chronic increase in pulmonary venous pressure.[34]

Anti-basement membrane antibody-induced glomerulonephritis (Goodpasture's syndrome) may produce indistinguishable pulmonary abnormalities in affected patients. Pulmonary hemorrhage may precede abnormal renal function by as much as 1 year in patients with Goodpasture's syndrome. Diffuse pulmonary hemorrhage may also occur in patients who are found to have immune complexes in alveolar walls on immunofluorescent studies of lung biopsy specimens. These are probably related to hypersensitivity reactions.

Patients who have had repeated episodes of pulmonary hemorrhage eventually have radiographic abnormalities similar to those of patients with chronic interstitial pneumonitis.

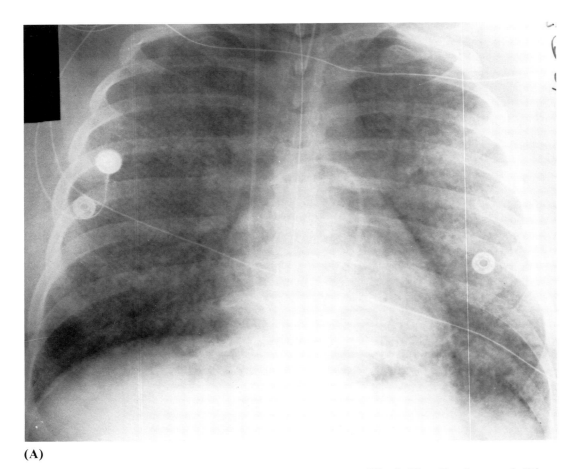

(A)

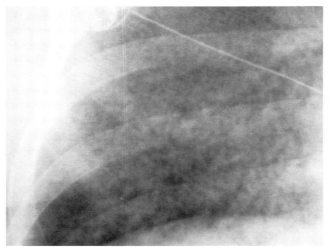

(B)

Fig. 9-10. Goodpasture's Disease

This woman had a brief febrile illness followed by hemoptysis, rapidly impaired pulmonary function, and hematuria. A lung biopsy showed intra-alveolar hemorrhage, and special stains were used to show classic linear depositions of immunoglobulins in the alveolar basement membranes.

(A) The chest film showed a marked profusion of small nodules throughout all portions of both lungs, although there are some relatively sparse zones at the extreme right base. The clinical and radiographic constellation is characteristic of Goodpasture's disease. However, intrapulmonary hemorrhage from any cause can produce an appearance indistinguishable from Goodpasture's disease, as can the edema and alveolar exudates that may accompany infections.

(B) Coned view of the right lower lung zone shows the appearance of the pulmonary lesions in greater detail.

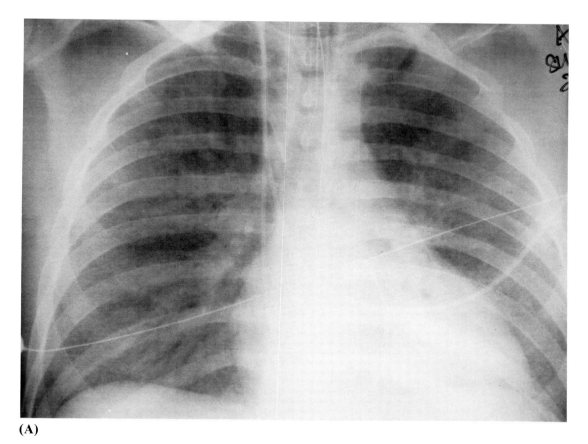

(A)

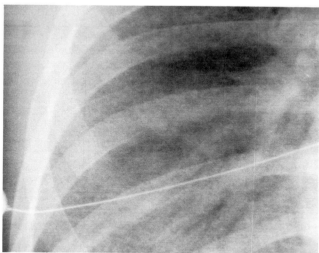

(B)

Fig. 9-11. Diffuse Alveolar Damage (Idiopathic)

(A) AP view of the chest of a 19-year-old man who had a recent flulike, febrile illness that was unresponsive to treatment. He developed rapid impairment of pulmonary function and renal failure.

Chest radiographs showed rapid progression of bilateral lung disease, which at first appeared patchy but over a few days became uniformly distributed. There is a profound loss of the images of medium and small vessels throughout both lungs and an increase in tissue density of the lungs.

(B) Coned view of the right lower lung zone shows the radiographic appearance in greater detail. I believe this appearance fits the description of "ground glass" as it is used by some observers. However, the background is composed of a multitude of closely packed, rather granular-appearing images.

Clinically this was thought to be another example of Goodpasture's disease. At lung biopsy the lesions were shown to be those of diffuse alveolar damage, but there was neither intra-alveolar hemorrhage nor evidence of vasculitis, nor was there any linear staining of the alveolar basement membranes by immunoglobulins. A renal biopsy also showed no evidence of basement membrane staining by immunoglobulins or any of the other characteristics of renal lesions associated with Goodpasture's disease. The precise etiology of this young man's illness may never be determined, but after a prolonged period in the intensive care unit he began to recover slowly. Although the images of this diffuse lung disease are not precisely the same as those shown in Fig. 9-10, the distribution is quite similar, and the radiographic spectrum of diffuse pulmonary hemorrhage encompasses this radiographic appearance. This case illustrates that a host of mixed interstitial and alveolar lesions may share a similar roentgenographic spectrum.

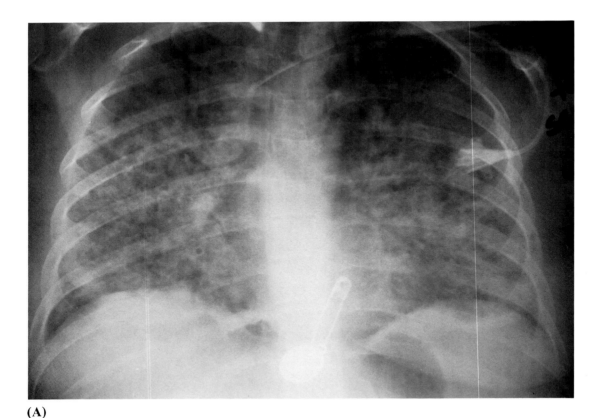

(A)

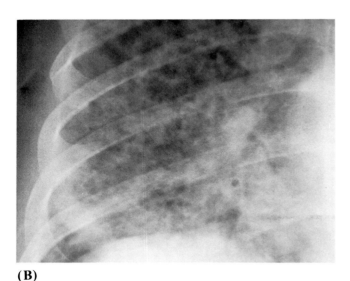

(B)

Fig. 9-12. Adult Respiratory Distress Syndrome

(A) AP film of the chest of a woman who had had extensive surgery for a recurrent carcinoma of the cervix and who subsequently suffered a prolonged period of sepsis. Within 3 days her chest film went from normal to this radiographic appearance. There is extensive bilateral lung disease characterized by inhomogeneity and a mixed pattern of ill-defined, irregular nodules of varying size as well as circumscribed radiolucencies and air bronchograms.

(B) Detail of the right lower lung zone. The patient's chest films over many days showed a monotonous repetition of these abnormalities with minor fluctuations. This behavior is characteristic of the pulmonary changes of adult respiratory distress syndrome (ARDS). Very often there is an initial appearance of mixed interstitial and alveolar edema, which commonly progresses to show so-called "air alveolograms," air bronchograms, ill-defined nodules of variable size, and patchy foci of inhomogeneous consolidation. The radiographic appearance may persist over many days while the patient is in the intensive care unit. There is a high rate of mortality, but some patients go on to show slow progressive clearing concomitant with clinical improvement. *(Figure continues.)*

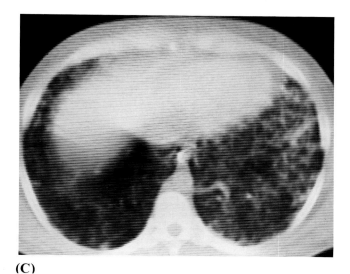

(C)

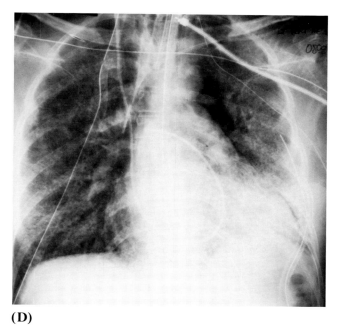

(D)

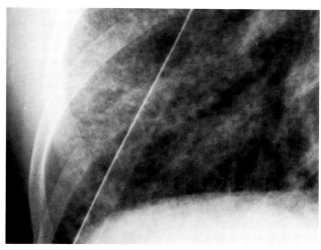

(E)

Fig. 9-12. *(Continued).* **(C)** CT scan through the lung bases of the same woman. This scan was obtained at the time of an abdominal scan done to rule out an abdominal abscess. It is a common routine to include the lung bases on abdominal CT scans. On the left you can see a diffuse network of small (about 5 mm to 1 cm) lucencies with well-defined soft tissue margins. This is a characteristic CT appearance of honeycombing, and even better detail would be shown on thinner sections. The lung is rather uniformly involved except for peripheral zones of lucency in the axillary regions that are consistent with focal emphysematous changes. Lung at the right base is less uniformly involved.

(D) PA view of another young woman who developed progressive respiratory failure coincident with a presumed viral syndrome. She did not survive prolonged treatment in the intensive care unit. The diffuse distribution of the pulmonary lesions is apparent.

(E) Coned view of the right lung base shows the character of the lesions in detail. What words would you use to describe this appearance?

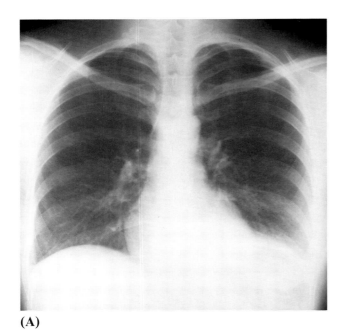

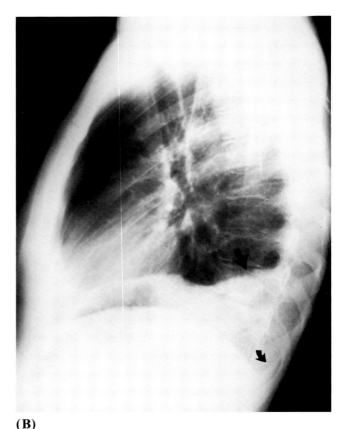

(A)   **(B)**

Fig. 9-13. Pulmonary Emboli and Pulmonary Infarction

This 34-year-old woman had recently been hospitalized for a presumptive viral syndrome and hemolytic anemia. She left the hospital feeling relatively well, but 3 days later she was awakened early in the morning with left pleuritic chest pain without cough or hemoptysis. She had some shortness of breath but no fever, chills, or myalgias. She was seen by a physician, who felt that she had a musculoskeletal problem and who gave her pain medication, which provided no relief. The following day she was seen by another physician, who recognized that she was in obvious pain, looked quite ill, and was dyspneic. On physical examination she had decreased breath sounds and a soft rub at the left base.

(A) PA film of the chest shows loss of the sharp image of the left hemidiaphragm, increased radiodensity at the left base, particularly in the retrocardiac region, and slight elevation of the left hemadiaphragm.

(B) Lateral view shows a zone of opacification completely filling the left posterior gutter. The opacity has a slightly convex contour toward the adjacent aerated lung (large arrow). There is also blunting of the extreme right posterior gutter, and a meniscoid image extends from the blunted angle up the posterior chest wall to at least the level of the next rib. This is the appearance of a small pleural effusion (curved arrow).

It may be difficult to decide how much of the abnormality on the left side is due to a parenchymal component and how much to a pleural component. This problem can usually be solved simply by obtaining a lateral decubitus view.

A focal area of consolidation in the base of the lung, with a major axis on the pleural surface and a convex contour toward adjacent aerated lung, is sometimes labeled "Hampton's hump." This appearance frequently is associated with pulmonary infarction, but is by no means specific for it. The question can be asked, however, why does the patient also have a small right pleural effusion? *(Figure continues.)*

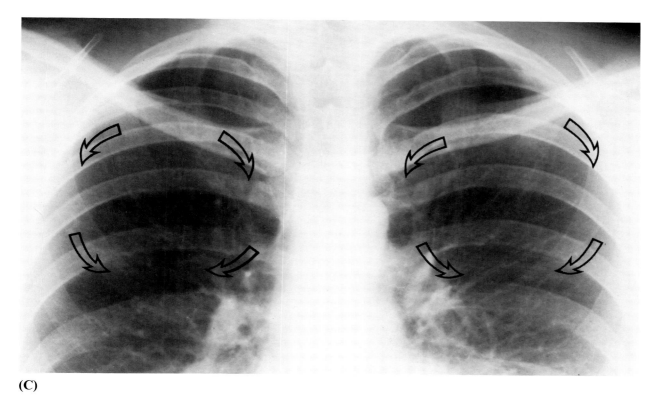

(C)

Fig. 9-13. *(Continued).* **(C)** Coned view of both upper lung zones reproduced with a different technique than Fig. A. The right upper zone appears slightly darker gray than the left. Recall that differences in gray tones between the sides of the chest are most commonly due to technical flaws. One important way to distinguish technical flaws from pathologic processes is to compare the size and concentration of vessel images on the two sides. Search and compare the lung zones within the circles of arrows. When there appears to be a true discrepancy in the vascular patterns of the two sides, the differences in overall radiodensity are more likely due to a pathologic process.

In this patient there is a clear discrepancy in vascular patterns. The vessels on the right are smaller in caliber and reduced in number compared to those on the left. The finding is subtle but definite. Pulmonary emboli are one of the causes of this discrepancy. (See Chs. 6 and 10 for other causes.)

A ventilation-perfusion lung scan was performed and showed a matching ventilation-perfusion defect involving most of the base of the left lower lobe. There was also an unmatched perfusion defect involving the apical segment of the right upper lobe and a minor perfusion abnormality in the peripheral portion of the posterior segment of the right upper lobe. These areas were normally ventilated. These unmatched defects are high-probability signs of pulmonary embolism. *(Figure continues.)*

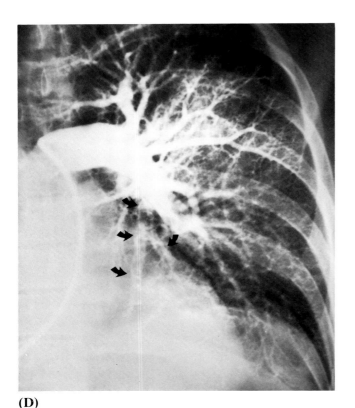

(D)

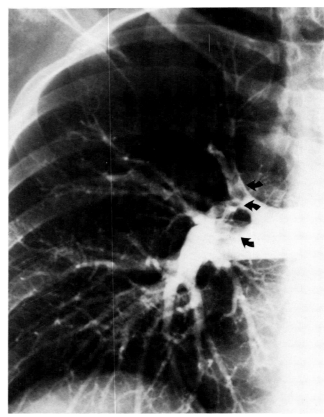

(E)

Fig. 9-13. *(Continued).* **(D)** Pulmonary arteriogram. There was a selective injection of contrast agent into the left pulmonary artery. A castlike filling defect is present in a pulmonary artery to the basilar segments of the left lower lobe (arrows). Enough contrast material enters the clot-filled peripheral branch vessels to permit their outlines to be seen.

(E) Right pulmonary arteriogram. Two large branches of the superior division of the right pulmonary artery are nearly completely filled with clot. Opacified blood passes around the margins of the clot (upper two arrows). There is also a large filling defect in the inferior division of the right pulmonary artery just past its origin (lowest arrow). These are characteristic angiographic appearances of intravascular blood clots.

This case illustrates several important radiographic features of pulmonary embolic disease.

1. Embolization with pulmonary infarction and embolization without pulmonary infarction frequently coexist in the same patient. Pulmonary emboli without infarction of the involved lung are responsible for the ventilation-perfusion mismatches seen on lung scans in these patients.
2. Ventilation-perfusion lung scans can be profitably used in the patient suspected of having pulmonary emboli even when there are zones of consolidation seen on the chest films, because other zones may contain emboli without associated infarction.
3. A small pleural effusion (such as is seen on the right side in this patient) may be present in patients with pulmonary emboli even in the absence of ipsilateral pulmonary infarction.
4. A zone of consolidation having the configuration of a "Hampton's hump" accompanied by even slight elevation of the ipsilateral hemidiaphragm and a small pleural effusion is highly suspicious for pulmonary infarction.
5. A zonal decrease in visible vascular shadows (Westermark's sign) is a significant indication of pulmonary embolism in the right clinical setting.

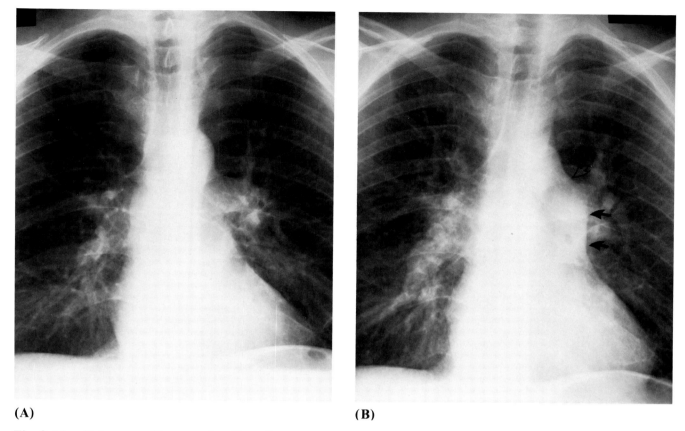

(A)   **(B)**

Fig. 9-14. Pulmonary Hypertension From Intravenous Drug Abuse

(A,B) Coned views of the chest made approximately 2 years apart in a patient who had developed severe pulmonary hypertension. At autopsy he was found to have extensive pulmonary arterial disease, probably the result of intravenous drug abuse. Evidence of talc was present in the thrombi examined under polarized light. The physiologic consequences are much the same as for a patient who has had multiple small pulmonary emboli episodically over a period of months or years.

Fig. B shows a marked increase in the size of the pulmonary arteries evidenced by change in the hila and cardiomediastinal silhouette. The pleural reflection between the aortic arch and the left pulmonary artery is less concave toward the lung in Fig. B than in Fig. A and has almost become straight. In addition, it extends higher onto the aortic arch, so that a portion of the aortic knob has been obscured. The mediastinal pleural reflection over the dilated main pulmonary artery is seen as a near-vertical edge (black arrows) in continuity with the pleural reflection over the left heart border.

Both hila show marked enlargement of vessels. Those that project end-on are particularly easy to recognize as increased in size. The vessels following the course of the major bronchi are also enlarged, but it would be possible to confuse their appearance with that produced by lymphadenopathy. The large end-on vessels, however, are the clue to the proper interpretation.

The immediate cause of death was infection and postinfectious complications secondary to AIDS.

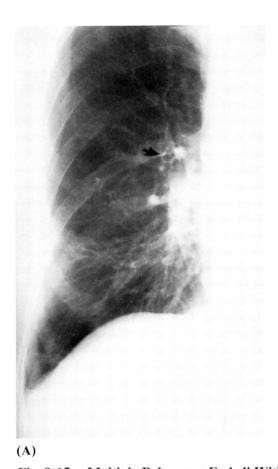

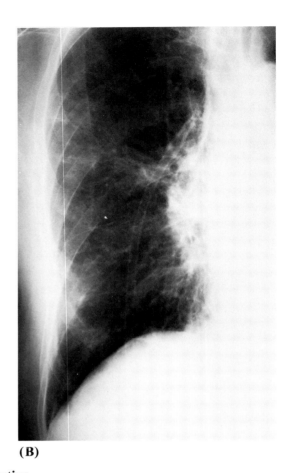

(A) **(B)**

Fig. 9-15. Multiple Pulmonary Emboli Without Pulmonary Infarction

This 70-year-old man had had an esophagogastrectomy for a carcinoma of the esophagogastric junction 5 months before the present admission. Ten days ago he became dyspneic while climbing stairs, and 2 days later noted shortness of breath while walking approximately 500 feet on a flat surface. The next day he saw his physician, who noted an irregular heartbeat and started the patient on digoxin. There was no improvement in the patient's symptoms, and 5 days later he was transferred by air ambulance. There was no history of hemoptysis, fever, chills, or chest pain.

On physical examination there were a few dry crackles at the right base and decreased breath sounds at the left base. The patient was hypoxemic (PO_2 48 mmHg) and had an abnormal EKG. There was no leg pain, swelling, or cramps. The patient was scheduled for a lung scan, and while in the Division of Nuclear Medicine he had an episode of marked respiratory distress. An EKG showed that he had developed an acute right bundle branch block. He was given a heparin bolus and oxygen and prepared for an emergency pulmonary arteriogram.

(A) Coned view of the right lung from a chest film made approximately 2 months following esophagogastrectomy. You can see the end-on projection of the anterior segmental bronchus of the right upper lobe (arrow), and immediately next to it a projection of its accompanying branch pulmonary artery is seen end-on. Caudally, you can see the end-on projection of another pulmonary artery branch.

(B) Coned view of the right lung at this admission. There has been a marked change in the appearance of the right hilum. The anterior segmental bronchus to the right upper lobe is still seen, but neither of the branch vessels seen in Fig. A are identifiable. Because of the marked distortion of the right hilum consequent to radiation treatment, it is not possible to say that this change is due solely to the presence of pulmonary emboli, but that possibility should be considered in this clinical setting. *(Figure continues.)*

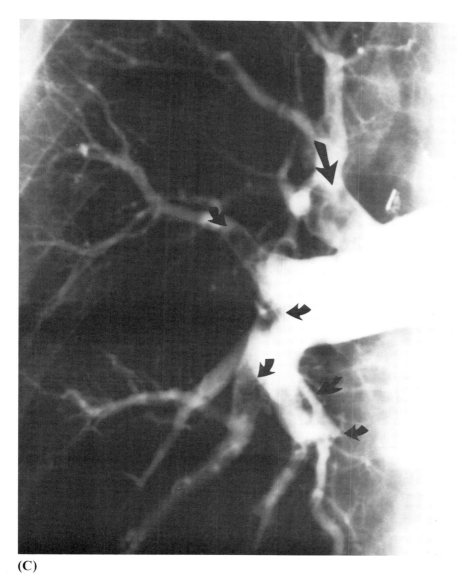

(C)

Fig. 9-15. *(Continued).* **(C)** Coned view of the opacified branches of the right pulmonary artery. Arrows point to numerous clots, which are seen as filling defects in the contrast column. Clusters of these filling defects are in the base of the superior branch of the right pulmonary artery (large arrow), and several emboli are seen in large tributaries of the interlobar branch of the right pulmonary artery (small, curved arrows). The branch to the lower lobe shows a fairly sharp cutoff (lowest arrow), and a few branches filled from just above the site of the cutoff project caudally like a pair of spindly legs.

This is an example of a patient with multiple pulmonary emboli but no radiographic sign of pulmonary infarction.

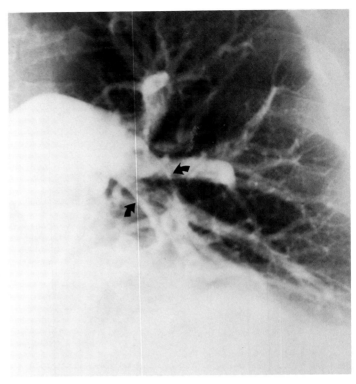

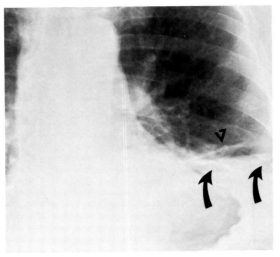

(A)   **(B)**

Fig. 9-16. Pulmonary Infarction and Probable Pneumonia

This 60-year-old man had a long history of arteriosclerotic coronary artery disease, previous myocardial infarction, and increasing angina on exertion. The angina had been worsening over the past 18 months. He was admitted for cardiac catheterization and coronary arteriography to evaluate him for possible coronary artery bypass surgery.

On admission the patient was in no acute distress. A chest film showed abnormalities of the left base that were interpreted as due to platelike atelectasis. An EKG showed signs of earlier myocardial infarctions. The patient underwent cardiac catheterization, following which he developed chest pain, cough, and fever. The cough was productive of thick sputum, and many polymorphonuclear leukocytes were found on microscopic examination. *Klebsiella pneumoniae* was cultured from the sputum in heavy growth.

The patient had repeated episodes of chest pain, which he considered to be that which he usually associated with angina. Within a few days, however, he began having blood-streaked sputum, and a repeat chest film showed further "atelectasis" in his left lower lobe. A ventilation-perfusion scan showed perfusion defects in both the right and left lower lobes. A pulmonary arteriogram showed large emboli in both the left lower and right lower lobe vessels.

(A) PA film of the chest coned to show the abnormalities at the left base. There is loss of sharp definition of the left hemidiaphragm, and there are thick (arrows) and thin (arrowhead) bandlike parenchymal abnormalities of a very nonspecific nature, such that a distinction among peripheral atelectasis, pneumonia, and pulmonary infarction cannot be made.

(B) Coned view of the left pulmonary arteriogram. A large embolus is seen as a lucent zone within the contrast column of the pulmonary artery branch supplying the left lower lobe (arrows). The size of the clot is striking compared to the caliber of the vessel.

Some questions remain unsettled: Was the pneumonia due to superinfection of the pulmonary infarction, or did the patient develop a pneumonia followed by pulmonary embolism because he was in congestive heart failure and at bed rest, or were his airways only colonized with *Klebsiella* and did he have no pneumonia at all? The patient was treated with appropriate antibiotics and heparin, and he recovered.

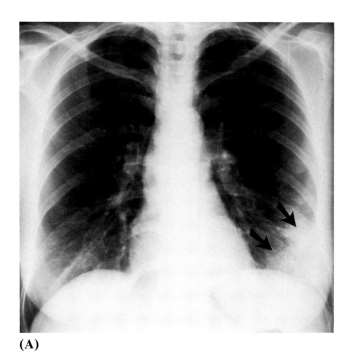 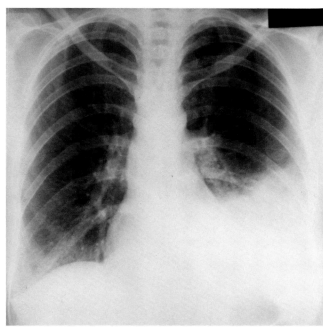

(A)   **(B)**

Fig. 9-17.   Pulmonary Infarction and Pneumonia

The patient is a 40-year-old woman who had left-sided pleuritic chest pain and shortness of breath on the evening before admission. She also had felt chilly and had a temperature of 100 degrees F. She had neither any cough nor any hemoptysis. She took some medication for pain relief and retired but during the night was awakened again with pleuritic chest pain.

Approximately 5 weeks before this episode the patient had had a vaginal hysterectomy for dysfunctional uterine bleeding. Since that time she had noted intermittent generalized anterior chest discomfort accompanied by episodes of shortness of breath.

On physical examination the patient was in acute distress with left pleuritic pain. Her temperature was 38 degrees C and respirations were 24 per minute. There was exquisite tenderness over the left posterior and anterior thorax with splinting of the left thorax and dullness with decreased fremitus and decreased breath sounds. There was tenderness in the region of the vaginal vault. The white blood cell count was 11,300 with 77 segmented forms, 17 lymphocytes, and 6 monocytes. Arterial PO_2 was 34.5 mmHg, and pH was 7.46.

A left thoracentesis was performed, revealing 2,000 white cells, of which 97 percent were mononuclear, and 2 million red cells, 15 percent of which were crenated. The protein was 4.7 grams percent, and glucose was 100 mg percent; lactic dehydrogenase was 610 units, and serum lactic dehydrogenase was 140 units. Sputum Gram stain revealed many gram-negative rods and gram-positive cocci as well as many polymorphonuclear leukocytes. The EKG was normal.

(A) PA view of the chest on the day of admission. It shows an area of consolidation peripherally in the left lower lobe (arrows). Lateral and decubitus views (not shown) revealed a small amount of pleural fluid. (Courtesy of Dr. R. Brown, Palo Alto, California.)

(B) PA view of the chest made the day after admission. There is a marked increase in the consolidation of the left lower lobe. A perfusion lung scan showed absent perfusion to most of the lower lobe and a smaller, peripheral perfusion defect in the left upper lobe. *(Figure continues.)*

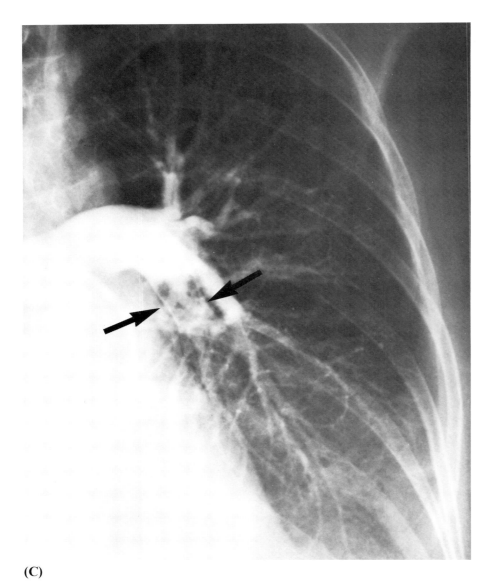

(C)

Fig. 9-17. *(Continued).* **(C)** Pulmonary arteriogram showing a large clot (arrows) practically filling the main arterial trunk to the left lower lobe. A zone of relative hypovascularity was also observed in the right upper lobe (not shown).

The initial sputum studies grew a *Haemophilus parainfluenzae.* The patient was treated with both anticoagulant and antibiotic therapy. She remained febrile, however, and in a few days subsequent sputum cultures showed a heavy growth of coagulase-positive staphylococci. Antibiotic therapy was then changed appropriately.

The large zone of consolidation seen at the left lung base is compatible with either a rapidly progressive pneumonia or an area of pulmonary embolism and infarction. Clinically, it is apparent that the patient had both a pneumonia and a pulmonary embolus with infarction. The case raises some interesting questions: (1) Were the multiple episodes of intermittent chest pain and shortness of breath following the hysterectomy due to repeated small pulmonary emboli without pulmonary infarction? (2) Did the area of infarction at the left base occur not only because there was obstruction of the pulmonary artery to this region, but also because there was infection in the lung? (3) Did the lung become infarcted because there was associated infection, or did the pulmonary infarct become secondarily infected?

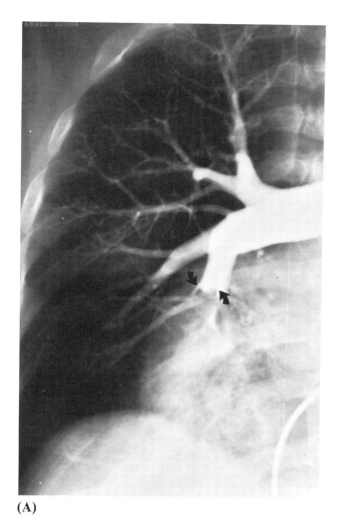

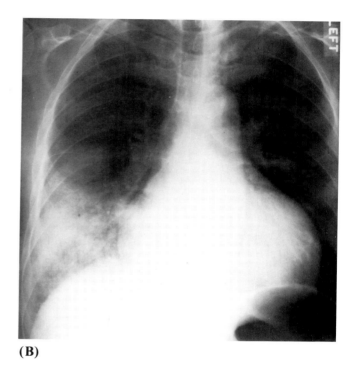

(A)

(B)

Fig. 9-18. Pulmonary Infarction

This 60-year-old man had had multiple myocardial infarctions in the previous 13 years and suffered from increasingly severe left heart failure with shortness of breath, dyspnea, orthopnea, paroxysmal nocturnal dyspnea, and continued chest pain. Six weeks before admission he noticed more acute changes with markedly increasing symptoms of left heart failure.

During his current hospitalization, he developed cough, fever, and hemoptysis. A ventilation-perfusion scan showed matched ventilation-perfusion defects on the right, but unmatched perfusion defects on the left.

(A) Opacification of the right pulmonary artery is seen following selective catheterization and injection of contrast material. There is total occlusion of the descending limb of the interlobar branch of the right pulmonary artery. Beyond the obstruction one can see an inhomogeneous consolidation in the lung superimposed on the heart in this slightly oblique projection. This consolidation due to infarction is indistinguishable from that accompanying pneumonitis. The consolidation also explains the matched ventilation-perfusion defects on the lung scan.

(B) Chest film made several days after Fig. A shows that there is still considerable inhomogeneous consolidation in the right lower lobe.

The pulmonary consolidation that occurs as a consequence of frank pulmonary infarction may take days and even weeks to clear. However, if there has been incomplete infarction and only transient bleeding into the lung, the intrapulmonary blood may clear very rapidly. Thus, if the diagnosis of pulmonary embolism has not been made, the patient may be mistakenly diagnosed as having had a pneumonia.

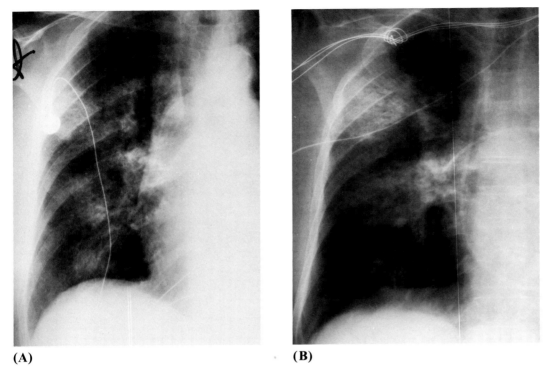

(A)　　　　　　　　　　　　　　(B)

Fig. 9-19.　Multiple Pulmonary Emboli and Incomplete Infarcts Simulating Pneumonia

(A,B) PA films (made 1 day apart) of the chest of a 75-year-old woman who had had an esophagogas-trectomy for esophageal carcinoma 2 months before. Her complicated postoperative course included respiratory problems requiring intubation, and a long period elapsed before she could be weaned from the respirator. Eventually her respiratory status stabilized. In accordance with the wishes of the patient and her family, she was discharged to home care. She was readmitted 4 days before the first film was taken because of persistent gastrointestinal difficulties, which led to dehydration. She was rehydrated but suffered increasing respiratory difficulty. Sputum cultures grew *Escherichia coli*. She was treated with antibiotics and initially her respiratory status improved. On the third and fourth hospital days she became progressively short of breath. She developed progressive acidosis that was unresponsive to treatment, and she suffered a cardiac arrest the same day the film in Fig. B was made.

(A) Poorly marginated, rounded foci of consolidation are seen in the upper, middle, and lower lung zones. **(B)** Film made approximately 24 hours later shows a significant increase in size of these zones of consolidation. Air bronchograms are seen in the consolidation in the axillary portions of the right upper lobe. Since Fig. B is more heavily exposed than Fig. A, the darker gray tone makes the lesions appear less dense even though they are increased in size.

The tip of a Swan-Ganz catheter is seen in the right pulmonary artery.

This rapid increase in consolidation of the lung is part of the expected behavior of pneumonias due to gram-negative infection. The fact that *Escherichia coli* was cultured from the sputum, however, does not necessarily establish it as the organism responsible for the pulmonary abnormalities. Patients who have been hospitalized, and particularly those who have been intubated, may become colonized by gram-negative organisms, and the pulmonary lesions they develop may or may not be related to the colonizing organisms.

At autopsy the patient was found to have massive bilateral pulmonary emboli, both recent and old. There were incomplete infarcts in the middle and upper lobes of the right lung. There was no inflammatory infiltrate to suggest a pneumonia.

This is an example of multiple pulmonary infarcts developing in a patient who had had a prolonged postoperative hospitalization with numerous complications. Although the radiographic findings are perfectly compatible with the diagnosis of pulmonary emboli and incomplete infarction, they are radiographically virtually indistinguishable from those produced by bacterial or fungal pneumonias.

10

Subacute and Chronic Noninfectious Lung Disease

This chapter considers those noninfectious pulmonary diseases that usually involve both lungs without any particular regard to anatomic segments. All of both lungs may be involved symmetrically, or there may be areas that appear more severely diseased than others. The abnormalities may show bibasilar, upper lobe, parahilar, or mantle (peripheral) predominance. The radiographic spectrum of these disorders includes examples where bilateral involvement is not apparent, but instead there is initial unilateral or focal disease. If the usual presentation is that of bilateral disease these conditions will still be included in this discussion.

The diagnosis of diffuse lung disease is usually pathologist dependent, and depending on the expertise, experience, and interests of those involved, the diagnoses can vary significantly. Therefore, an inquisitive skepticism is warranted, and it is important to consult with pathologists who devote much effort and have acquired much experience with the nuances that distinguish one entity from another.

Table 10-1 lists eight groupings of diseases and conditions that may present as noninfectious diffuse lung disease. Some of the entities (e.g., rheumatoid lung disease) can be included under more than one category. Pulmo-

nary parenchymal abnormalities associated with rheumatoid arthritis may appear much like those of usual interstitial pneumonitis, or they may present as nodules and have features of granulomatous lesions. You might also choose to place certain conditions under categories different from those I have chosen. For example, you may prefer to include chronic eosinophilic pneumonia with the hypersensitivity pneumonias. There is nothing special or unique about these groupings. They simply serve recall better than a listing of 50 or 60 ungrouped entities. If you have another method of accomplishing that, why change?

Pulmonary edema and pulmonary hemorrhage are also causes of diffuse bilateral pulmonary abnormalities on chest films, but they have already been discussed in Chapter 9. Nevertheless, they must be included in the differential diagnosis of diffuse lesions. Intrapulmonary hemorrhage may appear and resolve rather rapidly, as may pulmonary edema.

This material includes some uncommon diseases, but several rare ones (e.g., pulmonary lesions of Henoch-Schönlein purpura, Behçet's syndrome, idiopathic pulmonary ossification, and acute silicoproteinosis) are omitted.

TABLE 10-1. Subacute and Chronic Noninfectious Lung Disease

Chronic interstitial pneumonias
  Usual interstitial pneumonitis (UIP); see Table 10-2 for associated
    conditions
  Desquamative interstitial pneumonitis (DIP)
  Lymphocytic interstitial pneumonitis (LIP)
  Bronchiolitis obliterans and interstitial pneumonitis (BIP)
  Bronchiolitis obliterans and organizing pneumonitis (BOOP)
  Chronic eosinophilic pneumonia

Noninfectious granulomatous disease
  Sarcoid, including necrotizing sarcoid granulomatosis
  Histiocytosis X, eosinophilic granuloma
  Wegener's granulomatosis and variants
  Pneumoconioses
  Rheumatoid nodules

Hypersensitivity reactions
  Extrinsic allergic alveolitis due to organic dusts
  Reactions to drugs
  Reactions to blood transfusions
  Allergic bronchopulmonary aspergillosis

Unclassified
  Hemangiomatosis and lymphangiomatosis
  Alveolar proteinosis
  Lymphangioleiomyomatosis
  Tuberous sclerosis (same pulmonary lesions as lymphangioleio-
    myomatosis)
  Neurofibromatosis
  Alveolar microlithiasis
  Primary amyloidosis

Airways disease
  Emphysema
  Bronchitis
  Asthma
  Bronchiectasis
  Cystic fibrosis
  Immotile cilia syndrome

Pulmonary edema or hemorrhage[a]
  Acute hypersensitivity response
  Inhalation of toxic gases
  Aspiration of gastric juice of low pH
  Idiopathic pulmonary hemosiderosis
  Other causes of diffuse pulmonary hemorrhage
    Systemic lupus erythematosus, polyarteritis nodosa, and rarely
      other pulmonary vasculitides
    Thrombocytopenia from any cause
    Blunt chest trauma
    Goodpasture's syndrome
  Adult respiratory distress syndrome (ARDS)
  Fat embolism
  Narcotic (heroin) abuse

Neoplasms and lymphoproliferative disorders
  Malignant lymphomas and leukemias
  Bronchoalveolar cell tumors
  Intravascular bronchoalveolar cell tumors
  Kaposi's sarcoma
  Metastases
  Angioimmunoblastic lymphadenopathy
  Waldenström's macroglobulinemia
  Heavy chain disease

Conditions of infancy[b]

[a] See Chapter 9 for a discussion of these and the more usual causes of pulmonary edema or hemorrhage.
  [b] Not discussed in this text.

CLINICAL UTILITY OF PATTERN ANALYSIS

Much time can be spent arguing about the clinical utility of meticulous pattern analysis, but we all must use some form of pattern analysis whether we choose to call it that or not.[7,15] Some observers have developed pattern analysis to the level of an effective high art; the majority of more casual and less experienced observers have not. My impression, unsupported by any data, is that too many lesions characterized by inhomogeneity are considered "interstitial" when they are not. Much less commonly, lesions characterized by homogeneous opacity are considered "air space" or "acinar" lesions when they are not.

Even if pattern analysis could be used effectively by all, how significantly would differential diagnosis be influenced? For a given case of diffuse lung disease, a significant number of diagnostic possibilities will receive high rank-orders of probability, others will be ranked low, and occasionally one or two may be practically eliminated from consideration.[15] However, I cannot think of any pattern that is specific for any single cause, nor do the most avid proponents of pattern analysis make such claims. Therefore, careful correlation with clinical and laboratory data is required, and frequently lung biopsy is necessary to reach a definite diagnosis. Moreover, there are times when even histopathologic analysis and all the special tests that can be performed on a generous lung biopsy specimen yield nonspecific abnormalities that do not permit a precise diagnosis.

DISTINCTIONS BETWEEN INFECTIOUS AND NONINFECTIOUS LUNG DISEASE

When sufficient data are available it is relatively easy to distinguish pulmonary disease due to infection from pulmonary disease that is not. However, that distinction cannot be made from radiographic findings alone. Look at any article or text that provides lists for the differential diagnosis of lung disease; regardless of the radiographic pattern of the disease, the lists will include both infectious and noninfectious causes for the same pattern whether the disease is localized or diffuse. There are few exceptions.

Fortunately, the distinction between infectious and noninfectious pulmonary disease frequently can be made on the basis of clinical correlations and comparison with earlier films. In other cases the distinction simply cannot be made with enough assurance to permit good treatment planning. Some patients with subacute or chronic noninfectious lung disease may be toxic, febrile, and anemic, and have other signs and symptoms commonly seen in patients who have proven pulmonary infections. These patients often have known underlying malignancies or allergic responses to known and unknown antigens, which can cause pulmonary lesions similar to those of pulmonary infections. Proper treatment may not be forthcoming until biopsy has clarified the diagnosis.

INTEGRATING CLINICAL DATA

Commonly the initial diagnosis of diffuse noninfectious pulmonary disease is based on abnormalities seen on a chest film taken because the patient presented with respiratory symptoms.[3] Dyspnea is the commonest symptom. Cough (with or without sputum production), weight loss, fatigue, chest pain, and uncommonly hemoptysis are other, less common complaints. Even less frequently patients complain of fever or night sweats. A small but significant percentage of these patients complain of joint pains with or without any associated visible signs of joint disease such as swelling or erythema (Figs. 10-1 to 10-3).

In a minority of patients, diffuse pulmonary disease is first discovered because of abnormalities seen on a chest film taken as part of a routine examination or as part of a diagnostic workup for other disease. This is particularly true of patients with sarcoidosis and eosinophilic granuloma, and occasionally of patients with bronchoalveolar cell carcinoma, who may have no respiratory tract symptoms at the time of initial diagnosis.

Thoughtful analysis of the radiographic pattern and the distribution of the lesions in patients with diffuse lung disease is important in elaboration of the differential diagnosis.[15] However, the integration of the radiographic findings with clinical data can be even more useful. There are six questions the answers to which are extremely helpful:

1. Is the patient acutely "sick" or "not sick"?
2. Are there any known underlying or antecedent diseases or conditions, or has there been recent trauma?
3. What drugs or other treatments, including intravenous fluids, have been used or abused? Has there been a change in the drugs used in the recent past?
4. What are the details of a complete environmental history—living, working, travel, hobbies, habits, and pets? Has there been remote or recent exposure to others who have been sick?

5. What are the results of key laboratory studies—leukemoid reaction, anemia, neutropenia, eosinophilia, hematuria, abnormal immunoglobulins, blood gases, obstructive or restrictive defects on pulmonary function testing?
6. Are there certain physical findings (e.g., skin lesions, eye lesions, or bone or joint disease)?

Careful attention to the answers often will permit you to order the probabilities that a given patient falls into one or more of the eight categories in Table 10-1, and even to sequence the likelihood of specific diagnoses from most likely to least likely.

CHRONIC INTERSTITIAL PNEUMONIAS

Chronic interstitial pneumonias are an important subset of diffuse pulmonary diseases. Liebow and Carrington[21,22] have subdivided this subset into five entities based upon histopathologic characteristics. Roentgenographically, however, these subclasses have far more similarities than differences, and seldom can one reliably be distinguished from another on the basis of radiographic appearances alone. These subclasses have descriptive names:

1. Usual interstitial pneumonitis (UIP)
2. Desquamative interstitial pneumonitis (DIP)
3. Lymphocytic interstitial pneumonitis (LIP)
4. Bronchiolitis obliterans and interstitial pneumonia (BIP)
5. Giant cell interstitial pneumonia (GIP)

Of these, UIP is the most common; it has many other names such as idiopathic pulmonary fibrosis, chronic interstitial pneumonitis, fibrosing alveolitis, muscular cirrhosis of the lung, and Hamman-Rich syndrome. UIP begins with alveolar wall and capillary endothelial injury (Fig. 1). The largest single group of patients with UIP consists of those for whom the cause in unknown (idiopathic UIP).[13]

Radiographic Spectrum of UIP and DIP

The pulmonary lesions consist of fine and later coarse reticulonodular opacities. Lines and small or medium-sized irregular opacities generally predominate in the lower lung zones (Fig. 10-1) but are more widespread in patients with more severe disease (Figs. 10-2 and 10-3). Loss of detail of small vessels is also an early sign that I

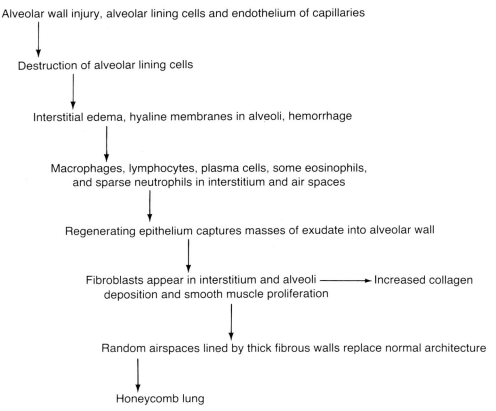

Fig. 1. The evolution of UIP. Various stages of the process are characteristically found in the same specimen along with zones of normal lung.

believe is perceived as a "ground glass" or hazy opacity by some observers. Comparison with earlier films may be required to appreciate this phase of disease. As the profusion of the lesions increases, medium-sized vascular images in the involved zones become ill defined or lost. There may also be thickening of peribronchial and perivascular tissues, and when lesions become more confluent, patchy zones of relatively homogeneous opacification become apparent.

In cases of DIP with a more cellular exudate, basilar zones of consolidation similar to those of bacterial or viral pneumonia may be present even initially. Some observers maintain that DIP is most likely an early phase in the evolution of UIP. Generally, UIP and DIP are radiographically indistinguishable. Perhaps pathologists also do not make the distinction consistently, since some local facilities where UIP is common have few biopsy-proven cases of DIP.

When the lesions of UIP progress there is a reduction in lung volume. Radiographically, the diaphragm re-mains elevated even at maximum inspiration.

If fibrosis continues, the lung architecture becomes more distorted, and progression to the diffuse honey-combing of end-stage lung disease may occur (Fig. 10-3). The late stages of many pulmonary lesions are character-ized histopathologically by extensive fibrosis with bron-chiolar dilatation and often proliferation of smooth muscle. The roentgenographic pattern is that of coarse ring shadows on the order of 5 to 10 mm in diameter occupying much of the lung and producing a honey-comb appearance. This has been called end-stage lung disease because it represents the final common stage in the evolution of lesions of diverse causes. At this stage it is often not possible to determine the nature of the origi-nal disease process.

Patients with chronic interstitial pneumonitis develop lung carcinoma with greater than expected frequency,[10] and at times the neoplasm may be occult, lost in the background of the diffuse lung disease (see Fig. 10-5).

UIP Pattern in Association With Other Clinical Entities

There is a group of patients with certain clinical syndromes — often grouped under the headings of collagen-vascular disease, connective tissue disease, or autoimmune disease — that may have UIP as a pulmonary manifestation of the disease process (Table 10-2; Figs. 10-4 to 10-6). Of this group, scleroderma and rheumatoid lung disease are the most likely to demonstrate UIP.

It should be understood that the UIP pattern is only a part of the radiographic spectrum of pulmonary lesions that may be seen with these conditions. For example, patients with systemic lupus erythematosus (SLE) may also have patchy areas of consolidation mimicking pneumonia but unassociated with any provable infection. In addition, pleural effusion with or without pericardial effusion is a more common abnormality in patients with SLE than is UIP. Patients with SLE may also have so-called lupus pneumonia or diffuse pulmonary hemorrhage, but these cases are rare.

Patients who have asbestosis may also show patterns indistinguishable from those of UIP or DIP. Similarly, graphite, talc, and diatomaceous earth pneumoconioses are also associated with the lesions of UIP[13] (Fig. 10-7).

Chronic pulmonary damage from inhalation of irritant gases or fumes such as O_2 in high concentration, chlorine, mercury vapors, or beryllium fumes may include the UIP pattern as part of the radiographic spectrum. Ingestion of toxic chemicals such as kerosene or Paraquat may also be associated with development of UIP.[21]

The chronic phase of pulmonary reactions to certain drugs such as hexamethonium, nitrofurantoin, methotrexate, busulfan, phenytoin, and bleomycin may also manifest as the UIP pattern. Drug-induced lung disease is discussed later in this chapter.

TABLE 10-2. Diseases and Conditions That May Have Lesions of UIP[13,21]

Connective tissue diseases
  Rheumatoid arthritis
  Scleroderma
  Dermatomyositis
  Polymyositis
  Systemic lupus erythematosus
  Mixed connective tissue disease

Pneumoconioses due to asbestos, graphite, talc, diatomaceous earth

Pulmonary injury
  Irritant gases and fumes
  Reaction to drugs
  X-irradiation
  Viral pneumonias
  Ingestion of toxic chemicals

Familial interstitial pneumonia

Chronic radiation damage to the lung may also have a histologic pattern similar to that of UIP, but the distribution of the abnormalities conforms to the radiation treatment portals and usually can be distinguished from the other causes of UIP on that basis alone.

Lymphocytic Interstitial Pneumonitis

LIP is a subclassification of chronic interstitial pneumonitis characterized by lymphoid cell infiltration of the interstitium of the lung (Fig. 10-8). It is apparently very difficult to distinguish LIP from malignant lymphoma involving the lungs on the basis of the histopathology alone. Distinctions among LIP, pseudolymphoma, and lymphocytic lymphoma based on immunochemical techniques may be more reliable. Patients with LIP often have symptoms of cough, chest pain, fatigue, low-grade fever, and weight loss. Three of the 13 patients in one series had Sjögren's syndrome.[17] Some type of gammopathy or autoimmune disease was frequently present, and 10 of the 13 had abnormal immunoglobulin levels. Five patients died primarily as a result of respiratory tract involvement.

Radiographically, the pulmonary patterns observed in patients with LIP are within the spectrum of patterns associated with UIP, such as a diffuse, fine or coarse reticulonodular pattern. Honeycombing may develop as a late complication.

Some patients develop conglomerate foci of consolidation varying in size from less than 1.0 cm to over 4.0 cm in diameter and resembling coarse nodules or small masses.

Patients with Waldenström's macroglobulinemia or angioimmunoblastic lymphadenopathy may show similar radiographic pulmonary lesions associated with lymphadenopathy, and patients with a diffuse form of pulmonary amyloidosis may do so as well. Some patients (e.g., Haitians and children with AIDS) may also develop LIP with or without manifest intrathoracic lymphadenopathy.

Bronchiolitis Obliterans

Bronchiolitis obliterans is characterized by obstruction of bronchioles and alveolar ducts by granulation tissue with destruction of peripheral airways and scarring.[24] Bronchiolitis obliterans may occur in a relatively pure form as judged by histopathology, but at other times there are also significant components of organizing pneumonia (bronchiolitis obliterans with organizing pneumonia, or BOOP).[24]

These histopathologic diagnoses, like those of other chronic interstitial pneumonias, seem to be pathologist dependent in that some specimens judged to be representative of idiopathic pulmonary fibrosis (UIP) may later be judged as indicative of bronchiolitis obliterans by the same or by another pathologist. Similarly a diagnosis of "organizing pneumonia" alone may be made at one time and "bronchiolitis obliterans with organizing pneumonia" (BOOP) at another, even though the same specimen is being analyzed. A mixture of these lesions in the specimen may account for some of these discrepancies.

Although not common disorders, BIP and BOOP occur over a broad age range from infancy to advanced age, with a male predominance. Malaise, fever, dyspnea, and cough with or without sputum production are the predominant symptoms. The majority of cases are idiopathic, but the abnormalities may be found as an aftermath or concomitant of viral, mycoplasma, bacterial, or fungal pneumonias, and they have also occurred after inhalation of toxic chemicals and gases. Some have coexisted with a variety of clinical entities such as heart failure, malignant lymphoma, leukemia, connective tissue diseases, allergic reactions, eosinophilic pneumonia, and bronchiectasis. Bronchiolitis obliterans due to chronic graft-versus-host disease has also been reported in bone marrow transplant recipients.[31] Early experience in heart-lung transplant recipients suggests that bronchiolitis obliterans may be an important manifestation of lung rejection. Clinically, it is detected by signs and symptoms and pulmonary function tests indicating airway obstruction. These usually precede roentgenographic evidence of diffuse disease.

The radiographic spectrum of bronchiolitis obliterans is broad[16,24]:

1. Nodular opacities may vary from granular to many millimeters in size (Fig. 10-9). When the primary pattern is that of small (2 to 3 mm), widely distributed nodules there is a likeness to miliary tuberculosis. Coarse, irregular nodules of varying size may be due to abnormal secretions in bronchiectatic foci proximal to obliterated peripheral bronchi (Fig. 10-10). Larger nodules may appear as patchy foci of consolidation, which can mimic pulmonary edema when they become confluent. Linear shadows in conjunction with small nodules may present a reticulonodular or lineonodular pattern similar to UIP.
2. Foci of opacification may occur with bibasilar, lobar, segmental, or diffuse distribution. These may regress and recur spontaneously (Fig. 10-11). Occasionally focal zones of opacification due to BOOP may be found even in asymptomatic individuals.
3. Hyperinflation without consolidation may be seen in patients who have survived the initial lung damage from toxic inhalation as well as in some of the

other conditions associated with bronchiolitis obliterans. Hyperinflation, however, is rare as the sole manifestation. Patients may have unilateral hypoperfusion due to a presumed postinfectious destructive bronchiolitis in childhood (Macleod's or Swyer-James syndrome), and the situation may not be diagnosed until adulthood. The involved lung is usually smaller than the uninvolved lung, and the ipsilateral pulmonary artery is small because of reduced blood flow. On expiration the radiographic signs of air trapping are accentuated. This would not occur if the primary disorder were due to an underdeveloped pulmonary artery.

4. The chest film has been reported to be normal in a few biopsy-proven cases of bronchiolitis obliterans.[13]

Giant Cell Interstitial Pneumonia

Giant cell interstitial pneumonia is a subclassification of interstitial pneumonitis originally based on analysis of five patients. It is distinguished from UIP by the presence of large, intra-alveolar, multinucleated cells (described as bizarre)[21] added to the more common cellular infiltrate of UIP.

GIP is a rare form of interstitial pneumonitis with no distinguishing clinical or radiologic features. It was at first considered to be idiopathic but later was related to inhalation of tungsten carbide dust.[35]

Chronic Eosinophilic Pneumonia

Chronic eosinophilic pneumonia can be considered as a distinct member of the chronic interstitial pneumonias or as a hypersensitivity pneumonia. A variety of other pulmonary lesions may be associated with a high percentage of eosinophils in the pulmonary exudate, and often, but not invariably, with blood eosinophilia as well. Among these are polyarteritis nodosa, allergic angiitis of Churg and Strauss, allergic bronchopulmonary aspergillosis, tropical pulmonary eosinophilia (associated with filaria infestation), and Löffler's syndrome.

Chronic eosinophilic pneumonia is of special interest because it can have a radiographic appearance that is nearly diagnostic.[12] Young and middle-aged adults are affected most commonly. Although females are more commonly afflicted than males, the difference is not great enough to have diagnostic significance. Some patients have a history of asthma or atopy and some do not. Most patients have significant blood eosinophilia (Fig. 10-12), but some do not (see Fig. 10-14). Some patients have acute febrile illnesses with cough, whereas others have subacute or chronic illness associated with cough and wheezing. Clinical symptoms respond rapidly to treatment with steroids, but radiographic clearing lags by a few days.

The *radiographic appearance* is frequently one of consolidation of lung about the periphery of the upper and middle lung zones, with fading off caudally (Fig. 10-12). This lesion distribution is so seldom due to other causes that some patients have been treated on the basis of the radiographic and clinical findings without biopsy confirmation. However, patients who have had mantle irradiation may have a similar distribution of radiation pneumonitis.

The cause of chronic eosinophilic pneumonia is usually unknown, but in some patients allergic pulmonary reaction to drugs (e.g., bleomycin[38] may be responsible (Figs. 10-13 and 10-14). Not all patients with chronic eosinophilic pneumonia have this characteristic distribution; some have radiographic changes similar to other chronic interstitial pneumonias. Some patients have recurrent episodes (Fig. 10-14).

Loeffler's syndrome is a benign syndrome of cough and malaise, usually of mild degree. Radiographically, patchy zones of consolidation show rapid fluctuations. Within a day, one area of consolidation can clear partially or totally while a new area appears elsewhere. The illness can last for 1 to 2 weeks, but complete recovery is the rule.

Correlations and Assessment of Severity

In general, there is little correlation between chest film appearances and distinctive histopathologic findings in the chronic interstitial pneumonias. Therefore, prebiopsy distinction of one from the others lacks precision. Cases of chronic eosinophilic pneumonia provide the exceptions.

Frequently there is a surprising discordance between lung function estimated from the degree of radiographic involvement and that measured by blood gas determinations and pulmonary mechanics (see Fig. 10-1). In general, the measured reductions of diffusing capacity and the increase in the alveolar-arterial O_2 pressure difference more accurately reflect the clinical severity of the pulmonary disease than does either the physical examination or the extent of radiographic abnormalities. Pathologic specimens in many cases of chronic interstitial pneumonias reveal more disease than would be estimated from the radiographic findings.

Carrington and Gaensler have reported that 7.7 percent of 508 patients undergoing biopsy for diffuse infiltrative lung disease had chest films that were considered normal even when severe disease was present in the biopsy specimen. This group included patients with UIP, DIP, sarcoid, BIP, allergic alveolitis, asbestosis, and lymphangioleiomyomatosis.[3]

It is general theory that the chronic interstitial pneumonias have an early stage of inflammatory alveolitis, during which there is exudation of a variety of inflammatory and immune effector cells. The response to treatment with corticosteroids is greatest during this stage and becomes less and less effective when the alveolitis has been replaced by fibrosis. Unfortunately there is no universally recognized variable, radiographic or clinical, that permits distinction between these histopathologic phases. Repeated lung biopsies to make the assessment are impractical. Some investigators place reliance on analyses of cell types retrieved from bronchial lavage and intensity of gallium-67 uptake on lung scans as a measure of alveolitis, but others do not.

NONINFECTIOUS GRANULOMATOUS DISEASES

The infectious granulomatous diseases caused by tubercle bacilli and the pathogenic fungi have been discussed in Chapter 5. Noninfectious granulomatous diseases comprise an important subset of conditions that may present radiographically as diffuse pulmonary disease.[4,5,12,20,25] Sarcoidosis, eosinophilic granuloma, Wegener's granulomatosis, a variety of pneumoconioses, and nodular rheumatoid lung disease are the main members of the noninfectious granulomatous disease group considered here. Granulomata may also be components of the pulmonary lesions of hypersensitivity pneumonitis. Wegener's granulomatosis and necrotizing sarcoidal granulomatosis may also be classified as pulmonary vasculitis.

Radiographic Appearances

Granulomatous nodules due to sarcoid, eosinophilic granuloma, silicosis, or coal worker's pneumoconiosis may be seen on chest films as nodules 1 to 3 mm in diameter, fairly discrete, rounded but often irregular in outline, and distributed widely throughout both lungs. In general, these nodules are very similar to one another in size. There may be true sparing of the apices (Fig. 10-15A to C) or the lateral bases (Fig. 10-15D) in some patients, which allows a tenuous distinction from miliary tuberculosis. Often, however, distinction from miliary tuberculosis or miliary dissemination of fungal infections is not possible. Much of the time, the distinction between infectious and noninfectious granulomatous disease presenting as a miliary pattern can be made from correlation of clinical and radiographic findings. In ill patients, however, that is often not possible, and some form of tissue biopsy is required to permit rational treatment.

Reticulonodular patterns are also part of the radiographic spectrum of noninfectious granulomatous disease. In some cases the nodules may be larger—on the order of several millimeters to 3 cm in diameter (Fig. 10-16). The spectrum also includes larger, rounded foci of opacity with sharp or unsharp margins and even air bronchograms. When due to sarcoidosis this pattern is often called "alveolar sarcoid" even though the lesions are likely due to extensive involvement of the interstitium and compression of alveoli rather than to alveolar filling (Fig. 10-17).

Patients with Wegener's granulomatosis frequently present with large nodules or zones of consolidation or even large masses (Figs. 10-18 and 10-19).

The nodular pulmonary lesions of silicosis or coal worker's pneumoconiosis may coalesce into zones of massive fibrosis[8] (Fig. 10-20). Progressive massive fibrosis (PMF) is manifest radiographically as large, irregular opacities most commonly seen in the upper zones bilaterally. Distortion of mediastinal contours, retraction of hila, and tenting of diaphragmatic contours due to contraction in volume of the involved lung may also be present. Pericicatricial emphysematous changes also occur about these conglomerate lesions. Pulmonary function is ordinarily well preserved in patients with coal worker's pneumoconiosis, but in those who progress to massive fibrosis, as in patients with silicosis, function is impaired. Sarcoidosis may cause radiographically similar massive lesions but does so uncommonly (Fig. 10-21).

Cavitation

Radiographically visible cavitation of lesions is questionable, if ever, in eosinophilic granuloma, rare in sarcoid, and common in Wegener's granulomatosis (see Fig. 10-18) and rheumatoid lung nodules. The coalescent lesions of PMF may cavitate because of aseptic necrosis or concomitant tuberculous infection. Caplan's nodules,[2] ranging from less than 1 cm to more than 4 cm in diameter, occur in the lungs of patients with rheumatoid arthritis and coal worker's or silica-related pneumoconioses. Caplan's nodules may cavitate but radiographically are indistinguishable from nodules that may be seen in the lungs of patients with rheumatoid arthritis and no known pneumoconiosis.

Cystic spaces, more like those seen with severe emphysema than true cavitation, may occur in association with marked distortion of lung architecture in late stages of noninfectious granulomatous disease (Fig. 10-22).

Distribution of Lesions

Although the parenchymal lesions of sarcoidosis are frequently diffuse, with sparing of the apices and lateral bases as previously noted, the spectrum includes patients whose lesions, radiographically at least, appear localized to one or both upper lobes. They can present as rather clustered nodular foci or foci of inhomogeneous consolidation (Fig. 10-23) as in patients with necrotizing sarcoid granulomatosis.[5]

Patient's with Wegener's granulomatosis may show area of segmental or subsegmental consolidation with or without associated nodules or cavitary masses. Air bronchograms may be seen in the zones of consolidation. A diffuse reticulonodular pattern also occurs but is unusual. A solitary nodule is also unusual for this entity as well as for sarcoid or eosinophilic granuloma. Patients with pseudolymphoma or lymphomatoid granulomatosis may show lesions similar to Wegener's granulomatosis, but they may not be true entities distinct from non-Hodgkin's lymphoma.

Patients with histiocytosis X or eosinophilic granuloma may show predominant disease in the upper lobes, with areas of emphysematous or cystlike lucencies as well, but lesions throughout both lungs are also common. The apices and extreme bases are frequently spared. A small percentage of patients with sarcoidosis or eosinophilic granuloma may suffer a progression of clinical symptoms. The pulmonary lesions can progress to a stage of diffuse honeycomb lung even after many years of a relatively benign clinical course. Patients with silicosis frequently show predominance of the small nodular lesions in the upper lobes.

Lymphadenopathy

Hilar and mediastinal lymphadenopathy is common in patients with sarcoidosis and silica-related pneumonoconioses and in patients with berylliosis. Hilar and mediastinal lymphadenopathy is unusual in the other noninfectious granulomatous diseases, with the possible exception of histiocytosis X in children.

Patients with sarcoidosis may present with hilar and mediastinal lymphadenopathy in the absence of any visible parenchymal disease, with hilar and mediastinal lymphadenopathy presenting simultaneously with radiographically apparent parenchymal disease (Fig. 10-24), or with radiographically apparent parenchymal disease but no detectable mediastinal or hilar lymphadenopathy. Some observers refer to these as stages 1, 2, and 3, respectively, or as stages 1, 2a, and 2b, reserving stage 3 for those patients who have extensive fibrosis. Although it is incorrect to say that anterior mediastinal nodes are not involved in sarcoidosis, it is true that *massive* anterior mediastinal nodal involvement—such as may occur in malignant lymphomas—is rare or does not occur in patients with sarcoidosis.

Adenopathy due to silicosis may show peripheral rims of calcification, which have been described as eggshell calcification, and this may also be seen in a small number of patients with sarcoid as well as other lesions, which have been discussed in Chapter 8.

HYPERSENSITIVITY REACTIONS

Hypersensitivity reactions to a variety of antigens were also briefly discussed in Chapter 9, because pulmonary edema may be a part of the radiographic spectrum acutely. Bilateral pulmonary lesions within the radiographic spectra of chronic interstitial pneumonitis and the noninfectious granulomatous diseases, however, are common in the subacute and chronic phases of hypersensitivity pneumonitis.

Extrinsic Allergic Alveolitis (Hypersensitivity Pneumonitis)

A large variety of organic dusts and fungal spores can act as inhaled antigens. A substantial variety of molds and fungal spores may be found in air circulating from contaminated air conditioners or humidifiers, or in association with certain farming operations or the processing of plant materials or food products. Avian proteins contaminate the air inhaled by bird fanciers (Fig. 10-25). The lists of these offending agents continue to grow to the point where it appears the *someone* will react to almost any organic dust.

In theory these inhaled antigens produce a precipitating antibody in susceptible hosts, which then interacts with complement in the pulmonary interstitium to produce a pathologic response in the lungs. Atopic patients may have an immediate asthma-like response provoked by inhalation of these antigens as well as delayed symptoms 4 to 6 hours later. Nonatopic patients generally have a delayed response. Symptoms in the delayed type of response usually consist of dyspnea without wheezing, and there may be accompanying fever and night sweats. Some patients also have malaise, anorexia, weight loss, headache, and even hemoptysis. Exposure to low levels of antigen may result in an insidious course, with signs and symptoms that patients frequently do not associate with the precipitating events.[37] Often the symptoms will abate when the patient is not subjected to the antigenic stimuli and recur when the stimulus is reencountered. At times there may be a history of onset of symptoms only when the patient has returned to the hostile environment

after a substantial absence (e.g., weeks to months) even though before the absence the patient recognized no symptoms while functioning in the same environment (Fig. 10-25).

Radiographic appearances vary. There may be multiple small, relatively discrete, widely disseminated nodules, often with sparing of the apices and bases. These small nodules may vary from barely recognizable to a few millimeters in size. There may also be a reticulonodular pattern and a pattern consisting of patchy foci of consolidation, which if unrecognized as to cause and untreated may become more massive (Fig. 10-25). Late changes of pulmonary fibrosis and honeycombing may develop much as in other causes of chronic interstitial lung disease. The differential diagnosis includes that of viral pneumonia and the other chronic interstitial pneumonitides as well as sarcoid and some of the pneumoconioses. At times the problem of diagnosis persists even after appropriate clinical and laboratory studies have been performed and even after lung biopsies have been obtained. The environmental history is critical in the diagnosis of these conditions. Treatment usually relies on removing the patient from the offending environment and the use of corticosteroids.

Allergic Bronchopulmonary Aspergillosis

Aspergillus organisms may provoke an allergic form of lung disease in susceptible patients. This is distinct from the invasive, destructive pneumonitis, vasculitis, and pulmonary infarction that *Aspergillus* can cause in patients with altered immunity, and from the saprophytic *Aspergillus* fungus balls that may develop in preexisting cavities.[14] In general, patients with allergic aspergillosis have a personal or family history of atopy or asthma, but this is not invariable. Usually, there is eosinophilia and a delayed hypersensitivity skin response to *Aspergillus* antigen. Patients also have precipitating antibodies against *Aspergillus* antigen and an immediate skin response to this antigen.

Characteristic radiographic abnormalities in this condition are associated with the presence of central bronchiectasis, that is, bronchiectasis that involves the proximal portions of the bronchi while the caliber and contours distally remain normal. These bronchi may become filled with mucoid impactions and may be seen as a series of lobulated, branching soft tissue opacities along the expected course of major bronchial branches. These stuffed bronchi have been called "gloved finger" contours (Fig. 10-26). Although involvement of upper lobes is common, lower lobes may be involved simultaneously or alone. When the dilated bronchi are not stuffed with mucus, they may appear as ring shadows on radiographs, or they may have air-fluid levels when only partly filled. Large zones of homogeneous consolidation may also be found in these patients. The lesions usually respond rapidly to corticosteroid therapy, but some patients with long-standing disease may develop scarring and gross distortion of lung architecture. Occasionally patients have been reported to have normal plain chest films but abnormal bronchograms, with the abnormalities best seen on post-tussig films.

Drug-Induced Lung Disease

The list of drugs known to be associated with or capable of inducing pulmonary disease in susceptible persons grows longer and longer, but the diagnosis still remains one of association and exclusion. The radiographic and histopathologic changes are often characteristic but still not diagnostic. The incidence of untoward reactions to offending drugs is low, but reactions occur with sufficient frequency to present diagnostic problems. Why some patients have a pulmonary reaction to a drug whereas others do not is unknown.

The drugs implicated can be classified into several groups: antibiotics, chemotherapeutic drugs, analgesics and narcotics, diuretics, anti-inflammatory agents, antihypertensive or antiarrhythmic agents, and antidepressants. In addition to these medications, patients may have reactions to blood transfusions or to oily medications chronically aspirated into the lungs. The interval between commencement of drug use and onset of pulmonary reaction is enormously variable—from hours to years. Some of the reactions appear to be dose dependent, as is the case with bleomycin and amiodarone, but the range of total dose before the onset of pulmonary disease may be broad.

The radiographic appearance[26] may vary from a subtle loss of detail of small vascular images at the lung bases (Fig. 10-27) to frank pulmonary edema. Reticulonodular opacities, patchy irregular consolidation, focal or widespread, some more marked at the lung bases, some more marked at upper zones (Fig. 10-28), and some showing combinations of these patterns, may also be seen. At times the distribution may be peripheral when the reaction is that of chronic eosinophilic pneumonia (see Figs. 10-13 and 10-14). Different patterns may predominate for certain drugs, but early and late components of these reaction patterns may vary for the same drug. Small pleural effusions may accompany the pulmonary reactions, and some drugs (e.g., antiepileptics) may be associated with hilar lymphadenopathy.

Treatment for drug-induced pulmonary disease primarily involves discontinuing the drug and sometimes the use of corticosteroids.

Unfortunately, the signs and symptoms of pulmonary reaction to drugs are frequently similar to those of pulmonary infections, and there is often a great reluctance to treat patients, especially those who are immunocompromised, with steroids until infection can be reasonably excluded. Such exclusion can seldom be accomplished without some type of biopsy.

Radiographic clearing of the acute phase may be dramatic but is often more gradual for subacute and chronic lesions. Death from pulmonary insufficiency may occur in a small percentage of patients, either acutely or after a subacute or chronic course.

Drug-induced pulmonary reactions in cardiac patients may mimic those of cardiogenic pulmonary edema but will not respond to diuretics. The pulmonary edema from blood transfusion reactions occurs within hours of the transfusion and is usually accompanied by hypoxemia, hypotension, and signs of hypovolemia; the use of diuretics in treatment would be detrimental (see Ch. 9).

Oxygen toxicity and radiation lung damage can cause pulmonary lesions histopathologically similar to those of reactions to drugs, but the latter are usually confined to known treatment portals whereas the former is diffuse but temporally related to treatment with high concentrations of oxygen.

When drug-induced pulmonary disease occurs in patients with a variety of malignant lymphomas, the radiographic appearances may be indistinguishable from those produced by rapid pulmonary progression of the lymphoma itself. Clinical signs and symptoms can also be similar, and distinction usually requires biopsy.

Lipoid Pneumonia

Lipoid pneumonia due to chronic aspiration of mineral oil used as cathartic, or of oil used in nose drops, is uncommon. Occasionally, however, these lesions are still found in elderly patients who give a history of taking mineral oil before retiring for sleep. While asleep, they aspirate oil that refluxes from the stomach. Similarly, oil may be aspirated by patients with a variety of swallowing disorders or neurologic deficits. I recall at least one patient who used oil to lubricate his tracheostomy stoma and developed a nodular zone of lipoid pneumonia in a lower lobe.

Radiologically, foci of oil pools surrounded by foreign body reaction appear as nodules or masses, solitary or multiple, showing either poorly defined or relatively sharp margins. They are mostly found in the lower or middle lobes or the lingula. At times the lesions may appear as consolidation of segments of lung as in pneumonia. Thickening of the interstitium may also result from accumulation of lipid-laden macrophages, which in turn produce a radiographic pattern of interstitial lung disease. Solitary masses of lipoid pneumonia simulate lung cancer; the fact that patients are often asymptomatic or have only nonspecific pulmonary symptoms is no help in differentiating between the two.

Lipoid pneumonia might better be considered as an irritant chemical pneumonitis than as a hypersensitivity reaction.

A form of endogenous lipoid pneumonia (cholesterol pneumonia, golden pneumonia) may occur peripheral to sites of obstruction of bronchi by neoplasm. When multiple small airways are obstructed, as may occur with infiltrating carcinomas or bronchoalveolar tumors, the associated chronic inflammation may be a substantial part of the radiographic image. Fluctuations in the inflammatory components from film to film (see Ch. 6) may mislead you into considering the lesion to be benign, particularly when the associated neoplasm is slow growing.

OTHER CAUSES OF CHRONIC NONINFECTIOUS LUNG DISEASE

Pulmonary Alveolar Proteinosis

Pulmonary alveolar proteinosis (PAP) is an uncommon, diffuse lung disease characterized by the presence of a periodic acid-Schiff positive-staining lipoprotein in the alveoli.[6] Theories of its pathogenesis implicate derangement of normal surfactant reprocessing, which results in decreased reuptake of surfactant by the alveolar lining cells and thus accumulation of the surfactant phospholipid in the alveoli. Accumulations of phospholipid have been found in alveolar spaces in association with focal interstitial pulmonary disease or with other systemic diseases such as leukemia or lymphoma. These may be considered part of the syndrome of "secondary alveolar proteinosis." The mechanisms of accumulation and derangements of metabolism may be similar to those of primary PAP, but in either case the precise cause is conjectural.

The most common and the major presenting symptom in patients with primary PAP is progressive dyspnea and limitation of physical activity. There may be associated cough, which is usually nonproductive or minimally productive. Clinically, the patients are seldom as ill as you would expect from their chest film appearances, and some are asymptomatic. Adults are more often affected than children, but cases have been reported even in infants.

The radiographic appearance may simulate that of pulmonary edema, with parahilar distribution of large

zones of consolidation. Some patients, however, show poorly defined patchy zones of opacity bilaterally, and these patchy foci may be very inhomogeneous. Septal lines may be visible, simulating an interstitial lung disease pattern when in fact the disease is primarily one of alveolar filling. Resolution may follow pulmonary lavage or may occur spontaneously (Figs. 10-29 and 10-30). There is, however, a significant mortality due to either progressive respiratory failure or complicating infection. A variety of opportunistic infections, such as cryptococcosis, nocardiosis, mucormycosis, mycobacterial infections, and histoplasmosis, have been reported in association with PAP. In most reported cases these infections have antedated the use of pulmonary lavage therapy.[6]

Lymphangioleiomyomatosis

Lymphangioleiomyomatosis is a rare pulmonary abnormality involving women in their reproductive and immediate postreproductive years, but isolated cases in postmenopausal women are known.[34] Abnormal quantities of smooth muscle are found in lymphatics and around alveolar septa and the walls of bronchi and blood vessels. Radiographically, there may be a reticulonodular appearance (Fig. 10-31), a fine honeycomb appearance, or other appearance of diffuse interstitial lung disease with the distinctive absence of reduction in lung volumes. Spontaneous pneumothoraces are frequent and may be often the event that first brings the patient to medical attention. Pleural effusions are common and are characteristically chylous (Fig. 10-32).

Patients with tuberous sclerosis may show radiographic and histopathologic abnormalities identical to those of lymphangioleiomyomatosis (Figs. 10-33 and 10-34). These may be accompanied by other stigmata of tuberous sclerosis or only with hamartomas of the kidneys.

Cystic Fibrosis (Mucoviscidosis)

Cystic fibrosis is a hereditary disease of infants and children. It is usually fatal, but with modern treatment methods increasing numbers of patients live to adulthood.[29] The fundamental defect involves abnormalities in the secretory functions of the exocrine glands. Progressive obstructive pulmonary disease and pancreatic insufficiency account for most of the clinical manifestations. Elevated levels of sodium chloride are found in sweat, and the clinical diagnosis depends on this analysis.

The lungs of patients with mucoviscidosis are damaged by plugs of mucus in the bronchial tree, which result in areas of peripheral atelectasis, obstructive pneumonitis, bronchiectasis, and mucoid impaction.[29] Pulmonary infection remains a constant threat. Staphylococcus and *Pseudomonas* sp. are common organisms responsible for pneumonia in these patients; other gram-negative pneumonias occur less commonly. Older patients may become colonized with *Aspergillus* and develop symptoms analogous to allergic bronchopulmonary aspergillosis. Radiographic abnormalities are reflections of the structural abnormalities and the ravages of repeated infection (Figs. 10-35 and 10-36). Patients with the immotile cilia syndrome and Kartagener's syndrome may show similar pulmonary radiographic abnormalities. Cilial malfunction is secondary in patients with mucoviscidosis. Hilar and mediastinal adenopathy caused by benign reactive changes due to chronic and recurrent pulmonary infection may be seen in some patients. Large central pulmonary arteries may develop in association with pulmonary hypertension. There is an increased incidence of pneumothorax associated with destruction of lung architecture.

OBSTRUCTIVE AIRWAYS DISEASE

Chronic obstructive pulmonary disease (COPD) is a clinically important subset of lung disease. Patients with COPD are a common source of referrals to physicians who specialize in disease of the chest. The name "chronic obstructive pulmonary disease" is considered poor medical terminology because it lumps together entities of diverse pathology. The clinical utility of the expression, however, makes it unlikely to be abandoned.[32]

Emphysema and Bronchitis

Pulmonary emphysema is defined in terms of its pathologic anatomy, and regardless of the nuances of different definitions there is general agreement that the definition includes enlargement of the air spaces peripheral to the terminal bronchiole. In the United States, destruction of alveolar walls is usually included as an integral part of the definition. Clinically, however, the patient with symptomatic emphysema has physiologic impairment due to chronic air flow obstruction.

Chronic bronchitis is defined in terms of its clinical presentation: an otherwise unexplained productive cough lasting at least 3 months for each of 2 successive years at a minimum.[32,36]

The clinical and physiologic abnormalities accompanying emphysema and chronic bronchitis overlap to

such a degree that it is extremely difficult to separate the contribution of each. They are therefore commonly considered under the heading of COPD. Within this classification, however, there are patients who primarily complain of dyspnea without significant cough and sputum production, and others whose symptoms are marked by cough and excessive sputum production. Hypoxemia and hypercapnia in the latter group are often in excess of those whose symptoms are predominantly those of dyspnea alone.

Pathologic specimens from both groups show emphysema and abnormalities of the airways, but the abnormalities of the large and the small bronchi are more severe in the patient with the symptoms of chronic bronchitis. Pathologic assessments of the lungs of patients who had emphysema, combined with studies of function, show that patients with measured severe chronic air flow obstruction have anatomic emphysema of moderate severity or worse. At the same time, some patients who anatomically have emphysema of moderate severity have no or mild air flow obstruction.[36]

The pathologic anatomy of emphysema is used to categorize and subclassify abnormalities. Centrilobular (centriacinar) emphysema is a form characterized by abnormalities in the proximal part of the acinus with selective distortion of respiratory bronchioles. Panacinar emphysema is characterized by a more uniform dilatation of the entire acinus. Mixtures of these forms also occur. Paraseptal emphysema involves the distal portions of the acinus, with a predominant distribution about the periphery of the lung including a distribution about interlobar fissures; it may be associated with apical bullous disease in young adults who have spontaneous pneumothoraces but are otherwise asymptomatic. Focal emphysema may also occur about areas of scarring in the lung.[32,36]

Centriacinar emphysema is more common in the upper parts of the lungs, and panacinar emphysema occurs in both the upper and lower zones but is somewhat more common in the lower portions of the lungs. It is likely that the severity of the emphysema and the proportion of the lung involved have more important clinical consequences than does the specific type of emphysema. Emphysema associated with α_1-antitrypsin deficiency is of the panacinar type.

Several different published series have attempted to correlate the radiographic diagnosis of emphysema with the extent of anatomic disease. The results have been discordant; both high and low correlations have been reported.[36] However:

1. In general, emphysema that is associated with clinical evidence of air flow obstruction and air trapping is more readily recognized radiographically than is anatomic emphysema that is not.

2. The majority of patients with severe anatomic emphysema will show radiographic abnormalities, but some will not.

3. Applying strict criteria to distinguish patients with mild to moderate emphysema from those without will improve the identification of those with emphysema. However, this will be accomplished by an increase in the incidence of false-positive diagnoses.

4. Chronic bronchitis, without signs of air trapping, cannot be diagnosed consistently on the basis of radiographic abnormalities. "Tramlines" (the radiographic appearance of thickening of bronchial walls paralleling the segmental and subsegmental bronchi) and thickening of the walls of bronchi seen end-on have been used by some as indications of chronic bronchitis, but their precise pathologic counterparts have not been clearly established. In some patients an unexplained prominence of bronchovascular markings has been described as a radiographic correlate of clinically manifest chronic bronchitis, but again the precise pathologic counterpart has not been elucidated. Furthermore, this appearance may be impossible to distinguish from the appearance of lung in heavy-set patients without clinical manifestations of bronchitis.

The radiographic hallmark of emphysema is that of "large-volume lungs" (Fig. 10-37). There are a variety of ways to define "large-volume lungs," but in general the following criteria suggested by George Simon are most functional for me.[33] At maximum inspiration only a small percentage of adults will move their diaphragm low enough so that any portion of the costochondral junction of the anterior seventh rib is seen above the diaphragm shadows on the chest film. This constitutes a functional definition of a low diaphragm (see Fig. 10-38). A flat diaphragm can be defined as one whose highest arc does not extend, on a perpendicular, at least 1 cm above a line connecting the ipsilateral costophrenic angle with the ipsilateral vertebral-phrenic angle. The same determination can be made from the lateral view by measuring the height of each hemidiaphragm from a line connecting the anterior and posterior extremities of the diaphragm. Of course, one seldom actually makes these measurements; rather the judgment of whether or not a diaphragm is flat is made from visual inspection.

Other signs of increased lung volume include an increase in the anterior clear space (i.e., the amount of lung that is seen projecting anterior to the cardiac silhouette and great vessels on the lateral view). Ordinarily this space is only 2 to 3 cm deep in the normal individual (measured from a point 3 cm below the sternomanubrial junction). In addition, the lower limit of this space is usually on the order of 7 cm or more above the diaphragm. In emphysema, however, this portion of aerated lung may extend as low as 3 or 4 cm above the diaphragm (Fig. 10-39).

In using these findings as variables in the diagnosis of pulmonary emphysema, it is of course important to use common sense, just as one would in the use of any isolated finding. For example, tall individuals such as one might find on a basketball team might all be expected to have low hemidiaphragms, although they assuredly do not have pulmonary emphysema. The other signs are also fallible but still useful in the appropriate clinical setting.

The heart in patients with emphysema is often described as being narrow and vertical, but this is probably a manifestation of the low position of the diaphragm, and it will not be seen in patients who have coincident hypervolemia associated with polycythemia or cardiomegaly of ischemic heart disease.

A reduction in the size and number of vessels in zones of emphysema is another radiologic variable. There also may be prominence of the central pulmonary vessels and a rapid tapering of peripheral vessels (Fig. 10-40). However, these findings are not present, unfortunately, in a significant proportion (roughly one-third to one-half) of patients with anatomically proven severe emphysema. Even in patients with widespread and severe radiographic abnormalities associated with pulmonary emphysema, there will be areas of lung that contain more large blood vessels than others, since obviously the cardiac output must be accommodated and portions of least-involved lung receive more blood flow.

Bullae may also be seen in patients with diffuse emphysema. They are usually multiple and may vary greatly in size (Figs. 10-37 and 10-39). Occasionally giant bullae occur, occupy large portions of a hemithorax, and cause severe pulmonary function impairment. Bullae may also occur in patients with paraseptal emphysema without symptoms or functional disturbances associated with chronic airflow obstruction (Fig. 10-41). For these patients the major consequence of the bullous disease is often recurrent pneumothorax.

The term "saber-sheath" trachea (see Ch. 8) has been applied to a characteristic deformity of the intrathoracic trachea that has been seen in association with pulmonary emphysema. In this condition the anteroposterior caliber of the trachea as seen on the lateral view is two or more times greater than the coronal diameter as seen on the PA view of the chest over the extent of the intrathoracic portion of the trachea. There are other causes of narrowing of the trachea, but these are usually circumferential.

Asthma

The majority of adults and children who have asthma have normal-appearing chest films when not suffering an attack. Asthma is defined as a condition characterized by increased sensitivity of the tracheobronchial tree to a variety of stimuli, resulting in episodic, reversible airway narrowing. During an attack there may be radiographic signs of air trapping, particularly in patients with severe or longstanding asthma. Thickening of bronchial walls and prominence of hilar vessels (the latter related to pulmonary hypertension) may also be seen on chest films of patients with severe and long-standing asthma.

Patients with partially obstructing neoplasms of the trachea and major bronchi may be misdiagnosed as having asthma becuase of wheezing heard on auscultation. Patients who have aspirated foreign bodies that impact in proximal bronchi also show signs of air trapping. Usually the episode of aspiration is remembered by the patient, but occasionally it is remote and forgotten.

Since pulmonary infection may precipitate an attack of asthma, chest films are often obtained when the patient presents for diagnosis and treatment, to rule out pneumonia as the cause of the acute episode.

Bronchiectasis

Bronchiectasis is an irreversible dilatation of bronchi. If bronchograms are performed on a patient during the convalescent phase of pneumonia, the bronchi supplying the involved lung may appear abnormally large and lose their normal, distally tapering configuration — very much as in true bronchiectasis. Yet if the study is repeated after complete resolution of the pneumonia, the bronchi have reverted to normal. This is one source of "reversible bronchiectasis," but others, unexplained as to cause, have also been documented.

Ectatic bronchi may appear as dilated tubular structures that do not taper but become wider as they extend peripherally. Lack of filling of obstructed distal side branches is the rule. This form is called cylindrical bronchiectasis. Some patients show a marked ballooning of the involved bronchi with extensive pruning of distal branches. This form is called cystic bronchiectasis (Figs. 10-42 to 10-44). There are intermediate and mixed forms as well, to which other names such as "varicose bronchiectasis" have been applied. The precise distinctions between bronchial abnormalities associated with severe chronic bronchitis and those due to cylindrical bronchiectasis are not clear. However, chronic bronchitis is usually considered a diffuse process whereas bronchiectasis is usually focal or multifocal in distribution. Patients with allergic aspergillosis (see section on "Hypersensitivity Reactions") show a rather unique form of bronchiectasis consisting of a proximal ballooning of the involved bronchi, which taper off to a more normal appearance distally.

Patients with bronchiectasis are bothered by excessive sputum production, which may be foul smelling when infected. Repeated pulmonary infections and bouts of hemoptysis are also common complaints. Although hemoptysis is seldom voluminous, in some patients with so-called dry bronchiectasis it may be the major symptom. Some patients only have minimal symptoms of chronic cough.

The cause of bronchiectasis in an individual patient is often unknown. In many patients it is probably a sequela of childhood pneumonia.[36] Tuberculosis was at one time a common cause of upper lobe bronchiectasis; it is now less common. Bronchiectasis can also develop peripheral to lesions that cause partial bronchial obstruction.

Patients with mucoviscidosis, the rare immotile cilia syndrome, and Kartagener's syndrome develop bronchiectasis frequently. It is likely that ineffective bronchial clearance mechanisms and consequent chronic infection play an important role.

Since bronchiectasis is usually a focal or multifocal process rather than a global disturbance of pulmonary structure, patients often have surprisingly little functional impairment. In patients with severe and extensive bronchiectasis, however, dyspnea may be a significant problem along with severe derangements of pulmonary function. The incidence and prevalence of bronchiectasis in populations with good access to medical care seem to be on a marked decline.

NEOPLASM

Patients with so-called "lymphangitic" spread of metastases (Fig. 10-45) or rapid increases in neoplasm burden, such as may occur in patients with malignant lymphoma (Fig. 10-46), mycosis fungoides, or small nodular metastases (Figs. 10-47 and 10-48), or patients with bronchoalveolar cell carcinoma may have radiographic abnormalities that overlap the spectrum of appearances of chronic pneumonias, infectious and noninfectious granulomatous disease, and drug-induced lung disease. Establishing the correct diagnosis usually requires biopsy (see Ch. 6).

CT IN THE EVALUATION OF DIFFUSE LUNG DISEASE

The precise role of CT in the assessment of diffuse lung disease is as yet unknown. The density discrimination inherent in the CT technique permits recognition of details of form and distribution of parenchymal lesions that are not apparent on chest films (see Figs. 10-33 and 10-34). Although very fine miliary lesions may be unrecognized on the usual 10-mm-thick sections, modern equipment permits the use of 1.5-mm-thick sections that provide significantly increased detail and are successful in imaging very small lesions.

A few studies have correlated CT findings of emphysema[9] and UIP (fibrosing alveolitis)[27] with chest film studies and pathology specimens. In cases of fibrosing alveolitis, CT scans showed the patchy nature of the disease process that would be anticipated from histopathologic study but is not always apparent on chest films. For example, chest films frequently show the bibasilar predominance of the lesions of UIP, but CT provides an additional dimension, showing that there is also a peripheral predominance even at the more heavily involved lung bases. Whether or not the distinctions will remain significant when larger numbers of patients have been studied is unknown.

CT may also be useful in distinguishing patients with large bullae, who may benefit from resection, from those that have diffuse emphysematous lungs that sometimes may mimic bullae.

There is little doubt that CT scans can be used to study the distribution and extent of pulmonary lesions in a manner that augments or exceeds the information obtained from plain-film studies (Fig. 10-49).[1,23] It is uncertain as yet whether the considerable additional information gained from CT scans of patients with diffuse lung disease is of sufficient benefit to warrant the cost when compared to the information already available from chest films, pulmonary function studies, and clinical assessments (see Fig. 10-10).

Although technique using thin slices may prove valuable in detecting low-signal lesions in patients with suspected diffuse lung disease whose chest films are negative or inconclusive, it is not practical to study the entire chest in this manner, principally because of the increased radiation dose required to obtain an adequate signal-to-noise ratio. Rather than survey the chest from apex to base it would probably be sufficient to obtain a few slices through the upper lung zones and a few through the lower lungs; six slices would serve as an adequate survey. Several investigators are exploring the clinical utility of this technique.

SUMMARY

1. The precise diagnosis of diffuse pulmonary disease frequently is not possible on the basis of radiographic appearance alone (where "precise diagnosis" means one that has such a high probability of

being correct that it permits optimum treatment planning without further investigation).
2. If we carefully integrate pertinent clinical data (see the six questions listed at the beginning of the chapter) with the radiographic analysis, the chance of our diagnosis being correct is increased. Even then, however, we will usually arrive at a differential diagnosis rather than a single diagnosis.
3. The inability to arrive at one precise diagnosis from the radiographic data may indeed be a weakness of the method, but the ability to generate a differential diagnosis is a decided strength, which frequently leads to the optimum choice and sequencing of other diagnostic studies to establish the correct diagnosis.
4. Some useful points for recall:
   a. UIP, DIP, and LIP, are often indistinguishable radiographically.
      (1) The lesions commonly show bibasilar predominance.
      (2) Patients are usually symptomatic when first seen, although older films obtained for comparison not uncommonly show lesser abnormalities at a time when the patient reportedly was asymptomatic.
      (3) In cases of UIP, when there is discordance between the apparent extent of disease seen radiographically and the magnitude of clinical signs (clubbing, cyanosis), symptoms (dyspnea), and pulmonary function disturbances (hypoxemia, restrictive defects, with or without obstructive components), it is often the clinical findings that are in excess of what would be predicted from the radiographic findings.
      (4) These conditions are usually idiopathic, but lesions of UIP may be found in patients with a variety of connective tissue diseases, such as scleroderma, dermatomyositis, and rheumatoid arthritis. Certain pneumoconioses (e.g., those caused by asbestos, diatomaceous earth, and talc) may also have lesions of UIP.
      (5) BIP and BOOP may also appear radiographically similar to UIP, although patients with BOOP may also have scattered, changing, irregular zones of consolidation that would be unusual for UIP.
   b. Chronic eosinophilic pneumonia may present as a bilateral, peripheral mantle of consolidation with heaviest concentrations in the upper lung zones. This configuration correlates highly (but imperfectly) with the specific diagnosis. Make sure the patient has not had radiation therapy to mantle ports.

c. The pulmonary lesions of sarcoidosis, eosinophilic granuloma of the lung, and certain pneumoconioses (e.g., berylliosis) may appear similar on chest films. A less common part of the radiographic spectrum of Wegener's granulomatosis (disseminated small to medium-sized nodules) may also resemble these conditions.

(1) When there is concomitant lymphadenopathy in the hila or the mediastinum, sarcoidosis is far more likely than either eosinophilic granuloma or Wegener's granulomatosis. Patients with berylliosis or silica-related pneumoconioses may also have such adenopathy, but can be distinguished by history of exposure. The absence of lymphadenopathy is of no distinguishing value.

(2) When there are multiple masses 3 cm or more in diameter and definite cavitation, Wegener's granulomatosis is far more likely to be the cause than is sarcoidosis or eosinophilic granuloma. Conglomerate masses may also occur late in sarcoidosis but rarely cavitate. Patients with silicosis may have conglomerate pulmonary masses that may also cavitate, but usually the history of silica-related industrial exposure is well known by the time these lesions evolve.

(3) Patients with non-Hodgkin's lymphoma may also present with multiple foci of consolidation appearing as coarse nodules or masses without evident hilar or mediastinal lymphadenopathy. Rarely, patients with LIP may also do so, and histopathologic distinction may be difficult.

(4) A substantial number of patients with sarcoid or eosinophilic granuloma have no symptoms in spite of extensive lesions seen on chest films. Pulmonary lesions in Wegener's granulomatosis may be found incidentally in patients whose clinical complaints are related to the skin, nose, sinuses, or kidneys, or they may first come to investigation because of hemoptysis. Pulmonary involvement without renal involvement is common.

(5) The diagnosis of pneumoconiosis depends on an accurate history review.

d. The diagnosis of pulmonary hypersensitivity reactions depends critically on an accurate environmental, habit, and hobby history.

e. Many conditions may progress to late-stage fibrosis (honeycombing), at which point the original condition may not be recognizable.

f. Patients with pulmonary lesions of lymphangioleiomyomatosis are women; they are usually, but not always, premenopausal when the diagnosis is first made.

(1) Preservation of lung volume in spite of extensive disease is the rule. However, patients with pulmonary sarcoid or eosinophilic granuloma may also show preserved lung volume.

(2) Pleural effusion (chylous) is common.

(3) Spontaneous pneumothorax is common.

g. Patients with alveolar proteinosis may have copious sputum, but this symptom is not common. Many patients have only progressive dyspnea on exertion. Treatment with steroids may promote pulmonary infection.

h. Patients with pulmonary hemorrhage usually have significant anemia. Hemoptysis is not invariable. Pulmonary hemorrhage, as observed radiographically, may clear rapidly after a single episode or slowly if the hemorrhage is recurrent.

i. Patients with severe chronic obstructive pulmonary disease usually have abnormalities on chest radiography whereas those with mild pulmonary function disturbances frequently do not.

(1) Patients with emphysema frequently have bullae.

(2) Patients with bullae do not always have COPD.

j. Neoplasm in the form of malignant lymphoma, diffuse metastases, bronchoalveolar carcinoma, or Kaposi's sarcoma may cause lesions similar radiographically to those of infections and other noninfectious diffuse lung disease.

k. Although this chapter is devoted to discussion of noninfectious diffuse lung disease, in clinical practice patients occasionally present with acute or subacute signs and symptoms such that the distinction between infection and noninfectious disease is not possible without invasive studies. This is particularly true in patients with:

(1) Lymphoma or leukemia

(2) Untoward reaction to therapeutic drugs

(3) Chronic eosinophilic pneumonia when the radiographic distribution of lesions is not of the characteristic pattern

(4) Transplant recipients who may be suffering from concomitant infection and rejection

(5) Patients with AIDS and Kaposi's sarcoma.

l. Pulmonary edema can mimic chronic lung disease. Whenever confronted with a problem of bilateral lung disease, pause and ask yourself whether the problem could be pulmonary edema. Usually, although not always, that question can be answered by judicious correlation with clinical data. This exercise might spare the patient unnecessary diagnostic studies.

BIBLIOGRAPHY

1. Bergin CJ, Müller HJ: CT of interstitial lung disease; a diagnostic approach. AJR 148:9, 1987
2. Caplan A: Certain unusual radiological appearances of the chest of coal-miners suffering from rheumatoid arthritis. Thorax 8:29, 1953
3. Carrington CB, Gaensler EA: Clinical-pathologic approach to diffuse infiltrative lung disease. Ch. 4. In Thurlbeck WM, Abell MR (eds): The Lung. Structure, Function, and Disease. Williams & Wilkins, Baltimore, 1978
4. Carrington CB, Gaensler EA, Mikas JP, et al: Structure and function in sarcoidosis. Ann NY Acad Sci 278:265, 1976
5. Churg A, Carrington C: Necrotizing sarcoid granulomatosis. Chest 76:406, 1979
6. Claypool WD, Rogers RM, Matuschak GM: Update on the clinical diagnosis, management, and pathogenesis of pulmonary alveolar proteinosis (phospholipidosis). Chest 85:550–558, 1984
7. Felson B: A new look at pattern recognition of diffuse pulmonary disease. AJR 133:183, 1979
8. Fitzgerald MX, Carrington CB, Gaensler EA: Environmental lung disease. Med Clin North Am 57:593, 1973
9. Foster WL, Pratt PC, Roggli VL, et al: Centrilobular emphysema: CT-pathologic correlation. Radiology 159:27, 1986
10. Fraire AE, Greenberg SD: Carcinoma and diffuse interstitial fibrosis of lung. Cancer 31:1078, 1973
11. Friedman PJ, Liebow AA, Sokoloff J: Eosinophilic granuloma of lung. Medicine 60:385, 1981
12. Gaensler EA, Carrington CE: Peripheral opacities in chronic eosinophilic pneumonia: photographic negative of pulmonary edema. Am J Roentgenol 128:1–13, 1977
13. Gaensler EA, Carrington CB, Contu RE: Chronic interstitial pneumonias. Clin Notes Respir Dis 10:3, 1972
14. Gefter WB, Epstein DM, Miller WT: Allergic bronchopulmonary aspergillosis: less common patterns. Radiology 140:307, 1981
15. Genereux GP: Pattern recognition in diffuse lung disease. A review of theory and practice. Med Radiogr Photogr 61:2, 1985
16. Gosink BB, Friedman PJ, Liebow AA: Bronchiolitis obliterans. Am J Roentgenol 117:816, 1973
17. Julsrud PR, Brown LR, Chin-Yang, et al: Pulmonary processes of mature-appearing lymphocytes: pseudolymphoma, well differentiated lymphocytic lymphoma, and lymphocytic interstitial pneumonitis. Radiology 127:289, 1978
18. Kirks DR, McCormick VD, Greenspan RH: Pulmonary sarcoidosis. Am J Roentgenol 117:777, 1973
19. Leavitt RV, Fauci AS: Pulmonary vasculitis. Am Rev Respir Dis 124:149, 1986
20. Liebow AA: The J. Burns Amberson Lecture— Pulmonary angiitis and granulomatosis. Am Rev Respir Dis 108:1, 1973
21. Liebow AA: Definition and classification of interstitial pneumonias in human pathology. Prog Respir Res 8:1, 1975
22. Liebow AA, Carrington CB: The interstitial pneumonias. p. 102. In Simon M, Potchen EJ, Le May M (eds): Frontiers of Pulmonary Radiology. New York, Grune & Stratton, 1969
23. Lien HH, Brodahl U, Telhaug R, et al: Pulmonary changes at computed tomography in patients with testicular carcinoma treated with cis-platinum, vinblastine and bleomycin. Acta Radiol [Diagn] (Stockh) 26:507, 1985
24. McLoud TC, Epler GR, Colby TV, et al: Bronchiolitis obliterans. Radiology 159:1, 1986
25. McLoud TC, Epler GR, Gaensler EA, et al: A radiologic classification for sarcoidosis. Physiologic correlation. Invest Radiol 17:129, 1982
26. Morrison DA, Goldman AL: Radiographic patterns of drug-induced lung disease. Radiology 131:299, 1979
27. Muller NL, Miller RR, Webb WR, et al: Fibrosing alveolitis: CT-pathologic correlations. Radiology 160:585, 1986
28. Olson LK, Forrest JV, Friedman PJ, et al: Pneumonitis after amiodarone therapy. Radiology 150:327, 1984
29. Pagtakhan RD, Reed MH, Chernick V: Cystic fibrosis in the adolescent and adult. J Thorac Imaging 1:41, 1986
30. Powers MA, Askin FB, Cresson DH: Pulmonary eosinophilic granuloma. Am Rev Respir Dis 129:503, 1984
31. Ralph DD, Springmeyer SC, Sullivan KM, et al: Rapidly progressive airflow obstruction in marrow transplant recipients. Possible association between obliterative bronchitis and chronic graft-versus-host disease. Am Rev Respir Dis 129:641, 1984
32. Reid L: Chronic obstructive lung disease. Ch. 40. In Fishman AP (ed): Pulmonary Diseases and Disorders. McGraw-Hill, New York, 1980
33. Simon G: Increased transradiency and altered vessel pattern in emphysema. p. 154. In Simon G: *Princi-*

ples of Chest X-Ray Diagnosis. 4th Ed. Butterworths, London, 1973

34. Sinclair W, Wright JS, Churg A: Lymphangioleiomyomatosis presenting in a postmenopausal woman. Thorax 40:475, 1985
35. Spencer H: Pathology of the Lung. 4th Ed. p. 798. Pergamon Press, Oxford, 1985
36. Thurlbeck WM, Henderson JA, Fraser RG, Bates DV: Chronic obstructive lung disease. Medicine 49:81, 1970
37. Unger GF, Scanlon GT, Fink JA, et al: A radiologic approach to hypersensitivity pneumonias. Radiol Clin North Am 11:339, 1973
38. Yousem SA, Lifson JD, Colby TV: Chemotherapy-induced eosinophilic pneumonia. Chest 88:103, 1985

Atlas

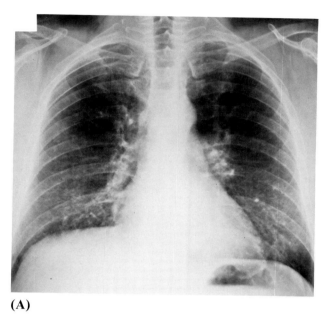

(A)

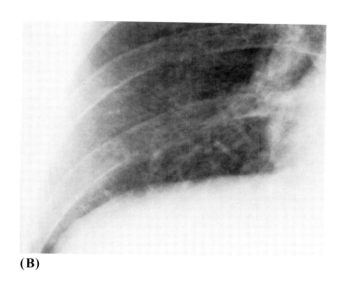

(B)

Fig. 10-1.   Usual Interstitial Pneumonitis

This 43-year-old man noted the onset of fatigue and decreased exercise tolerance approximately 6 months ago. He did not have cough or significant shortness of breath. His activity levels fluctuated over the next few months. Approximately 2 months before presenting he noted fatigue, malaise, myalgias, and arthralgias of his wrists, elbows, and shoulders. He had smoked for approximately 25 years (25 to 30 packs/year).

On physical examination there were bibasilar rales that persisted after coughing. He had moderately severe clubbing of the fingers and toes, which he felt had been present as long as he could remember but had gotten worse over the past 10 years. Pulmonary function studies confirmed the presence of a moderate restrictive defect with a reduction of diffusing capacity, but normal arterial blood gases.

An open biopsy of the right lower lobe was performed. Histopathologic analysis showed striking interstitial fibrosis with marked thickening of alveolar walls and proliferation of smooth muscle within the interalveolar septa. Plump alveolar cells were also noted to fill alveolar spaces. Only a few lymphocytes and plasma cells were present focally in the interstitium. The biopsy was interpreted as showing interstitial fibrosis (UIP).

(A) PA film of the chest made before the lung biopsy. It shows predominately bibasilar abnormalities of a fine reticular pattern.

(B) Coned view of the right base shows the detail of this abnormality to better advantage. Notice first that whereas medium-sized vessels can be seen medially just above the diaphragm, the very small vessel images are lost within the fine reticulation throughout the entire region shown. This is one of the characteristic appearances of UIP, either idiopathic or associated with a variety of diseases that are listed in Table 10-2. If one does not recognize the loss of the small vessel images, it is quite possible to erroneously interpret this film as normal.

Although this patient was not very ill, the magnitude of the clinical findings and the abnormal pulmonary function studies are greater than one might expect from the abnormalities seen on the chest film. This disparity is a common feature of UIP.

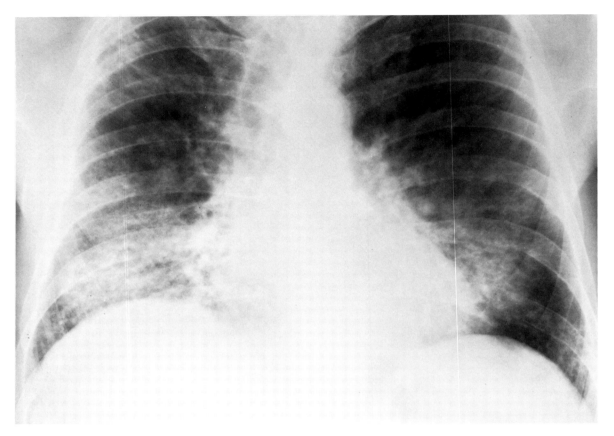

Fig. 10-2. Severe UIP

The patient was a 59-year-old man complaining of progressive shortness of breath over 6 to 8 months. His exercise tolerance became limited to walking one block. In addition, he had a dry cough and hoarseness and had lost 10 pounds over the past 6 months. He had smoked 4 packs of cigarettes a day for 20 years, but at the time of this examination he had not smoked for the past 20 years. He had clubbing of the fingers and cyanosis of the lips. There was also ankle edema. Pulmonary function studies showed combined restrictive and mild to moderate obstructive defects, which improved with bronchodilator therapy. He also had hypoxemia, hyperventilation, and uneven distribution of venti-lation. A lung biopsy showed interstitial fibrosis (UIP). There was no substantial clinical response to treatment with prednisone, and on follow-up study a year later the patient had developed frank cor pulmonale.

This PA film of the chest shows florid disease with increased opacification in the lower portions of both lungs. Abnormalities extend up toward the apices in a peripheral distribution on the right side and to a lesser extent on the left. It is difficult to characterize the lesions in the heaviest zones of opacification, but along the periphery you can see ill-defined nodules that vary only slightly in size. There is a reticular background consisting of irregular linear and very small ring-shaped opacities. Faint air bronchograms are seen within the denser zones of consolidation. A chest film 3 years earlier showed only disseminated, scattered, irregular small nodules on the order of 5 mm in diameter and few linear opacities. There was much less disease than is seen on the present study.

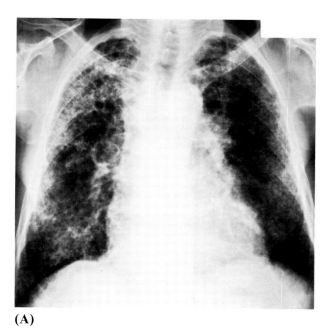

(A)

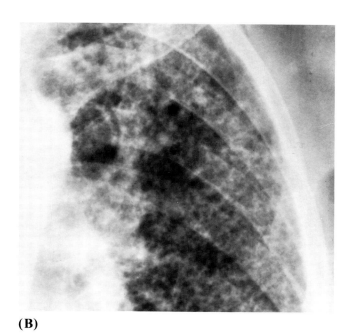

(B)

Fig. 10-3. End-Stage UIP—Honeycomb Lung Phase

This 70-year-old man complained of increasing dyspnea over the past year. He had less than a one-block exercise tolerance and had lost 20 pounds. One week before admission he began to produce copious amounts of sputum, and he also noted ankle edema. He had been a cigarette smoker with a productive cough (intermittently purulent) for 20 years. He had a history of bronchitis and bronchiectasis as a teenager, but the exact findings on which those diagnoses were based were not known.

(A,B) Chest films show marked abnormalities involving both lungs. On PA view (Fig. A) the abnormalities appear more severe on the right side than on the left, but a coned view of the left midlung zone (Fig. B) shows that the left lung is also very severely involved. There are rounded lucencies 1 cm in diameter, more or less, with fairly thick soft tissue "jackets." These radiographic abnormalities are characteristic of honeycomb lung.

(C) Tomogram shows diffuse honeycombing and emphysematous bullae medially. They are seen as fairly large, circumscribed areas of radiolucency (arrows). In fact, one bulla, superimposed on the right hilum on the full PA view, simulates a thin-walled cavity.

So-called end-stage lung disease represents the late stages of chronic lung disease, commonly UIP but occasionally the late effects of sarcoidosis, eosinophilic granuloma, hypersensitivity pneumonitis, or other conditions.

The patient died in acute respiratory failure. His lungs at postmortem examination showed honeycombing with extensive replacement of lung architecture by fibrous tissue. There was also emphysema and bronchiectasis.

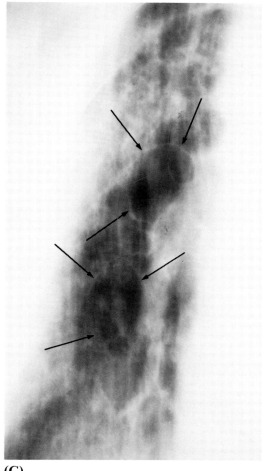

(C)

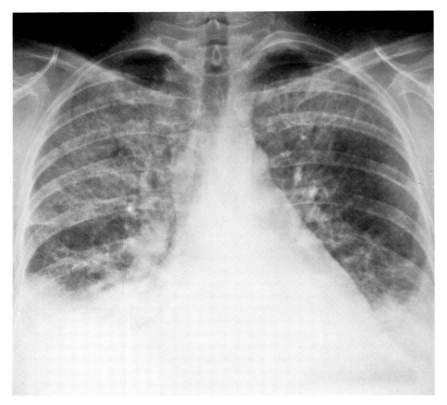

Fig. 10-4. Rheumatoid Lung Disease

The patient is a 54-year-old woman with a long history of rheumatoid arthritis complicated by dermatitis, inflammatory muscle disease, and hemolytic anemia. She had extensive dermatitis as well as marked changes of rheumatoid arthritis in the hands. On the basis of clinical findings and positive serologic tests, the diagnosis of an overlap syndrome of rheumatoid arthritis with features of lupus erythematosus and dermatomyositis was made.

Approximately 2 months before this admission the patient noted the onset of dyspnea on exertion as well as episodes of sweats with fevers as high as 102° F. She became short of breath at rest. On physical examination she appeared to be in moderately severe respiratory distress. There were bilateral inspiratory rales. Her PO_2 was 55 mmHg on room air and PCO_2 was 32 mmHg. She underwent an open-lung biopsy.

The biopsy specimen showed histopathologic changes of chronic interstitial pneumonia (UIP) with areas of fibrosis and honeycombing as well as a superimposed organizing acute interstitial process. The numerous plasma cells and lymphoid follicles in the biopsy specimen were felt to be consistent with the diagnosis of rheumatoid arthritis. The initial culture of the lung biopsy specimen grew a single non-lactose-fermenting *Pseudomonas,* which was thought to be a contaminant, but because of her severe illness, it was decided to treat the patient with carbenicillin and gentamicin. She was later treated with high doses of steroids and showed marked improvement in her respiratory symptoms, her blood gases, and her radiographic abnormalities.

The chest film shows extensive bilateral pulmonary disease. There are zones of opacification in the right upper lung as well as in the left subclavicular region. Linear and small nodular opacities are seen in areas of relative sparing in the left midlung zone and in the right lower parahilar region. Intense zones of opacification (ground glass?) at the bases obscure the definition of the diaphragm. Air bronchograms are clearly visible on the original films. There are also small pleural effusions.

Pulmonary lesions associated with rheumatoid arthritis are usually within the radiographic spectrum of UIP. However, in some patients nodules several centimeters in diameter, similar to those of Caplan's syndrome,[2] may be the dominant pattern.

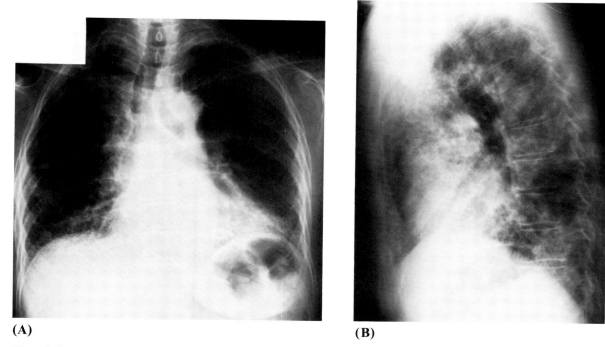

(A)   (B)

Fig. 10-5. Unclassified Connective Tissue Disease, UIP, and Occult Squamous Cell Carcinoma

This 63-year-old woman had a 9-year history of chronic, nonproductive cough accompanied by bibasilar pulmonary abnormalities on chest films. Three years ago an acute arthritis began in the metatarsal heads and later spread to the wrists, shoulders, and knees. This was accompanied by weakness of the proximal muscles, especially of the shoulder girdle and the legs. Even after a number of serologic studies, skin and muscle biopsies, and immunoelectrophoresis studies, it was not possible to clearly classify the nature of her connective tissue disease. It was felt that she had features of rheumatoid arthritis as well as polymyalgia rheumatica.

Pulmonary function tests showed features of both restrictive and obstructive lung disease. Over the last 2 years the patient had suffered progressive deterioration of pulmonary function with increase in cough, sputum, and dyspnea on exertion. A variety of regimens were employed with intermittent improvement and subsequent exacerbation of symptoms.

(A) Chest film made approximately 9 days before the patient's death. It is a heavily exposed film that shows the predominance of the pulmonary abnormalities in the lower portions of the lungs. (Examine the portion of lung superimposed on the right diaphragm and the retrocardiac portion of the left lower lobe.) On the original films, however, there is evidence of extensive disease in the form of ill-defined reticulonodular opacities extending throughout the greater part of both lungs. The basilar abnormalities show evidence of honeycombing, and there is some reduction in volume of the lower lobes. Faint air bronchograms show approximation of segmental bronchi particularly well in the left lower lobe.

(B) Lateral view confirms the presence of extensive disease throughout the lungs rather than simply at the bases. Notice the widespread effacement of vessel images.

Pathologic study of the lungs showed diffuse bilateral pulmonary interstitial fibrosis (UIP) with bronchiolectasis (honeycomb lung). Both lungs showed marked rigidity, retained their shape, and were capable of standing freely on their bases. Microscopically, in an area of the lingula where there were honeycomb changes, there was also a squamous cell carcinoma. It had origins in spaces lined by atypical epithelial proliferation. The size of the carcinoma, unfortunately, was not given, nor was it recognized on gross examination.

The development of atypical epithelial proliferation and an increased incidence of carcinoma associated with honeycomb change has been reported, but the patients are usually males with a substantial smoking history.[10]

Even in retrospect I do not think it is possible to make the diagnosis of a carcinoma in the lingula from these radiographs. In fact, comparison with a chest film 3 months earlier showed very little change in the distribution or severity of this patient's lung disease.

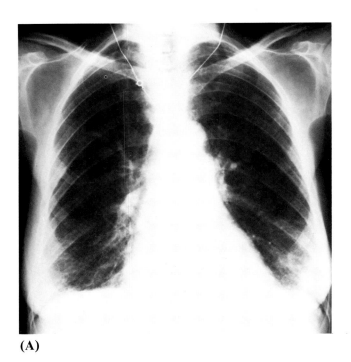

(A)

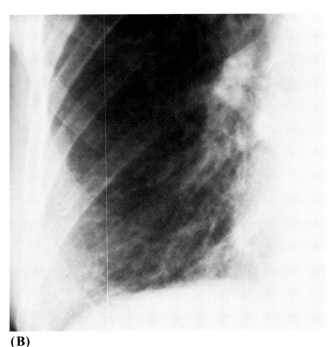

(B)

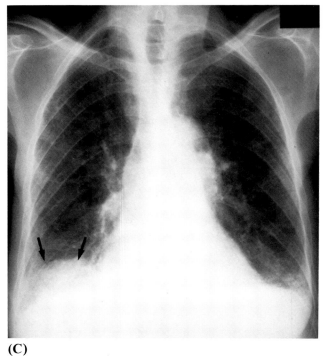

(C)

Fig. 10-6. Scleroderma, UIP, and Development of Bronchogenic Carcinoma

This 65-year-old woman had had scleroderma with esophageal and pulmonary involvement for 23 years. On physical examination she had alopecia, increased ankle pigmentation, telangiectases, sclerodactyly, palmar nodules, thin facial features (nose, lips, and ears), and Raynaud's phenomenon.

(A) PA film of the chest made approximately 5 years before the present admission. It is heavily exposed to show the bibasilar distribution of the patient's chronic interstitial pneumonitis.

(B) Coned view of the right base shows a series of small ring shadows laterally as well as effacement of vascular detail both laterally and medially. This appearance is consistent with a reticulonodular pattern and focal honeycombing.

(C) Chest film made at the current hospital visit. In addition to the interstitial lung disease, there is the rounded dome of a new mass at the right base (arrows). *(Figure continues.)*

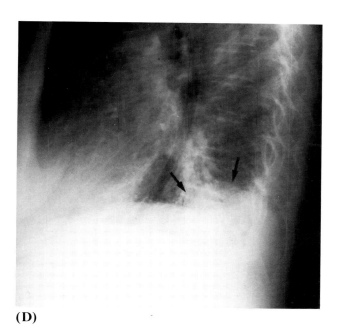

(D)

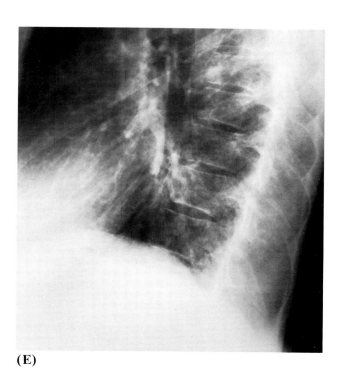

(E)

Fig. 10-6. *(Continued.)* **(D)** Lateral view of the chest shows the edge of a soft tissue mass far posteriorly (arrows) corresponding to that seen on the right side of the PA view.

(E) Lateral view of the chest taken 5 years earlier demonstrates that the mass was not present at that time.

(F) Tomogram through the lesion at the right base shows the outlines of the mass to better advantage. *(Figure continues.)*

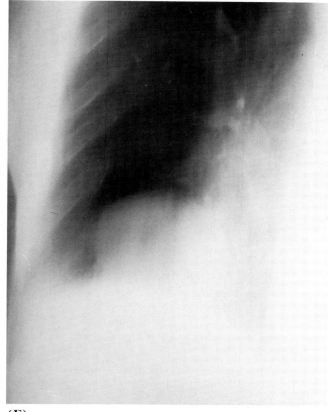

(F)

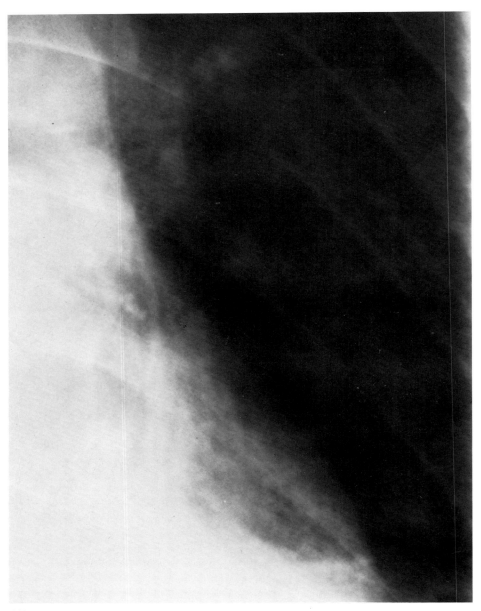

(G)

Fig. 10-6. *(Continued.)* **(G)** Coned view of the left base at the time of the present study shows peribronchial and perivascular thickening due to chronic interstitial pneumonitis.

This distribution of thick bands of soft tissue paralleling bronchovascular bundles is part of the radiographic spectrum of lesions that may be seen with any chronic interstitial pneumonitis. It can also be seen in patients with pooling of secretions on bronchi and consequent atelectasis of segments or subsegments of lung.

At the time of the last chest film, the patient still had symptoms only of dyspnea on exertion. An aspiration needle biopsy of the mass showed that it was a malignant tumor. The patient's pulmonary function status, although abnormal, was still considered adequate to permit a lobectomy. The patient was operated upon, and a diagnosis of undifferentiated carcinoma or carcinosarcoma was made from histopathologic study of the resected neoplasm. Two nodes along the intrapulmonary course of the right lower lobe bronchovascular bundle were positive for metastases. The lung away from the neoplasm showed extensive interstitial fibrosis, metaplasia of alveolar lining cells, and honeycombing, all of which were consistent with UIP associated with scleroderma.

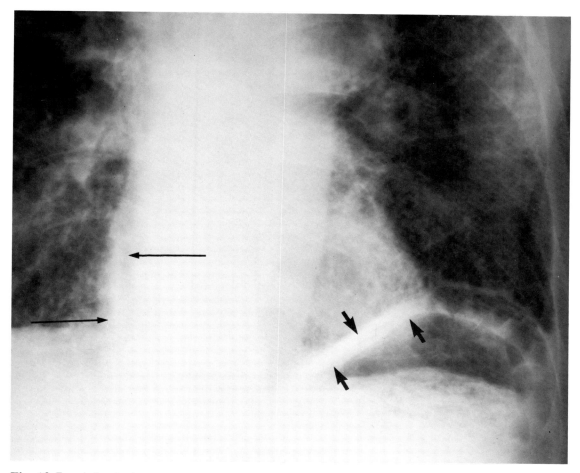

Fig. 10-7. Asbestosis

This film shows bilateral reticulonodular opacities that are indistinguishable from the lesions of UIP shown in the previous examples. There are thick linear pleural calcifications, however, which are a classic appearance of calcified pleural plaques due to asbestos (arrows). The combination of pleural plaques and parenchymal lesions of UIP support the diagnosis of asbestosis.

Pulmonary parenchymal lesions due to asbestosis are indistinguishable from those of UIP or DIP radiographically and often histopathologically unless asbestos bodies are also seen.

Pleural plaques may occur without radiographic evidence of parenchymal lung disease. The chest manifestations of asbestos exposure — pleural effusion, pleural thickening, pleural plaques, and pulmonary asbestosis — may occur alone or together at long intervals after initial exposure. Malignant mesothelioma has a high correlation with asbestos exposure but is not exclusively related.

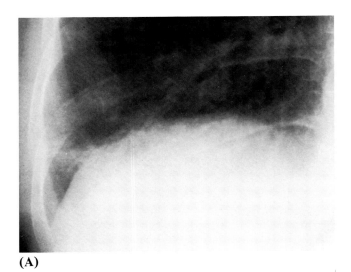

(A)

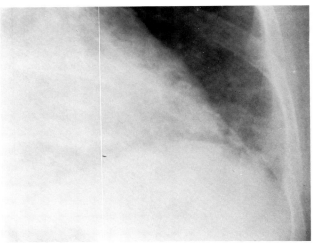

(B)

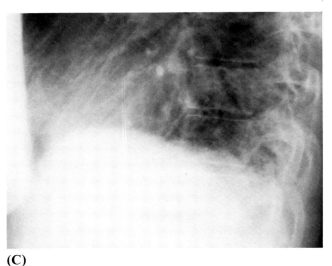

(C)

Fig. 10-8. Sjögren's Syndrome and LIP

This 38-year-old white female first presented with complaints of fatigue, low-grade fever, dry eyes, minor lymph gland enlargement, dry cough, mild diarrhea, and joint pain affecting the proximal interphalangeal (PIP) and metacarpophalangeal (MCP) joints and the wrist joints. The symptoms had begun approximately 9 months earlier.

Physical examination revealed mild lymphadenopathy, dryness of the eyes, bibasilar rales over both lungs, and mild palpable synovitis over the PIP, MCP, and wrist joints.

Laboratory values were as follows: lactic dehydrogenase 397, serum glutamic-oxaloacetic transferase 80, aldolase 28, creatine phosphokinase 965, and thyroxine 2.5; fluorescent antinuclear antibodies test was negative, C3 was negative, latex fixation was negative, protein electrophoresis was normal, skin tests (PPD, histoplas-min, coccidioidin, mumps, and streptokinase-streptodornase) were all negative, and esophageal motility was normal. Pulmonary function tests showed some restrictive defects and reduced diffusing capacity.

A lung biopsy showed fibrosing obliterative bronchiolitis and lymphocytic infiltration of the bronchioles. The diagnosis of LIP was made. There was also lipid pneumonia secondary to obstruction by degenerating macrophages. The clinical, laboratory, and pathologic findings were consistent with Sjögren's syndrome.

The patient was started on prednisone 60 mg daily and showed continued improvement of pulmonary function and return to normal SGOT, LDH, and aldolase values.

(A,B) Coned views of the right and left lung bases, respectively. Note on the right the reticular appearance and the very small nodules, which are best seen in the area superimposed on the diaphragm dome and the adjacent costophrenic angle. Similar lesions on the left are best seen lateral to the cardiac apex, because the heart obscures the details of the retrocardiac portions of the left lower lobe.

(C) Coned lateral view of the base shows the reticular pattern best in the retrocardiac and posterior gutter regions.

The syndrome described by Sjögren in 1933 consists of keratoconjunctivitis sicca, xerostomia, and recurrent swelling of the parotid glands with occasional manifestations in other organ systems. Indeed a substantial number of patients with rheumatoid arthritis and approximately 30 percent of patients with LIP have Sjögren's syndrome.[21] In addition to joint involvement, renal and pulmonary involvement have been noted. Involvement in all organ systems is characterized by a lymphocytic and plasma cell infiltrate. This patient illustrates the reticular pattern of lung involvement, which is indistinguishable radiographically from UIP.

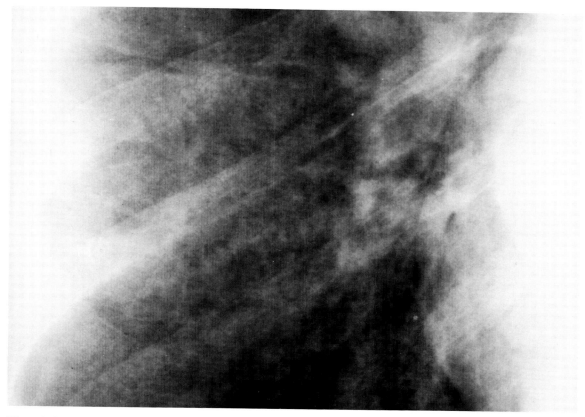

Fig. 10-9. Bronchiolitis Obliterans

Approximately 5 months ago this 47-year-old woman had a febrile illness associated with a sore throat and pain in her right knee, foot, and ankle. Empirical treatment with ampicillin and later tetracycline was unsuccessful. Throat culture grew only normal flora. She developed a diffuse rash presumably related to tetracycline, which was discontinued. Over the next several months she suffered from intermittent low-grade fevers, a high sedimentation rate, leukocytosis, and chest pain on deep inspiration. Multiple tests including a bone marrow aspirate were nondiagnostic. Her low-grade fevers persisted and she developed polyarthritis. She was referred because of progressive dyspnea and pleuritic chest pain.

She had moderately severe respiratory distress with a respiratory rate of 44 per minute and blood gases of PO$_2$ 52 mmHg, PCO$_2$ 33 mmHg, and pH 7.47 while breathing room air.

This coned view of the right lower lung zone is representative of the diffuse disease present throughout both lungs. There is loss of detail of small and medium-sized vessels in a background pattern of granular and very finely reticular opacities.

A transbronchial biopsy showed histopathologic changes of bronchiolitis obliterans. Foci of bronchiolitis obliterans may be found in biopsy specimens of cases of UIP but do not represent the predominant pathology as seen in cases of bronchiolitis obliterans per se.

The radiographic pattern is one that is part of the spectrum of BIP but is totally nonspecific and could be seen with any of the chronic interstitial pneumonias.

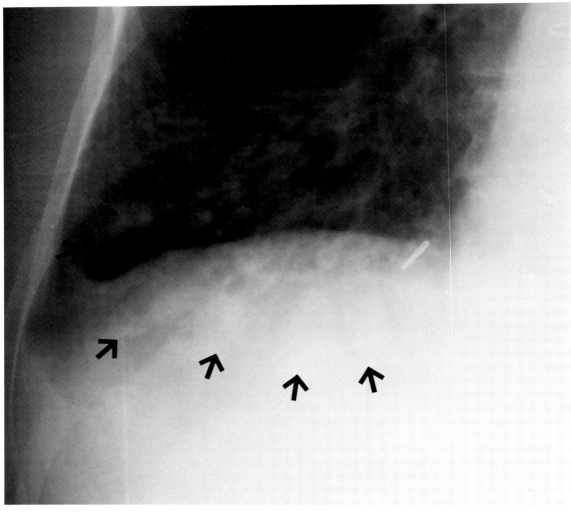

(A)

Fig. 10-10.   Bronchiolitis Obliterans in a Heart-Lung Transplant Recipient

This man is the recipient of a heart-lung transplant who subsequently developed clinical signs and symptoms of air flow obstruction.[1]

Radiographically, the most florid abnormalities were seen at the right base, with patchy and less conspicuous abnormalities present elsewhere in the lungs.

(A) Coned view of the right lung base. Poorly defined, irregular nodular foci of consolidation are clustered caudally (arrows). Linear and smaller nodular foci are also present in the right lower lobe. *(Figure continues.)*

Fig. 10-10. *(Continued).* **(B)** Lateral view shows similar lesions (arrows) and linear tracks parallel to bronchial walls.

(C) CT scans show thick-walled ring images of dilated bronchi, their adjacent vessels, and partially filled lumina. The frame at top left also shows a few thick-walled bronchi parallel to the plane of the scan (open arrowhead); these correspond to "tramline" images representing thick-walled bronchi on chest films of patients with chronic bronchitis or bronchiectasis.

The diagnosis of bronchiolitis obliterans was confirmed histopathologically. The abnormalities seen on these illustrations are those of bronchiectasis proximal to extensive bronchiolitis obliterans.

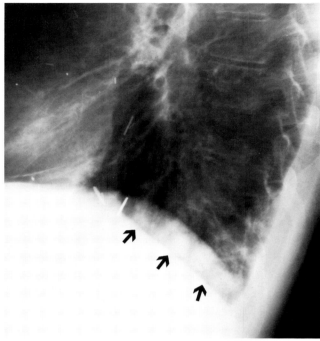

(B)

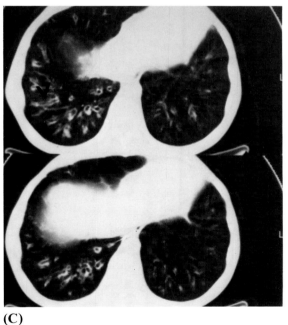

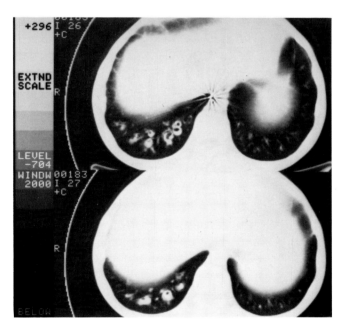

(C)

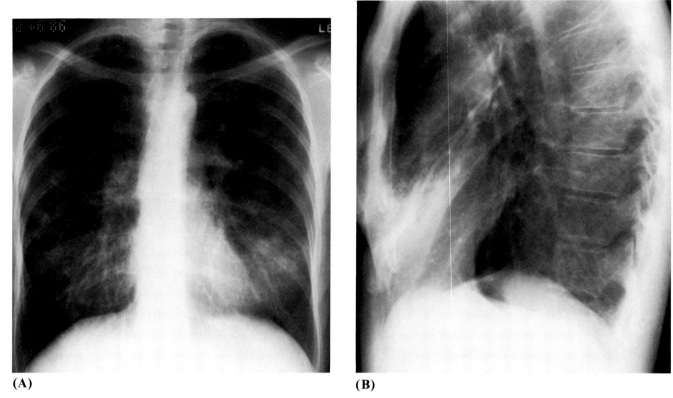

(A)   **(B)**

Fig. 10-11.   Bronchiolitis Obliterans and Probable Hypersensitivity Pneumonitis

This 45-year-old woman was in good health until the onset 4 months ago of fevers, chills, night sweats, fatigue, and a cough productive of green sputum. She was admitted to another hospital where a chest film was made and reported to show a "right-sided pulmonary infiltrate." She was treated with erythromycin and later cefaclor (Ceclor) without benefit.

Upon referral she had persistent symptoms. Her cough was less productive, but she had marked exertional dyspnea. She had lost 17 pounds over the last 3 months. She had had no significant industrial exposure; no other drugs had been used. She had traveled to Europe more than a year before her symptoms began. She did have a parakeet in her home, but she had no known allergies other than a vaguely remembered reaction to sulfa as a child.

On examination she was in no acute distress but had a dry, hacking cough. Respirations were 22 per minute. There were coarse breath sounds throughout both lungs with inspiratory wheezes on the left. The examination otherwise uncovered no abnormalities. Her white blood cell count was normal.

A left lung biopsy was done via a minithoracotomy approach. Histopathologic changes of bronchiolitis obliterans were evident along with microgranulomas and a cellular infiltrate suggesting a hypersensitivity pneumonitis.

(A,B) PA and lateral views of the chest show a poorly marginated zone of consolidation in the lingula, which is well shown anterior to the lower half of the left major fissure on the lateral view. *(Figure continues.)*

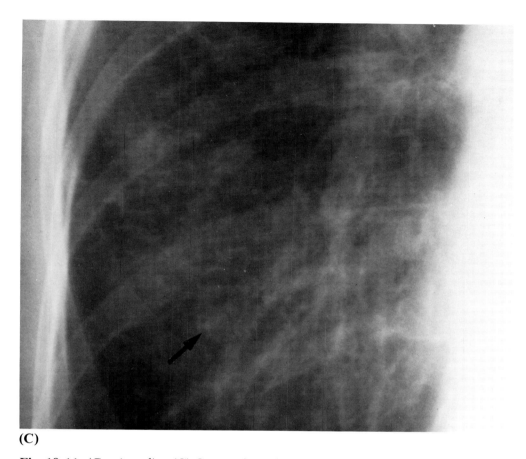

(C)

Fig. 10-11. *(Continued).* **(C)** Coned view of the right middle and lower lung zones. There is efface-ment of small vessels and a series of subtle, confluent ring shadows, which vary slightly in size and are under 1.0 cm in diameter. These can be seen best by viewing the illustration under bright light. An arrow points to a prominent nipple shadow (see below).

Bronchiolitis obliterans may be a component of the pulmonary reaction in cases of hypersensitivity pneumonitis. The radiographic appearances may be analogous to those of UIP, but frequently there are also irregular opaque zones that may fluctuate in extent on films made from days to weeks apart, especially when there is a substantial component of nonspecific obstructive pneumonitis.

The patient was treated with steroids and the parakeet was removed from the home. She responded both clinically and radiographically to these measures.

Notice the prominent nipple shadow, whose inferolateral margins are well defined whereas the superomedial margins are not, as is common when nipples are seen on chest radiographs. In this woman, the nipple shadow is projected in the midclavicular line of the anterior fourth interspace. It is important to distinguish nipple shadows from pulmonary nodules. This can be done by obtaining stereoscopic PA chest films with metallic nipple markers in place or by fluoroscopy.

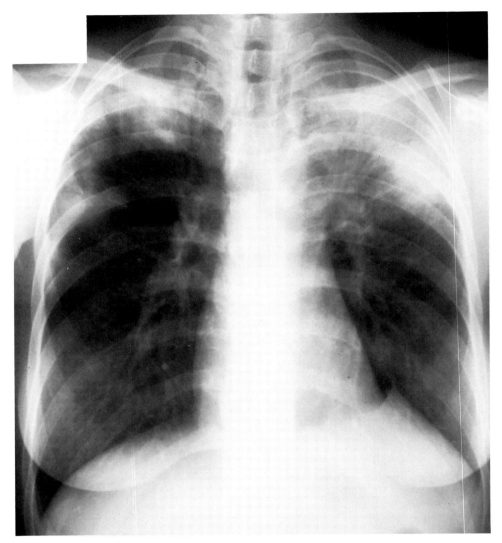

Fig. 10-12. Chronic Eosinophilic Pneumonitis

This 29-year-old woman complained of cough, shortness of breath, and fever. Her white blood cell count was over 22,000/mm³ with 31 percent eosinophils. Over the next few days this changed to 59 percent eosinophils. She was treated with a brief course of erythromycin and had had ampicillin before that. A general chemistry and electrolyte panel was normal. Sputa were negative for acid-fast bacilli and fungi on stain. Stool specimens for ova and parasites were negative.

The chest film shows moderately extensive opacification in a peripheral or mantle distribution about the upper lung zones. There is some central extension on the left but parahilar sparing on the right. This distribution is characteristic of chronic eosinophilic pneumonia. An air bronchogram effect on the left side is seen as tubular, gray, branching structures within the zones of pulmonary consolidation. There is tenting of the left hemidiaphragm due to contraction in volume of the left upper lobe.

Because of the characteristic radiographic pattern and the fact that the patient did not wish to have a bronchoscopy or biopsy, she was started on treatment with prednisone. There was prompt relief of symptoms, clearing of the radiographic abnormalities, and a marked reduction in the eosinophilic count.

In retrospect the patient recalled an episode of upper respiratory infection and recurrent cough over the preceding 3 months. She also related that she had been visiting friends who had a parakeet. It is a matter of conjecture as to whether or not these episodes are related.

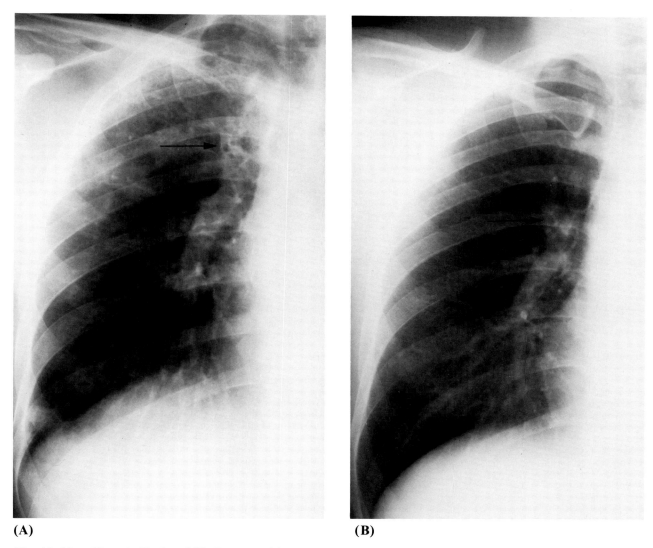

(A)   **(B)**

Fig. 10-13.   Chronic Eosinophilic Pneumonitis Associated With Bleomycin Chemotherapy

This man was receiving chemotherapy for carcinoma of the testis. He developed a persistent cough following the fourth cycle of treatment. Bleomycin was one of the drugs in his treatment regimen: it is one of the chemotherapeutic agents known to be associated with the development of chronic interstitial pneumonitis. Up to this time he had received a total dose of 280 mg of bleomycin.

(A) Coned view of the right lung after the onset of the cough. There is an inhomogeneous zone of patchy consolidation in a mantle involving the apex and the subclavicular region, with a small patch visible just above the right costophrenic angle. Abnormalities in a similar distribution were present on the left.

(B) The same areas 5 months before. Compare the appearance of the lung that is projected over the upper five posterior interspaces on Figs. A and B and notice the striking change. In addition to the patchy consolidation, there is contraction in volume of the right upper lobe. The bronchus seen end-on in Fig. B (arrow) has been drawn cephalad and medially by the contracting right upper lobe. (Compare its change in position relative to the anterior and posterior ribs on the two films.)

The mantle distribution pattern of this consolidation is one known to occur with chronic eosinophilic pneumonia, the proven diagnosis in this case. Reaction to drugs is one of the known causes of this type of pneumonia. Bleomycin-induced chronic eosinophilic pneumonia may occur at lower cumulative doses than does the more usual UIP-like bleomycin-induced chronic interstitial pneumonitis, which ordinarily predominates at the lung bases.

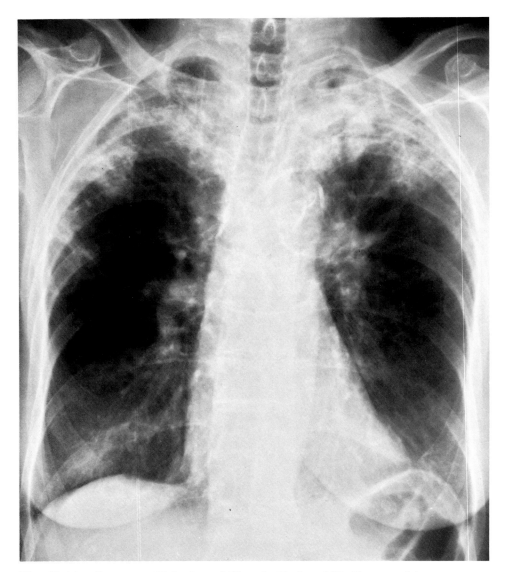

Fig. 10-14. Recurrent Episodes of Chronic Eosinophilic Pneumonitis

This elderly woman developed fever, cough, and dyspnea. All sputum smears and cultures were negative for pathogens. No eosinophilia was present, nor were eosinophils found in the sputum. Because of the patient's age and the characteristic radiographic pattern of chronic eosinophilic pneumonitis, she was begun on a trial of steroid medication. She had a rapid, favorable response, both clinically and radiographically, beginning approximately 12 hours after initial treatment. The steroids were tapered off. She then had a flare-up of symptoms. The steroids were restarted, remission followed, and the steroids were again tapered. Again she had a recurrence and the cycle was repeated. She denied taking any other medicines. Finally, her chest physician discovered that she had been using a vaginal cream, which recently had been changed to one that contained sulfanilamide. When she discontinued the use of this preparation, on advice of the chest physician, she had a complete and sustained remission of symptoms and radiographic lesions.

Recurrent episodes of chronic eosinophilic pneumonia are not rare. Whether they are all consequent to hypersensitivity to an unidentified allergen is unknown. (Courtesy of Drs. Norman Rizk and Richard Kramer, Palo Alto, California.)

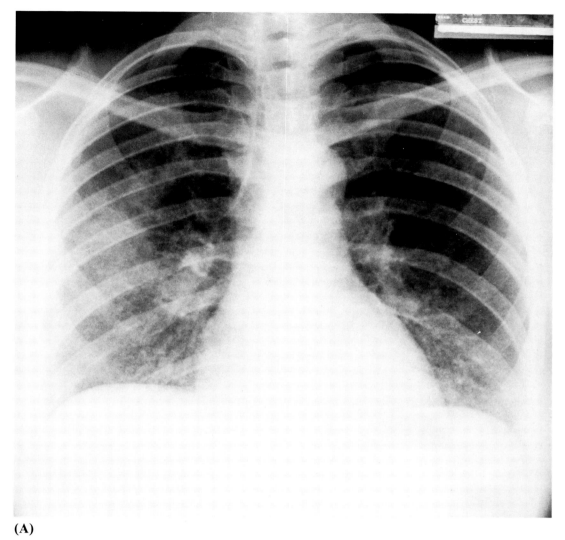

(A)

Fig. 10-15. (A – C) Sarcoidosis With a Miliary Appearance

This 40-year-old black woman had a history of intermittent fever, malaise, and chills for approximately 5 months associated with a moderate weight loss. A few weeks before Figs. A and B were taken she first developed a dry, hacking cough.

Her brother died of tuberculosis 2 years ago, and she was exposed to a nephew with active tuberculosis at about the time her own symptoms began. She has had persistently negative skin tuberculin tests, no unusual occupational exposure or travel history, and no exposure to household pets.

On examination she was in no acute distress. Her temperature was 100°F, and respirations were 18 per minute. There were a few scattered inspiratory rales at the right lung base and an ejection murmur along the left sternal border. There were no other significant physical findings.

Pulmonary function tests were compatible with early restrictive lung disease, but blood gas determinations were normal. Skin tests were positive for streptokinase-streptodornase, dermatophyton, and mumps, but negative for PPD, coccidioidin, and histoplasmin. Sputum smears for acid-fast bacilli (AFB), fungi, and other pathogens were negative on repeated study, although the results of AFB cultures were pending.

(A) PA chest film shows a bilateral, granular-appearing pattern that is more marked at the bases, extends cephalad to the infraclavicular regions, and spares the parahilar zones and the apices. *(Figure continues.)*

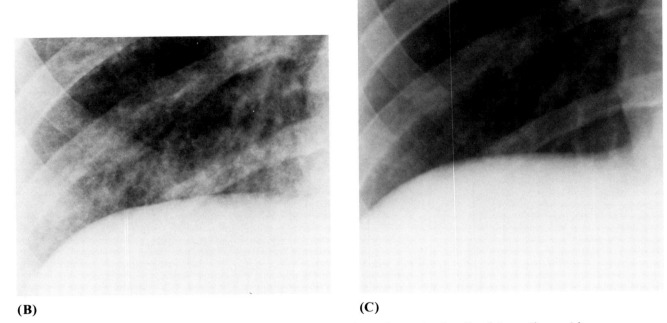

(B)   **(C)**

Fig. 10-15. *(Continued).* **(B)** Coned view of the right lung base shows the details of the radiographic appearance.

(C) Coned view of the right lung base of a chest film made 7 years earlier.

In Fig. B there is effacement of small peripheral vessels, and even the larger vessels have lost their sharpness of outline.

The prime diagnostic considerations were noninfectious granulomatous disease (particularly sarcoid) and infectious granulomatous disease (particularly tuberculosis). Tuberculosis was favored over the other infectious granulomatous diseases simply because it was the most common in the community where the patient lives.

A transbronchial lung biopsy was obtained. Multiple noncaseating granulomas were present, and the tissue was negative for microorganisms on special staining and on culture. Liver biopsy also showed multiple granulomata. A diagnosis of sarcoidosis was made. Subsequently the patient began to show signs of spontaneous improvement without any specific treatment.

The histopathologic diagnosis of sarcoid is nonspecific. The presence of noncaseating granulomas in tissue is essential to substantiate the clinical diagnosis, but it is important to culture biopsy specimens whenever they are obtained, and to use special stains to study the tissue for bacteria and fungi. Vasculitis and necrosis (but not caseation) may be found in association with the variant known as necrotizing sarcoidal granulomatosis.

A good industrial exposure history is also necessary since chronic berylliosis can mimic sarcoidosis, both histopathologically and radiographically. *(Figure continues.)*

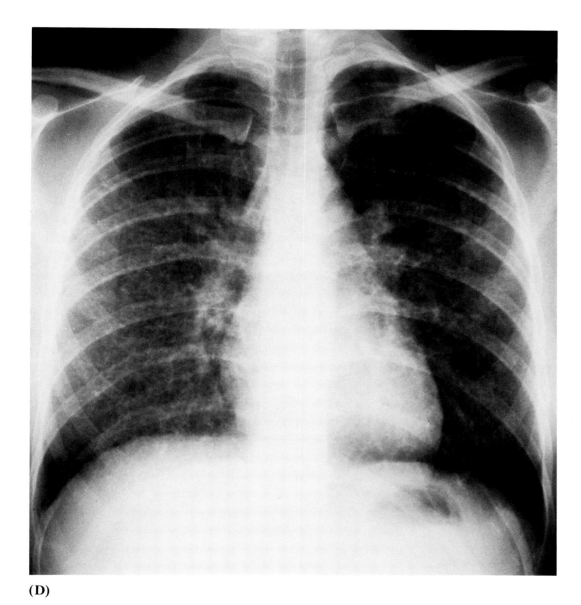

(D)

Fig. 10-15. *(Continued).* **(D,E) Eosinophilic Granuloma of the Lung**

This 27-year-old woman had enjoyed excellent health until approximately 6 months ago when she noted the onset of shortness of breath. This coincided with a respiratory infection marked by coughing and wheezing, which she thought persisted longer than usual.

On examination there were bibasilar inspiratory wheezes that did not clear with coughing. The patient stated that she was aware of the wheezing when she took a very deep breath. The physical examination was otherwise normal.

A bronchoscopy with brushings and biopsies was nondiagnostic. She then had a minithoracotomy. The biopsy specimen showed multiple small nodules, both subpleurally and surrounding bronchioles. They were composed largely of histiocytes, which were associated with scattered infiltrates of eosinophils. A diagnosis of the eosinophilic granuloma subclass of histiocytosis X was made.

(D) PA film of the chest shows very small, scattered, irregular opacities and reticulation distributed throughout both lungs. There is relative sparing of the extreme costophrenic angles, but the lesions extend all the way up into the apices. *(Figure continues.)*

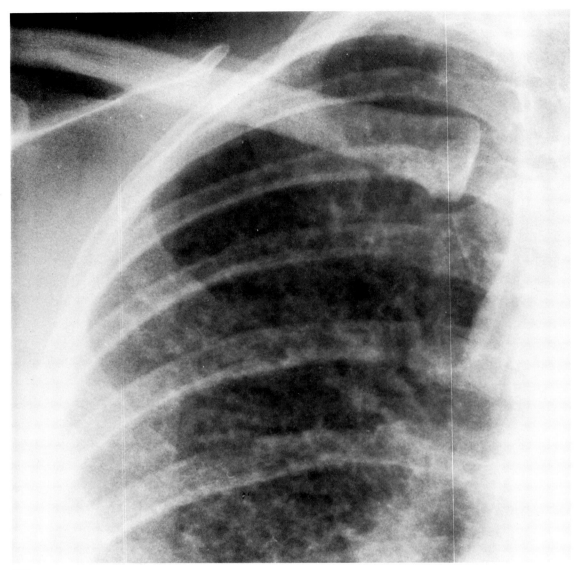

(E)

Fig. 10-15. *(Continued).* **(E)** Coned view of the right upper lobe shows the irregular nature of these small opacities and demonstrates the effacement of the small vessels in the periphery of the lung. The reticulation produces an appearance of small (less than 1 cm in diameter) cystic spaces interspersed among the small, irregular nodules.

This radiographic appearance is part of the spectrum of eosinophilic granuloma of the lung, but it is also part of the spectra of the other noninfectious granulomatous diseases. From the radiographic findings alone it would also not be possible to exclude the possibility of infectious granulomatous disease.

Notice the well-preserved lung volumes.

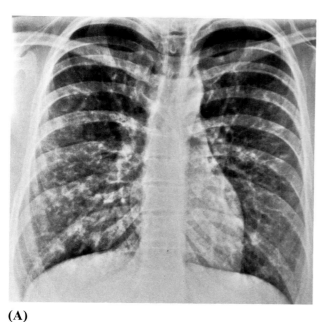
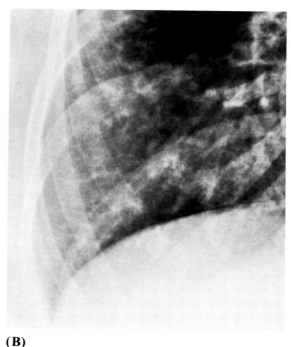

(A)   **(B)**

Fig. 10-16.   Eosinophilic Granuloma of the Lung in an Asymptomatic Woman

This 26-year-old woman had no signs or symptoms of pulmonary disease.

(A) PA film. There are abnormalities rather evenly distributed throughout both lungs except for sparing of the extreme apices.

(B) Coned view of the right base shows detail. Small, irregular opacities or small, irregular nodules with short linear peripheral extensions are interspersed with short, curved linear opacities. Most of the nodules are a few millimeters in diameter, but a few measure almost a centimeter. This is a biopsy-proven case of eosinophilic granuloma of the lung.

Eosinophilic granuloma is a clinically indolent member of the group of entities included under the name histiocytosis X.[11,30] The disease can occur at any age from childhood on, with a peak incidence in the age range of 20 to 40 years. A significant portion (approximately 20 percent) of patients are asymptomatic despite extensive radiographic abnormalities. Those who are symptomatic usually suffer nonspecific symptoms common to pulmonary disease in general: cough (usually nonproductive, but occasionally with hemoptysis), fever, malaise, weight loss, and dyspnea. Lung volumes in these patients may also be preserved, as in some patients with pulmonary sarcoidosis or lymphangioleiomyomatosis, but this would be unexpected in patients with UIP who had advanced lesions on radiography. There is a frequent history of cigarette smoking in adults with eosinophilic granuloma of the lungs.[11]

The lesions of eosinophilic granuloma may clear spontaneously or progress slowly and produce patterns of interstitial fibrosis, with formation of blebs and bullae or cystic-appearing structures, particularly in the upper lobes. Spontaneous pneumothorax is a known consequence of pulmonary eosinophilic granuloma, but also of many other types of disseminated lung disease. Although generally considered a benign disease, as many as 40 percent of patients may develop significant functional impairment. Late progress (after 25 years) to advanced interstitial fibrosis resulting in death has been reported.[30]

The lung alone may be involved, or there may be lesions in the bones or in the pituitary gland with clinically manifest diabetes insipidus.

Notice incidentally the conspicuous costal cartilages passing obliquely cephalad toward the sternum from the costochondral junctions of the fourth through the seventh rib. They are visible because of the technique of the reproduction and because they are well calcified. Although there is much interindividual variation, it is uncommon for these cartilages to be so well calcified at this age.

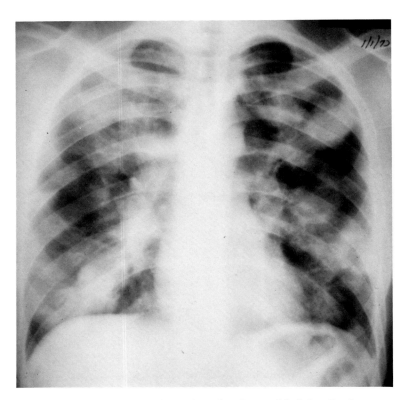

Fig. 10-17. Pulmonary Sarcoid With Large Nodular Lesions

This 23-year-old black man presented with a 3-day history of left-sided pleuritic chest and abdominal pain. He had no cough, hemoptysis, fever, or chills, and he had taken no drugs other than Tylenol. He was well until approximately 2 weeks before admission when he developed frontal headaches and decreased exercise tolerance with dyspnea noted on marked exertion. On physical examination he was well developed, muscular, and in no acute distress. Respirations were 18 per minute and regular. On auscultation there were scattered rales noted in both lungs. Erythrocyte sedimentation rate was 23, and multiple sputum cultures revealed only normal flora. Blood cultures were also negative. PO_2 on room air was 76 mmHg, PCO_2 38 mmHg, and pH 7.43.

Pulmonary function studies showed considerable reduction in lung volumes consistent with severe restrictive lung disease, and there was also a component of obstruction manifest by reduced flow rates, which were only minimally improved with bronchodilators.

The chest radiograph shows bilateral large nodular opacities. (Do you perceive these as nodules or as rounded or oval zones of consolidation?) Some of those in the right lower lung have become confluent. The hila appear abnormal, but it is difficult to determine whether this is hilar adenopathy or superimposition of nodular masses in the lung in front or behind the hila. If it were critical to establish the presence or absence of hilar and mediastinal lymphadenopathy, either tomography, CT, or MRI could be done. However, it was decided to do a limited thoracotomy and biopsy. The tissue diagnosis was noncaseating granulomas consistent with sarcoidosis.

Multiple large nodular opaque zones are a known but uncommon component of the radiographic spectrum of sarcoidosis. Sarcoidosis should be considered in the differential diagnosis because of the patient's age, race, and disproportionately mild symptoms in conjunction with extensive disease. However, other noninfectious granulomas, particularly Wegener's granulomatosis, could not reliably be ruled out. Pulmonary metastases (e.g., from a testicular tumor) in this age group should also be considered. Pulmonary infection of this magnitude would rarely present such a mild clinical picture. Rarely, large nodular lesions may be seen in patients with histoplasmosis who have surprisingly few symptoms, but even then the lesions are not this numerous.

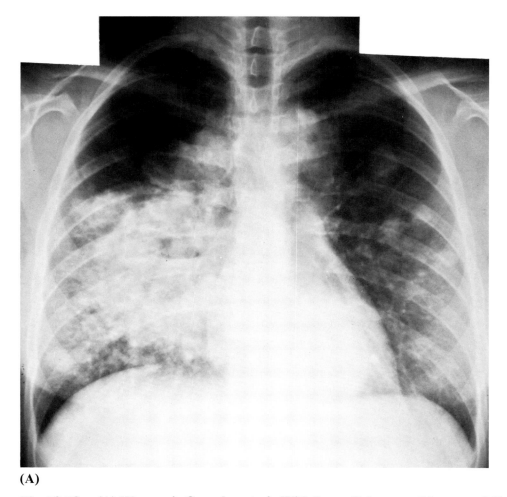

(A)

Fig. 10-18.   (A) Wegener's Granulomatosis With Large Pulmonary Masses and Cavitation

This 20-year-old woman was well until approximately 10 months before admission, when she was noted to have palpable purpura, fever, arthritis, and rectal bleeding. At that time she was felt to have Henoch-Schönlein purpura. She was treated with prednisone and intermittently with azathioprine (Imuran). During this time she also had intermittent hemoptysis. She was later admitted with increasing shortness of breath, hacking cough, and fever. There was no renal dysfunction or proteinuria.

The chest film shows bilateral multiple nodular opacities that vary in size. Large masses are present in the right lower lung and in the left lower lobe behind the heart. An air-fluid level (medially in the posterior seventh interspace) can be seen within the cavitating mass on the right side. There are also interspersed small (approximately 5 mm) nodules in both lungs. There is sparing of the apices, the subclavicular regions, and the extreme lateral bases. The pulmonary abnormalities pervade the hilar and paramediastinal regions, making it difficult to evaluate the presence or absence of lymphadenopathy.

A lung biopsy showed lesions of Wegener's granulomatosis. The patient was treated with cyclophosphamide (Cytoxan) and high-dose steroids and was discharged from the hospital.

Although this patient is clearly one whose immune mechanisms are altered both by her disease and by the fact that she had received treatment with steroids and Imuran, it is most unusual to have this much pulmonary infection in a patient who does not appear more critically ill. Infection with the ubiquitous fungi or *Nocardia* in an altered host, when present in this magnitude, would be expected to be accompanied by more severe symptoms than this patient had. Nevertheless, since there was no noninvasive way to completely exclude infection, and since treatment involved increasing the dose of steroids, the lung biopsy was done. *(Figure continues.)*

Fig. 10-18. *(Continued).* **(B) Wegener's Granulomatosis With Infection**

Seven days after discharge the patient in Fig. A returned complaining of cough productive of foul-smelling sputum. Her chest film now shows further cavitation of many lesions. The cavities can be seen as irregular lucent zones within the consolidations.

Progressive cavitation of the pulmonary lesions of Wegener's granulomatosis may be a response to treatment. However, in a patient with increasing cough, fever, and foul-smelling sputum, the likelihood of secondary infection must be strongly considered. Dark brown mucus was seen in the patient's sputum, and cultures showed a high percentage of *Staphylococcus aureus.* Other bacteria were interpreted as normal flora. The diagnosis of anaerobic organism pneumonia cannot be made from sputum cultures since these organisms are part of the normal oral flora, but the foul smell of the sputum supports the presumption that the patient also had pulmonary infection with anaerobes. Whether the increasing cavitation in the pulmonary lesions is due to superinfection or to response to the necrotizing granulomas to treatment, or both, still cannot be ascertained. The patient was treated with appropriate antibiotics and responded.

Wegener's granulomatosis is a systemic disease that can involve many organ systems.[19] Most commonly there is involvement of the lungs and kidneys. The nose and paranasal sinuses are also commonly involved, and there may be involvement of the skin, the ears, the brain, and the joints. In the limited form of Wegener's granulomatosis there is no associated glomerulonephritis, and pulmonary involvement is usually dominant. Although an uncommon condition, Wegener's granulomatosis is still one of the more common causes of pulmonary vasculitis. It occurs at all ages but is most common in older males. The pulmonary involvement may be asymptomatic or may be associated with cough, malaise, fever, dyspnea, and hemoptysis. Other signs and symptoms depend on the organ systems involved.

The radiographic spectrum of pulmonary Wegener's granulomatosis is broad and includes:

1. Nodules, either the countable or the uncountable variety, with or without cavitation (solitary nodules are less common as a presenting radiographic finding, but do occur)
2. Patchy zones of consolidation indistinguishable from those of bacterial, viral, fungal, or obstructive pneumonias (obstruction can result from endobronchial lesions)
3. Conglomerate masses of varying sizes, with or without associated cavitation
4. Reticulonodular opacities
5. Varying combinations of all of the above lesions.

Hilar or mediastinal adenopathy is seldom manifest on chest films.

As cavitary lesions respond to treatment they may become thin walled and indistinguishable from bullae. Secondary infection of cavities with *Staphylococcus aureus* or mixed anaerobes is a known complication.

In children and young adults the clinical signs and symptoms of Wegener's granulomatosis may lead to a misdiagnosis of Henoch-Schönlein purpura.[19] In addition, lesions of tuberculosis and the pathogenic fungi may be histologically similar in appearance to the extravascular lesions of Wegener's granulomatosis. It is critical, therefore, that biopsy specimens be cultured when they are obtained and that special stains be used to rule out these infectious causes.

Before the advent of modern treatment, Wegener's granulomatosis was usually a fatal disease, with death resulting from either renal failure or infection or occasionally overwhelming hemorrhage from pulmonary cavities. Modern treatment has had a markedly favorable influence on prognosis.

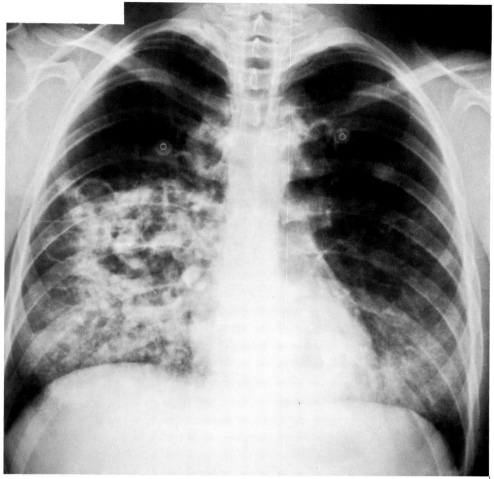

Fig. 10-18. (B)

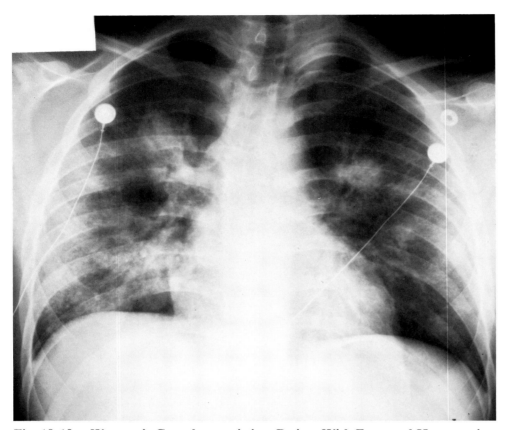

Fig. 10-19. Wegener's Granulomatosis in a Patient With Fever and Hemoptysis

This 17-year-old patient had a short history of fevers, wheezing, and a cough productive of several teaspoons of clear sputum mixed with dark brown blood. A week before admission he had gone to a walk-in clinic. A chest film was reported to show bilateral pulmonary abnormalities. He was treated with erythromycin, which was subsequently changed to amoxicillin. His fever and hemoptysis increased and he became progressively weaker. He had a long history of chronic sinusitis and rhinitis that had become worse over the past several weeks. On physical examination the patient was well developed, acutely ill, tachypneic (30 respirations per minute), and febrile (38.5°C rectal). Arterial blood gas analysis showed that the patient was hypoxemic (PO_2 65 mmHg). He was also anemic.

Necrotizing granulomas and necrotizing vasculitis, consistent with Wegener's granulomatosis, were seen on a lung biopsy specimen. Special stains for acid-fast bacilli and fungi were negative. Cultures of the specimen for bacterial and fungal pathogens were negative.

Patchy zones of consolidation on the right and nodules on the left are seen on the chest film. Air bronchograms are visible in the zones of consolidation about the upper portions of the right hilum and in a smaller zone of consolidation about the periphery of the upper left hilum. Small nodular opacities (measuring in millimeters) were also seen in the periphery of the right lung and scattered throughout the left lung, but they do not show well on this reproduction.

One of the critical distinctions to make in patients with disseminated lung disease is whether or not the abnormalities are due to infection or to noninfectious disease. This is critical because steroids are frequently used to treat noninfectious, nonneoplastic disseminated pulmonary diseases of different etiologies. There is understandably a great reluctance to use steroids in the treatment of lung disease when there is the possibility of disseminating infection. Non-Hodgkin's lymphoma of the lung could also produce a similar radiographic appearance and would receive different treatment.

This patient was treated with steroids and Cytoxan and had a gratifying response. To date there has been no clinical evidence of renal involvement.

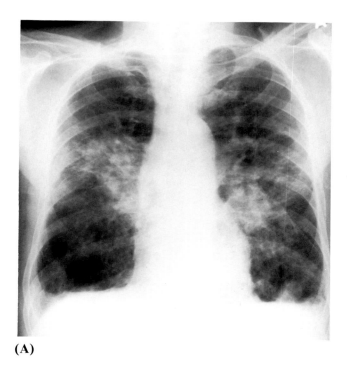

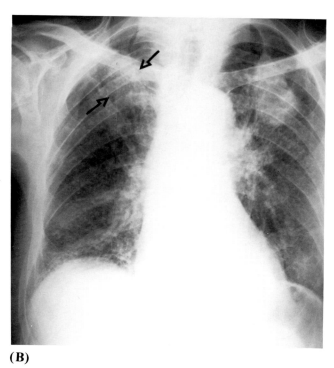

(A)

(B)

Fig. 10-20.　(A) Silicosis

This 74-year-old man had a 20-year history of exposure to silica from cutting firebricks. He had dyspnea, progressive shortness of breath, and essential hypertension.

The film shows characteristic changes consisting of multiple small (measuring in millimeters), fairly discrete nodules predominating in the upper zones. On this reproduction, however, they are overshadowed by larger conglomerate nodules of progressive massive fibrosis adjacent to the upper right hilum and to the lower aspect of the left hilum. The overall conformation of the chest is also consistent with the presence of emphysema.

(B) Coal Worker's Pneumoconiosis

This patient was a coal miner for 28 years. Unfortunately, his present pulmonary functional status is unavailable. His chest film, however, shows myriad small (millimeter-sized), barely discrete, rounded nodules distributed throughout both lungs. In addition, in both upper lung zones there are masslike zones of consolidation. That on the left side has more discrete margins than the lesion in the right subapical region (arrow). These are consistent with zones of progressive massive fibrosis (PMF).

Small, fairly discrete, rounded nodules may be seen in the lungs of patients with silicosis, and they are fre-

quently more numerous in the upper lung zones. They may also present as indistinguishable nodules in patients with coal worker's pneumoconiosis. In patients with silicosis, the nodules are manifestations of granulomas or hyaline nodules, and there is associated scarring. In coal worker's pneumoconiosis, on the other hand, the nodules correlate with the presence of dust macules, which are accumulations of macrophages and coal dust about the margins of peripheral bronchioles associated with only minimal scarring of pulmonary parenchyma. In general, the degree of pulmonary dysfunction does not correlate well with the profusion of these nodules as seen radiographically. However, patients with silicosis, presumably because of the associated scarring, are much more likely to have symptoms than patients with simple coal worker's pneumoconiosis. Both types of pneumoconiosis may be complicated by zones of PMF, in which case symptoms of chronic lung disease are usually present. PMF may occur anywhere in the lung but is more common in the upper lung.

When the masslike lesions of dense fibrosis (PMF) are unilateral and solitary, they are virtually impossible to distinguish radiographically from neoplasm. The PMF lesions can enlarge progressively and contain foci of necrosis.

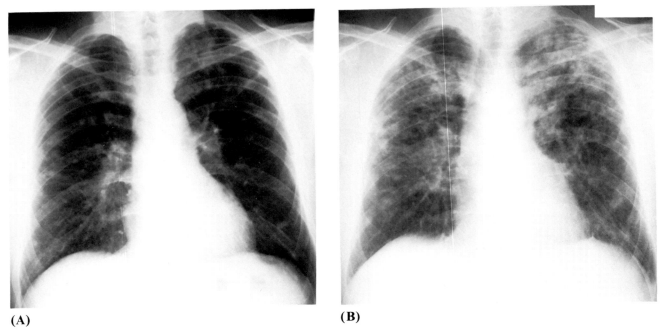

(A)   (B)

Fig. 10-21. Progressive Pulmonary Lesions of Sarcoidosis

This 49-year-old man had a diagnosis of sarcoidosis based on the finding of noncaseating granulomas in a lymph node retrieved at mediastinoscopy 4 years before the film shown in Fig. A. At that time he was asymptomatic but apparently had hilar adenopathy on a chest film. His pulmonary function tests were normal. Three years later he noticed a right submandibular swelling. A local biopsy again revealed noncaseating granuloma in a right neck lymph node and in the right submaxillary gland.

(A) Multiple, fairly discrete (5 to 10 mm) nodules with unsharp margins are seen scattered throughout both lungs. There is some coalescence of nodules in the left apex, and there are scattered linear strands in the left upper lobe. At this time (4 years after the initial diagnosis) he had a mild, dry cough but normal pulmonary function. Over the next few years he had gradual worsening of his dry cough related to taking deep breaths. He had a slow decline in total lung capacity with mild obstruction and progression of abnormalities on chest films.

He was started on prednisone treatment with subjective and objective improvement, but after a few months it was necessary to taper and discontinue the prednisone because of objectionable side effects.

(B) Chest film taken 33 months after Fig. A. There has been an increase in size of the scattered nodules, much more coalescence in both upper lobes, and some honeycombing as well. There is contraction in volume of the left upper lobe with upward retraction of the left hilum and tenting of the left diaphragm. These are changes of a chronic scarring process; they are part of the spectrum of late abnormalities that may occur in some patients with sarcoid but may also be seen with other chronic lung diseases.

The patient was still able to continue his strenuous work, but his cough had worsened and he had increased fatigability. Pulmonary function tests showed evidence of mild restrictive and obstructive disease. He was treated with steroids in low dosage.

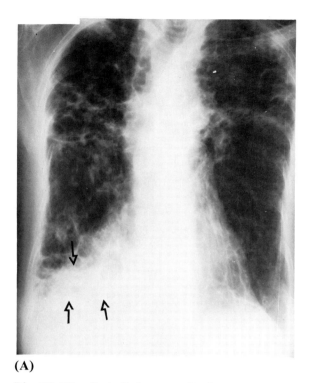

(A)

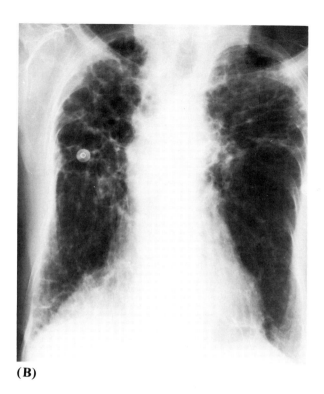

(B)

Fig. 10-22. Late Pulmonary Lesions of Sarcoidosis

This 83-year-old white woman complained of increasing shortness of breath and exertional dyspnea. She had had a chronic cough with production of moderate amounts of white sputum especially in the mornings for the past 12 years.

Twenty years ago she had been hospitalized with shortness of breath, pedal edema, and erythema nodosum (a nonspecific reaction of the skin that may be seen in conjunction with a variety of systemic diseases, including sarcoidosis and some of the infectious granulomatous diseases, especially coccidioidomycosis). She also reportedly had hilar adenopathy on chest films. A Kveim test was positive, and a liver biopsy was positive for noncaseating granulomas. Stains for microorganisms were negative and a PPD was negative. A diagnosis of sarcoidosis was made, and the patient was treated with steroids for 6 months with complete resolution of symptoms.

A month before the chest film shown in Fig. A the patient had pulmonary function tests consistent with mixed obstructive and restrictive disease. Results of blood gas tests on room air were PO_2 63 mmHg, PCO_2 35 mmHg, bicarbonate 23.4, and pH 7.43.

(A) PA film shows contraction in volume of the upper lobes and extensive cystic or bullous changes throughout both lungs. There is also an area of consolidation, consistent with pneumonitis, at the extreme right base (arrows). Her temperature was 38.2°C and respi-

rations were 36 per minute. There was minimal dullness with decreased breath sounds at the bases and rales and bronchi on the right. Her PO_2 on room air was now 45 mmHg. Sputum cultures were negative, but the patient was treated with antibiotics and the fever rapidly abated. Her shortness of breath, however, was only minimally improved.

(B) PA film taken 3 months later shows clearing of the acute pneumonia at the right base, but there is a persistent opacity due to a prominent right pericardiac fat pad. The extensive abnormalities throughout the remainder of both lungs show little change. There is persistent distortion of the trachea, which buckles to the right as a result of the unequal contraction in volume of the upper lobes.

These abnormalities are late changes that may occur in the lungs of patients with noninfectious granulomatous disease, particularly sarcoid and eosinophilic granuloma. Biopsy of the lungs at this stage shows characteristic changes of severe UIP, and the granulomatous components may not always remain recognizable. Death, due to respiratory failure in the late stages of sarcoidosis, probably occurs in fewer than 10 percent of all cases.[18]

This case also illustrates how much easier it is to recognize pneumonia superimposed on chronic lung disease when earlier films are available for comparison. Otherwise, it is often not possible to distinguish acute consolidation from chronic lesions.

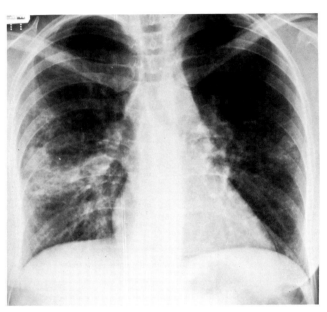

(A)

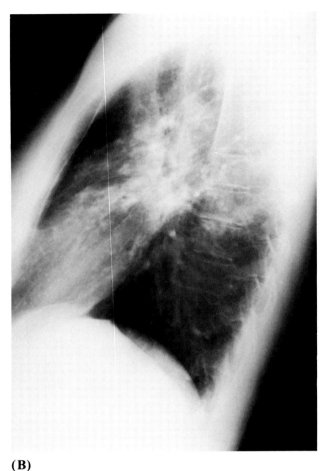

(B)

Fig. 10-23. Necrotizing Sarcoid Granulomatosis

This 30-year-old woman had signs and symptoms of a pituitary tumor. The abnormalities seen on the chest film were incidental findings. The patient had no signs or symptoms of lung disease.

(A) PA view. Clusters of poorly defined nodules under 1 cm in diameter are seen in the axillary regions of both midlung zones. They are more extensive on the right side, but the larger more opaque area is in part caused by postoperative reaction at the biopsy site.

(B) The histopathology was consistent with necrotizing sarcoid granulomatosis.[5,20] The histologic differential in the case, however, included infection. Cultures of the sputum and of the biopsy specimen itself were negative for pathogens, including viruses. Multiple special stains for fungi, acid-fast bacilli, and other bacteria showed no microorganisms.

Necrotizing sarcoid granulomatosis is characterized by a histologic pattern of sarcoid-like granulomas, prominent vasculitis, and variable necrosis.[5] Radiographically, bilateral pulmonary nodules of variable size (up to 4.0 cm) are most common, but unilateral or single-nodule presentations also occur. A miliary pattern has also been reported. Hilar adenopathy may be present or absent. The clinical course is generally benign and patients are often asymptomatic. When present, symptoms are those of nonspecific chest disease.

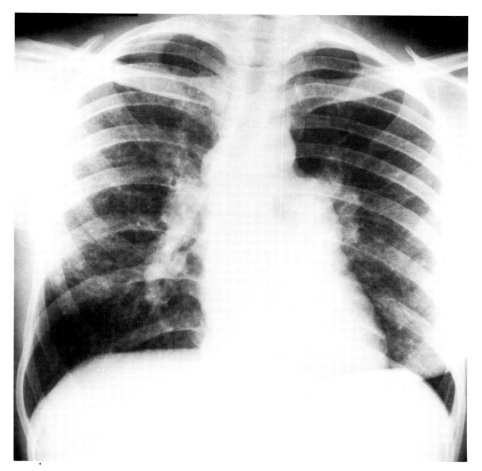

Fig. 10-24. Hilar and Mediastinal Lymphadenopathy in Sarcoidosis

This 28-year-old woman had a mastectomy for intraductal carcinoma of the breast 3 years ago and for the past year has noticed increasing fatigue. Her PA chest film shows mediastinal, bilateral hilar, and right paratracheal adenopathy. This combination of adenopathies is common in patients with sarcoidosis. Small pulmonary nodules are present in the midlung zones, more markedly on the right.

Although the radiographic findings fit well with sarcoidosis, metastases from breast carcinoma or malignant lymphoma could not be eliminated from consideration. The patient's Kveim test was positive, and a right scalene node biopsy showed noncaseating epithelioid granulomas compatible with sarcoid.

Unfortunately, noncaseating granulomata may also be found as incidental abnormalities in the tissues of patients with known infectious granulomatous diseases and with certain malignancies such as carcinoma of the breast, lymphoma, melanoma, and even carcinoma of the lung. Therefore, the positive Kveim test is very important for this patient, and careful follow-up studies are also indicated.

Spontaneous remission is frequent in all stages of sarcoid, but it is most common in those who have hilar and mediastinal lymphadenopathy as the sole radiographic manifestation. In those with manifest parenchymal disease in addition to the lymphadenopathy, the spontaneous remission rate is lower, but still appreciable, whereas in patients who have parenchymal disease in the absence of detectable mediastinal and hilar lymphadenopathy the spontaneous remission rate is still lower. Patients may be asymptomatic at any of these stages, but those with predominant hilar and mediastinal lymphadenopathy may have fever and cough, whereas those with parenchymal disease may have a decrease in diffusing capacity and a decrease in lung volume. Patients with sarcoidosis may present with hypercalcemia and hypercalciuria.

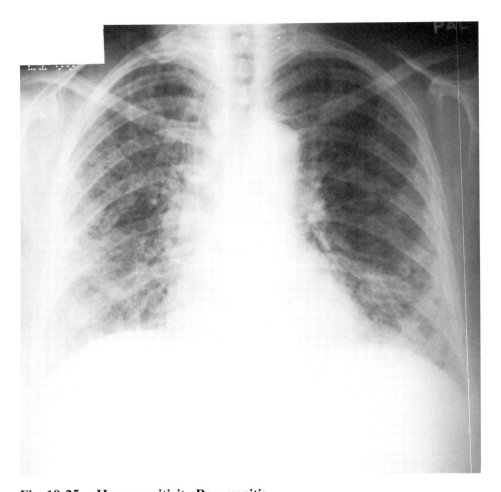

Fig. 10-25. Hypersensitivity Pneumonitis

This 45-year-old woman was in good health until she returned from a vacation. Then she developed dyspnea, malaise, aches, and intermittent fevers to 104°F.

Her chest film shows diffuse pulmonary abnormalities with irregular nodular and linear components that coalesce in places to form larger irregular, foci. A chest film made 6 days earlier showed similar lesions.

The patient was a bird conservationist who cared for well and sick birds. Because she developed her symptoms upon returning to her usual environment from a prolonged vacation, the diagnosis of hypersensitivity pneumonitis was considered, and a transbronchial lung biopsy was done.

The biopsy showed a mixed intra-alveolar and interstitial inflammatory process composed of macrophages, lymphocytes, and rare acute inflammatory cells. Eosinophils were not prominent. There were both well-formed and poorly formed granulomata, all without evidence of caseation. There were also mild parabronchial fibrosis and features of bronchiolitis obliterans. There were no histopathologic changes to suggest viral infection, and no microorganisms were identified on special stains. The findings were considered those of a nonspecific granulomatous pneumonitis consistent with hypersensitivity pneumonitis. The patient later also tested sensitive to bird serum on a gel diffusion test.

Hypersensitivity pneumonitis consequent to inhalation of a large variety of organic dusts and animal excreta or dander is a well-known disorder. The intriguing question is why so few people develop hypersensitivity pneumonitis when so many are exposed to these antigens. Furthermore, why do many subjects who test positive to these antigens never develop any clinical manifestations of this sensitivity?

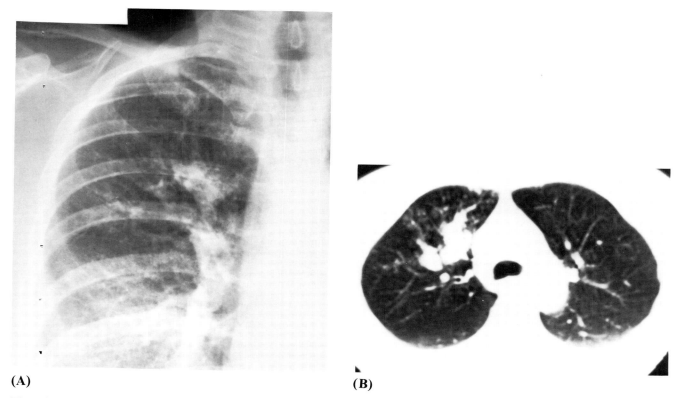

(A)   **(B)**

Fig. 10-26.   Bronchopulmonary Allergic Aspergillosis

This 47-year-old woman was in good health until approximately 6 months ago. Then she noticed increasing fatigue accompanied by intermittent cough and a feeling as though she had a chest cold. She did not pay much attention to these symptoms until approximately 1 month ago, when she visited her physician. She had a chest film and was referred.

Her pulmonary function tests and blood gases were normal. She had neither any signs of asthma nor any eosinophilia.

(A) Coned view of the right upper and midlung zones. There is an abnormal branching opacity that extends into the lung from the upper portions of the right hilum. This appearance of "stuffed bronchi" is one of the characteristic ways in which allergic bronchopulmonary aspergillosis may present radiographically. However, any endobronchial lesion causing chronic partial obstruction and retention of secretions in peripheral bronchi could produce the same picture (see Ch. 6). The surrounding portions of the lung remain expanded because of collateral air flow via the pores of Kohn, the canals of Lambert, and small-airway communications.

(B) CT scan. Distended, distorted, mucus-filled bronchi are seen branching in the anterior portions of the right upper lobe. Histopathologically this lesion had characteristic features of allergic bronchopulmonary aspergillosis. There was mucoid impaction of the involved bronchi with a mixture of necrotic alveolar exudate, Charcot-Leyden crystals, and hyphae of *Aspergillus.*

Commonly, patients with allergic aspergillosis have a history of atopy or asthma, but that is not invariable. Usually there is eosinophilia. Although numerous eosinophils were found in the specimen, this patient had no blood eosinophilia.

The diagnosis of allergic bronchopulmonary aspergillosis can be suggested from characteristic radiographic findings, and the organisms may be recovered from bronchoscopy specimens. The lesions usually respond rapidly to steroid therapy. (Fig. B courtesy of Dr. P.N. Schield, San Ramon, California.)

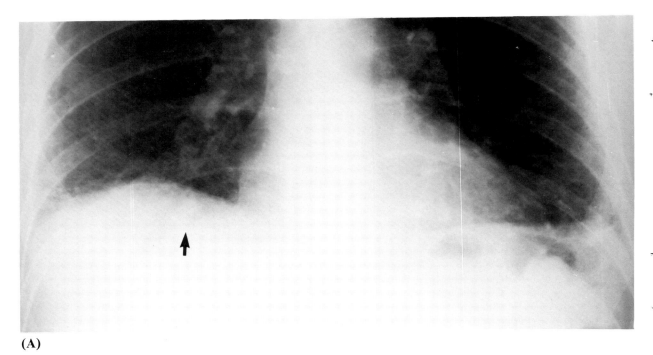

(A)

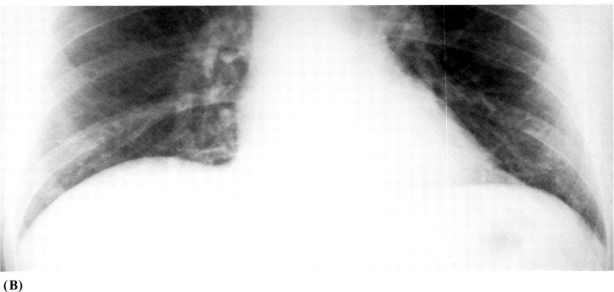

(B)

Fig. 10-27. Bleomycin Pulmonary Toxicity

This man had received chemotherapy for a testicular carcinoma; bleomycin was one of the drugs used.

(A) Coned view of the bases after completion of chemotherapy. Vessels at both bases have lost sharpness of outline, and the ordinarily sharp lung-diaphragm interfaces are lost. There are nodular opacities at the bases varying in size from a few millimeters to over 1 cm in diameter. The larger nodules are projected beneath the dome of the right diaphragm (arrow). The lateral aspect of the left diaphragm is effaced by opacities in adjacent lung along with focal pleural reaction. These findings are common elements within the spectrum of bleomycin-induced lung disease.

(B) Coned view of the lung bases taken approximately 5 months before Fig. A. Both hemi-diaphragms are sharply defined in the absence of any disease in the adjacent lung. The small, irregular, nodular densities present in the lung bases in Fig. A are not present in Fig. B, at which time the patient was not suffering from bleomycin toxicity.

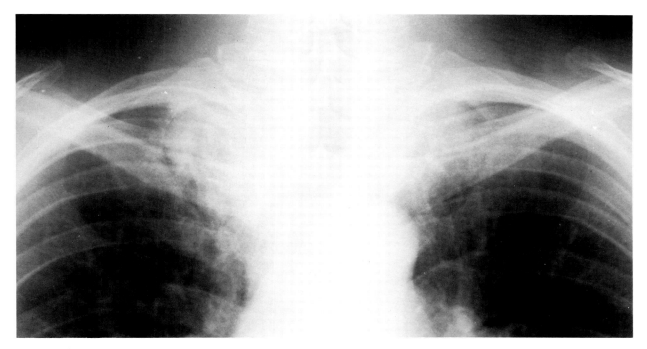

Fig. 10-28. Amiodarone Pulmonary Toxicity

The patient is a 51-year-old man with a history of severe arteriosclerotic cardiovascular disease since the age of 38 years. After a coronary artery bypass graft operation many years ago he had a long symptom-free interval. At present he is incapacitated by progressive coronary artery disease. Treatment with amiodarone was required to control severe arrhythmias while the patient awaited a donor heart for transplantation.

This coned view shows intense consolidation medially in both the apical and subapical lung zones. These regions were clear on pretreatment baseline films. The radiographic appearance is characteristic of pulmonary reaction to amiodarone. Frequently, however, there is a need to rule out infection, particularly tuberculosis. Although apical opacities due to tuberculosis are common, they would rarely be so symmetrical at the time of initial disease presentation.

Bilateral upper lobe zones of consolidation, sometimes in a distribution resembling that of chronic eosinophilic pneumonia, is one radiographic pattern of amiodarone-induced lung disease. Other reported patterns include patchy foci of consolidation, both homogeneous and inhomogeneous, in either the upper or the lower lobes or both; zones of dense consolidation; and "interstitial disease." Pulmonary lesions have occurred 1.5 to 12 months after first use of the drug. When present, symptoms are those common to many types of pulmonary disease. Radiographic regression may be slow after use of the drug is stopped and may not be complete.[28]

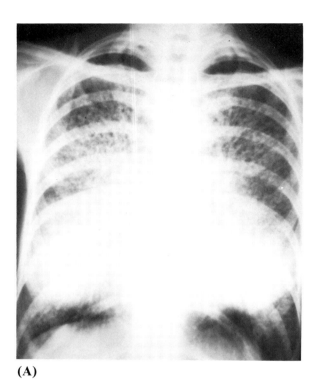

(A)

Fig. 10-29. Pulmonary Alveolar Proteinosis

This 42-year-old woman had a history of six episodes of pneumonia and two episodes of bronchitis requiring hospitalization during her lifetime. In recent years she has been well and had negative chest film results.

Three months before Fig. A was taken she developed progressive shortness of breath, a nonproductive cough, orthopnea, and paroxysmal nocturnal dyspnea. She has had no fever. Her PO_2 on room air was in the low 40s (mmHg).

(A) PA film shows bilateral pulmonary abnormalities with relative sparing of the extreme apices and bases. The increase in radiodensity of the lower zones is due in part to projection of the patient's dense breasts, accentuated by the techniques used to produce this illustration. You can evaluate the roentgenographic details of the lesions in the upper lung. There is a series of juxtaposed ring shadows with relatively thick, unit-density walls and radiolucent centers. The appearance is reminiscent of, but not identical to, the radiographic images of honeycombing. However, this patient has biopsy-proven alveolar proteinosis, which is essentially an airspace-filling disease process.

(B) Coned view of the upper portions of the right lung is shown on the left; for comparison, a coned view from a chest film made approximately 10 months earlier is shown on the right. Even on the earlier film there are small nodular opacities peripherally and along the paths of vessels, but there has been much disease progression in the interval.

The patient did not improve on conservative treatment. She then had lung lavage, first on the left and later on the right. The return lavage fluid was the color of skim milk. Following the second lavage her PO_2 increased to over 70 mmHg, and there was clearing on her chest radiograph. The patient felt significantly improved.

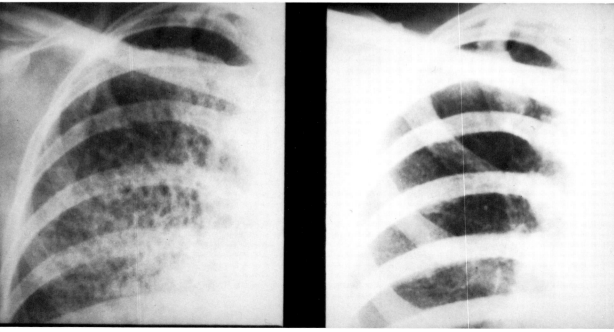

(B)

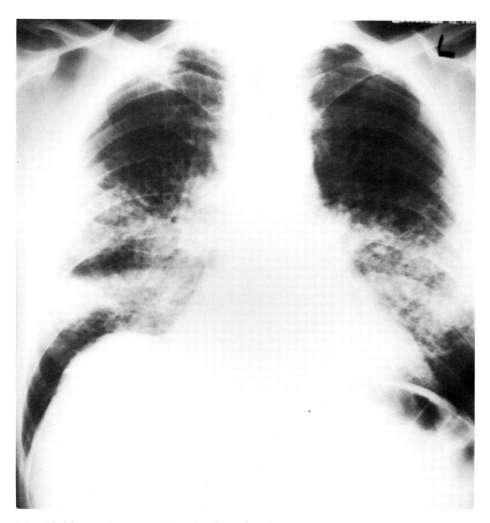

Fig. 10-30. Pulmonary Alveolar Proteinosis

PA view of the chest of a 52-year-old man with a history of episodic pain in the region of his anterior trachea, accompanied by a sensation of shortness of breath made worse by deep inspiration. Because of abnormalities seen on a chest film 2 years ago he had an open-lung biopsy in his local hospital. The specimen was reportedly normal. Nevertheless, he was treated with prednisone and experienced improvement of his symptoms until he suffered side effects from the steroids. He remained relatively asymptomatic until 3 months before admission, when he suffered a recurrence of the same symptoms, which did not respond to steroids. On admission, the patient was short of breath with even slight exertion, and his neck pain was quite bothersome.

On physical examination he appeared somewhat cyanotic. On chest auscultation there were occasional tubular breath sounds on expiration and a few coarse rales at the bases. Blood gas analysis results (on room air) were PO_2 52 mmHg, PCO_2 32.5 mmHg, HCO_3 22, and pH 7.45.

There are bilateral large central foci of inhomogeneous consolidation, within which multiple juxtaposed small, rounded foci of radiolucency are evident. There is sparing of the periphery of the lung. In the lateral projection (not shown) the distribution of the pulmonary abnormalities was again found to be heaviest centrally. Alveolar proteinosis was diagnosed by lung biopsy.

Frequently the lesions in pulmonary alveolar proteinosis have a distribution much the same as those of pulmonary edema of renal failure: the so-called "butterfly" or "bat's wing" distribution.

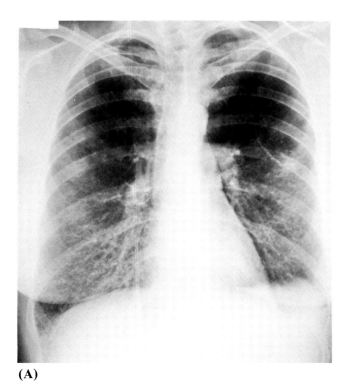

(A)

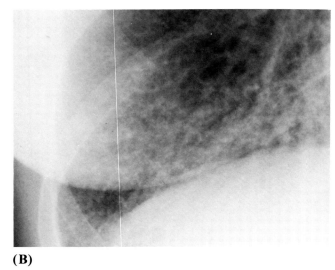

(B)

Fig. 10-31. Lymphangioleiomyomatosis

The patient is a 39-year-old woman who noticed progressive dyspnea on exertion over a period of 5 years. She had had severe asthma as a child, but since the age of 14 she has been without symptoms.

Her pulmonary function studies now show hypoxemia, preserved lung volumes, and moderately severe obstructive defects. She has a daily cough productive of approximately 1 teaspoon of thick white to pale yellow sputum.

The histopathologic diagnosis of lymphangioleiomyomatosis was made from an open-lung biopsy specimen.

(A) PA view of the chest shows profuse but subtle bilateral pulmonary abnormalities with relative sparing of the medial portions of the upper lung zones. The arclike thin-band shadow lateral to the left hilum is due to a series of staples at the site of the lung biopsy. The left hemidiaphragm has lost its sharp marginal contour and appears slightly high, simulating a pleural effusion. This appearance is probably due to pleuritis consequent to the lung biopsy.

(B) Coned view of the right lower lung shows myriad poorly marginated, overlapping nodular opacities with effacement of small vessel images. In addition, cystic-appearing spaces (black) can be seen nestled between larger vessel branches.

The radiographic patterns of lymphangioleiomyomatosis may be indistinguishable from those of UIP. However, in lymphangioleiomyomatosis preservation of lung volumes is the rule, whereas patients with UIP with comparable amounts of visible disease show a reduction in lung volumes. The reticulonodular pattern of lymphangioleiomyomatosis may be generalized or may be more prominent in the lung bases. Cystic changes are present in the lungs, pathologically varying in size from millimeters to centimeters. These may impart a pronounced cystic appearance radiographically.

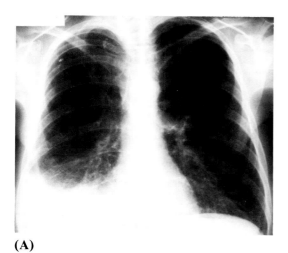

(A)

Fig. 10-32. Pulmonary Lymphangioleiomyomatosis, Chylous Pleural Effusion, and a Pelvic Mass

This 35-year-old woman has pulmonary lymphangioleiomyomatosis. The patient reported having had a chest film 4 years earlier that showed bibasilar scarring. A right supraclavicular lymph node biopsy at that time was normal, and a gallium scan was normal. Pulmonary function tests showed a marked diminution in diffusing capacity. A clinical diagnosis of sarcoidosis was apparently made. One year ago the patient was operated on because of a pelvic mass that had increased in size over a period of about 6 years. Two weeks after this surgery she noticed abdominal swelling, and 1 month later she noted increasing dyspnea on exertion. She was admitted to another hospital where a right pleural effusion and ascites were noted. Fluid from a thoracentesis was chylous. The histopathology of the pelvic mass was considered characteristic of lymphangioleiomyomatosis.

For the 3 months preceding these studies the patient had experienced shortness of breath and recurrent right pleural effusions with thoracenteses producing 2 to 3 liters of chylous effusion 2 to 3 times per week. She has also lost 25 pounds in the past 6 months. On physical examination the patient was in respiratory distress with a respiratory rate of 30 per minute. She was afebrile. She had hypoxemia and also hypoproteinemia.

(A) PA view of the chest shows the distribution of the pulmonary and pleural abnormalities.

(B,C) Coned views of the right and left lower lung, respectively. Pleural effusion obscures much of the right lung base, but the lung that is visible shows a loss of definition of small-vessel images. On the left side the abnormalities are not at all striking, but again there is an effacement of the details of the small-vessel images. Even the medium-sized vessels, particularly those that project just lateral to the left heart border, show a loss of sharpness of outline. *(Figure continues.)*

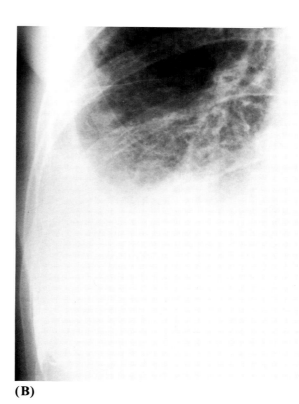

(B)

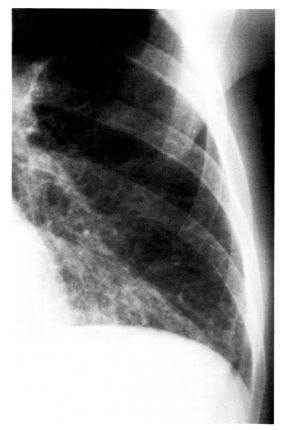

(C)

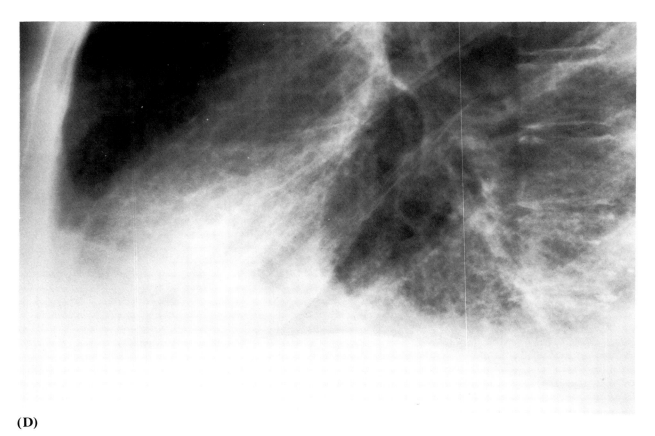

(D)

Fig. 10-32. *(Continued).* **(D)** Lateral view of the lung bases. Here the pulmonary abnormalities are more easily appreciated. In addition to effacement of all of the small vessels at the bases there are linear and curvilinear opacities with foci of honeycombing or pseudohoneycombing of the lower lung. Pulmonary abnormalities may often be seen more readily on the lateral view of the chest since the abnormalities of both lungs are superimposed. However, these interstitial abnormalities can also be seen on critical study of B and C.

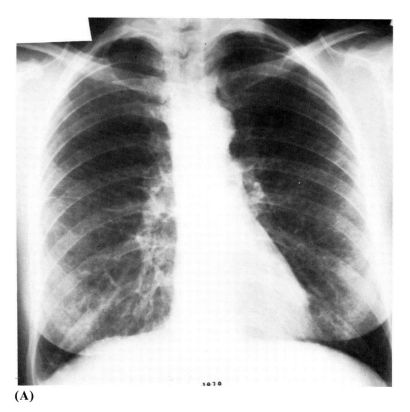

(A)

Fig. 10-33. Tuberous Sclerosis With Pulmonary Lesions of Lymphangioleiomyomatosis

(A,B) PA and lateral chest films, respectively, of a middle-aged woman with known tuberous sclerosis. She was being seen in consultation because of hematuria and a known hamartoma of the kidney.

In the lower lung zones you can see ill-defined small nodular opacities about the periphery. Toward the center there are some subtle radiolucent or cystic-appearing zones. In the lung behind the upper sternum on the lateral view there is a loss of vascular detail and there are some irregular nodular and linear opacities. There is also a rather subtle appearance of cystic structures, some of which are fairly large, on the order of 2 cm or more. The patient was in no respiratory distress, and no pulmonary function studies were done at this time.

The lung bases were included on an abdominal CT series (Fig. 10-34), which was done to evaluate the patient's renal hamartoma.

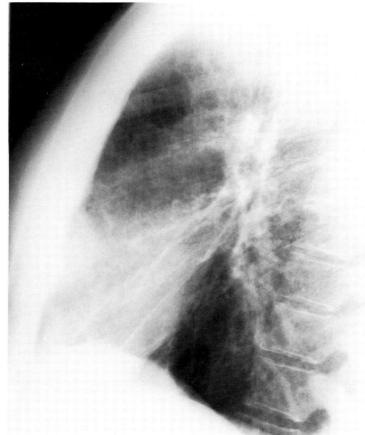

(B)

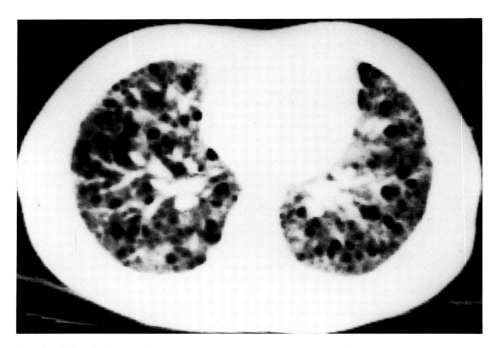

Fig. 10-34.   CT of Pulmonary Lymphangioleiomyomatosis

CT scan through the lung bases reveals marked distortion of lung architecture. Circumscribed, cystic-appearing lesions occupy both lung bases. Most of the branching, near-white structures seen are due to blood vessels, but some of the more flame-shaped, near-white opacities along the periphery of the lung are probably caused by thickened interlobular septa, which produce a nodular appearance. Although the chest film is not normal, the discrepancy in magnitude of the lesions between the CT scan and the chest films is striking. This is a good example of how the enhanced density discrimination afforded by the CT technique can permit the display of abnormalities that are subtle at best on the chest film. The pulmonary lesions of tuberous sclerosis are the same as those of lymphangioleiomyomatosis.

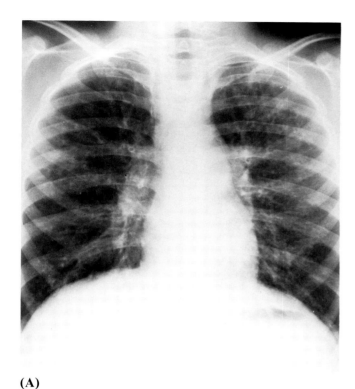

(A)

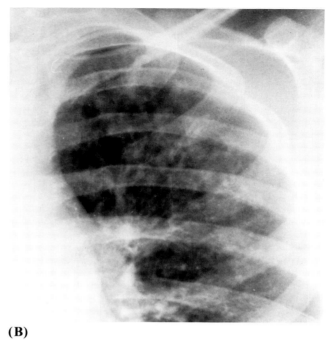

(B)

Fig. 10-35. Cystic Fibrosis

This young man has long-standing cystic fibrosis.

(A) PA view. Both lungs show diffuse abnormalities consisting of linear, nodular, or circumscribed ring images. Some of the latter are fairly discrete, whereas others are subtle because their walls are not seen through 360 degrees.

The hilar shadows have lost their normal contours. They show rounded marginal arcs that do not correlate with the size of the vessels seen to emanate from them.

In addition, the mediastinum is wide, and the pleural reflection between the left pulmonary artery and the aortic arch is slightly convex to the lung. These findings are compatible with the presence of hilar and mediastinal lymphadenopathy, which may be seen in patients with mucoviscidosis because of chronic and recurrent pulmonary infection.

Notice the thickness of the walls of the proximal bronchi seen end-on. For example, there is one on the right that is superimposed on the posteromedial end of the sixth rib, and one on the left that is projected beneath the cortex of the posteromedial aspect of the sixth rib.

(B) Coned view of the left upper lobe. Fairly straight linear shadows parallel the bronchi as they emanate from the upper left hilum. The rounded lucencies of dilated peripheral bronchi and bronchioles are also visible. Those projecting into the posterior fourth and fifth interspaces are seen best. This radiographic appearance is characteristic of cystic fibrosis (mucoviscidosis), and the linear shadows ("tramlines") produced by thickened bronchial walls are most commonly seen in persons with severe chronic bronchitis and bronchiectasis. In addition, there are scattered small, ill-defined, nodular opacities.

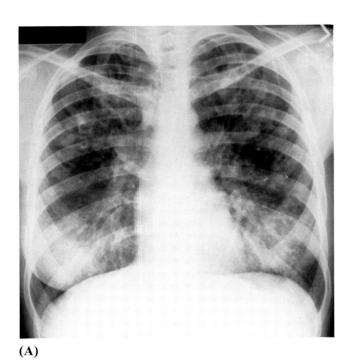

(A)

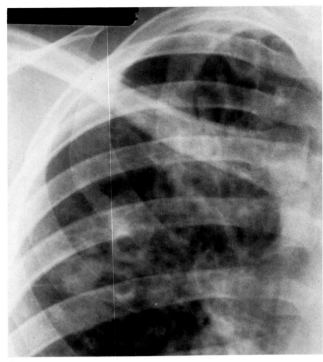

(B)

Fig. 10-36.   Cystic Fibrosis With Bronchiectasis

(A) In both upper lobes in this young woman there are clusters of ringlike lesions, some of which have rather thick walls.

(B) Coned view of the right subclavicular zone shows better detail. In addition to the thick-walled rings there are clusters of smaller, thin-walled ring shadows. Similar findings are present on the left side. These "holes" are typical changes seen in the lungs of patients with cystic fibrosis after they have had repeated infections and have developed bronchiectasis. Some of the unit-density material seen in these bronchiectatic cavities is due to retained secretions and mucus plugs or impactions. This patient has more severe pulmonary involvement than the patient seen in Fig. 10-35.

Both hila are distorted and appear larger than normal. The distortion is due in part to contraction in volume of the more severely damaged portions of the upper lobes with consequent retraction of the hila. In addition, it is likely that there is hilar adenopathy. Hilar adenopathy probably represents a benign reactive change consequent to the chronic or repeated infections (*Staphylococcus aureus* and *Pseudomonas* sp.) from which these patients suffer.

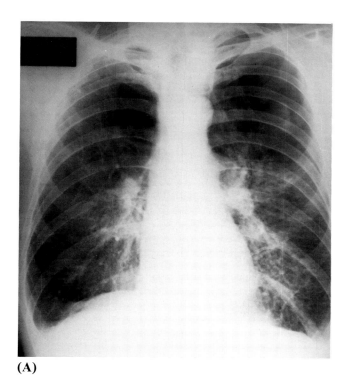

(A)

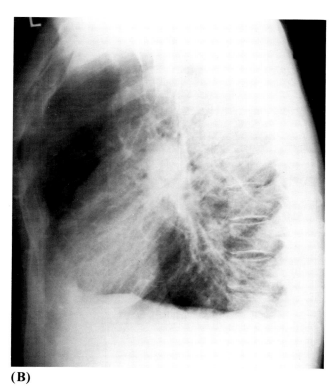

(B)

Fig. 10-37. Pulmonary Emphysema

(A,B) PA and lateral views of the chest, respectively, of a man with severe, long-standing pulmonary emphysema. On the PA view large areas of both upper lobes and the midlung on the right side are devoid of normal vessels. In the left upper lobe a large bulla extends from the apex down to the posterior sixth rib. Superimposed on it, at the level of the posterior fifth interspace, there is amorphous soft tissue density of an undetermined nature. On the right side, bullae are also seen in the upper and midlung zones. They can be identified by the areas devoid of pulmonary vessels as well as by their thin, curvilinear walls. As is usual, the entire circumferences of the bullae are not seen, but only those thicker arcs projected in tangent are visible.

The diaphragms are flat. The costophrenic angles are blunted as a result of projection of the slips of origin of the diaphragm from the lower ribs.

Both hila show large pulmonary arteries, which are frequently seen in patients with this degree of chronic obstructive pulmonary disease. They are usually manifestations of pulmonary hypertension.

In the left lower lobe there is mottling, and a cluster of small, nodular lesions is seen on both the PA and the lateral view. This is due to a coincidental pneumonia, which cleared with antibiotic therapy. In patients with emphysema, however, it may be very difficult to distinguish pneumonia from areas of pulmonary edema, since the patients will have pulmonary edema only in the portions of the lung that are still well perfused. Since the emphysematous zones do not participate, the distribution of edema is often atypical.

On the lateral view the diaphragms are seen to be flattened, and there is a considerable increase in the size of the retrosternal "clear space." Emphysematous lung is present between the mediastinum and the anterior chest wall.

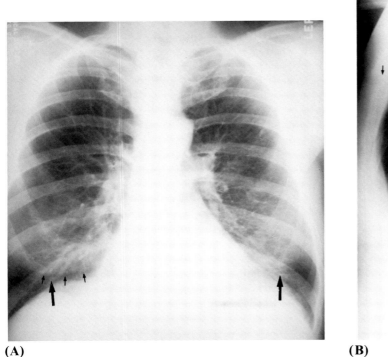

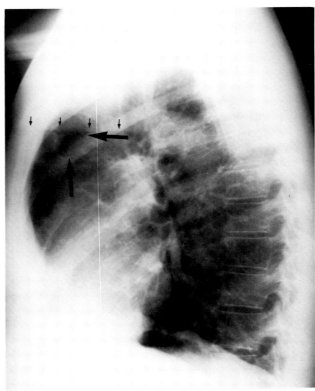

(A)   **(B)**

Fig. 10-38.   Large-Volume Lungs With Few Signs of Air Trapping

(A) PA view. Large arrows point to the anterior ends of the seventh ribs bilaterally. Other than the low positions of the hemidiaphragms there are few other signs of air trapping or of emphysema. The hilar vessels are slightly large in relationship to the peripheral vessels, but there are no zones of hyperlucency seen in either lung. The pectoral shadows are heavy in this man and account for the lighter gray that is seen in the region of the anterior fifth and sixth interspaces on both sides. On the right side you can even make out the faint inferior margin of prominent pectoral soft tissues that simulate breast tissue (small arrows).

The right upper lung zone appears more radiolucent than the left, but this is probably a technical artifact. If you compare the film density of the extrathoracic portions of the film you can see that there is also a darker gray tone on the right side than there is on the left.

(B) Lateral view. Here again, the findings of air trapping are not striking, but there is some increase in the radiolucency of the retrosternal and retrocardiac portions of the lung. In addition, there is evidence of a bulla (large arrow) in the retrosternal region. Again, the hilar vascular shadows are large. The edge of the soft tissues of the patient's arms (small arrows) are superimposed upon the mediastinum either because of improper positioning by the technologist or because the patient could not or would not raise his arms up over his head.

If the patient were fluoroscoped and asked to perform a vital capacity maneuver, signs of air trapping during the expiratory phase would be accentuated. Likewise, a chest film obtained at the end of a fast expiration could be used to compare with a film at maximum inspiration in order to detect signs of air flow obstruction (i.e., reduction of diaphragmatic excursion and deficient increase in the radiodensity of the lungs at end-expiration).

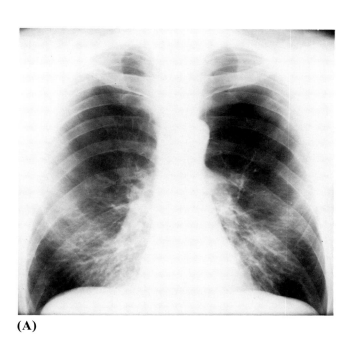

(A)

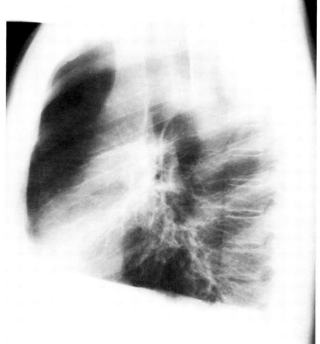

(B)

Fig. 10-39. Bullectomy for a Patient With Emphysema

(A,B) PA and lateral views of the chest, respectively, of a 51-year-old man with a history of progressive decrease in activities because of shortness of breath. All forms of medical treatment brought no relief.

The patient's vital capacity was 4.53 liters (88 percent of normal). His forced expiratory volume at 1 second was less than 37 percent of the predicted value and did not improve with bronchodilator medication. His functional residual capacity was 128 percent of the predicted value.

(A) PA view shows a marked loss of vessels in the left upper lung from the level of the left pulmonary artery all the way to the apex. On the right side there is a similar paucity of pulmonary vessels, but some vessels are rather sharply defined by surrounding hyperexpanded lung. These vessels are thinner than normal and lack peripheral branches. The hilar vessels are large bilaterally, and there is an approximation of vessels throughout the lower lung zones due to an increase in lower zone blood flow and diminished flow to the upper zones. There is also some lower lung compression from the hyperexpanded emphysematous lung above.

(B) Lateral view shows a marked increase in the depth, length, and radiolucency of the retrosternal portions of the lung, which extend caudally almost to the level of the diaphragm. This appearance is characteristic of emphysematous lungs, which expand to fill the anterior portions of the chest and encroach upon the mediastinum. Although the contour of the diaphragm on the PA view is within the limits of normal, on the lateral view the diaphragms have a markedly flattened appearance. The diaphragms are low in position on both the PA and the lateral view.

In spite of the evidence of generalized chronic obstructive pulmonary disease it was elected to offer the patient the option of having bullectomies performed in order to remove the nonfunctioning portions of the emphysematous upper lobes and allow for the possibility of increased pulmonary function by reducing the volume of this dead space. The bullectomies were first performed on the left side. Postoperatively the patient noticed a significant improvement in functional status. Bullectomies were then performed on the right side, and the patient noted further improvement. After the surgery he had improved exercise tolerance, improved vital capacity, and improved flow rates.

It is often difficult to determine which patients with obstructive airway disease will benefit from surgery. Those who have large emphysematous bullae with radiologic evidence of compression of well-perfused adjacent lung seem to do best.

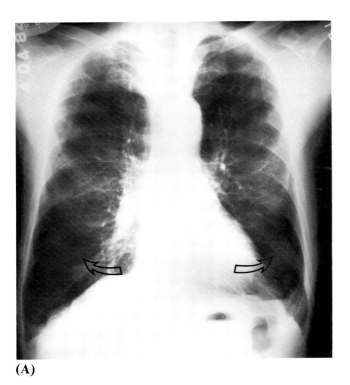

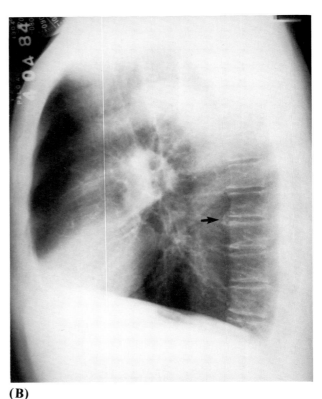

(A)   **(B)**

Fig. 10-40.   Emphysema and Overexposed Films

(A) PA view. Both hemidiaphragms are low in position. Arrows point to the anterior ends of the seventh ribs. The ribs are difficult to see because the patient is osteopenic and the ribs are deficient in bone mineral. In addition, for a variety of technical reasons, it is very common for patients who have pulmonary emphysema to have chest films made that are overexposed. The AP chest dimension is often increased in patients with emphysema, and the exposure calculation used does not take into account that the increased size is due to the presence of emphysematous lung, not muscle or fat. Automatic sensing devices to determine film exposure partly correct for the error.

The lateral aspects of both hemidiaphragms have lobulated contours because of the projection of slips of origin of the diaphragm from the anterior ribs.

On this PA view the parahilar portions of both lungs show pulmonary vessels well, but the upper lobes bilaterally show a significantly diminished vascular pattern, and those vessels seen medially are much smaller in caliber than normal. Laterally at both lung bases there is a diminution of blood vessels, more so than is accounted for by the overexposure alone. If the blackness were due only to overexposure, and you had the original film, you could use a bright light to bring out the images of the vessels. In the case of emphysema and diminished vessels, the bright light cannot show what is not there.

The hila are both large in comparison to the vessel branches that emanate from them. There is rapid tapering of the pulmonary arteries as is common in patients with emphysema.

(B) Lateral view. The diaphragms are quite flat. The film is not overexposed, judging from the appearance of the vertebral column and the image of the thoracic aorta. There is still an increased radiolucency in the retrosternal region, and the part of the lung that projects in front of the mediastinum extends quite low toward the diaphragm. There is also an increased lucency in the retrocardiac region above the diaphragm in front of the descending aorta. Large central vessels are also seen on this lateral view.

Notice incidentally the spurs on the vertebral bodies and the presence of a bridging syndesmophyte (arrow) at one of the lower thoracic interspaces.

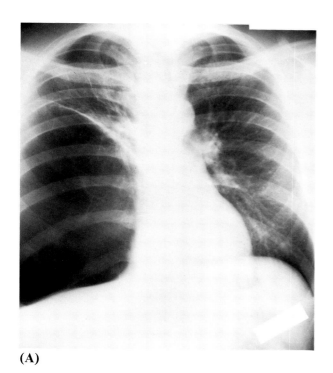

(A)

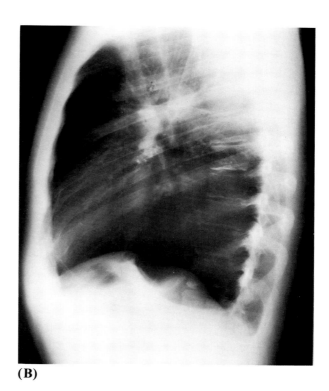

(B)

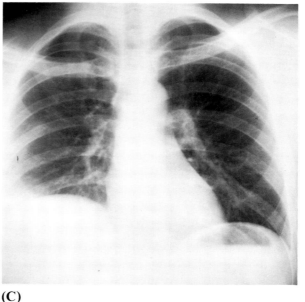

(C)

Fig. 10-41. Large Bulla Without Chronic Obstructive Pulmonary Disease

This is an active 25-year-old man who had noted occasional mild right lower anterior chest pain of 2 or 3 months' duration. Approximately 2½ weeks before admission he noted the onset of dry cough and right anterior chest pain. He had no limitations of activity and no dyspnea. A ^{99m}Tc perfusion lung scan was performed. Perfusion of the left lung was normal, but only the upper lung zone and the apex were perfused on the right.

At thoracotomy a giant bulla attached to the right lower lobe of the lung was excised. This bulla displaced the heart and mediastinum into the left chest and displaced the liver and diaphragm down to approximately the twelfth rib. The bulla was a sac approximately 16 cm in diameter. It was composed of a thin (less than 1.0 mm), translucent membrane of unremarkable fibrous tissue with no inflammation or granulomatous lesions in the wall. Sections of the adjacent lung parenchyma included with the specimen showed no abnormality.

(A) PA view shows the very large air-filled sac occupying the lower two-thirds of the right hemithorax. The bulla compresses the lung medially and superiorly and depresses the right hemidiaphragm.

(B) On lateral view an area of increased radiolucency occupies the distribution of the lower lobe posteriorly and inferiorly, extending well up into the region of an elevated right hilum. The right diaphragm forms a sharply caudal arc under the bulla.

(C) PA view of the chest a short time after thoracotomy and resection of the bulla. The lung has returned to a normal configuration. There is still considerable pleural thickening along the right lower lateral chest wall after the recent surgery. The distribution of blood vessels throughout both the right and the left lung is within normal limits, and there is no radiographic evidence of diffuse pulmonary emphysema. (Courtesy of Dr. James Mark, Stanford, California.)

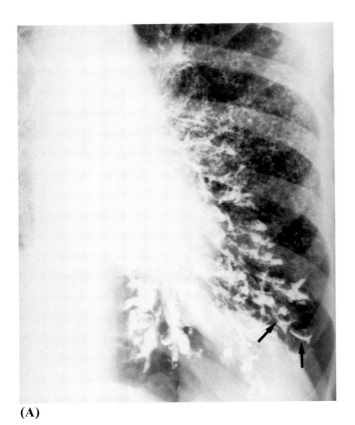

(A)

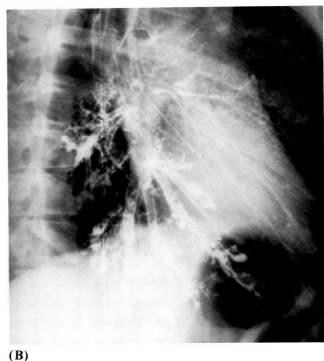

(B)

Fig. 10-42. Saccular Bronchiectasis

(A,B) Coned views of a bronchogram of a 15-year-old boy with severe bronchiectasis of the left lower lobe. **(A)** In this AP projection the bronchi that are projected beyond the heart show rather bizarre distortions. There are markedly dilated bronchi from which the small peripheral branches have been pruned. This appearance is due to peripheral saccules of bronchiectasis that are partly filled with secretions. Contrast material finds its way only around the periphery of these retained secretions (arrows).

(B) In this left posterior oblique projection the segmental bronchi in the left lower lobe are separated from each other. All of the left lower lobe bronchi, including the branches to the superior segment, are involved. A particularly prominent, rounded collection of contrast material within a saccular bronchial deformity is seen superimposed on the gas in the fundus of the stomach. Another, more caudal collection is seen as a rim of contrast material about a lucent center. There are only faint outlines of the bronchi of the lingula and the upper lobe, since these have largely emptied at the time of filming.

On the PA view you can see a reticulonodular appearance of the contrast material in the peripheral portions of the lingula. This is contrast material that is retained in the bronchioles. It has an appearance reminiscent of the reticular lesions of diffuse interstitial lung disease. Yet this material is entirely within the airways.

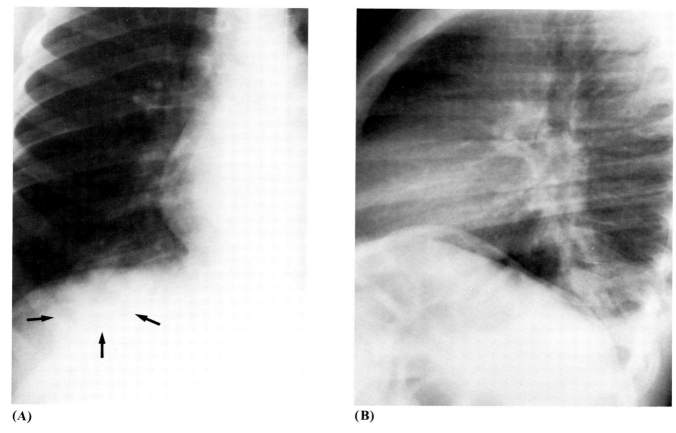

(A)   **(B)**

Fig. 10-43. Bronchiectasis on Plain Films

(A,B) Coned PA view of the right lung and lateral view of the chest of a child whose parents noticed she was bringing up a rather foul-smelling sputum. There is inhomogeneous consolidation of the basal segments of the right lower lobe, with some reduction in volume.

(A) On PA view a cluster of round and oval radiolucencies (arrows) is seen in the consolidation, which is projected caudal to the dome of the right diaphragm.

(B) On lateral view only, some air bronchograms are seen in the consolidation.

The radiographic appearance, in conjunction with the history, is strongly supportive of the diagnosis of bronchiectasis, probably due to an untreated episode of pneumonia in infancy. A bronchogram is hardly necessary to confirm the diagnosis but should be done to map other possible but unrecognized areas of bronchiectasis in either lung if surgery is being considered.

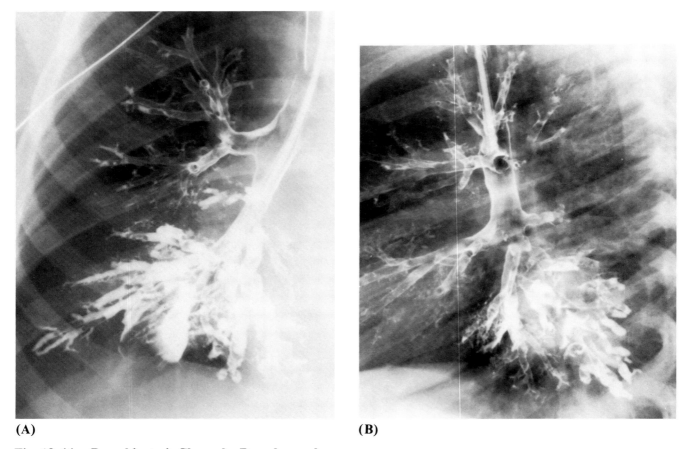

(A)   **(B)**

Fig. 10-44.   Bronchiectasis Shown by Bronchography

(A,B) AP and lateral views, respectively, of the bronchogram performed on the patient in Fig. 10-43. There is gross distortion of the basilar segmental bronchi, which show loss of tapering, extensive marginal irregularities, saccular dilatations, and nonfilling of small branches. The anterior basal segment is least involved. The superior segmental bronchus of the left lower lobe is only partly filled. Bronchi to the middle and upper lobes are coated rather than filled with contrast, and their peripheral branches are only beginning to be filled. The bronchographic study eliminates pulmonary sequestration from the differential diagnosis, since the segmental bronchi communicate normally with the lower lobe bronchus.

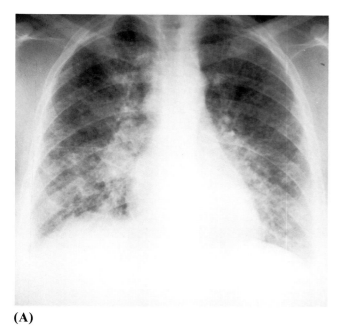

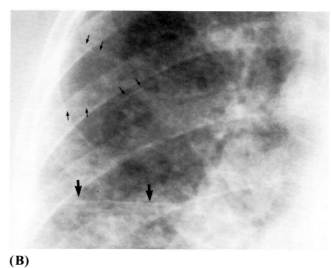

(A)   **(B)**

Fig. 10-45.   Diffuse Lymphangitic Metastases or Unusual Bronchoalveolar Carcinoma

This patient is a 33-year-old woman who was in good health until approximately 2 months before these radiographs were taken. She had a complicated history of upper extremity venous thrombosis and clinical signs and symptoms of pulmonary emboli.

She was referred the first time she noted a small hemoptysis. Because of her clinical history, documented venous thrombosis, and low arterial PO_2, the possibility of multiple pulmonary emboli was considered and a pulmonary arteriogram was performed. Small emboli were present in branch vessels of the right lower lobe.

(A) PA film of the chest shows pulmonary abnormalities, which are heavily concentrated in the lower lung zones. There are small pleural effusions (confirmed on other films) seen as blunting of the costophrenic angles. In addition, however, the hila are large and slightly lobulated, and there is a focal convexity on the right side of the mediastinum in the region of the azygos vein and node.

(B) Coned view of the lung lateral to the right hilum. There is slight thickening of the minor interlobar fissure (large arrows), and a few septal lines can be seen, faintly, in the lateral portions of the right midlung zone (small arrows). There is a background of small, irregular nodules, which obscure the vascular shadows.

The few small emboli found in the right lower lobe arterial branches would not account for the magnitude of these abnormalities. Either metastasis from an unknown primary tumor or bronchoalveolar carcinoma was considered a more likely cause.

A lung biopsy showed adenocarcinoma within lymphatic spaces, and a small, organizing pulmonary artery thromboembolus was seen as well. The biopsy suggested mucin-producing adenocarcinoma. No signs or symptoms relating to a primary malignant neoplasm at some other site were elicited, and further radiologic studies also revealed no primary site.

Although it is an unusual occurrence, bronchoalveolar cell carcinoma can spread through lymphatic spaces. Most commonly it spreads through the airways. Therefore, the diagnosis remains uncertain as to whether this is a primary bronchoalveolar cell tumor with an unusual mode of spread, or metastatic adenocarcinoma from an undetermined primary site.

Hilar and mediastinal lymphadenopathy may be associated with lymphangitic metastases but are by no means necessary to make that diagnosis. Many cases of confirmed lymphangitic spread of metastases to the lungs are not associated with recognizable lymphadenopathy on chest films.

In retrospect it is likely that the patient's original symptoms were related to a superior vena cava syndrome.

Fig. 10-46. Malignant Lymphoma Simulating Infection

Ten days before these films were made this patient developed severe shortness of breath and was admitted to a nearby hospital. She had a PO$_2$ of 72 mmHg on room air and a temperature of 101 degrees F, and chest films showed bilateral pulmonary abnormalities. She was treated for 6 days with erythromycin and oxygen, and was discharged home on intravenous erythromycin and oxygen. She improved for a short time, but on the evening of readmission she noticed a marked increase in shortness of breath. She was admitted with a temperature of 102°F, respirations 32 per minute, and a PO$_2$ of 47 mmHg on room air. Clinically, there was concern that the patient had an overwhelming infection with an organism such as *Legionella.*

After preliminary studies, fiberoptic bronchoscopy and bronchoscopic biopsy were done. The patient developed a pneumothorax on the right and a chest tube was placed.

Biopsy specimens of the lung showed histologic and immunologic features of large cell malignant lymphoma with T cell phenotype. No pathogens were present in cultures of multiple body fluids or in the lung biopsy specimens.

(A) Supine frontal film taken shortly after the first bronchoscopy and right chest tube placement. There are extensive bilateral pulmonary abnormalities with relative sparing of the apices and the extreme bases.

The tip of the endotracheal tube is at the orifice of the left main bronchus, and its position was changed. There is a Swan-Ganz catheter in place with its tip in the interlobar branch of the right pulmonary artery. The wires and the rounded, dense opacities are EKG leads. A zone of radiolucency, completely devoid of vessels or nodules, is seen below the dome of the right diaphragm. A large pneumothorax under the lung appears this way on AP films made with the patient supine. Arrows mark the caudal margin of the right pleural space. (See also Chapter 3.)

(B) Coned view of the left lung base shows multiple, poorly marginated, ill-defined nodules measuring 5 mm to 1 cm with small, interspersed radiolucencies. A more diffuse consolidation with faint peripheral air bronchograms is seen superimposed on the heart.

This radiographic appearance is part of the spectrum of pulmonary involvement by non-Hodgkin's malignant lymphoma. There may be extensive parenchymal disease without visible hilar or mediastinal adenopathy. It is uncommon but well recognized. These severe symptoms, however, are unusual at the time of initial diagnosis and are more likely to accompany recurrent disease after unsuccessful treatment. Patients with disseminated pulmonary involvement with non-Hodgkin's lymphoma occasionally present with signs and symptoms that mimic acute infections. Naturally, they do not respond to antibiotic therapy. A lung biopsy is required to establish the diagnosis even when a correct presumptive diagnosis has been made before biopsy.

Diffuse pulmonary infection due to a variety of viruses could also cause this roentgenographic appearance but would be unusual in an adult with normal immune mechanisms at a time of no known community epidemic. A similar appearance could be due to bronchoalveolar cell tumor, but the presentation mimicking acute infection would be unlikely. Pulmonary alveolar proteinosis or even pulmonary edema per se could present a similar radiographic appearance, but the clinical data do not fit with either of those possibilities.

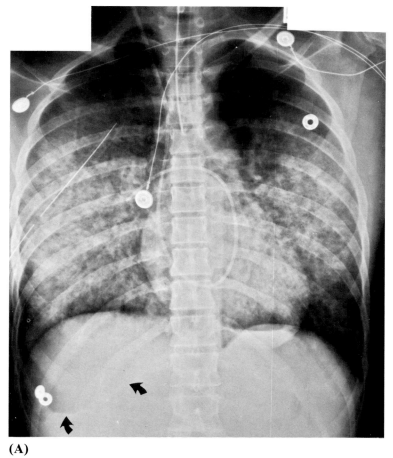

(A)

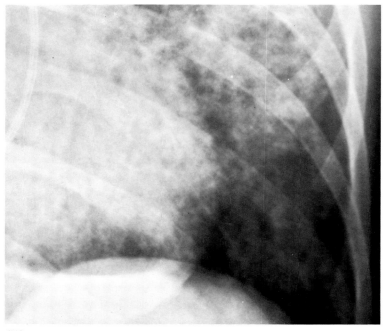

(B)

Fig. 10-46

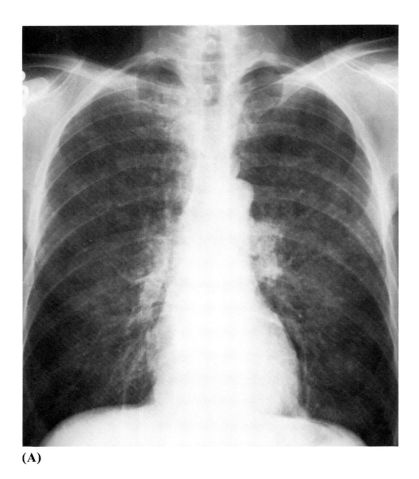

(A)

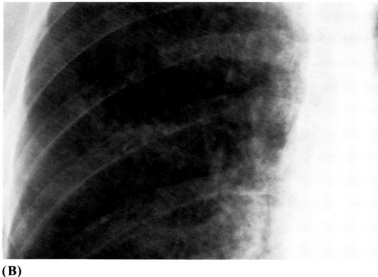

(B)

Fig. 10-47. Metastases From Melanoma

This man has extensive metastases throughout the pulmonary interstitium from a malignant melanoma.

(A) PA view shows innumerable, small (several millimeters), irregular opacities distributed throughout both lungs. They are fairly uniform in size, although a few seem slightly larger (about 1 cm). The hila are large, and there is probable adenopathy on the left at least.

(B) Coned view of the right midlung showing the irregular contours of the small nodules. Although these are foci of metastatic neoplasm, they closely resemble the granulomatous nodules that may be seen in both noninfectious and infectious granulomatous lung disease.

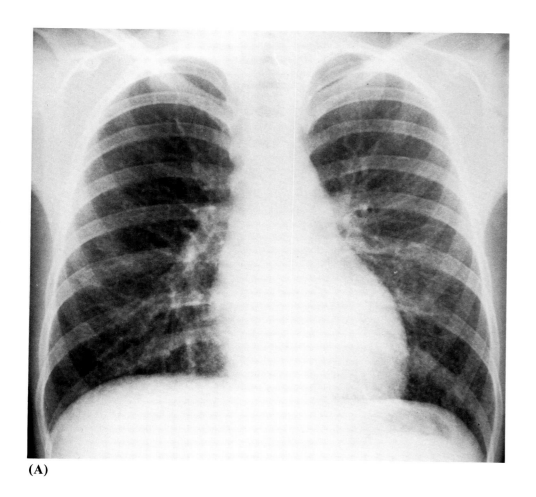

(A)

Fig. 10-48. Miliary Metastases From Thyroid Carcinoma

(A) PA film of a 10-year-old girl with known metastases from a carcinoma of the thyroid. There are miliary nodular metastases throughout both lungs.

(B) Coned view of the right base showing the small (2 to 3 mm) nodules distributed rather evenly throughout all portions of the lung. There is no sparing of even the extreme bases. This radiographic appearance raises concern about the possibility of miliary tuberculosis, histoplasmosis, or coccidioidomycosis. The fact that the patient is afebrile and has extensive disease seen on chest film, yet has little in the way of symptoms, practically removes tuberculosis and the other infectious granulomatous diseases from first-order consideration. The uniform involvement of all portions of both lungs is unusual for sarcoid or eosinophilic granuloma but does not exclude them. Since the patient has had a known thyroid carcinoma, a radioiodine scan could be used to assess the uptake of the pulmonary lesions and establish the diagnosis. This was done.

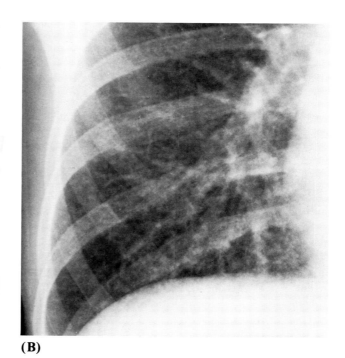

(B)

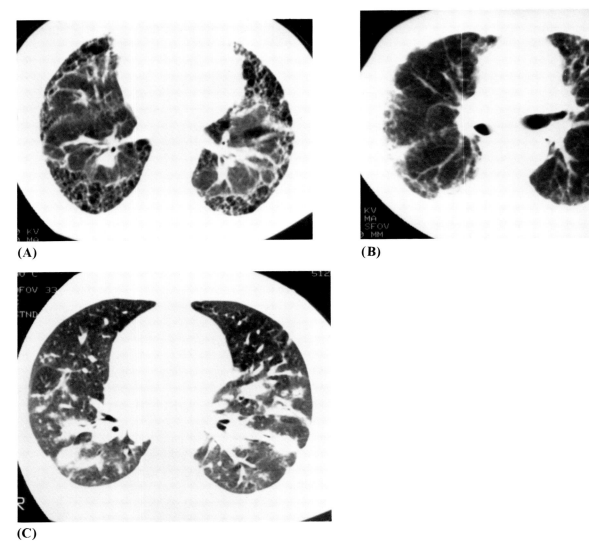

(A)

(B)

(C)

Fig. 10-49.   Distribution Of The Lesions Of Diffuse Lung Disease In The Transverse Plane

(A) Thin section CT scan through the lower lobes of a patient with UIP. The pulmonary abnormalities predominate in the periphery of the lungs and are seen here as a mantle of small circumscribed radiolucent spaces reminiscent of a honeycomb structure. The predominantly peripheral distribution is striking. On PA and lateral views of the chest, it is not possible to show this type of peripheral distribution because of the superimposition of the lesions from front to back and side to side.

(B) Thin section CT scan through the mid-lung zones of another patient with UIP. Again, the peripheral distribution of the predominant lesions is quite striking. Patchy foci of honeycombing are interspersed in peripheral areas of amorphous opacity.

(C) Thin section CT scan through the lower lung zones of a patient with proven sarcoid. In this example, the opaque zones have a predominant distribution along the course of bronchovascular bundles. This is one of the known CT appearances of pulmonary sarcoid. The finding is not specific for pulmonary sarcoid, but under the appropriate clinical circumstances, sarcoid would be the prime diagnostic consideration. The distribution of these parenchymal changes is strikingly different from the peripheral abnormalities of UIP seen in Figs. A and B. (Courtesy of Dr. Colleen J. Bergin.)

11

Blunt Chest Trauma

Trauma is a major cause of death in the United States, and chest trauma alone or in combination with other organ system damage is responsible for a high proportion of those deaths.[3]

Automobile occupants, pedestrians, and motorcycle riders comprise the bulk of patients who sustain serious chest injuries as the result of accidents. People who have fallen, been beaten, or been crushed in a variety of ways comprise an additional but smaller number of accident victims with serious chest injury. Chest radiographs play an obvious role in the diagnosis of injuries from major chest trauma and frequently are among the very first radiographic studies to be obtained after initial clinical evaluation. Whenever possible, PA and lateral views should be obtained with the patient upright, and additional films in different projections should be obtained to clarify uncertainties that arise from the initial interpretation. Unfortunately, the first chest film obtained is often made with the patient supine because severe injuries preclude assumption of the erect or even the sitting position. However, most patients can be filmed in lateral decubitus positions, which greatly assist in the assessment of pleural fluid or pneumothorax when views of the erect patient cannot be obtained.

It is helpful to analyze blunt chest trauma in terms of components affecting the thoracic cage, the lungs and pleura, the mediastinal contents, and the diaphragm. These distinctions are artificial in that excessive force causes simultaneous injuries to a multitude of tissues to which it is applied, but they are useful for purposes of organization.

MECHANISMS OF INJURY

There is much speculation about the mechanisms of injury in blunt chest trauma. Even with the limited data obtained from deceleration and impact studies using humans, models, and animals, precise reconstruction of all the forces acting during any specific accident is not possible. Components of shearing secondary to differential deceleration, impact (often multiple sequential impacts), contrecoup, bursting, and crushing forces may all be acting at various times during the violent phase of activity. There is also evidence that jagged edges of rib fractures may cause cutting injury to adjacent lung or vessels.

FRACTURES OF THE RIBS

Practically every known intrathoracic complication of blunt trauma has been reported to occur in the absence of rib fracture. That may be so, but rib fractures can be elusive. A complete radiographic study of the ribs consists of films in AP, PA, and oblique projections using radiographic techniques entirely different from those used for chest radiography. Additional coned views of regions where signs, symptoms, and physical findings indicate a high likelihood of injury complement the routine views. Seldom are these films obtained in the se-

The bulk of the text and illustrations for this chapter is taken from "Non-penetrating Thoracic Trauma: Emphasis on Plain Film Findings," *Postgraduate Radiology* 4:5–37, 1984, with permission of the editor and publisher.

verely, acutely traumatized patient because of the presence of other, more compelling injuries. Often the first chest radiograph obtained is an AP view with the patient supine. Rib fractures on this examination may not be recognized even when a laborious, rib-by-rib search is conducted. It is common, after days or weeks have elapsed, to see radiographic signs of callus and deformities of ribs at fracture sites that defy recognition even on rescrutiny of the first films obtained. Alternatively, reevaluation of those first films may show, in retrospect, fractures that were missed because of attention drawn to other, more pressing abnormalities. It is not unusual, even in cases of severe trauma, to recognize one or two rib fractures at the time of first examination, and then on serial films made over the next several days while the patient is in intensive care to recognize more and more fractures that become apparent as a result first of demineralization and subsequently of callus formation. Even minor differences in projection can bring some fractures out of obscurity and simultaneously hide others (Fig. 11-1).

Therefore, the fact that no rib fractures are seen does not mean that none are present. Displacement of the fragments at the fracture site makes it easier to see rib fractures. Lack of fragment displacement, however, permits underestimation of the degree of maximum dislocation that occurred before the fragments returned to their resting position.

Conn, Hardy, Fain, and Netterville[7] analyzed more than 637 cases of blunt chest trauma and studied the distribution of rib fractures in 532 (84 percent). If one plotted the number of fractures on the vertical axis and the number of the involved rib on the horizontal axis, the plot would have a nearly bell-shaped curve with its high points occurring at the sixth and seventh ribs on the right and the sixth through the eighth on the left. At the extreme ends, however, there would be some distortion of the curve for the right side, as the first rib was fractured about three times more often than the twelfth. Curiously, on the left side this discrepancy was minor.

Fractures of multiple ribs, and particularly multiple fractures of multiple ribs, may lead to the condition known as flail chest, in which involved portions of the chest show paradoxical motion with respiration. In some patients this phenomenon may not be evident on first appraisal, but it becomes so as physiologic derangements consequent to pooling of secretions in the bronchi and evolution of areas of atelectasis lead to increased muscular effort for breathing. These patients are frequently treated by tracheal intubation or tracheotomy to permit the use of volume respirators. It is arguable whether the flail phenomenon or the attendant pulmonary contusion is more responsible for the apparent ventilatory impairment.[36]

Several analyses have been made to determine whether fractures of the highest ribs have predictive value for the coincident presence of major vascular injuries.[12,23,30–32,39,42,44] I interpret the data to indicate that whereas many patients with thoracic vascular injuries do have fractures of the first and second ribs and frequently others as well, only a minority of patients with fractures of upper ribs (about 14 percent) have confirmed major vascular injuries. Nevertheless, this minority is large enough to warrant serious consideration of angiographic study of the aorta and great vessels in these traumatized patients.

The possibility of damage to adjacent lung, viscera, or vessels is the most important consideration in patients with rib fractures. Splenic injury from fractures of the lower ribs on the left or liver injury from fractures of lower ribs on the right must also be seriously considered.

Even uncomplicated rib fractures, however, may impair respiratory function because of pain and splinting of the chest wall. In the elderly or in patients with low cardiorespiratory reserves, close observation is important, along with pain control, to prevent further deterioration due to atelectasis. In addition, follow-up chest roentgenograms a few days after injury may be worthwhile to look for delayed hemothorax.

Fractures of costal cartilages are not recognizable on chest films. They may contribute to the flail chest phenomenon and probably to other visceral injury as well.

OTHER FRACTURES

Fracture of the sternum is often difficult to detect on a chest film. On films made in frontal projections with the patient supine, a fractured sternum would rarely be seen. Any patient who has sustained multiple rib fractures is likely to have a sternal fracture as well. A sternal fracture may be suspected clinically because it is painful. On the lateral view of the chest, even a subtle, minimally displaced sternal fracture may be recognized when there is an adjacent soft tissue mound due to extrapleural hematoma (Fig. 11-2). Sternal fractures are important because they cause pain, contribute to the paradoxical motion of flail chest if present, and raise the possibility of pericardial or myocardial damage.

Fractures of thoracic vertebrae seem to contribute to serious problems less frequently than does damage to many other thoracic structures. Nevertheless, they may contribute to pain, may have associated paravertebral masses due to hematoma, and may be responsible for vascular or neurologic damage, especially when accompanied by dislocation (Fig. 11-3).

PULMONARY CONTUSION

Lung contusion is the commonest sign of pulmonary injury seen radiographically after blunt trauma. There is an increase in radiodensity of the involved area, with loss of the images of small vessels even on films that are exposed well. The loss of the vessel images permits localization of the lesions to the lung rather than to the overlying pleura or chest wall. These solitary or multiple foci of patchy consolidation usually do not conform to anatomic segments. Damage to large areas of lung or coalescence of patchy foci may produce a diffuse consolidation that simulates, but rarely duplicates, lobar consolidation (Fig. 11-1A and 11-4). There may also be linear and peribronchial components.

The vast majority of pulmonary contusions will be seen on chest films made within a few hours of injury. A small proportion, however, may not be apparent for up to 48 hours, or original lesions may progress for up to 48 hours. Resolution usually begins within 48 to 72 hours, and in mild cases clearing may be complete within 24 hours. However, gradual clearing over as many as 8 days has been reported.[33]

The pathologic counterpart of the radiographic lesion is intra-alveolar hemorrhage and edema and hemorrhage into the interlobular septa.[33]

The clinical manifestations are varied. There may be no symptoms and no physical signs. There may be ecchymoses of the chest wall that correlate strikingly with the location of consolidation seen on chest films. On the other hand, the lung lesions may be remote from the region of chest impact — the so-called contrecoup effect. Dyspnea, shortness of breath, hyperpnea, and chest pain may be present, and decreased breath sounds, wheezes and rales, and low-grade fever may be found on physical examination. Significant hemoptysis is uncommon.

Disparity between the magnitude of the radiographic abnormality and the clinical or pathophysiologic disturbance may be remarkable.[14] In some cases, a significant hypoxemia precedes the appearance of radiographic abnormalities by 6 to 24 hours. Radiographic evidence commonly leads to underestimation of physiologic impairment and only rarely to overestimation. CT studies of the chest in a small number of patients following blunt chest trauma have also shown more extensive pulmonary lesions than would be predicted from chest radiographs made at approximately the same time.[35] In experiments with rhesus monkeys, autopsies showed large areas of significant pulmonary contusion that were not seen radiographically.[9]

Fortunately, uncomplicated pulmonary contusion responds to rational supportive measures. However, animal experimental data indicate that the contused lung is at high risk to become edematous or infected. Radio-graphic lesions that progress or appear more than 72 hours after trauma are generally not due to uncomplicated lung contusion. Pulmonary infection, pulmonary edema from any cause, and the nonspecific but life-threatening complications of the adult respiratory distress syndrome must be considered.

TRAUMATIC PNEUMATOCELES (CYSTS) AND HEMATOMAS

Traumatic pneumatoceles and hematomas are some of the more unusual but intriguing lesions seen in the lungs after trauma. They result from tears of lung parenchyma and may be accompanied by other signs of injury, such as pneumothorax and hemothorax. Some are detected on films made within an hour of trauma and may be the most obvious abnormality seen (Fig. 11-5A). Others, buried within a sea of lung contusion, may not be visible until there has been clearing of surrounding hemorrhage and edema (Fig. 11-5B).

Lung lacerations may appear as small masses (hematomas). When their content liquefies and is coughed up, a fluid level may become visible. Some lacerations may appear initially as thin-walled cystic spaces. The walls of others may appear quite thick because of bleeding, edema, and atelectasis in adjacent lung. Their size is variable, but lesions as large as 14 cm have been described. They may be solitary, multiple, or even multiloculated. Resolution over a period of days to months without specific treatment is the rule. Sometimes an air-filled space may become solid in appearance and remain as a pulmonary nodule. Complications are rare.[10] Recurrent pneumothorax occurs, but is infrequent.

FAT EMBOLISM

There is little doubt that fat embolism occurs after major chest trauma, particularly when there are also fractures of the long bones. The existence of this entity is substantiated by pathologic changes observed in a small but significant minority (about 5 percent) of patients dying of major trauma.[13] Clinical diagnosis is extremely difficult, and the radiographic appearance of the pulmonary lesions is not specific. The precise source of the embolic fat globules is still disputed. Marrow fat as well as altered emulsions of bloodstream fat may be responsible.[18] The full-blown clinical spectrum of radiographic diffuse pulmonary opacity, skin petechiae, central nervous system dysfunction, ophthalmologic changes, and altered blood pH occurs rarely. Radiographically, the pulmonary abnormalities resemble those of increased capillary permeability edema. Patchy opacities may antedate confluent, diffuse pulmonary opacification. In the absence of the full-blown clinical syndrome, the radiographic pulmonary lesions are indistinguishable from noncardiogenic pulmonary edema, oxygen toxicity, so-called shock lung, or disseminated infection. In mild cases, pulmonary lesions may not be seen radiographically. Fortunately, with present management, the majority of clinically suspected cases resolve without sequelae after symptoms of short duration. Some patients that were clinically considered fatalities due to fat embolism were found on autopsy examination to have died of undetected hypovolemic shock.[13]

The signs and symptoms may appear shortly after trauma or may be delayed for a period of days. Tests for the presence of fat in the blood or urine are considered unreliable.

ATELECTASIS

In patients who have sustained severe chest trauma, atelectasis may result from aspiration of gastric contents or foreign bodies, splinting and pooling of secretions, formation of mucus plugs, or the presence of blood clots within the airways. Occasionally, no cause for atelectasis is found on bronchoscopy. Undoubtedly, all of the mechanisms involved underestimate the role of surfactant insufficiency in the genesis and perpetuation of atelectasis (Fig. 11-6). In a small number of patients, CT detected more instances of atelectasis than were seen on corresponding chest films.[35]

PNEUMOTHORAX

Pneumothorax following blunt chest trauma is common, and its radiographic appearance is no different from that of pneumothorax from any other cause. However, chest films are frequently made with the patient supine; air in the pleural space then collects anteromedially and caudally. Pneumothorax under the lung base can be identified by recognizing the fine line of visceral pleura that separates the lung from the adjacent lucency of the pneumothorax (see Fig. 11-4). The pneumothorax outlines the pleural surface under the more anterior middle lobe on the right side or the lingula on the left side. When it is difficult to tell with confidence that you are dealing with a pneumothorax under the lung as opposed to a pneumoperitoneum with air under a thin hemidiaphragm, a decubitus film with the suspect side uppermost will permit accurate distinction. Small pneumothoraces may not be visible on films made with the patient recumbent. Small pneumothoraces have been

seen with CT (see Fig. 11-3C) that were not visible on films made at about the same time.[35] Since small pneumothoraces may cause little physiologic impairment, their detection may not be critical. Surveillance films at short intervals will serve to detect those pneumothoraces that become larger because of a persistent air leak. However, in patients who are to receive positive-pressure assisted ventilation or general anesthesia, it is important to know in advance that even a small pneumothorax is present because rapid expansion of the pneumothorax can occur under those circumstances.

Tension pneumothorax obviously requires urgent correction but is seldom a diagnostic problem. Pneumothorax in cases of blunt trauma has been seen in the absence of recognizable rib fracture. The mechanism of pneumothorax formation is discussed in Chapter 3.

PNEUMOMEDIASTINUM

Pneumomediastinum most commonly results from air that escapes from ruptured peripheral alveoli and extends medially into the mediastinum via perivascular sheaths. In these instances, the pneumomediastinum does not require any treatment other than that indicated to manage the often-associated pneumothorax. In cases of blunt chest trauma, pneumomediastinum may also be seen consequent to fractures of the airway or, rarely, to esophageal rupture.

Pneumomediastinum may be recognized radiographically because streaks of air are seen in the mediastinal soft tissues, and occasionally large collections of air may be seen superimposed on the heart (Fig. 11-7). Air streaks may also be seen in the soft tissues of the neck and supraclavicular region. Small amounts of air in the mediastinum may be very difficult to recognize and must be deliberately searched for, especially on AP chest films made with portable equipment. CT scans have shown that pneumomediastinum may be present when not detectable, even in retrospect, on accompanying plain films.[35] Occasionally, air along the medial aspects of the lung in a pneumothorax may simulate mediastinal air, but the error is usually avoided by recognizing the manifestations of the pneumothorax along the convexities of the lung as well.

HEMOTHORAX AND HEMOPNEUMOTHORAX

Small amounts of blood may be seen in the pleural space even after simple rib fracture. Hemothorax and hemopneumothorax are common complications of blunt chest trauma and were present in slightly fewer than one-fourth of a series of 637 patients.[7] Hemothorax may be present far more frequently than those figures indicate. It would be detected more often if films in the lateral decubitus position were obtained, if good-quality PA and lateral chest films could be obtained with the patient upright, or if CT scans were used more frequently.

Radiographically, it is not possible to distinguish one type of pleural fluid from another—that is to say, exudates from transudates or blood from chyle. When large quantities of fluid are seen in the pleural space following trauma, it is safest to consider the fluid to be blood until proven otherwise. Bleeding vessels of the chest wall or the great vessels of the mediastinum are a more likely source than pulmonary laceration. Careful monitoring of the amount and rate of evacuation of blood from the pleural space by catheter drainage is necessary to determine whether immediate thoracotomy is indicated to isolate and control bleeding sites. Although it is estimated that fewer than 5 percent of patients with thoracic injuries require emergency thoracotomy, when uncontrolled bleeding or uncontrolled air leaks are encountered such surgery is lifesaving (Fig. 11-8).[34,40] Intrathoracic bleeding may also be seen as extrapleural hematoma or as a loculated pleural fluid collection.

CT examination is sensitive in the detection of pleural fluid. In many instances the bloody nature of the fluid is predictable because the attenuation coefficients of fresh blood, as opposed to transudates, are such that CT numbers of 70 to 80 Hounsfield units may be recorded.[35]

INJURIES OF THE THORACIC AORTA AND THE GREAT VESSELS

The vast majority of people who sustain lacerations of the thoracic aorta or the great vessels as the result of thoracic trauma die before they reach the emergency room. For that substantial minority who do reach the hospital alive, accurate assessment of the site of major vessel disruption is critical. It is estimated that if the diagnosis of major arterial disruption were missed at this point, up to 90 percent of those who survived would be dead within 4 months. There are cases, however, in which calcified pseudoaneurysms are first recognized on films made many years after the responsible injury (Fig. 11-9).

Chest Film Findings

Several authors have analyzed their data seeking some constellation of findings that would predict the presence of major vascular injuries, or at least permit critical

choice as to which patient requires angiographic examination and which does not (Figs. 11-10 to 11-12). However, even in busy trauma centers, it may take up to a decade to accumulate 50 cases. Much of this information has been brought together by Fisher, Hadlock, and Ben-Menachem in a thoughtful review, which also contains a comprehensive bibliography.[11] The following is a list of commonly sought chest film findings in patients with potential aortic and brachiocephalic vascular injuries:

1. Widening of the superior mediastinum
2. Loss of sharpness or obscuring of the aortic arch
3. The apical cap sign
4. Deviation of the trachea to the right
5. Downward displacement of the left main bronchus
6. Deviation of a nasogastric tube to the right
7. Enlarged or abnormal aortic contour
8. Left hemothorax
9. Partial obscuring of the descending aorta
10. Displaced left paraspinal interface
11. Displaced right paraspinal interface.

The incidence of these findings was compared in two groups of patients who had suffered blunt chest trauma. In one group, lacerations of the aorta or the brachiocephalic vessels was demonstrated by angiography; the other group had no angiographically demonstrable injury to these vessels. Only three signs occurred with statistically significant increased frequency in the angiographically positive group. Those signs related to displacement of the trachea, the esophagus (judged by nasogastric tube position), and the left main bronchus. However, even these signs occurred with sufficient frequency (between 20 and 30 percent) in the angiographically negative group that they offered little in terms of specificity.

Marsh and Sturm also studied plain-film findings in patients with blunt chest trauma and found a high incidence of the first five signs (they used 8.0 centimeters as maximal mediastinal width at the level of the aortic knob on supine films at 100 cm TFD). They also added a sixth sign, opacification of the clear space between the aortic arch and the left pulmonary artery. All six signs were also seen, with lesser frequency, in patients with chest trauma and no aortic rupture. Furthermore, each sign may be invalidated by nonspecific coincident factors such as poor inspiration, rotation of the patient, atelectasis or lung contusion effacing adjacent mediastinal contours, or extrapleural apical hematomas from upper rib fractures (producing the apical cap sign independent of aortic tear).[25,42] This list does not include other signs such as fractures of the upper ribs, associated injuries other than thoracic, and anterior displacement of the trachea.

Milne et al.[27] analyzed their experience with aortic tear and emphasized the effacement or widening of the paratracheal stripe in more than 95 percent of their cases. They also showed that the image of the azygos vein is usually not seen after such major vascular injury, whereas it is commonly prominent on AP films of the supine patient when widening of the superior mediastinum is physiologic.

In another series of 86 cases of blunt chest trauma, 13 patients were shown to have traumatic aortic tears.[24] Analysis of these cases showed that there were no aortic tears found in any case that showed all four of the following negative findings:

1. No esophageal deviation (judged from the position of the nasogastric tube)
2. No tracheal deviation (to the extent that the left wall of the trachea is projected to the right of the T4 spinous process on a nonrotated film)
3. No loss of sharpness of the aortic arch contour
4. No loss of sharpness of the descending aortic contour.

Clinical Findings

The clinical signs and symptoms associated with major vascular injuries are also quite variable. One of the most common, retrosternal or interscapular pain, is reported in only 26 percent of patients.[21] Dyspnea, stridor, and hoarseness may also be presenting symptoms. Upper extremity hypertension with increased pulse amplitude may be a striking finding in patients who have sustained aortic lacerations, but unfortunately it is present in fewer than half of the reported patients. A midscapular murmur may also be noted. Anuria and paraplegia have been reported, but infrequently.

In patients who have sustained lacerations of the brachiocephalic vessels there may be a difference in pulse amplitude between the extremities, but absence of this sign is of no significance. In patients who have sustained lacerations of the innominate artery there may be displacement of the nasogastric tube to the left, and patients who have sustained fracture dislocations of the thoracic spine may have traumatic rupture of the aorta at that level. Unfortunately, more than one-third of patients reported in the literature had no external evidence of thoracic injury at the time of the initial physical examination. Thoracic aortic laceration has even been reported to occur in patients whose initial chest films were considered normal.[21] Follow-up chest films over the next few hours or days, however, may show some of the signs discussed.

There is little question that angiographic study is required to establish the diagnosis of intrathoracic arteriovascular laceration whenever exsanguinating hemorrhage does not force the issue of emergency thoracotomy. Although tears at the aortic isthmus are the most common injury, other sites in the ascending or the descending aorta can be involved separately or (rarely) concurrently, and tears of the brachiocephalic or subclavian vessels may not be distinguished from aortic laceration without angiographic examination.

Personnel at major trauma centers base the decision of whether or not to perform angiography on an analysis of their own experience. However, at least two responsible investigators endorse the very conservative approach that aortography should be performed on any patient who has sustained a high-speed, decelerating injury or blunt trauma to the chest, whether or not there is external evidence of thoracic injuries or clinical findings or changes in the chest roentgenogram.[11,21] This would probably mean that more than 100 patients would undergo angiograms in order to detect a life-threatening injury in one or two. Requiring the presence of some minimal radiographic sign would probably mean that at least 10 or 15 angiograms out of 100 could be expected to be positive. In any event, angiography requires talented personnel to perform the study and to interpret the results.

Lacerations of the internal mammary or intercostal arteries may cause exsanguinating hemorrhage, and lacerations of the great veins of the thorax may cause life-threatening bleeding. Over the last several years at Stanford University Hospital there have been at least two such cases. One was a man who sustained tears of the junction of the right subclavian and right innominate veins that required emergency thoracotomy for control of bleeding, with no other major vascular injury associated (Fig. 11-8). The other was a woman who suffered an avulsion of the azygos vein from the superior vena cava. An emergency thoracotomy was required for control of bleeding. She also had a laceration of the right subclavian artery demonstrated on an arteriogram, but repair of that lesion had to be postponed for several days. It is presumed that many of the mediastinal hematomas that prove to have no associated arterial lacerations demonstrated on angiogram result from venous bleeding that is self-limited.

Rarely, a patient presents with a history of recent trauma, an abnormal mediastinum on chest films, and a negative arteriogram and is subsequently proven to have a neoplasm (e.g., malignant lymphoma) as the cause of the abnormality.

TEARS OF THE MAJOR AIRWAYS

Disruption of major airways is basically caused by one of three mechanisms: compression of the lower trachea and main bronchi against the spine; shearing forces accompanying sudden deceleration and rotation of the lung laterally at the moment of chest compression; and bursting forces occurring with violent compression of the airways when the glottis is closed.

In closed chest trauma, the vast majority of airway tears occur within a few centimeters of the tracheal carina, predominantly in the major bronchi and much less frequently in the distal trachea. A small minority of tears occur in the lobar bronchi. The injury may cause complete transection of the tube or partial disruption as a result of fracture of cartilage or mucosal tear.[5]

The spectrum of radiographic and clinical findings extends from the highly suggestive to the astonishingly cryptic. The former category includes the patient with pneumomediastinum (see Fig. 11-7), air in the soft tissues of the thorax and neck, a large pneumothorax, an uncontrollable air leak after chest tube placement, hemoptysis, cyanosis, dyspnea, pain, cough, and shock. Unfortunately, this hypothetical conjunction of radiographic data and clinical signs and symptoms is rare. Too often, the pneumothorax does respond to chest tube suction, the lung reexpands, and the comforting illusion of a controlled air leak due to torn lung displaces the concern over the possibility of major airway trauma.[2,16] In other cases, a pneumomediastinum is not seen on the chest film, nor is there air in the soft tissues. Some patients have disarmingly few symptoms or have concomitant injuries whose clinical manifestations overwhelm those of the airway injury. Even hemoptysis may be explained away by the discovery of bleeding from lacerations of the oral or nasal mucosa. The very rarity of serious bronchial injury undoubtedly contributes to its misdiagnosis.

Patients with major airway tears that present initially with little radiographic or clinical evidence may have the diagnosis delayed until lung atelectasis, with or without attendant signs of infection, is discovered. In the majority of cases of delayed diagnosis it is the late discovery of atelectatic lung that leads eventually to the correct diagnosis[5] (Fig. 11-13).

An explanation of this wide spectrum of clinical and radiographic presentation may be found in the following possibilities: If the connective tissue sheath about the site of bronchial injury—even in the event of complete transection—remains intact, an air leak into mediastinum or pleural space will not occur. If the tear is small, occlusion may be achieved by organizing thrombus, and the leak may stop; hence, catheter drainage of a pneumothorax may succeed, and pneumomediastinum may resolve spontaneously. If the tear is central, pneumomediastinum may occur without pneumothorax, and if the tear is peripheral, pneumothorax may occur without pneumomediastinum.

There may be an alternative explanation for the lack of radiographically apparent pneumothorax or pneumomediastinum in some of these patients. Experience with CT of the chest has shown that small pneumothoraces and small amounts of mediastinal air may be recognized when they defy identification on chest films even in retrospect. The same is true of small to moderate-sized pleural effusions when the CT study is compared to portable films of the chest with the patient supine. Since supine AP chest films taken with portable equipment are the usual form of radiographic examination in patients after major trauma, it is likely that a number of instances of small pneumothorax, pneumomediastinum, and pleural effusion go unrecorded.

Bronchoscopy is the method of choice for establishing the diagnosis of major airway tear, but the true nature or extent of the airway injury may not be detected even on repeat study. Bronchography or tomography (Fig. 11-13B) may contribute to diagnosis in those equivocal cases. Surgical correction is usually carried out as soon as feasible. Diagnosis is frequently delayed, however, until the patient presents days, months, or even years later with atelectasis of the lung secondary to bronchostenosis resulting from scarring. Successful late repair depends on whether or not infection with bronchiectasis and pulmonary fibrosis has intervened. Successful repairs years after injury have been recorded. In addition, there are rare instances in which small bronchial tears were recognized but were treated only by catheter drainage of the pleural space, because the attendant physical and physiologic impairment was not compelling enough to override the demands for correction of other concurrent injuries; these patients apparently healed without sequelae.[2]

Fractures of the upper ribs are frequently present in patients with fractures of the trachea or major bronchi; they are remarkably frequent in patients over the age of 30 years.[5] The opposite conclusion, however, that fractures of the intrathoracic airways are frequent in patients with fractures of the upper ribs, cannot be supported.[7] In addition, in children and young adults, airway injury is present in the absence of recognizable rib fracture.[5]

One sign of ruptured bronchus is described as characteristic: a collapse of the lung away from the hilum and mediastinum. This occurs when the lung is tethered only by its vascular pedicle.[22,28] Regardless of the specificity of this appearance, it is so rare as to be a curiosity.

Airway tears at more than one location rarely may be found and are even more difficult to diagnose correctly. Torsion of the lung about its axis, so that the base occupies the apex of the chest, is another rare consequence of chest trauma. Theoretically, torsion can be recognized by noting a discrepant vascular pattern.[8]

RUPTURE OF THE ESOPHAGUS

This is a rare but devastating injury in patients who have survived blunt chest trauma long enough to obtain medical care. Mortality from esophageal rupture is high even when the diagnosis is made promptly, and higher when diagnosis is delayed. The very rarity of the injury contributes to the difficulty of diagnosis. Conn, Hardy, Fain, and Netterville[7] found only one case of esophageal injury and one case of tracheoesophageal fistula in an analysis of 637 cases of blunt chest trauma. Worman, Hurley, Pemberton, and Narodick[43] reviewed the English literature and found only 27 cases reported since 1900, to which they added 3 cases of their own garnered from 15 years of records. There was a striking difference in survival between those patients who suffered esophageal tears alone and those who developed tracheoesophageal fistula. Ten of the 12 patients who developed tracheoesophageal fistula survived, even though there usually was a delay of months before repair. On the other hand, of the 15 patients with rupture of the thoracic esophagus due to either blunt thoracic trauma or blunt abdominal trauma, 12 died. Two died in spite of repair within 24 hours, and 10 were only discovered at autopsy.

The diagnosis is difficult because of a lack of specific signs and symptoms, but dyspnea and cyanosis out of proportion to the injury are frequent. Chest films may show air in the mediastinum with or without associated pneumothorax or hemopneumothorax (the left side more than the right). Air may also be found in the soft tissues of the neck. Pneumomediastinum may be unrecognized on portable chest films if the amount of air present is small, and air in the neck in small quantities may also go unnoticed on physical examination. Patients who live for a few days may show radiographic evidence of pyopneumothorax or empyema. Death is due to those complications in association with gangrenous mediastinitis.

In patients who are to some degree mobile after chest trauma, it would be simple to perform contrast studies of the esophagus. In those who are comatose or whose mobility is severely restricted by traction devices, the examination is difficult to perform well. Fluoroscopy should be used, which invariably means transporting the patient to the x-ray department. A small quantity of water-soluble contrast can be administered by swallow or by tube. The bolus must be observed fluoroscopically as it passes through the entire esophagus, since traumatic laceration can occur in the upper, middle, or lower third. If no contrast is seen to escape from the esophagus, it is reasonable to switch to a barium mixture. Barium is much easier to swallow. Peristaltic waves should be followed fluoroscopically to look for small tears. If the patient can only be examined while supine, the anterior wall of the esophagus may escape critical evaluation except during the passage of a moderately large bolus. A cross-table lateral view will show that the barium passes down the posterior portions of the esophageal lumen while a layer of air passes down anteriorly, hence the lumen may be filled with barium only during the passage of the contraction wave. Contrast escaping into the mediastinum or the pleural cavity establishes the diagnosis. Fluoroscopy serves to identify the site of the leak and to call a halt to the further administration of contrast. Perforations of the lower esophagus have a higher mortality rate than those of the cervical esophagus.[37] Simultaneous airway tear and esophageal tear has been reported.[20]

CARDIAC TAMPONADE

Patients with severe cardiac injuries usually do not survive. However, there are reports of successful repair of myocardial laceration using "finger in the hole" obturation in the emergency room or while transporting the patient to the operating room. Obviously no detour is made to obtain chest films.

Myocardial contusion probably occurs more commonly than it is diagnosed, because if not extreme it seems well tolerated.[1,38] Diagnosis is dependent on EKG changes, although radionuclide cardiac studies would likely be revealing were they used more often.

Pericardial effusions or hemopericardium can be suggested from chest films if the fluid accumulation is large or increasing on serial films (Fig. 11-14). However, in acute cardiac tamponade, the volume of pericardial fluid required to result in seriously impaired cardiac filling is often small. The pressure-volume curve of the pericardium indicates that excess pericardial fluid will be accommodated up to a certain point, above which only a small additional increment will result in tamponade. I believe that 100 to 200 ml of excess pericardial fluid, and perhaps lesser amounts, may cause tamponade acutely. The difference in size of the apparent "cardiac" silhouette may be no more than one would expect from comparing a supine film of the chest with an upright film (Fig. 11-15), and that has been the case: The patient suffering from tamponade has a film made while supine, and an earlier film for comparison, usually from a happier time, is in the upright position. Cardiac echography is much more sensitive than chest radiography in detecting increased pericardial fluid. At no time should a cardiac size "within the limits of normal" on a chest film deter one from pursuing the suspected diagnosis of cardiac tamponade. This is particularly so in a patient whose state of shock is disproportionate to that expected from the amount of blood loss. Furthermore, patients who are severely hypovolemic may show neither the radiographic nor the clinical signs of increased venous pressure.

RUPTURE OF THE DIAPHRAGM

Rupture of the diaphragm with blunt trauma occurs much more often on the left than on the right side. The liver presumably spares the right diaphragm from the effects of a sudden increase in abdominal pressure. Rarely, rupture is bilateral or central, with herniation of abdominal contents into the pericardium. Combined thoracoabdominal trauma, with the abdominal component paramount, is a common antecedent of diaphragmatic rupture. Associated pelvic fractures are common. The incidence of diaphragmatic tear in those patients who reach the hospital is difficult to estimate because more of these lesions are missed at initial evaluation than are discovered.[19] The majority of these injuries occur as a result of automobile accidents, but some are due to falls or other injuries causing severe compression of the abdomen or the chest.

Symptoms fall into two distinct groups. Some patients have critical problems shortly following the trauma as a result of disturbed cardiorespiratory function associated with large herniation of abdominal contents into the pleural space. Rents in the diaphragm commonly are in excess of 10 cm in length. Other patients have no symptoms or have other overwhelming injuries, so that the diaphragmatic tear is not recognized. Significant associated injuries are found in the vast majority of patients with diaphragmatic rupture.[15,41] In those patients in whom the diagnosis is delayed, there may be either no symptoms; vague, recurrent gastrointestinal or cardiorespiratory symptoms, which may be aggravated by eating; or left upper quadrant pain. Acute symptoms secondary to bowel obstruction may appear long after the original injury, and if strangulation occurs the patient may be desperately ill.[4,26]

Radiographic findings are variable. Diaphragmatic tear may occur without associated hernia initially, in which case the chest film findings may be minimal or limited to nonspecific hemothorax. Fractured ribs are reported in fewer than half of these patients, usually on the same side as the rupture, occasionally on the opposite side, or bilaterally. Sometimes the diagnosis can be suggested from a chest roentgenogram that shows the aberrant course of a nasogastric tube that has entered a herniated stomach.

In cases diagnosed late, the plain-film findings may be indistinguishable from those of eventration of the diaphragm. Carter, Guiseffi, and Felson[6] have described the following roentgenographic findings in cases of traumatic diaphragmatic hernia:

1. An archlike shadow resembling an abnormally high diaphragm, often on both PA and lateral films (Fig. 11-16A and B).
2. Extraneous shadows such as gas bubbles, homogeneous densities, or other abnormal markings extending above the anticipated level of a normal diaphragm
3. Shift of the heart and mediastinal structures to the right when the left diaphragm is torn (depends on the volume of encroaching viscera and fluid in the chest)
4. Disc atelectasis in adjacent lung.

The diagnosis can be confirmed by barium contrast studies when these are not contraindicated by signs of bowel strangulation (Fig. 11-16C). When barium enters the herniated portion of the gut, the efferent and afferent loops will appear constricted where they pass through the diaphragmatic tear. If either limb is obstructed, the barium column will come to an abrupt, tapered end at that site. Fluoroscopy may also show absent or decreased motion of the simulated diaphragm. The herniated viscus may contain no gas, and when there is strangulation, large amounts of bloody fluid may be present. Misdiagnosis can result in dangerous drainage attempts.

Left-sided hernias may include omentum, stomach, and colon most commonly, small bowel less commonly, and liver and kidney uncommonly. The liver is the organ that most commonly herniates on the right side, but colon, omentum, gallbladder, and rarely stomach or small bowel have also been reported.[15] The herniated liver may precisely simulate the more common condition of eventration of the diaphragm (Fig. 11-17A and B). Radionuclide studies may support the diagnosis of liver herniation (Fig. 11-17C), but occasionally pneumoperitoneum has been induced for diagnosis. Incomplete delineation of the undersurface of the diaphragm on properly positioned films supports the diagnosis in those cases in which the hernia contents occlude the opening so that gas does not enter the thorax as usually expected.[29]

The majority of patients with diaphragmatic rupture show some chest roentgenographic abnormality initially, but Wise, Connors, Young, and Anderson[41] have reported two patients with normal chest films who sustained lacerations of the diaphragm of 5 and 8 cm, respectively, from blunt trauma.

The overall mortality from diaphragmatic hernia is on the order of 7 percent, but among those who undergo surgery because of bowel strangulation the mortality increases to 40 percent. Obstruction and strangulation may occur early or late.

CT IN THE ASSESSMENT OF BLUNT CHEST TRAUMA

CT is an attractive examination method because so many organs can be examined by one study if the patient is stable and time is not a critical factor. The anatomic display in the axial plane provides detailed information about the chest wall and the intrathoracic contents while the patient rests in the supine position. Some of the information could be obtained radiographically but would require multiple projections, which frequently involve changing the patient's position. This can be difficult for the severely injured patient. CT studies of the head or the abdomen can also be added to the study of the chest (or vice versa) without moving the patient.

There is ample evidence that CT studies are more sensitive than chest films in detecting pleural fluid, pericardial fluid, pneumothorax, pneumomediastinum, and the extent of pulmonary contusion and atelectasis. This is especially so when comparison is made with chest films obtained with the patient supine.

CT examination may also show vertebral fractures, sternal fractures, rib fractures, sternoclavicular dislocations, and fractures of the scapula that are not apparent when initial examination is limited to the AP chest film of the supine patient. CT can also distinguish mediastinal hematoma from mediastinal fat or from dilated, tortuous, or anomalous great vessels.

The diagnosis of aortic laceration has been made by CT examination.[17] However, whether or not CT would establish the diagnosis of aortic tear or laceration of the great vessels arising from the aortic arch with the consistency achieved by angiography is unknown. CT is not, to my knowledge, being used to replace angiography in evaluation of trauma victims suspected of having major vascular injury. The relatively focal nature of traumatic aortic laceration presents a greater challenge to CT examination than does the more common and more extensive lesion of aortic dissection unrelated to trauma.

It is unlikely that CT could consistently detect the site of an esophageal or bronchial tear as opposed to establishing the presence of pneumomediastinum or mediastinal fluid collection. Conventional contrast studies could adequately detect these injuries if they were properly considered. The very rarity of esophageal or airway lacerations and their co-occurrence with other serious injuries that demand attention are often responsible for failure in diagnosis.

SUMMARY

1. Blunt chest trauma is an important cause of morbidity and mortality at all ages.

2. Chest films (PA and lateral) should be obtained with the trauma victim erect or sitting whenever possible.

3. AP chest films of the supine patient can be supplemented by lateral decubitus views to assess for pleural fluid (centered on the side down) and pneumothorax (centered on the side up), which may not be apparent on the supine AP view.

4. Post-traumatic rib fractures are common but often missed on the initial study. The associated injuries are more important than the rib fractures per se.

5. Pulmonary contusion is the most common radiographic sign of pulmonary injury. The chest film may show patchy zones of opacification or confluent opacity, unilateral or bilateral. Progression of the lesions after 72 hours is likely to be due to pulmonary edema of other cause, infection, or adult respiratory distress syndrome.

6. Laceration of lung may appear as a hematoma (mass or nodule) or as a cystic-appearing space (pneumatocele). These may be present early (hours after trauma) or may only become apparent as surrounding contusion clears. Slow resolution without specific treatment is the rule.

7. Fat embolism usually can be diagnosed reliably only when the full-blown syndrome is present.

8. Atelectasis of segments, lobes, or an entire lung may be due to the usual causes or may have no detectable cause.

9. Pneumothorax after trauma is common. The detection of even a small pneumothorax is important for patients who are to have mechanical ventilatory assistance or general anesthesia.

10. Pneumomediastinum after trauma is common and usually due to rupture of peripheral air spaces and dissection of air along perivascular sheaths into the mediastinum. Other causes are rare, but pneumomediastinum may reflect a catastrophic event such as rupture of the esophagus.

11. Hemothorax after blunt trauma is common. Initially it is most important to assess the rate of bleeding to determine whether emergency thoracotomy is required for control. Massive hemothorax is readily apparent on a supine chest film, but a small amount of blood in the pleural space is not.

12. Injuries of the thoracic aorta and great vessels are important causes of death in victims of blunt chest trauma. Several plain-film findings have been used to predict major intrathoracic vascular injury with varying degrees of success. Angiographic examination is required for definitive radiographic diagnosis.

13. Tears of major airways are very uncommon and frequently go unrecognized until late sequelae are present. Pneumothorax unresponsive to catheter

drainage, persistent pneumomediastinum, and hemoptysis are highly suggestive but inconstant findings.

14. Esophageal rupture due to blunt chest trauma is
rare, frequently missed on initial assessment, and
often fatal. Pneumomediastinum and pneumothorax are nonspecific and inconstant findings.
When they are combined with dyspnea and cyanosis
out of proportion to other injuries, the suspicion of
esophageal rupture is high.

15. Cardiac tamponade may be present even when the
cardiomediastinal silhouette does not appear enlarged.

16. Rupture of the diaphragm is more often missed than
diagnosed after combined thoracoabdominal
trauma. Contrast studies of the bowel are useful to
show signs of bowel herniation into the chest when
plain-film findings simulate those of an elevated diaphragm.

17. CT studies of patients after blunt chest trauma are
useful because much information can be gained
with little inconvenience to the patients, provided
the patient is stable.

    a. Fluid (presumably blood) is more easily detected
    in the mediastinum, the pleural space, and the
    pericardium. The same is true of the detection of
    air in those spaces.

    b. Important fractures of the thoracic cage may be
    seen on CT that are not recognized on chest
    films.

18. CT does not replace angiography in the diagnosis of
major vascular injury in the chest.

BIBLIOGRAPHY

1. Anderson AE, Doty DB: Cardiac trauma. J Trauma 15:237, 1975

2. Bates M: Rupture of the bronchus. p. 142 In Williams WG, Smith RE (eds): Trauma of the Chest (The Fourth Coventry Conference). John Wright and Sons, Bristol, 1977

3. Baxt WG, Moody P: The impact of a rotorcraft aero-medical emergency care service on trauma mortality. JAMA 249:3047, 1983

4. Bernatz PE, Burnside AF, Claggett OT: Problems of the ruptured diaphragm. JAMA 168:877, 1958

5. Burke JF: Early diagnosis of traumatic rupture of the bronchus. JAMA 181:682, 1962

6. Carter NB, Giuseffi J, Felson B: Traumatic diaphragmatic hernia. Am J Roentgenol 65:56, 1951

7. Conn H, Hardy JD, Fain WR, Netterville RE: Thoracic trauma: analysis of 1022 cases. J Trauma 3:22, 1963

8. Daughtry DC. Traumatic torsion of the lung. N Engl J Med 256:385, 1957

9. Erickson DR, Shinozaki T, Beekman E, Davis JH: Relationship of arterial blood gases and pulmonary radiographs to the degree of pulmonary damage in experimental pulmonary contusion. J Trauma 11:689, 1971

10. Fagan CJ: Traumatic lung cyst. Am J Roentgenol 97:186, 1966

11. Fisher RG, Hadlock F, Ben-Menachem Y: Laceration of the thoracic aorta and bracheocephalic arteries by blunt trauma. Report of 54 cases and review of the literature. Radiol Cl in North Am 19:91, 1981

12. Fisher RG, Ward RE, Ben-Menachem Y, et al: Arteriography and the fractured first rib: too much for too little. AJR 138:1059, 1982

13. Fuschig P, Bruckle P, Blumel G, Gottlob R: A new clinical and experimental concept of fat embolism. N Engl J Med 276:1192, 1967

14. Hankins JR, Attar S, Turney SZ, et al: Differential diagnosis of pulmonary parenchymal changes in thoracic trauma. Am Surg 39:309, 1973

15. Harley HRS: Traumatic diaphragmatic hernia due to blunt injury. p. 80. In Williams WF, Smith RE (eds): Trauma of the Chest (The Fourth Coventry Conference). John Wright and Sons, Bristol, 1977

16. Harvey-Smith W, Bush W, Northrop C: Traumatic bronchial rupture. AJR 134:1189, 1980

17. Heiberg E, Wolverson MK, Sundaram M, et al: CT in aortic trauma. AJR 140:1119, 1983

18. Herndon JH, Risenborough EJ, Fischer JE: Fat embolism: a review of current concepts. J Trauma 11:673, 1971

19. Hill LD: Injuries of the diaphragm following blunt trauma. Surg Clin North Am 52:611, 1972

20. Hood RM, Sloan HE: Injuries of the trachea and major bronchi. J Thorac Cardiovasc Surg 38:458, 1959

21. Kirsh MM, Behrent DM, Orringer MB, et al: The treatment of acute traumatic rupture of the aorta. Ann Surg 184:308, 1976

22. Kumpe DA, Oh KS, Wyman SM: A characteristic pulmonary finding in unilateral complete bronchial transection. Radiology 110:704, 1970

23. Livoni JP, Barcia TC: Fracture of the first and second ribs: incidence of vascular injury relative to type of fracture. Radiology 145:31, 1982

24. Marnocha KE, Maglinte DDT: Plain-film criteria for excluding aortic rupture in blunt chest trauma. AJR 144:19, 1985

25. Marsh LG, Sturm JT: Traumatic aortic rupture: roentgenographic indications for angiography. Ann Thorac Surg 21:337, 1976

26. Mattila S, Jarvinen A, Mattila T, Ketonen P: Traumatic diaphragmatic hernia (report of 50 cases) Acta Chir Scand 143:313, 1977
27. Milne ENC, Murray TJ, Pistolesi M, et al: The vascular pedicle and the vena azygos. Part III. In trauma—the "vanishing" azygos. Radiology 153:25, 1984
28. Oh KS, Fleischner FG, Wyman SM: Characteristic pulmonary finding in traumatic complete transection of main-stem bronchus. Radiology 92:371, 1969
29. Peck WA: Radiologic features of hernia into the right pleural cavity. Am J Roentgenol 78:99, 1957
30. Phillips EH, Rogers WF, Gasper MR: First rib fractures: incidence of vascular injury and indications for angiography. Surgery 89:42, 1981
31. Pierce GE, Maxwell JA, Boggan MD: Special hazards of first rib fractures. J Trauma 15:264, 1975
32. Richardson JD: Chest wall fractures. p. 31. In Trinkle JK, Grover FL (eds): Management of Thoracic Trauma Victims. JB Lippincott, Philadelphia, 1980
33. Stevens E, Templeton AW: Traumatic nonpenetrating lung contusion. Radiology 85:247, 1965
34. Sturm JT, Points BJ, Perry JF: Hemopneumothorax following blunt trauma to the thorax. Surg Gynecol Obstet 141:539, 1975
35. Toombs BD, Sandler CM, Lester RG: Computed tomography of chest trauma. Radiology 40:733, 1981
36. Trinkle JK: Flail chest—facts and fancies. p. 39. In Williams WG and Smith RE (eds): Trauma of the Chest (The Fourth Coventry Conference). John Wright and Sons, Bristol, 1977
37. Vessal K, Montali RJ, Larson SM, et al: Evaluation of barium and gastrografin as contrast media for the diagnosis of esophageal ruptures or perforations. Am J Roentgenol 123:307, 1975
38. Watson JH, Bartholomae WM: Cardiac injury due to nonpenetrating chest trauma. Ann Intern Med 52:871, 1960
39. Wilson JM, Thomas AN, Goodman PC, Lewis F: Severe chest trauma. Morbidity implication of first and second rib fracture in 120 patients. Arch Surg 113:846, 1978
40. Wilson RF, Murray C, Antonenko DR: Nonpenetrating thoracic injuries. Surg Clin North Am 57:17, 1977
41. Wise L, Connors J, Young H, Anderson C: Traumatic injuries to the diaphragm. J Trauma 13:946, 1975
42. Woodring JH, Fried AM, Hatfield DR, et al: Fractures of first and second ribs: predictive value for arterial and bronchial injury. AJR 138:211, 1982
43. Worman LW, Hurley JD, Pemberton AH, Narodick BG: Rupture of the esophagus from external blunt trauma. Arch Surg 85:333, 1962
44. Yee ES, Thomas AN, Goodman PC: Isolated first rib fracture: clinical significance after blunt chest trauma. Ann Thorac Surg 32:278, 1981

Atlas

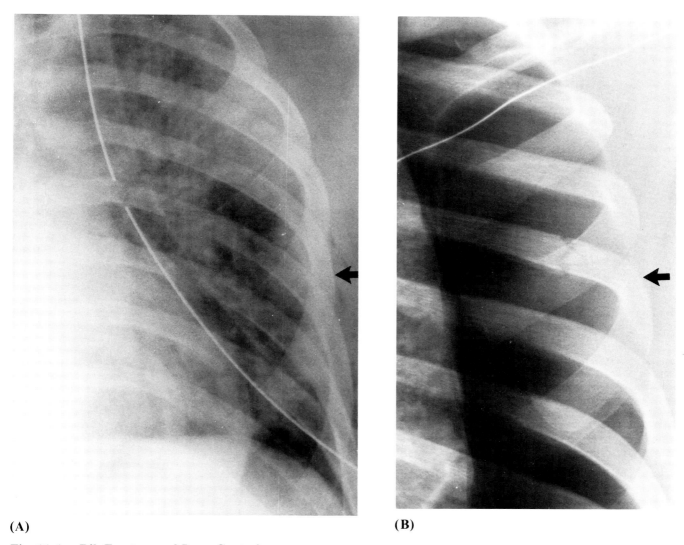

(A)

(B)

Fig. 11-1. Rib Fracture and Lung Contusion

(A) Severe lung contusion obscures a fracture of the posterior sixth rib (arrow).

(B) The fracture becomes easy to see on a film taken after pneumothorax has developed (arrow). Severe contusion has been reported in the absence of rib fracture but may be responsible for masking the fracture lines when the rib fragments return to a near-anatomical position. Arrows point to the sixth rib. The fracture in Fig. B is easily seen because the pneumothorax has caused the lung to move away from the fracture site so that no confusing pulmonary opacity is superimposed, and because the projection of this film is slightly different from that of Fig. A. (Film for Fig. A courtesy of Dr. James Crane, San Jose, California.)

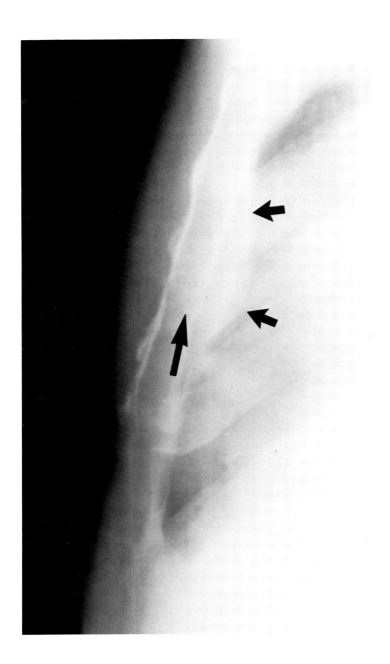

Fig. 11-2. Retrosternal Hematoma From Fracture of the Sternum

There is a retrosternal soft tissue mound produced by an extrapleural hematoma (short arrows) due to a barely perceptible fracture of the body of the sternum (vertical arrow).

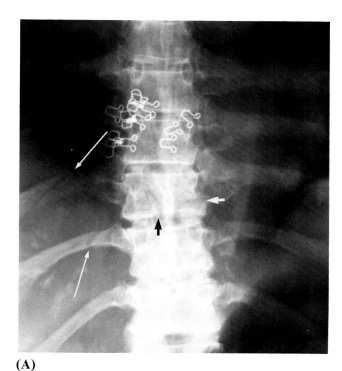

(A)

Fig. 11-3. (A,B) Vertebral Fracture from Blunt Trauma

This woman fell off the roof of her garage while attempting to trim some vines.

(A) Coned AP view of the lower thoracic spine. T12 is not entirely included in the lower most portion of the film. T9 has been fractured and multiple fragments are seen (short arrows). In addition, there are fractures of the posterior right ninth and tenth ribs (long arrows). The lateral view (not shown) showed some reduction in the height of T9, but no additional abnormalities.

(B) CT scan through the level of T9. There is a severely comminuted fracture of the body of T9. Although this is clearly present on the spine films, the severe disruption and fragmentation of the vertebrae are shown more graphically on CT. In addition, there is evidence of a small left pleural effusion (ef), and the image of the descending thoracic aorta (A) is surrounded by an abnormal soft tissue density (presumably blood). There is also an abnormal paraspinal soft tissue density on the right side, probably due to hemorrhage. There is a very small bony fragment in the spinal canal.

The white opacity at the center of a starburst artifact pattern represents a nasogastric tube in the distal esophagus.

In the evaluation of fractured vertebrae, CT offers the advantage of displaying the spinal canal in the axial plane so that disruption of its bony margins are more easily recognized than they are on plain-film images. In addition, fragment displacements in the sagittal plane are much more easily seen on CT than on spine film studies.

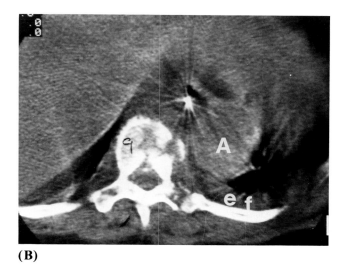

(B)

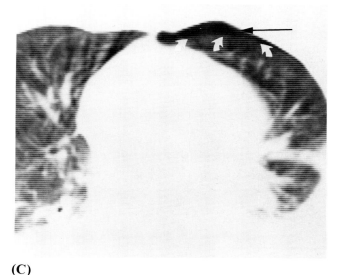

(C)

(C) Small Pneumothorax Seen on CT Scan

CT slice from the lower third of the chest, displayed at settings that show lung detail. There is a small pneumothorax (black arrow) on the left that was not visible on the AP chest film made with the patient supine.

The air in the pneumothorax rises anteriorly in this supine patient and is seen as a black crescent between the anterior chest wall and the thin layer of visceral pleura over the lung (white arrows), which is slightly retracted from the chest wall. Since this crescent presents en face to the x-ray beam when a chest film is made with the patient supine, the thin anterior rim of pneumothorax can go unrecognized. When there is sufficient air in the pneumothorax to move the lung off of the diaphragm (Fig. 11-4) or away from the lateral chest wall, the pneumothorax may be seen even on a chest film of a supine patient.

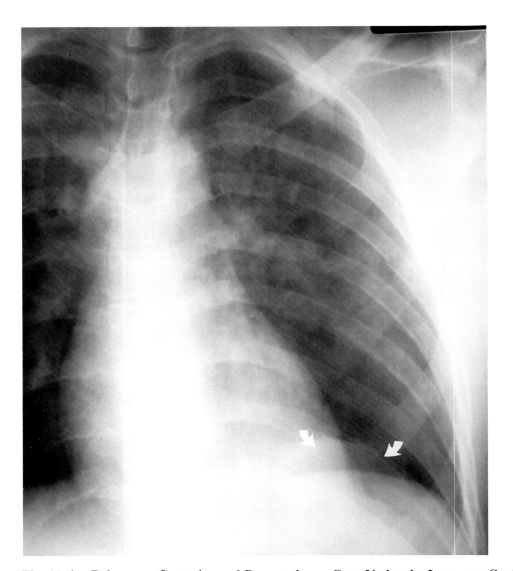

Fig. 11-4.   Pulmonary Contusion and Pneumothorax Seen Under the Lung on a Supine Film

Initial film of a young man shortly after he had been in a severe automobile accident. The vessels throughout the left lung have lost their sharp outlines as a result of extensive pulmonary contusion. Bleeding into the lung will cause an appearance quite like that of pneumonia or pulmonary edema. It is the association of the abnormality with trauma and its relatively nonsegmental distribution that favors the diagnosis of lung contusion.

There is a pneumothorax under the left lung (arrows), which was confirmed by a left-side-up decubitus view. No pneumothorax is seen over the convexities of the lung. The film was made with the patient supine because a hip fracture prevented him from standing or sitting. He also sustained a fracture of the clavicle and a fracture of the left first rib, which cannot be seen on this reproduction. A fracture of the posterior fifth rib, however, can be seen.

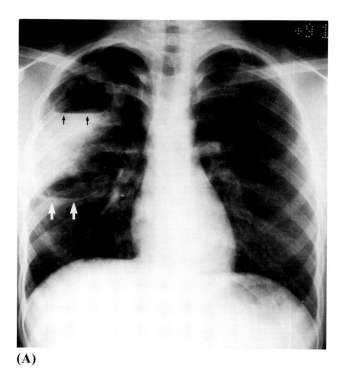

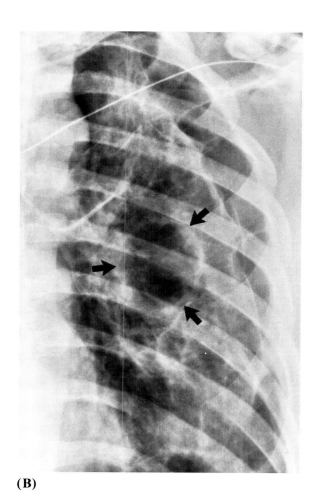

(A)   (B)

Fig. 11-5.   Post-Traumatic Pneumatocele

(A) This young girl had a horse fall on her. Chest film shows a large zone of opacification accompanied by two large areas of circumscribed radiolucency that have fluid levels (arrows). This is a part of the radiographic spectrum of pulmonary injuries due to blunt chest trauma.

The opaque zone is consistent with a hemorrhage secondary to a tear of lung parenchyma, and the pseudocavities are circumscribed pockets of air in the interstitium of the lung also due to tearing of lung parenchyma. The air pockets may be present on the initial film or may not become apparent for a few days at which time the clearing of surrounding intrapulmonary hemorrhage permits them to be seen.

The lesions in this case slowly resolved over several months and at last examination there was only a small residual mass with no residual cavities at the trauma site.

(B) Same patient as seen in Fig. 11-1. A circumscribed, cystic-appearing space (arrows) has emerged from formerly contused lung many days after the original trauma. Notice that there is also recurrent pneumothorax and partial lung collapse. In retrospect, the pneumatocele can be seen as a rounded zone of radiolucency lateral to the left hilum in Fig. 11-1A.

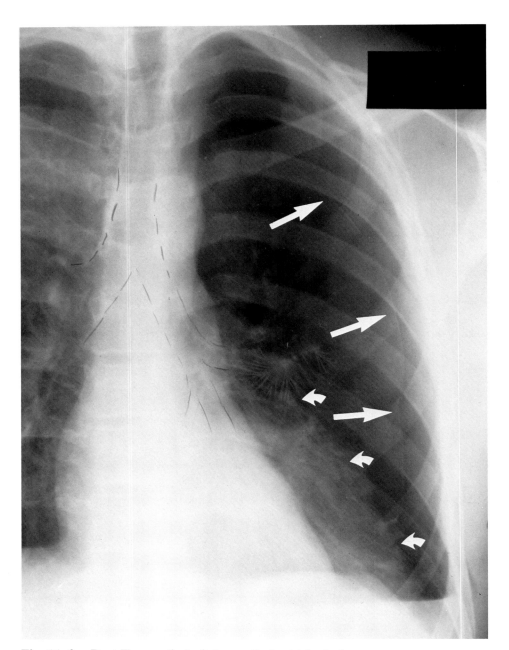

Fig. 11-6. Post-Traumatic Left Lower Lobe Atelectasis

This young man suffered multiple injuries in an automobile accident. He had several rib fractures and a fractured clavicle as well as a hip fracture. The initial chest film showed evidence of left lung contusion and pneumothorax. A film a few hours later showed left lower lobe atelectasis.

This film shows caudal deviation of the left main and upper lobe bronchi, depression of the left pulmonary artery, and medial displacement of the left lower lobe bronchus. There is a moderately large pneumothorax (straight arrows), and a fluid level (probably blood) is present at the left base. The atelectasis cleared after respiratory therapy.

The lower trachea and major bronchi are outlined by dashes. Air bronchograms were visible in the left lower lobe on the original films. The margins of the atelectatic left lower lobe are outlined by short, curved arrows.

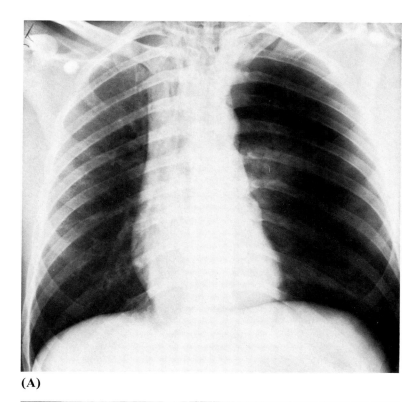

(A)

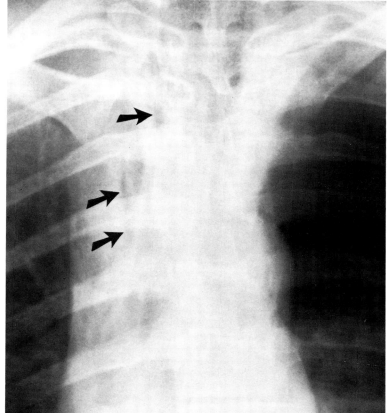

(B)

Fig. 11-7. **Pneumomediastinum and Left Pneumothorax Due to Bronchial Injury**

A young man was crushed between a truck and a wall.

(A) Initial chest film shows a pneumomediastinum and a large left pneumothorax.

(B) Coned view shows the air streaks in the mediastinum (arrows). These streaks are fairly subtle but clearly do not belong in the normal mediastinum. The pneumothorax responded to tube drainage and the pneumomediastinum resolved (see Fig. 11-13). (Courtesy of Dr. James Mark, Stanford University Medical Center, Stanford, California.)

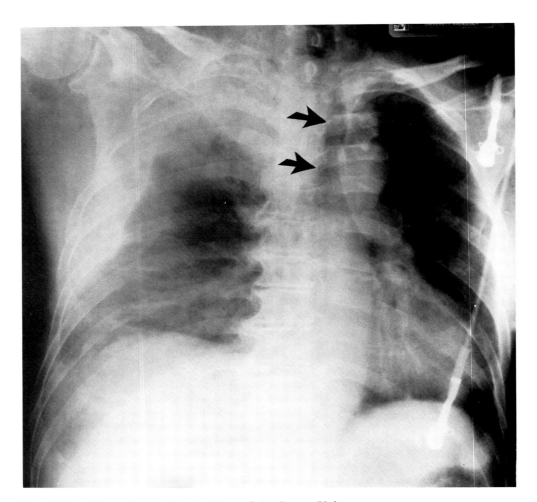

Fig. 11-8.   Hemothorax Due to Tear of the Large Veins

Supine chest film of a man who sustained severe blunt chest trauma. There is a large mantle of fluid over the superior and lateral aspects of the right chest. The shift of the trachea (arrows) and the mediastinal contents to the left is more than can be accounted for by rotation. The right paratracheal stripe and the azygos vein are not visible. The appearance of the abnormality is consistent with the presence of a large loculated or extrapleural component of fluid extending from the mediastinum around the chest wall.

A right chest tube was inserted, and there was a persistent, rapid drainage of bloody fluid. The patient was taken to the operating room without further radiographic study, and a laceration of the right subclavian-innominate vein junction was repaired. No other major vessel injury was found. A small hemopericardium was drained.

Multiple rib fractures are seen bilaterally on the original films. There were more visible rib fractures on the left side than on the right.

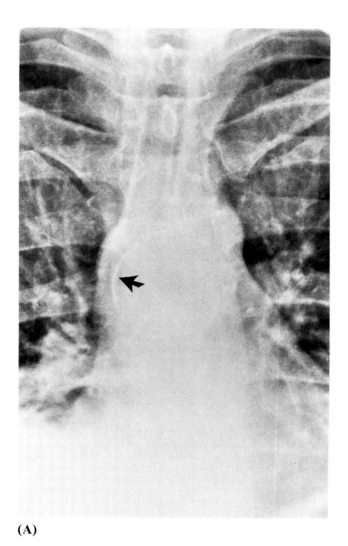

(A)

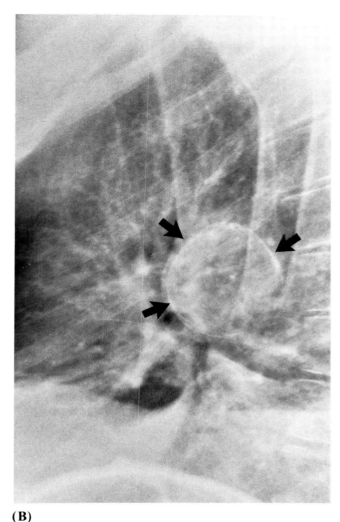

(B)

Fig. 11-9.   Late Diagnosis of Pseudoaneurysm of the Aorta

(A) Coned view of the mediastinum of a patient who was in a severe auto accident 30 years before. A curved band of calcification is seen superimposed on the mediastinum (arrow).

(B) Lateral view shows the calcified rim (arrows) of a pseudoaneurysm of the descending thoracic aorta beyond the level of the isthmus. It was confirmed on an angiogram.

(C) CT scan shows the calcified pseudoaneurysm and its encroachment on the tracheal carina. There were remarkably few symptoms related to the aneurysm despite its distortion of the airway. The patient was admitted because of the onset of symptoms suggesting that the aneurysm was leaking. The CT scan shows a posterior pleural pocket (anterior to p), which contains a chest tube (medial to t) in its axillary portion and air in its posterior portion. There is also a large, undrained pleural pocket anteriorly (P). The patient had a bacterial em-

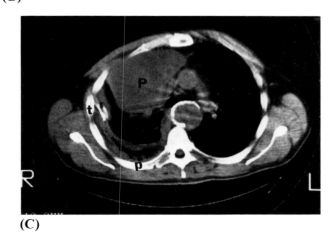

(C)

pyema, which was unrelated to the aneurysm and which responded to further drainage and antibiotic therapy. The patient was advised to have his aorta repaired when his empyema resolved.

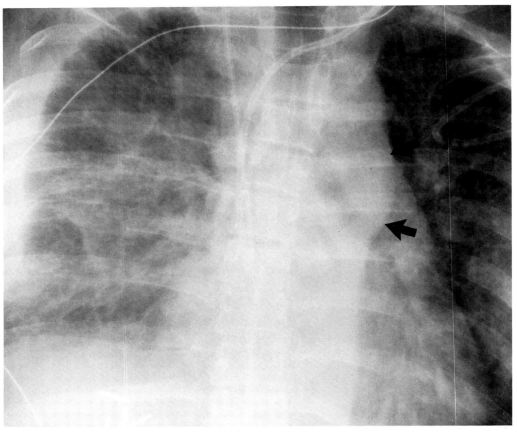

(A)

Fig. 11-10.   Late Diagnosis of Aortic Transection

This 43-year-old woman was involved in a head-on automobile collision. She was taken to the emergency room of a local hospital. She was stuporous and had a systolic blood pressure of less than 70 mmHg. A laparotomy was performed because of evidence of massive intra-abdominal bleeding.

She had an astonishing array of injuries, the most important of which included severe lacerations of the liver, avulsion of the gallbladder, rupture of the spleen, avulsion of the right ovarian vein, avulsion of multiple lumbar veins, renal contusion, pericecal hematoma, and multiple extremity fractures. Her postoperative course was remarkably complicated by sepsis, coagulopathy, hepatic encephalopathy, and jaundice with abnormal liver function tests.

(A) Supine AP, film of the chest taken approximately 5 weeks after the accident shows a moderately large right pleural effusion and an abnormal mediastinum. The superior mediastinum is wide, and there is an abnormal bulge in the contour of the descending aorta (arrows). The left main bronchus is depressed. Despite their late discovery, these abnormalities were considered highly suspect for aortic laceration. *(Figure continues.)*

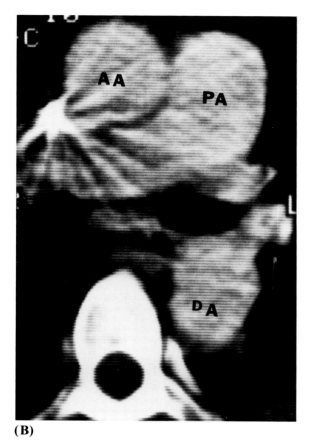

(B)

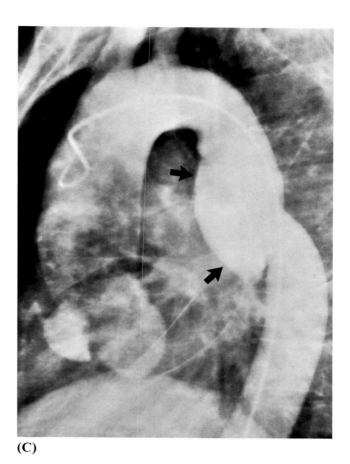

(C)

Fig. 11-10. *(Continued).* **(B)** Portion of a dynamic CT scan of the chest several seconds following a bolus of intravenous contrast injection. The film is coned to the area of the heart and vessels at the level of the left main bronchus. There is still a portion of the contrast bolus in the superior vena cava just anterior to the right pulmonary artery. There is a series of streak artifacts radiating outward. The descendıng aorta (DA) behind the left main bronchus has an abnormal elongated oval contour, but no laceration was seen on this or adjacent cuts (AA, ascending aorta; PA, pulmonary artery). This was not a conclusive study, and an aortogram was done.

Fig. 11-10. **(C)** Film from the patient's aortogram shows a false aneurysm (arrows) at the site of laceration of the proximal descending thoracic aorta. Following control of infection at other sites, the patient had a successful aortic repair. There was complete transection of the aorta, which was circumferential through both the intima and the media. The false aneurysm was contained only by adventitia and adjacent pleural reaction.

The patient also had a right upper quadrant abdominal abscess, which probably accounted for the right pleural effusion.

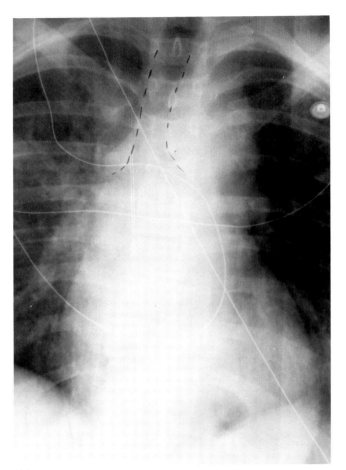

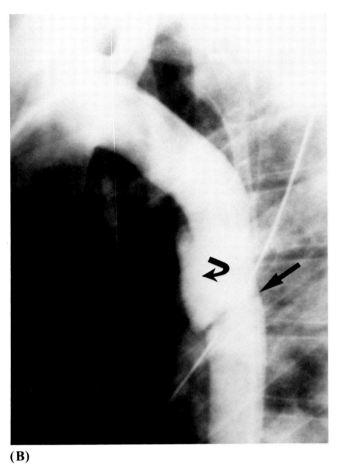

(B)

(A)

Fig. 11-11. Traumatic Aortic Laceration With Tracheal Shift

This man suffered severe injuries in an automobile accident (rapid deceleration). **(A)** The chest film was made with the patient supine. In this position the mediastinum is usually significantly (about 20 percent) wider than it is when the patient is upright, and this complicates the analysis of the film. However, multiple injuries are frequently present and require that the patient remain supine.

The mediastinum, measured at the expected level of the aortic arch, was more than 8.5 cm in width. The sharp image of the transverse portion of the aortic arch is lost. The wide left side of the mediastinum has a convex bulge over the aorto pulmonic window. The mediastinal pleural reflection over the left subclavian artery is deviated laterally and has no concavity toward the left lung. The image of the descending aorta is effaced. The left paraspinal stripe, however, could be seen. Dashes outline the trachea, which is shifted to the right so that its left wall is superimposed on the spinous processes of T3 and T4. This shift cannot be explained on the basis of rotation of the patient, judging from the position of the medial ends of the clavicles relative to the spine. These abnormalities are highly suggestive of a mediastinal bleed. The azygos vein, however, can still be seen in the right tracheobronchial angle. An aortogram was done.

(B) Frame from the aortogram. There is an interruption of the smooth contours of the descending thoracic aorta at a level just beyond the location of the ligamentum arteriosum. There is a traumatic aneurysm (curved arrow) at the site of an aortic laceration. The torn, retracted intima is seen as a thin lucent band (straight arrow). The continuity of the aorta depends on the tenuous support provided by the adventitia and the unopacified hematoma that surrounds the site of injury. This is a common site of aortic tear due to deceleration injury.

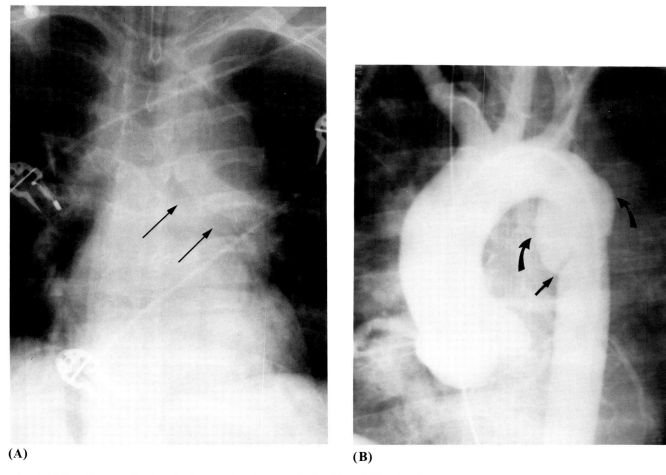

(A)   **(B)**

Fig. 11-12.   Traumatic Aortic Laceration Without Significant Tracheal Shift

This woman suffered severe injuries in an automobile accident.

(A) Coned view of the mediastinum taken from a chest film made with the patient supine. The mediastinum, at the expected level of the aortic arch, measures in excess of 9.5 cm. There is effacement of the image of the aortic knob, lateral displacement of the mediastinal pleural reflection over the region of the aortopulmonic window, effacement of the image of the descending thoracic aorta, and depression of the left main bronchus (arrows). There is also a wide right paratracheal band with loss of the sharp interface between the mediastinal pleural reflection over the superior vena cava and the right upper lobe. The azygos vein is not seen. The trachea is not significantly displaced. This film displays many but not all of the radiographic signs of mediastinal bleeding due to blunt chest trauma. An aortogram was performed.

(B) Frame from the patient's aortogram. There has been a laceration of the descending thoracic aorta in the region of the ligamentum arteriosum. A traumatic aneurysm has formed (curved arrows). Torn, retracted intima is seen as a lucent band (straight arrow). Continuity of aortic blood flow is maintained by the adventitia of the aorta and the unopacified hematoma about the laceration. Since many aortic lacerations are complete transections, it is not surprising that a high percentage of these patients do not live long enough to reach the emergency room.

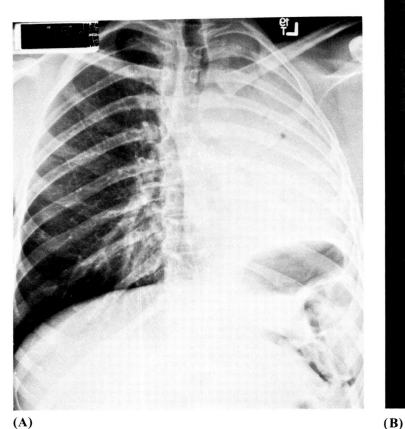

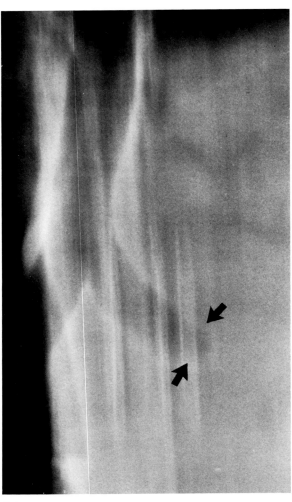

(A)   **(B)**

Fig. 11-13.   Traumatic Tear of the Left Main Bronchus

(A) This is the same young man who was seen in Fig. 11-7. Over several days he developed progressive atelectasis of the left lung, which did not respond to bronchoscopy. Fig. A was taken at the time of referral. There is now atelectasis of the left lung. An air bronchogram is clearly present on the original film.

(B) Tomogram shows an abrupt end to the air column of the left main bronchus (arrows), and a bronchial disruption was confirmed at bronchoscopy. A successful repair of the left main bronchus was performed. (Courtesy of Dr. James Mark, Stanford University Medical Center, Stanford, California.)

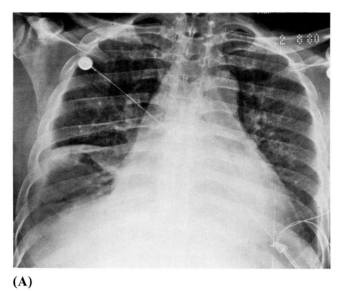

(A)

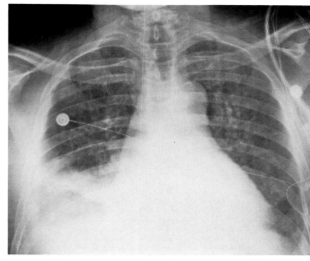

(B)

Fig. 11-14. Pericardial Tamponade

(A) This man was in a severe automobile accident the day before this film was taken. Because his mediastinum was judged to be widened, he was referred. An angiogram showed no arterial laceration. The film was taken with the patient supine and is a semilordotic projection. Notice the tentlike appearance of the mediastinal boundaries. This was considered suspicious for pericardial fluid. There is also right pleural fluid and left lower lobe atelectasis.

(B) Film of the same patient 1 day later. It was not taken in the lordotic position, and the tentlike appearance of the mediastinum is less apparent. The cardiac silhouette is still too large. Although increased pericardial fluid was considered probable, there were no apparent physiologic deficits.

(C) Four days after Fig. B was taken, the cardiac contour has changed but is not much larger in transverse diameter. Now the patient has developed an increased central venous pressure, a decreased systolic pressure, and muffled heart sounds. After preliminary pericardiocentesis of 300 ml, he had a mediastinotomy, and approximately 300 ml of blood clot and serosanguineous fluid was removed from the pericardial sac. This case illustrates how pericardial fluid can increase up to a point on the pressure-volume curve at which a small additional increment can cause tamponade.

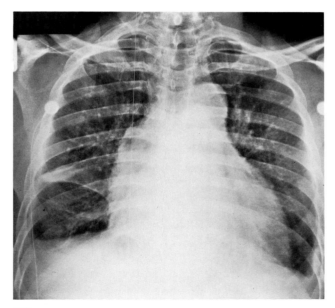

(C)

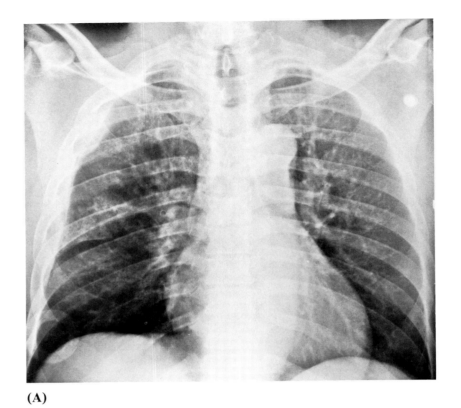

(A)

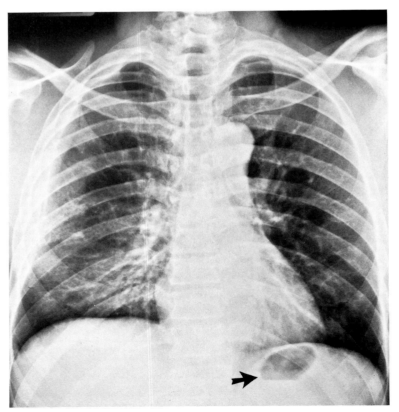

(B)

Fig. 11-15. Change in Appearance of the Heart on Upright and Supine Chest Films

(A) Supine view of the chest of a man who had suffered blunt chest trauma.

(B) Upright view of the chest on the same day. Notice the striking difference in apparent cardiac size due simply to the difference in posture. The right-sided pleural fluid changes configuration very little between views, suggesting the presence of extrapleural or loculated fluid. It probably represents a moderate hemothorax secondary to rib fractures. The fluid level in the stomach (arrow) confirms that the film was made with the patient upright.

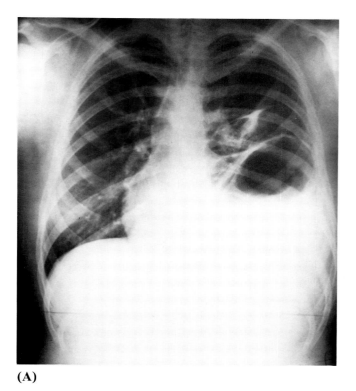

(A)

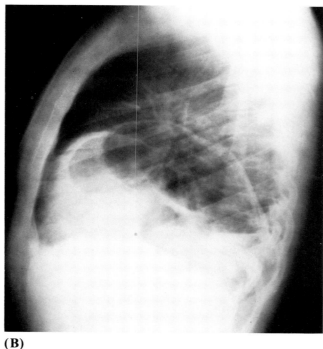

(B)

**Fig. 11-16.   Late Diagnosis and Repair of a Laceration
of the Diaphragm**

(A,B) PA and lateral films, respectively, made a long
time after this young man had been in a serious motorcycle accident. He denied any significant symptoms but
reluctantly admitted to minor distress after large meals.
There are obvious bowel shadows under what is either an
eventration of the left diaphragm or herniation into the
chest. There is also some subsegmental atelectasis of adjacent lung.

   (C) Contrast study of the gastrointestinal tract shows a
large amount of bowel herniated into the left chest. A
successful repair of a diaphragmatic laceration was performed. (Courtesy of Dr. James Mark, Stanford University Medical Center, Stanford, California.)

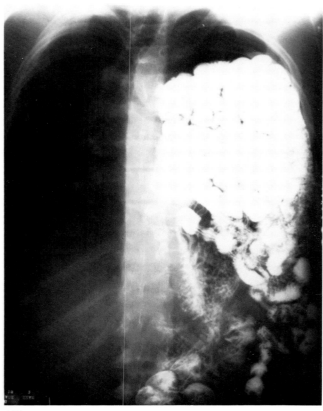

(C)

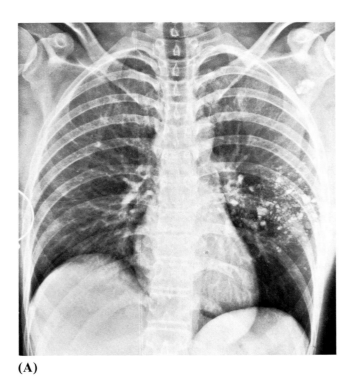

(A)

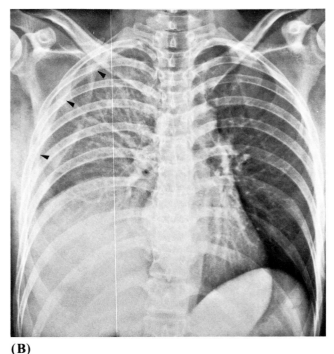

(B)

Fig. 11-17.   Herniation of Liver Through a Laceration of the Right Diaphragm

(A) This equestrian fell from her horse. The horse fell on her and she sustained a fracture of the pelvis. This is her initial chest film. The right hemidiaphragm is elevated. The opaque material over the left chest and scapula represents dirt and gravel.

(B) The same woman's chest film a day later. Now there is a characteristic appearance of a moderately large amount of pleural fluid on the right—an overall increase in radiodensity produced by a layer of fluid posteriorly. A mantle of fluid also is seen adjacent to the ribs (arrowheads). The medial edge of the right scapula is projected as an arc medial to the arrowheads.

On the original films, a minimally displaced fracture of the anterior end of the right eighth rib was also visible. A diagnosis of diaphragmatic rupture with herniation of liver was suggested.

(C) Radionuclide scan shows deformity of the right lobe of the liver secondary to herniation. The patient was experiencing only mild distress from this lesion, so it was elected to delay definitive repair for a few days until she recovered from other injuries. At thoracotomy, the herniated but undamaged right lobe of the liver was easily reduced, and a large diaphragmatic rent was repaired.

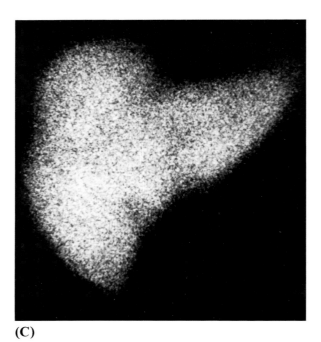

(C)

Index

Page numbers followed by *f* represent figures; those followed by *t* represent tables.